Oxford Textbook of

# Creative Arts, Health, and Wellbeing

# Oxford Textbooks in Public Health

**Oxford Textbook of Infectious Disease Control**
A Geographical Analysis from Medieval Quarantine to Global Eradication
Andrew Cliff and Matthew Smallman-Raynor

**Oxford Textbook of Spirituality in Healthcare**
Edited by Mark Cobb, Christina Puchalski, and Bruce Rumbold

**Oxford Textbook of Violence Prevention**
Epidemiology, Evidence, and Policy
Edited by Peter D. Donnelly and Catherine L. Ward

**Oxford Textbook of Zoonoses**
Biology, Clinical Practice, and Public Health Control
Second Edition
Edited by S.R. Palmer, Lord Soulsby, Paul Torgerson, and David W. G. Brown

# Free personal online access for 12 months

Individual purchasers of this book are also entitled to free personal access to the online edition for 12 months on Oxford Medicine Online (<http://oxfordmedicine.com/>). Please refer to the access token card for instructions on token redemption and access.

Online ancillary materials, where available, are noted at the end of the respective chapters in this book. Additionally, Oxford Medicine Online allows you to print, save, cite, email, and share content; download high-resolution figures as PowerPoint® slides; save often-used books, chapters, or searches; annotate; and quickly jump to other chapters or related material on a mobile-optimized platform.

We encourage you to take advantage of these features. If you are interested in ongoing access after the 12-month gift period, please consider an individual subscription or consult with your librarian.

# Oxford Textbook of

# Creative Arts, Health, and Wellbeing

## International perspectives on practice, policy, and research

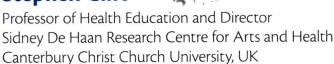

**Edited by**

**Stephen Clift**
Professor of Health Education and Director
Sidney De Haan Research Centre for Arts and Health
Canterbury Christ Church University, UK

**Paul M. Camic**
Professor of Psychology and Public Health and Research Director
Salomons Centre for Applied Psychology
Canterbury Christ Church University, UK

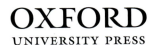

OXFORD
UNIVERSITY PRESS

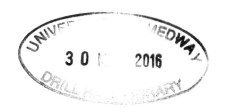

# OXFORD
UNIVERSITY PRESS

Great Clarendon Street, Oxford, OX2 6DP,
United Kingdom

Oxford University Press is a department of the University of Oxford.
It furthers the University's objective of excellence in research, scholarship,
and education by publishing worldwide. Oxford is a registered trade mark of
Oxford University Press in the UK and in certain other countries

First Edition published in 2016

Impression: 1

Published in the United States of America by Oxford University Press
198 Madison Avenue, New York, NY 10016, United States of America

British Library Cataloguing in Publication Data
Data available

Library of Congress Control Number: 2015933916

ISBN 978–0–19–968807–4

Printed in China by
Asia Pacific Offset Ltd

# Foreword

The last few years have seen a major shift in how we view the role of the creative arts in improving public health. Two decades ago you would rarely have seen reference made to arts and health in the same sentence, whereas now they are inextricably linked. This important book could not be more timely as it draws together the many strands of arts and health, sharing the growing empirical evidence and knowledge about the efficacy of a wide range of arts programmes in improving health together with a variety of inspiring case studies to show the real difference that the creative arts can make to the lives of individuals.

The Royal Society for Public Health (RSPH) has long been a strong proponent of the capacity of the arts to improve health and wellbeing, and it has done much to identify and promote the excellent creative programmes that are happening across the UK. The RSPH's annual Arts and Health Awards shine a bright light on outstanding UK projects, recognizing organizations and individuals who have made significant contributions to research and practice. The journals and education programmes of the RSPH have focused on the growing arts and health movement, and it is hugely gratifying that public health professionals, national and local government, and the public now recognize the contribution that the arts can make to a healthier society.

The editors of this book, themselves leading academics and advocates for the role of the arts in improving health, have brought together an extraordinary group of eminent contributors. Academics and practitioners from across the globe highlight the international nature of the field and the benefits the arts can bring to health. These contributions show that the creative arts have a positive effect on health and wellbeing across the lifespan, benefitting young, working age, and older people as well as across different settings including hospitals, schools, community centres, the workplace, care homes, and prisons.

This book underlines the importance of the evidence base to validate the impact that the creative arts can have on supporting society. From a public health perspective the challenge is no longer whether the arts have a beneficial impact but whether resources spent on arts initiatives will have more impact and deliver a better return on investment than other projects. The role of the arts in improving the public's health has gone mainstream, and we will all be the better for it.

*Shirley Cramer*
Chief Executive, Royal Society for Public Health

# Acknowledgements

The editors are hugely grateful to Caroline Smith, our commissioning editor at Oxford University Press (OUP), for her support for the idea of this textbook as part of OUP's Textbooks in Public Health series from the initial planning stages and throughout the process of getting the book together. Our thanks also go to James Cox, for assisting with the editing process, to Bridget Johnson for her skilled copy editing and to Saranya Manohar, for help during the production phase.

We are delighted also to have had enthusiastic encouragement throughout from Shirley Cramer, Chief Executive of the Royal Society for Public Health and Institute of Healthcare Management, and Dr Heather Davison, Director of Education and Development. Our special thanks to Shirley for providing a Foreword to this textbook.

We want also to thank all of the contributors to this text, who individually have shared their expertise and experience in their own specialist areas, and who collectively have contributed to providing a global overview of developments in the new field of creative arts, health, and wellbeing, which none of us could provide alone. The whole is surely greater than the sum of the parts.

We acknowledge the support we have received from Canterbury Christ Church University and from all of our colleagues who have assisted and expressed their interest in the progress of this book.

On a personal note, our partners Lynda and Larry have provided moral support throughout and are no doubt happy that the task is now complete!

But finally, and not least, this project would never have come to fruition without the dedicated, skilled, and always efficient support we have had from Lian Wilson, our editorial assistant. We thank you most warmly for all you have contributed to making this textbook a reality.

# Endorsements

'Professor Clift and Professor Camic have been at the forefront of developing the evidence base for the link between the arts, health, and wellbeing to support public policy in this emerging field.'

Rt Hon Lord Howarth of Newport
Co-Chair, All Party Parliamentary Group on Arts
Health and Wellbeing, London, UK

'This volume is destined to become the handbook for anyone interested in the bourgeoning field of arts and health. Grounded in research from top international researchers across a wide range of art forms, the Oxford Textbook of Creative Arts, Health, and Wellbeing presents a rich, theoretically grounded and practically applicable understanding of the landscape of this important field.'

Jean E. Rhodes, Frank L. Boyden
Professor, Department of Psychology
University of Massachusetts, USA

'A comprehensive, persuasive, and truly international outlook on the public health resources offered by the arts, in many different clinical and cultural contexts. The evidence base is growing, so culture and the arts can no longer be neglected.'

Lars Ole Bonde
Professor of Music Therapy, Aalborg University, Denmark,
*and*
Professor of Music and Health
The Norwegian Academy of Music, Norway

'This excellent textbook reveals that creativity abounds across art-forms and health settings, and significant change is afoot. Professor Clift and Professor Camic's book is timely as the National Health Service looks for new approaches, and prevention and social prescribing rise up the health agenda.'

Tim Joss
Chief Executive of AESOP Arts and Society, UK

# Contents

**List of Abbreviations**  *xiii*

**List of Contributors**  *xv*

## PART 1
### Creative arts and human health and wellbeing: setting the scene

1 **Introduction to the field of creative arts, wellbeing, and health: achievements and current challenges**  *3*
Stephen Clift and Paul M. Camic

2 **The arts and healing: the power of an idea**  *11*
Eleonora Belfiore

3 **The fifth wave of public health and the contributions of culture and the arts**  *19*
Phil Hanlon and Sandra Carlisle

4 **The social determinants of health, empowerment, and participation**  *27*
Jessica Allen and Matilda Allen

5 **Case study: Southbank Centre London and the social utility of the arts**  *35*
Shân Maclennan

6 **The means to flourish: arts in community health and education**  *41*
Mike White

7 **Community cultural development for health and wellbeing**  *49*
Paul M. Camic

8 **Epidemiological studies of the relationship between cultural experiences and public health**  *55*
Töres Theorell and Fredrik Ullén

9 **Psychophysiological links between cultural activities and public health**  *65*
Töres Theorell

10 **The role of qualitative research in arts and health**  *73*
Norma Daykin and Theo Stickley

11 **Ethical issues in arts-based health research**  *83*
Susan M. Cox and Katherine M. Boydell

## PART 2
### National and international developments in practice

12 **Seeking a common language: the challenge of embedding participatory arts in a major public health programme**  *95*
Marsaili Cameron, Richard Ings, and Nikki Crane

13 **Arts for health in community settings: promising practices for using the arts to enhance wellness, access to healthcare, and health literacy**  *103*
Jill Sonke and Jenny Baxley Lee

14 **Arts in healthcare settings in the United States**  *113*
Jill Sonke, Judy Rollins, and John Graham-Pole

15 **Arts in healthcare in Uganda: an historical, political, and practical case study**  *123*
Kizito Maria Kasule, Kizito Fred Kakinda, and Jill Sonke

16 **Siyazama in South Africa: Zulu beadwork, HIV/AIDS, and the consequences of culture**  *129*
Kate Wells

17 **Arts and health in Australia**  *135*
Gareth Wreford

18  Addressing the health needs of
    indigenous Australians through creative
    engagement: a case study  *145*
    Jing Sun and Nicholas Buys

19  Arts and health initiatives in India  *151*
    Varun Ramnarayan Venkit, Anand Sharad
    Godse, and Amruta Anand Godse

20  A role for the creative arts in addressing
    public health challenges in China  *163*
    Jing Sun and Nicholas Buys

21  Culture and public health activities
    in Sweden and Norway  *171*
    Töres Theorell, Margunn Skjei Knudtsen,
    Eva Bojner Horwitz, and Britt-Maj Wikström

22  Talking about a revolution: arts, health,
    and wellbeing on Avenida Brasil  *179*
    Paul Heritage and Silvia Ramos

23  Case study: 'I once was lost but now
    am found'—music and embodied arts
    in two American prisons  *187*
    André de Quadros

24  Case study: lost—or found?—in translation.
    The globalization of Venezuela's El Sistema  *193*
    Andrea Creech, Patricia A. González-Moreno,
    Lisa Lorenzino, and Grace Waitman

PART 3
Creative arts and public health across
the life-course

25  Creativity and promoting wellbeing in children
    and young people through education  *201*
    Jonathan Barnes

26  The value of music for public health  *211*
    Gunter Kreutz

27  Addressing the needs of seriously
    disadvantaged children through the
    arts: the work of Kids Company  *219*
    Camila Batmanghelidjh

28  The power of dance to transform the
    lives of disadvantaged youth  *227*
    Pauline Gladstone-Barrett and Victoria Hunter

29  The arts and older people: a
    global perspective  *235*
    Trish Vella-Burrows

30  Case study: engaging older people in creative
    thinking—the Active Energy project  *245*
    Loraine Leeson

31  Group singing as a public health resource  *251*
    Stephen Clift, Grenville Hancox, Ian Morrison, Matthew
    Shipton, Sonia Page, Ann Skingley, and Trish Vella-Burrows

32  Intergenerational music-making: a vehicle for
    active ageing for children and older people  *259*
    Maria Varvarigou, Susan Hallam, Andrea
    Creech, and Hilary McQueen

PART 4
Creative arts and public health in
different settings

33  The arts therapies: approaches, goals,
    and integration in arts and health  *271*
    Amy Bucciarelli

34  Museums and art galleries as settings
    for public health interventions  *281*
    Helen J. Chatterjee

35  Case study: creativity in criminal justice
    settings—the work of the Koestler Trust  *291*
    Tim Robertson

36  Quality of place and wellbeing  *299*
    Bryan Lawson and Rosie Parnell

37  Creative arts in health professional education
    and practice: a case study reflection and
    evaluation of a complex intervention to
    deliver the Culture and Care Programme at
    the Florence Nightingale School of Nursing
    and Midwifery, King's College London  *309*
    Ian Noonan, Anne Marie Rafferty, and John Browne

38  Case study: singing in hospitals—bridging
    therapy and everyday life  *317*
    Gunter Kreutz, Stephen Clift, and Wolfgang Bossinger

39  Case study: the value of group drumming for
    women in sex work in Mumbai, India  *325*
    Varun Ramnarayan Venkit, Anand Sharad
    Godse, and Amruta Anand Godse

Index  *331*

# List of Abbreviations

| | |
|---|---|
| ABHR | arts-based health research |
| ABR | arts-based research |
| ACAH | Australian Centre for Arts and Health |
| ACNI | Arts Council Northern Ireland |
| ADHD | attention deficit hyperactivity disorder |
| AHCC | Arts in Healthcare Certification Commission |
| AHI | Arts Health Institute |
| AIA | American Institute of Architects |
| AIPFCC | Australian Institute for Patient and Family Centred Care |
| ANAH | Australian Network for Arts and Health |
| AOPP | Arts and Older People Programme |
| BPG | Brooklyn Parkinson Group |
| CABE | Commission for Architecture and the Built Environment |
| CAC | Community Arts Committee |
| CASP | Critical Appraisal Skills Programme |
| CC | corpus callosum |
| CCD | community cultural development |
| CCE | continuing care establishment |
| CCHSs | [Aboriginal] Community Controlled Health Services |
| CDN | Cultural Development Network [Melbourne] |
| CECAT | Creative Expression Centre for Arts Therapy [Perth, Australia] |
| CMC | Cultural Ministers Council |
| CMH | Centre for Medical Humanities [Durham University] |
| COPD | chronic obstructive pulmonary disease |
| CORE | Clinical Outcomes in Routine Evaluation |
| CRC | [UN] Convention on the Rights of the Child |
| CSDH | [WHO] Commission on the Social Determinants of Health |
| DCMS | [UK] Department of Culture, Media, and Sport |
| DA | discourse analysis |
| DALY | disability adjusted life-year |
| EU | European Union |
| FA | fractional anisotropy |
| FDA | Foucauldian discourse analysis |
| FEV | forced expiratory volume |
| FIC | Freedom in Creation |
| fMRI | functional magnetic resonance imaging |
| FVC | forced vital capacity |
| GAAH | Global Alliance for Arts and Health |
| GDP | gross domestic product |
| GNI | gross national income |
| HADS | Hospital Anxiety and Depression Scale |
| HDI | human development index |
| HOPE | Hubs for Older People's Engagement |
| HPA | hypothalamic–pituitary–adrenocortical |
| HRV | heart rate variability |
| IBS | irritable bowel syndrome |
| ICH | Institute for Creative Health |
| ICT | information and communication technology |
| IDI | Infectious Disease Institute |
| IoP | Institute of Psychiatry at King's College, London |
| IRIS | Indigenous Risk Impact Screen |
| LCACE | London Centre for Arts and Cultural Exchange |
| MBSR | mindfulness-based stress reduction |
| MMDG | Mark Morris Dance Group |
| MOMA | [New York] Museum of Modern Art |
| MRC | Medical Research Council |
| MTFs | military treatment facilities |
| NA | narrative analysis |
| NaCuHeal | nature–culture–health |
| NAHF | National Arts and Health Framework [Australia] |
| NCCA | National Center for Creative Aging |
| NEA | National Endowment for the Arts |
| NEF | New Economics Foundation |
| NGO | non-governmental organization |
| NHS | National Health Service |
| NICE | National Institute for health and Care Excellence |
| NICoE | National Intrepid Center of Excellence |
| NML | National Museums Liverpool |
| NOMS | National Offender Management Service |
| NSW | New South Wales |
| Ofsted | Office for Standards in Education |
| PADA | People with AIDS Development Association |
| PANAS | Positive Affect–Negative Affect Scale |
| PAR | Participatory action research |
| PD | Parkinson's disease |
| PNE | psychoneuroendocrinology |
| PWD | people with dementia |
| QAIHC | Queensland Aboriginal and Islander Health Council |
| QoL | quality of life |
| RCT | randomized controlled trial |
| REB | research ethics board |

| | | | |
|---|---|---|---|
| RMIT | Royal Melbourne Institute of Technology | UNAIDS | Joint United Nations Programme on HIV/AIDS |
| SDH | social determinants of health | UNESCO | United Nations Educational, Scientific and |
| SGRQ | St George's Respiratory Questionnaire | | Cultural Organization |
| SLCN | speech, language, and communication needs | UNICEF | United Nations Children's Fund |
| SMTC | Sampoorna Music Therapy Centre | USDHHS | US Department of Health and Human Services |
| SPREAD | Sustaining Partnerships to Enhance Rural | VAMCs | Veterans Administration Medical Centers |
| | Enterprise and Agribusiness Development | VAMPS | Veshya AIDS Mukabla Parishad, Sangli |
| | [Rwanda] | VAS | visual analogue scale |
| SPSS | Statistical Package for Social Science | WCCLF | World Centre for Creative Learning Foundation |
| TASO | The AIDS Support Organization | WEHI | Walter and Eliza Hall Institute [Melbourne] |
| UCL | University College London | WEMWBS | Warwick–Edinburgh Mental Wellbeing Scale |
| UF | University of Florida | WHO | World Health Organization |
| UFCAM | UF Center for Arts in Medicine | WRNMMC | Walter Reed National Military Medical Center |

# List of Contributors

**Jessica Allen**
UCL Institute of Health Equity and UCL Research Department
of Epidemiology and Public Health
University College London
London, UK

**Matilda Allen**
UCL Institute of Health Equity
University College London
London, UK

**Jonathan Barnes**
Sidney De Haan Research Centre for Arts and Health
Canterbury Christ Church University
Canterbury, UK

**Camila Batmanghelidjh**
Kids Company
London, UK

**Eleonora Belfiore**
Centre for Cultural Policy Studies
University of Coventry UK and Warwick Commission
on the Future of Cultural Value
University of Warwick
Coventry, UK

**Wolfgang Bossinger**
Singing Hospitals International Network
Ulm, Germany

**Katherine M. Boydell**
Professor of Mental Health
The Black Dog Institute
University of New South Wales
Sydney
NSW, Australia

**John Browne**
Composer, UK

**Amy Bucciarelli**
UF Health Shands Arts in Medicine
University of Florida
Florida, USA

**Nicholas Buys**
Menzies Health Institute Queensland
Griffith University
Gold Coast Campus
Parkland, Australia

**Marsaili Cameron**
PublicServiceWorks
London, UK

**Paul M. Camic**
Salomons Centre for Applied Psychology
Canterbury Christ Church University
Tunbridge Wells, UK

**Sandra Carlisle**
Rowett Institute of Nutrition and Health
University of Aberdeen
Aberdeen, UK

**Helen J. Chatterjee**
UCL Museums and Public Engagement
University College London
London, UK

**Stephen Clift**
Sidney De Haan Research Centre for
Arts and Health
Canterbury Christ Church University
Canterbury, UK

**Susan M. Cox**
Maurice W. Young Centre for Applied Ethics
and School of Population and Public Health
University of British Columbia
Vancouver, Canada

**Nikki Crane**
Independent consultant
currently Head of Arts Strategy for Guy's and
St Thomas' Charity
London, UK

**Andrea Creech**
The UCL Institute of Education
London, UK

**Norma Daykin**
Centre for Arts as Wellbeing
University of Winchester
Winchester, UK

**André de Quadros**
School of Music
Boston University
Boston, USA

**Pauline Gladstone-Barrett**
Dance United
London, UK

**Amruta Anand Godse**
FLOW: Social Sciences Research for Health
and Wellbeing
Pune, India

**Anand Sharad Godse**
FLOW: Social Sciences Research for Health
and Wellbeing
Pune, India

**Patricia A. González-Moreno**
Faculty of Arts
Autonomous University of Chihuahua
Chih., Mexico

**John Graham-Pole**
College of Medicine
University of Florida
Florida, USA

**Susan Hallam**
The UCL Institute of Education
London, UK

**Grenville Hancox**
Sidney De Haan Research Centre for Arts and Health
Canterbury Christ Church University
Canterbury, UK

**Phil Hanlon**
Institute for Health and Wellbeing
University of Glasgow
Glasgow, UK

**Paul Heritage**
People's Palace Projects
School of English and Drama
Queen Mary University
London, UK

**Eva Bojner Horwitz**
Department of Public Health and
Caring Sciences
Uppsala University
Uppsala, Sweden

**Victoria Hunter**
University of Chichester
West Sussex, UK

**Richard Ings**
Independent consultant
currently working for Arts Council England
London, UK

**Kizito Fred Kakinda**
College of Engineering
Design, Art and Technology
Makerere University
Kampala, Uganda

**Kizito Maria Kasule**
School of Industrial and Fine Art
Makerere University
Kampala, Uganda

**Margunn Skjei Knudtsen**
Chief Physician for Public Health
Levanger County
Levanger, Norway

**Gunter Kreutz**
Institute of Music
Carl von Ossietzky University of Oldenburg
Oldenburg, Germany

**Bryan Lawson**
School of Architecture
University of Sheffield
Sheffield, UK

**Jenny Baxley Lee**
University of Florida
Florida, USA

**Loraine Leeson**
School of Art and Design
Middlesex University and Faculty of Media
Arts and Design
University of Westminster
London, UK

**Lisa Lorenzino**
Schulich School of Music
McGill University
Montreal, Canada

**Shân Maclennan**
South Bank Centre
London, UK

**Hilary McQueen**
The UCL Institute of Education
London, UK

**Ian Morrison**
Sidney De Haan Research Centre for Arts and Health
Canterbury Christ Church University
Folkstone, UK

**Ian Noonan**
Department of Mental Health Nursing
King's College London
London, UK

**Sonia Page**
Sidney De Haan Research Centre for Arts and Health
Canterbury Christ Church University
Folkstone, UK

**Rosie Parnell**
School of Architecture
University of Sheffield
Sheffield, UK

**Anne Marie Rafferty**
Florence Nightingale School of Nursing and Midwifery
King's College
University of London
London, UK

**Silvia Ramos**
Centre for Studies of Public Security and
   Citizenship (CESeC)
University of Candido Mendes
Rio de Janeiro, Brazil

**Tim Robertson**
Koestler Trust
London, UK

**Judy Rollins**
Rollins and Associates
Washington, DC, USA

**Matthew Shipton**
Sidney De Haan Research Centre for Arts and Health
Canterbury Christ Church University
Folkstone, UK

**Ann Skingley**
Sidney De Haan Research Centre for Arts and Health
Canterbury Christ Church University
Folkstone, UK

**Jill Sonke**
Center for Arts in Medicine
University of Florida
Florida, USA

**Theo Stickley**
School of Health Sciences
University of Nottingham
Nottingham, UK

**Jing Sun**
Menzies Health Institute and School of Medicine
Griffith University
Queensland, Australia

**Töres Theorell**
Stress Research Institute and Department of Neuroscience
Karolinska Institutet
Stockholm, Sweden

**Fredrik Ullén**
Department of Neuroscience
Karolinska Institutet
Stockholm, Sweden

**Maria Varvarigou**
Canterbury Christ Church University
Canterbury UK
The UCL Institute of Education
London, UK

**Trish Vella-Burrows**
Sidney De Haan Research Centre for Arts and Health
Canterbury Christ Church University
Folkstone, UK

**Varun Ramnarayan Venkit**
FLOW: Social Sciences Research for Health and Wellbeing
Pune, India

**Grace Waitman**
Washington University
St Louis
Missouri, USA

**Kate Wells**
Department of Visual Communication Design
Durban University of Technology
Durban, South Africa

The late **Mike White**
(Formerly of) Centre for Medical Humanities
Durham University
Durham, UK

**Britt-Maj Wikström**
Akershus College and Oslo University
Oslo, Norway

**Gareth Wreford**
New South Wales
Department of Family and Community Services
Sydney, Australia

# PART 1

# Creative arts and human health and wellbeing: setting the scene

1 **Introduction to the field of creative arts, wellbeing, and health: achievements and current challenges** *3*
Stephen Clift and Paul M. Camic

2 **The arts and healing: the power of an idea** *11*
Eleonora Belfiore

3 **The fifth wave of public health and the contributions of culture and the arts** *19*
Phil Hanlon and Sandra Carlisle

4 **The social determinants of health, empowerment, and participation** *27*
Jessica Allen and Matilda Allen

5 **Case study: Southbank Centre London and the social utility of the arts** *35*
Shân Maclennan

6 **The means to flourish: arts in community health and education** *41*
Mike White

7 **Community cultural development for health and wellbeing** *49*
Paul M. Camic

8 **Epidemiological studies of the relationship between cultural experiences and public health** *55*
Töres Theorell and Fredrik Ullén

9 **Psychophysiological links between cultural activities and public health** *65*
Töres Theorell

10 **The role of qualitative research in arts and health** *73*
Norma Daykin and Theo Stickley

11 **Ethical issues in arts-based health research** *83*
Susan M. Cox and Katherine M. Boydell

# CHAPTER 1

# Introduction to the field of creative arts, wellbeing, and health: achievements and current challenges

Stephen Clift and Paul M. Camic

## The growth of interest in arts and health

This volume is the first of its kind to offer a global perspective on the value of the creative arts in relation to health and wellbeing. Historically speaking, the role of the arts and artists in society has been the subject of debate and controversy since classical times—from the reflections of Plato and Aristotle in Ancient Greece to the recent series of BBC Reith Lectures by the controversial, socially engaged yet playful UK artist Grayson Perry—and the more challenging, politically informed and even dissident work of artists throughout the world (Klantan et al. 2011).

The idea that the creative arts have a direct role in the care of people suffering from illness and in promoting recovery also has a long history and appears in cultures throughout the world. However, it is only since the beginning of the twentieth century that serious attention has been given to the potential of the arts in therapeutic and healthcare interventions, especially on a psychological level. The development of practice, reflection, and evaluation, and the role of the arts in the broader context of community wellbeing and health promotion is even more recent, developing and gaining ground over the last 60 years. This book appears at a crucial and opportune time for the field of arts, wellbeing, and health—a time marked by a considerable development in interest and activity worldwide, concerns about the future growth and sustainability of arts for health practice, and the need for robust and credible evidence on which to base future developments and investment in this field.

The editors of this volume have played a small part in these developments over the last 15 years, not least by establishing in 2009 a dedicated peer-reviewed scientific journal in this field, *Arts & Health: An International Journal for Research, Policy and Practice* (*Applied Arts and Health*, edited by Dr Ross Prior, first appeared in 2010). A range of other academic journals also specifically address the value of creative arts therapies and the significance of community arts practice in supporting health and wellbeing, as well as the increased recognition of the importance of the arts and humanities in the training of medical and healthcare professionals of all kinds. These journals portray the growth, diversity, and vitality of practice and research in the field of creative arts, wellbeing, and health in recent years; however, they are specialist academic sources and it is now time for a more accessible publication to appear. The present textbook endeavours to provide a broad overview of the field, highlighting recent developments in arts for health practice and research throughout the world.

In addition to the increasing number of publications in this field, growth is also demonstrated by the number of well-established national and regional arts for health organizations, particularly in English-speaking countries (e.g. Australia, Canada, New Zealand, and the United Kingdom) and across Europe and Scandinavia (see Box 1.1 for some weblinks). Such organizations are invaluable for the purposes of networking and sharing on an organizational and individual level, training and resource development to support capacity and delivery, and advocacy and lobbying to build a case for expansion of the sector and securing funding. Box 1.1 gives some examples of the underpinning philosophy, mission, and reach of these organizations. The Global Alliance for Arts and Health provided substantial leadership to the field in the United States, but unfortunately this network closed in late 2014 due to financial difficulties. Nevertheless, we still include details of the objectives it pursued.

The substantial international growth of interest in the field of arts and health is also clearly represented in the number of international conferences that have been held on arts and health. Box 1.2 lists a selection of international conferences from the spring of 2013 to the end of 2014. Conferences in English-speaking countries predominate, but this list also reflects significant interest in this field in Finland, Israel, Lithuania, and Uganda.

## What is health?

Throughout this volume individual contributors address the issue of defining health and what is perhaps the more contested concept of human wellbeing and flourishing. In some chapters reference

**Box 1.1**  Principal networks for arts and health

### Arts and Health Australia

Arts and Health Australia (AHA; <http://www.artsandhealth.org/about-us.html>) was established to enhance and improve health and wellbeing within the community through engagement in creative activities. It provides guidance on research and strategic development, hosts conferences, and provides training. The arts and health field covers primary and acute care, aged care, community health, and health promotion. Arts and Health Australia:

- advocates arts and health practice in primary care and community health
- demonstrates the effectiveness of the arts in health promotion
- showcases the value of the humanities in medical education and the wellbeing of clinicians and healthcare professionals
- networks with people working in healthcare, arts, education, and the community
- connects with international counterparts on development in practice and research
- facilitates policy change at all levels of government to stimulate the growth of arts and health initiatives in Australia
- supports scientific research and evaluation of arts and health programmes

### Arts Health Network Canada

The primary purpose of Arts Health Network Canada (AHNC; <http://artshealthnetwork.ca/>) is to increase public awareness, understanding, and appreciation of the contributions of arts-based initiatives to individual and community health, as well as to Canada's public healthcare system. AHNC aims to bring arts and health activities into the mainstream, integrated in the fabric of communities and healthcare services so that the arts and cultural activities are embraced as integral in meeting the health and social needs of all Canadians. AHNC engages arts/health users, organizations, decision-makers, and the broader public to understand and support the connections between health and arts-based activities. Arts Health Network Canada:

- supports connection, dialogue, and information-sharing through a comprehensive knowledge repository on arts and health in Canada
- encourages the development of local and provincial networks of individuals and organizations interested and working in arts and health
- raises awareness of the individual and community health and wellness benefits of arts-based activities and helps increase support for Canadian arts and health initiatives
- collaborates with researchers and the community to assess the effectiveness of arts-based health initiatives
- draws on experiences and research conducted in Canada and around the world to expand knowledge about effective arts and health programmes and practices

### Global Alliance for Arts and Health (United States)

The Global Alliance for Arts and Health (formerly the Society for the Arts in Healthcare) was a not-for-profit organization based in Washington, DC which ceased to operate in late 2014. Until that time it was the largest and one of the most long-standing arts and health organizations internationally. Its focus was on practice development, supporting policy initiatives, and training. It also provided sponsorship of the journal, *Arts & Health*. The Alliance when it operated sought to:

- demonstrate the valuable roles the arts can play in enhancing the healing process
- advocate for the integration of the arts into the environment and delivery of care within healthcare facilities
- assist in the professional development and management of arts programming for healthcare populations
- provide resources and education to healthcare and arts professionals
- encourage research on the beneficial effects of the arts in healthcare
- Clearly this organization will be sadly missed by practitioners and researchers in the United States and more widely throughout the world.

### National Alliance for Arts, Health and Wellbeing (England)

The National Alliance for Arts, Health and Wellbeing (<http://www.artshealthandwellbeing.org.uk>) was established in 2012 with the support of Arts Council England. It brings together regional arts for health organizations from across England to offer a national voice for arts and health. The Alliance has developed a Charter for Arts, Health and Wellbeing, and their website profiles current practice and research in England. The National Alliance:

- provides a clear and focused voice to articulate the role that creativity can play in health and wellbeing
- offers a repository for arts and health practice and research
- advocates on behalf of the arts and health sector to policy-makers in central and local government
- encourages the use of the arts by health and social care providers
- aspires to raise standards in drawing on the creative arts in the healthcare sector

Source: data from Arts and Health Australia, 'About' (<http://www.artsandhealth.org/about-us.html>), accessed October 2014; Arts Health Network Canada, 'About: priorities' (<http://artshealthnetwork.ca/about/priorities>), accessed October 2014; Arts and Health Alliance, 'About' (<https://www.artsandhealthalliance.org/about/>), accessed October 2014; National Alliance for Arts, Health and Wellbeing, 'What is Arts in Health?: National Alliance for Arts, Health and Wellbeing' (<http://www.artshealthandwellbeing.org.uk/recent-developments/national-alliance-arts-health-and-wellbeing>), accessed October 2014.

**Box 1.2** Recent international conferences on arts and health

The Arch of Arts in Health International Conference, Haifa, Israel, March 2013

Culture, Health and Wellbeing International Conference, Bristol, UK, June 2013

The Art of Good Health and Wellbeing, 5th Annual Arts and Health Conference, Sydney, Australia, November 2013

Music, Mind and Health, Melbourne, Australia, November 2013

Art Goes Work—Wellbeing for You, Helsinki, Finland, December 2013

Enhancing Lives through Arts & Health, Global Alliance for Arts & Health, Texas, USA, April 2014

The Role of Arts in Living Well with Dementia, Creative Arts Dementia Network, Oxford UK, April 2014

Art and Mental Health. Creative Partnership—Policy and Practice, Vilnius, Lithuania, April 2014

The Creative Age: Exploring Potential in the Second Half of Life, National Center for Creative Aging, Washington, USA, June 2014

Arts in Medicine for Global Communities Intensive, Kampala, Uganda, June 2014

3rd International Conference of the International Association for Music & Medicine, Toronto, Canada, June 2014

Singing, Wellbeing and Health—International Symposium, London UK, September 2014

6th Annual Arts and Health and Wellbeing Conference, Arts and Health, Melbourne, Australia, November 2014

is made to the World Health Organization's (WHO) definition of health, formulated in 1946 and enshrined in the preamble to the WHO constitution. This states that:

'Health is a state of complete physical, mental and social wellbeing and not merely an absence of disease or infirmity'

WHO (1946)

Given the centrality of a definition of health to work of the WHO, and the need for a formulation that is relevant and meaningful across all of the world's cultures, one might expect that this definition was arrived at following extensive consultation and debate. This is far from being the case, however. In an interview published in 1988, Dr Szeming Sze, a member of the Chinese delegation to the conference which drafted the Charter of the United Nations and a 'founding father' of the WHO, explained, in response to the question, 'How did you arrive at a consensus on the definition of health?', how the definition came about:

'A lot of people did not think that we should define health in the Constitution of WHO. I only got involved because I found myself on the subcommittee on the preamble in the Technical Preparatory Committee. I think there were three of us—Dr Brock Chisholm from Canada (who became the first Director-General of the WHO), Dr Gregorio Bermann from Argentina and myself; it was a pleasant little group and we had some interesting academic discussions.

Chisholm, being a psychiatrist wanted to mention mental health, and I thought we should put something in that emphasised the importance of the preventive side of health. That's how we came up with the wording in the Constitution that defines health as not merely the absence of illness.'

Sze (1988, p. 33)

Although the definition has repeatedly come under scrutiny since 1946, and there have been periodic calls for it to be revised, extended, and even abandoned altogether, it has stood the test of time and has not been amended. The WHO after all is the World *Health* Organization and not the World *Medical* Organization, so the definition has the strength of being positively worded, multidimensional, and holistic. Some commentators suggest that the definition is too idealistic and unrealizable, and are often critical of the word 'complete'. An alternative reading of this word, however, can be that all elements of physical, mental, and social wellbeing should be considered together; the definition does not necessarily imply 'perfect' health, only that an absence of physical disease in and of itself does not mean that a person's overall wellbeing can be assumed.

The most recent example of recurrent debate is provided by a report from an international conference in The Netherlands in 2010 called to examine the need for a revised definition of health to reflect changing global health realities (Huber et al. 2011). Huber and colleagues identify a number of possible problems with the existing definition. First they suggest that it 'unintentionally contributes to the medicalisation of society' by supporting 'the tendencies of the medical technology and drugs industries, in association with professional organisations to redefine diseases, expanding the scope of the healthcare system'. Secondly, they point to the enormous demographic and epidemiological changes that have occurred since the late 1940s, leading to increased numbers of older people in populations around the world and greater burdens of chronic ill-health. Thirdly, they suggest that the existing definition does not lend itself very readily to validated and reliable measurement. The solution offered by the combined intellectual resources of the conference was a move from the static character of the WHO definition to a more dynamic view:

'The discussion of the experts at the Dutch conference [. . .] led to broad support for moving from the present static formulation towards a more dynamic one based on the resilience or capacity to cope and maintain and restore one's integrity, equilibrium, and sense of wellbeing. The preferred view on health was 'the ability to adapt and self manage'.'

Huber et al. (2011, p. 2)

In many respects, however, the account by Huber et al. revisits a line of development that the WHO itself has pursued over many years: to establish international consensus on the definition and scope of health promotion; to devise instruments for the assessment and measurement of health (e.g. the development of quality-of-life questionnaires; The WHOQOL Group 1998); and, most recently, to address the nature and assessment of wellbeing (WHO Regional Office for Europe 2013).Since the mid 1960s the WHO has been central to the development and growth of a common international framework for health promotion. Starting with the Ottawa Charter in 1968, a series of declarations has given rise to a common understanding of the multiple determinants of health, wellbeing, and illness and the most appropriate strategies needed to improve population health—through policy, the development of person-centred community health services, and health education. The central feature of the Ottawa Charter is a definition of health promotion, which reiterates the WHO definition of health but goes beyond it in recognizing health as 'a resource for everyday life':

'Health promotion is the process of enabling people to increase control over, and to improve, their health. To reach a state of complete physical mental and social wellbeing, an individual or group must be able to identify and realize aspirations, to satisfy needs, and the change or cope with the environment. Health is, therefore, seen as a resource for everyday life, not the objective of living. Health is a positive concept emphasizing social and personal resources, as well as physical capacities. Therefore, health promotion is not just the responsibility of the health sector, but goes beyond health life-styles to wellbeing.'

WHO (1986)

The Ottawa Charter builds on this definition of health promotion, by specifying the routes through which health promotion can be achieved:

◆ build healthy public policy
◆ create supportive environments
◆ strengthen community actions
◆ develop personal skills
◆ reorient health services

In addition, several of the guiding principles expressed in the Ottawa Charter can be readily translated into the best practices seen in the arts and health field:

'The overall guiding principle for the world, nations, regions and communities alike is the need to encourage reciprocal maintenance—to take care of each other, our communities and our natural environment.'

[. . .]

'Work and leisure should be a source of health for people. The way society organizes work should help create a healthy society. Health promotion generates living and working conditions that are safe, stimulating, satisfying and enjoyable.'

[. . .]

'Health promotion works through concrete and effective community action in setting priorities, making decisions, planning strategies and implementing them to achieve better health. At the heart of this process is the empowerment of communities, their ownership and control of their own endeavours and destinies.'

WHO (1986, pp. 2–3)

An informative archive film on the development of the Ottawa Charter, its historical context, and philosophical underpinnings can be viewed on the WHO website (WHO 2011).

## The role of evaluation and research

Along with the growth of interest in the contribution of the creative arts to healthcare and health promotion there has been increased attention to evaluation and research. This is essential not only in documenting the nature of arts practices for health, but also in understanding how involvement in creative activity can positively influence wellbeing and health and for assessing outcomes over time. The central questions from a health perspective are the extent to which creative activity and engagement with the arts work to promote health and assist in the treatment of specified health conditions, and also whether such interventions are cost-effective. The application of research findings in helping to establish a basis for evidence-based practice in the field of arts for health is also an important issue.

One approach to evaluating arts for health interventions draws upon the methodological principles embodied in the so-called 'hierarchy of evidence' widely adopted in medical and health sciences. This essentially promotes the value of controlled trials for establishing causal connections between interventions and objective measureable outcomes, together with the synthesis of robust experimental findings through systematic reviews and meta-analysis. More and more research is appearing in which randomized controlled trial methods and systematic reviews have been applied to the field of arts for health, emulating a longer track record of experimental approaches and systematic reviews in the field of creative arts therapies, the outcomes of which served to test the validity of these approaches—not always with positive outcomes for practitioners.

There is a need for more rigorous controlled studies which can help to build a robust evidence base for arts and health, but an experimental, quantitative approach is not without its critics. For example, Sagan (2014) reflected on the challenges in assessing the value of engaging with the visual arts for wellbeing and health:

'In some ways, 'evidencing' the impact of visual arts activity on mental wellbeing, the area in which I work, is much like the proverbial nailing of jelly to a wall. It brings together the confounding difficulties of what is still felt to be a mysterious process (making art) and the disputed qualities of what constitutes creativity with the contested and evolving nature of our knowledge about mental wellbeing and our dissatisfaction with the instruments for measuring it. We also contend with the political discomfort of reductionism, instrumentalism and the pitfalls of delivering only what can be counted.'

Another critic of an 'empirical' approach in arts and health research, demanding controlled designs and measureable outcomes, is White (2014):

'Arts in health is at a fork in the road. The hard-paved route, The Empirical Highway, leads to probable damnation by way of austerity culture, a narrowing definition of accredited practice, and evidence calls that are signalled through a medical model of health. Those who venture on this path will find their creativity randomised, controlled and trialled. The other route, which I term The Lantern Road, tracks its progress through reflective practice, has lit beacons of new traditions in participatory health promotion, and affirms relationship-based working as the way to a sustainable vision of community-based arts in health supported by interdisciplinary research.'

Such reflections by highly experienced and esteemed practitioners in creative arts therapy and community arts development, respectively, must be taken seriously; indeed they make important points, while also highlighting concerns often expressed by artists about the legitimacy of applying scientific methodologies to creative endeavours. After all it was D. H. Lawrence who observed that the botanist in dissecting and naming the parts of a flower destroys it and fails to understand the beauty of the whole.

In fact, however, even in the medical and health sciences, there are dissenting voices regarding the applicability of 'the medical model', the idea of a hierarchy of evidence, and the view that randomized trials are capable of answering all questions of importance in the assessment of interventions. There is also increasingly widespread acceptance of the need for mixed-method approaches, in which qualitative evidence is used to supplement and deepen the evidence that comes from attempts to measure and quantify.

The UK Medical Research Council (MRC), for example, recognizes that social interventions are generally multifaceted in nature and has offered guidance on the evaluation of such complex interventions (Craig et al. 2008). In MRC terms initiatives in which the creative arts are drawn on to promote wellbeing and health in community settings or to improve outcomes in the context of healthcare with patient groups count as such complex interventions, and MRC guidance has made a very significant contribution to furthering more sophisticated evaluation in the arts and health field. It is also important, as Petticrew and Roberts (2003) emphasize, to appreciate a close link between the questions research seeks to answer and the methods that are most appropriate for answering those questions. Rather than a hierarchy of evidence, they suggest, we should think in terms of a typology of methods. The following scheme is suggested on the basis of the general principles they outline:

◆ Where we are interested in the acceptability and appropriateness of an activity, and participant satisfaction, qualitative studies including questionnaires, interviews, and focus group discussions would be appropriate.

◆ Where we want to understand the process of delivery of an intervention, and assess the skills of a facilitator or artist, qualitative studies would again be most appropriate drawing on observations, reflective journals, and feedback from participants.

◆ Where the longer-term effects of cultural and creative participation are of interest, a large-scale epidemiological study involving clear outcomes and statistical controls may be revealing.

◆ Where the safety and risks associated with interventions need to be assessed, pilot studies with appropriate indicators are needed.

◆ Where the efficacy, effectiveness, and cost-effectiveness of interventions are the focus of interest, then experimental studies with suitable controls and clear health outcomes are required.

◆ Where we wish to draw together all the available evidence on a particular kind of creative arts intervention and its health outcomes, then systematic mapping, reviewing, and even a Cochrane review are needed.

A recent UK initiative, Aesop, has developed a useful framework for arts and health research (Fancourt and Joss 2015). Created on the basis of wide consultation with health science methodologists, arts and health researchers, and artists, the framework provides a tool for researchers evaluating and planning research studies in the arts and health field.

The purpose and function of the framework is explained as follows (Aesop 2014):

'This Framework creates a link between arts activity and health research. Arts in health research can be confusing and misunderstood by those working in the arts and in health, artists, reviewers, researchers and funders. For reviewers of research proposals, it is neither fish nor fowl, falling between the humanities and sciences and using methodologies that may be unfamiliar and queried by at least half the reviewers. Funders need to know what good methodology should look like in the field but have no reference point. Equally artists do not necessarily understand what is required in order to develop robust, publishable research findings and existing

researchers in the field simply want to ensure that their proposals are understood, have validity and get funding.'

'Without a common methodological framework in which all parties have confidence, arts in health research will continue to languish at the fringes of health research. The arts may have the potential to play a particular role in the prevention and management of long term conditions, currently the subject of much greater focus, and it would be disappointing for the arts not to be able to contribute to this agenda or other health agendas for lack of a common methodological framework, understood and respected by all. This framework takes you through the various steps in a developing an arts intervention in health and associated research study, and invites you to score your intended project.'

## Why have we seen this growth of interest in arts and health?

As we have already mentioned, the growth of interest in the therapeutic value of the arts is relatively recent. The Global Alliance for Arts and Health Conference celebrated its 25th anniversary in 2014, but as Box 1.2 illustrates, the annual conferences in Australia have a shorter history and the Culture, Health and Wellbeing Conference in Bristol in 2013 was the first of its kind in the United Kingdom. It remains to be seen whether this interest can be sustained and developed, and it will be for future historians to reflect on the factors and influences accounting for this growth of interest at the tail end of the last millennium and into the twenty-first century.

In an inspiring and wide-ranging keynote address to the Bristol conference, Alan Howarth (2013), a member of the UK House of Lords offered his view of the wider political, economic, and social context which may explain why there is movement towards the creative arts as resources to support and promote wellbeing and health. Howarth referred to 'the pathology of the west' driven by forces such as a classical economic model of human nature, an increasingly ascendant biomedical view of health, growing social inequalities, and the rise in use and abuse of digital technologies:

'The view of human nature taken by so-called classical economics, the economics of the free market, that people are all self-seeking utility maximisers, is false and degrading. After forty years of intellectual hegemony we have brought into being societies, and indeed a world, riven by inequalities, as seen in health and morbidity statistics. One in three people in our society experiences mental illness. The new Diagnostic and Statistical Manual catalogues a vast variety of mental disorders, but proposes that these are more biological than psychosocial in origin—a proposition rightly disputed by the British Psychological Society. In Britain more than 9000 people with mental illness are detained each year in police custody and treated as suspected criminals.'

'The banalities of the media and the ubiquity of porn and violence in entertainment coarsen relationships. Societies infatuated with technology and wealth neglect traditional wisdom and disrespect their elderly. The politics of money has issued in disastrous economic mismanagement. The poorest are bearing the heaviest burden of that failure, with immediate consequences for their health. Vast expenditures on the military and weapons have left ravaged conflict zone, injury and disease across the world. Gross disrespect for nature has jeopardized even the survival of the human societies'.

Howarth went on to say:

'I have spoken about the pathology of the west, not because I think arts in health practitioners can solve all the problems of the west, but because this is the context of political culture and still prevailing values into which you make your interventions. You, no doubt, in your day-to-day work take a less grandiose and more pragmatic view of what you are about, and I applaud you for that. Nonetheless, what you are about expresses a choice of values as well as techniques. You, as heretics and radicals, are challenging dominant values and conventional policies.'

Further drivers must also be that everywhere in the world populations are getting older, and with greater life expectancy has come an increased prevalence of non-communicable, chronic disease, including the growing challenges of long-term obesity, substance dependences, and dementias and other neurodegenerative conditions. Coupled with this is the recognition not only that medicine is limited in what it can offer in support of people with chronic and progressive illnesses for which there is no cure, but also that the provision and quality of health and social care services face an uncertain future in an age of economic austerity. Increasingly, it is recognized that the growing challenges of public health cannot be tackled solely by healthcare systems at the stage of treatment and care, but have to be addressed in a coordinated way by governments, statutory services, civil society, and the private sector, with a commitment also to primary prevention, health protection, and health promotion. Initiatives to educate and support people in taking responsibility for their own health and the self-management of long-term conditions are also important.

It is clear, however, from the details in Box 1.1 that the strongest interest and practical initiatives in creative arts in health can be found in affluent English-speaking countries. And while the US-based Society for Arts in Healthcare renamed itself the Global Alliance for Arts and Health (before its subsequent closure), there is a substantial question mark over whether the creative arts can make a contribution in the context of the global realities of population health, given the principal drivers of poor health in poorer countries around the world and the growing inequities in health both across and within countries. This is an issue which Clift et al. (2010) addressed directly in an editorial of the journal *Arts & Health* in response to the publication of the report of the WHO Commission on the Social Determinants of Health led by Sir Michael Marmot (CSDH 2008).

Clift et al. (2010) ask whether the idea that the creative arts have a role in promoting health is 'an elitist luxury available only to the already advantaged' or whether, in the wider scheme of things, pursuit of the arts for health agenda is 'an irrelevant distraction, offering little or nothing to the task of tackling major sources of ill health, suffering and premature death in the world' (Clift et al. 2010, p. 3).

The arts may indeed have the power to improve wellbeing and quality of life given that basic physical, emotional, and social needs are met, but can they really engage with the fundamental drivers of current health inequities? The report of the WHO Commission is replete with statistics which are difficult to grasp, reflecting the scale of the public health challenges facing the vast bulk of the world's growing population today. Today (2015) these statistics may be different—almost certainly they will be worse:

◆ 1 billion people in the world live in slums, without clean running water and sanitation (CSDH 2008, p. 4)

◆ 40% of the world's population survive on $2 per day (p. 31)

◆ worldwide, 10 million children die each year before their fifth birthday (p. 50)

◆ half a million women die each year during pregnancy and child-birth from want of adequate healthcare (p. 94)

◆ 126 million children are working in hazardous conditions (p. 35) and nearly 6 million children are in bonded labour (p. 74)

◆ four in every five people worldwide lack social security coverage (p. 84)

It is important to recognize the political, economic, and social realities which actually determine the poor health outcomes for most of the world's population today, and to have a proper sense of proportion and humility in claiming a role for the creative arts in addressing such issues, and perhaps in a small way making a difference in promoting health and wellbeing under the most difficult and challenging circumstances. And this is not just in the poorer countries of the world. As Marmot so strikingly shows through his work, in all countries we find a clear social gradient, with the less advantaged strata in all societies having poorer health and shorter healthy life expectancies.

Clift et al. (2010) nevertheless express surprise that in the whole of the WHO Commission report there is not a single reference to the creative arts as having some relevance in addressing current health challenges—especially given that the report could have profiled some examples of initiatives from around the world in which 'the power of the arts has a key role in tackling health inequalities'. Clift et al. (2010) cite three examples of how the arts can work in this way, illustrated by cases from South Africa, India, Uganda, Venezuela, and Brazil:

◆ International campaigning, fundraising, and advocacy—for example the central role of music in the international initiative to raise awareness of the blight of poverty and the scourge of HIV/AIDS in Nelson Mandela's *46664* campaign.

◆ Community social action and education for health—for example inspiring community performing arts projects such as the Darpana Academy of Performing Arts in Gujarat, India working to train young people as peer educators, or the role of women in promoting awareness of AIDS in traditional East African communities through singing (Barz 2006).

◆ Challenging cultures of poverty, violence, and drug use through skill development and empowerment—for example through the nationwide El Sistema project in Venezuela or the work of Gruppo Cultural AfroReggae working with young people in the favelas of Rio de Janeiro.

Clift et al.'s editorial was the starting point for the current text, and we will conclude this introductory chapter by outlining the structure and content of this volume.

## The structure and content of this volume

A key claim of this text is that the arts, culture, and creative engagement can all offer resources in everyday life to help promote health and wellbeing in a holistic manner, and that the arts are assets which can be drawn upon in culturally appropriate ways in countries throughout the world to help address pressing health challenges. The arts are not a panacea—and there may be many issues for which they have limited relevance. But the arts at heart are about creativity and problem-solving, and above all about helping to create both meaning and a sense of beauty in all of our lives.

The volume is structured in four parts. Part 1 provides important contextual contributions, locating current perspectives in arts and health within the history of debates about the nature and value of the arts in society, but also offering perspectives from the history and current concerns of the field of public health. Given that the aim here is to explore the value of the creative arts for wellbeing and health, we are attempting the formidable task of bridging, integrating, and perhaps reconciling the generally separate worlds of 'the arts' and 'medicine and healthcare'—and in a more general sense addressing the divide between 'arts and humanities' and 'natural science'. Accordingly, it is important to provide a historical and philosophical view from the perspective of the arts for readers coming to this volume from a medical or wider health background. For those with a grounding in arts and humanities it is important to introduce historical perspectives on the development of public health, as well as current thinking about the broader political, economic, social, and cultural determinants of both disease and ill-health, but also, more positively, health and wellbeing. Important methodological and ethical issues are also explored in this part.

Part 2 reviews or presents examples of arts for health initiatives in selected countries throughout the world, and also gives concrete case studies of particular initiatives. We have tried to ensure a wide global coverage and not limit presentations to work undertaken in affluent English-speaking countries. So alongside broad reviews of developments in the United States, Australia, Sweden, and Norway, there are overviews of arts for health initiatives in India and China and case studies from Uganda, Brazil, and Peru. A particularly striking example is included of how a community music initiative for young people developed in Venezuela, El Sistema, has inspired similar projects in countries around the world.

Part 3 takes its lead from the work of the WHO Commission on the Social Determinants of Health to highlight the need to think about health across the whole of the life course. Chapters address the value of participation in the creative arts from the early years of life through to old age, including the way in which the creative arts can be an effective vehicle for intergenerational projects which bring children and older people together. Case studies again add depth and a concrete perspective on how the visual and performing arts can help address very challenging realities of socio-economic deprivation, abuse and neglect, and a lack of educational opportunities in the lives of children and young people. The value of creative activity for the wellbeing of older people facing challenges of long-term health conditions, social isolation, and loneliness is also explored.

Part 4 takes as its starting point a key element of the WHO approach to health promotion, namely the need to think about the impact of settings on health, and also the opportunities that different social settings offer for impacting positively on health. Foremost among such setting are schools for children and young people, other educational settings catering for older students and adults, and health and social care settings, such as hospitals and residential care homes. Other settings addressed include US prisons, rehabilitation centres for young women rescued from the sex industry in India, and public galleries and museums in the United Kingdom.

Medicine, healthcare, and public health are increasingly driven by scientific evidence. They are also deeply moral enterprises concerned with human wellbeing and dignity. But there is a third dimension to human life and experience beyond the scientific concerns for objectivity and knowledge and the ethical concerns for values and what is right and good. That third dimension is aesthetic, with its concerns for pleasure, enjoyment, and beauty (Clift 2012). These three concerns—what is true, what is good, and what is beautiful—are identified by Gardner (2011) as central to the educational enterprise and should be at the heart of any balanced curriculum. Medicine and public health are fields with a clear ethical base and are driven by evidence, but more and more practitioners and researchers are beginning to see a role for aesthetic dimensions in our understanding of health and wellbeing. We hope that this text will help to show how far we have come in this endeavour, and will offer inspiration for yet further developments in this exciting and diverse field.

## References

Aesop (2014). Aesop 1: A framework for developing and researching arts in health programmes. Available at:<http://artsinhealth-framework. org/ [see under filmed interviews for the views of Professor Sally MacIntyre].

Barz, G. (2006). *Singing for Life: HIV/AIDS and music in Uganda.* London: Routledge.

Clift, S. (2012) Creative arts as a public health resource: moving from practice-based research to evidence-based practice. *Perspectives in Public Health,* **132,** 120–127.

Clift, S., Camic, P., and Daykin, N. (2010). The arts and global health inequities. *Arts & Health: An International Journal for Research, Policy and practice,* **2,** 3–7.

Craig, P., Dieppe, P., Macintyre, S., Michie, S., Nazarath, I., and Petticrew, M. (2008). Developing and evaluating complex interventions: the new Medical Research Council guidance. *British Medical Journal,* **337,** a1555.

CSDH (2008). *Closing the Gap in a Generation: Health Equity Through Action on the Social Determinants of Health.* Geneva: World Health Organization. Available at: <http://www.who.int/social_determinants/final_report/csdh_finalreport_2008.pdf>Gardner, H. (2011). *Truth, Beauty and Goodness Reframed: Educating for the Virtues in the 21st Century.* New York: Basic Books.

Howarth, A. (2013). Arts, health and wellbeing – personal reflections and political perspectives. *Address to Culture, Health and Wellbeing International Conference, Bristol, 25 June 2013.* Available at: <http://www.artsforhealth.org/news/LordHowarthBristolSpeech250613. pdf>

Huber, M., Knottnerus, J.A., van der Horst, H., et al. (2011). How should we define health? *British Medical Journal,* **343,** 1–3.

Klantan, R., Hübner, M., Bieber, A., Alonzo, P., and Jansen, G. (2011). *Art & Agenda: Political Art and Activism.* Berlin: Gestalten.

Petticrew, M. and Roberts, H. (2003). Evidence, hierarchies, and typologies: horses for courses. *Journal of Epidemiology and Community Health,* **57,** 527–529.

Sagan, O. (2014). Position statement in advance of the Elusive Evidence conference, York St John University, 10 June 2014.

Sze, S. (1988). WHO: from small beginnings. *World Health Forum,* **9,** 29–34.

The WHOQOL Group (1998). The World Health Organization quality of life assessment (WHOQOL): development and general psychometric properties. *Social Science and Medicine,* **46,** 1569–1585.

White, M. (2014). *Asking the Way—Directions and Misdirections in Arts in Health.* Commissioned and published by ixia, the public art think tank, 14 April 2014. Available at: <http://www.publicartonline.org.uk/downloads/news/Asking%20the%20Way%20-%20Mike%20White.pdf>

WHO (1946). Preamble to the Constitution of the World Health Organization as adopted by the International Health Conference, New York, 19–22 June, 1946; signed on 22 July 1946 by the representatives of 61 States (*Official Records of the World Health Organization,* no. 2, p. 100) and entered into force on 7 April 1948.

WHO (1986). *Ottawa Charter for Health Promotion, 1986.* Available at: <http://www.who.int/healthpromotion/conferences/previous/ottawa/en/>

WHO (2011). 25 years of Ottawa Charter. Available at: <http://www.euro.who.int/en/about-us/governance/regional-committee-for-europe/past-sessions/sixty-first-session/multimedia/video-25-years-of-ottawa-charter>

WHO Regional Office for Europe (2013). *The European Health Report 2012: Charting the Way to Wellbeing.* Copenhagen: WHO Europe.

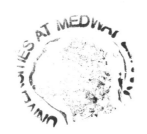

# CHAPTER 2

# The arts and healing: the power of an idea

Eleonora Belfiore

## Introduction to the arts and healing

One of the most original developments in public policies for the support and funding of the arts in post-war Britain (although the phenomenon is hardly limited to Britain) is arguably the increased prominence of the conviction that engagement and participation in the arts can have beneficial effects on health and individual wellbeing. From its beginnings in the late 1980s, with the first pilot projects that deployed the arts for community health development and in a primary-care setting, 'arts in health' has developed into a distinct component of arts practice attracting increasing levels of funding (White 2009). In Britain, interest in the connection between arts (as well as sport) and health flourished from 1997 onwards in the era of the New Labour administration, when it became part of the broader strategies to achieve social inclusion and 'neighbourhood renewal' (Stickley and Duncan 2010).

This is hardly surprising, since a commitment to social inclusion and an ethics of social justice have both been central to the arts and health movement (Clift 2012). As Mike White (2009, p. 4) explains: 'Through sustained programmes of participatory arts, shared creativity can make committed expressions of public health, simultaneously identifying and addressing the local and specific health needs in a community. This is what distinguishes arts in health work from art therapies and connect into social inclusion work'. And yet, back in 2002, at the height of the New Labour administration, the London Health Commission published a pamphlet pointedly entitled *Culture and Health: Making the Link*, which lamented the neglect that up until then had surrounded the connection between cultural activities and social and personal wellbeing, and the 'little attention given to understanding how cultural policy impacts on the health of communities and how it can contribute to achieving health objectives' (London Health Commission 2002, p. 3).

Today the picture appears very different. The late 1990s saw the first concerted ministerial attempts to coordinate the activities of the UK Department of Culture, Media, and Sport (DCMS) and the Department of Health. Such attempts were behind the establishment, by the Department of Health, of a Review of Arts and Health Working Group, whose work culminated in *A Prospectus for Arts and Health* jointly published by the Department of Health and Arts Council England in 2007. The prospectus purported to 'show that the arts can, and do, make a major contribution to key health and wider community issues' (ACE 2007, p. 2), and presented itself as 'a celebration of the role of arts and health' (ACE 2007, p. 7):

> 'This prospectus demonstrates the value of arts and health work in a range of settings. The wealth of evidence and good practice examples illustrates the benefits right across the spectrum of arts and health, including improving clinical and therapeutic outcomes, helping users to express, contain and transform distress and disturbance, creating a less stressful environment for patients, service users, staff and visitors, increasing the understanding between clinicians and the people for whom they care, bettering public health, developing and delivering more patient-focused services, and improving the experience for all.'
>
> ACE (2007, p. 8)

A publication by Arts Council England in 2014, entitled *The Value of Arts and Culture to People and Society*, identified 'health and wellbeing' as one of the four key areas in which the arts can generate public value, alongside the economy, the social sphere, and education. Never before had the health impacts of the arts featured so prominently in a policy document of a general arts funding body with a clear strategic nature. This shows how mainstream the support of arts and health activity has now become within British cultural policy discourse, at least at the rhetorical level (whether financial support will also grow proportionately remains to be seen).

A similar enthusiasm has been shown by members of the medical community (although, as we will see, this is not a universally shared or consensual position). For instance, in 2002, Richard Smith, then editor of the prestigious *British Medical Journal*, penned an editorial entitled 'Spend (slightly) less on health and more on the arts—health would probably be improved', which semi-seriously contended that 'diverting 0.5% of the healthcare budget to the arts would improve the health of people in Britain' (Smith 2002, p. 1433). He further elaborated his argument thus:

> 'The arts don't solve problems. Books or films may allow you temporarily to forget your pain, but great books or films (let's call them art) will ultimately teach you something useful about your pain. [. . .] If health is about adaptation, understanding, and acceptance, then the arts may be more potent than anything that medicine has to offer.'
>
> Smith (2002, p. 1433)

## Arts and health: the evidence question

There is a degree of agreement among practitioners in the field as well as academic observers that there is, cumulatively, sufficient evidence of the beneficial health effects of arts participation and arts-based public health intervention to justify both the growing volume of this strand of work and public expenditure on it (Secker et al. 2007; Clift 2012). Nevertheless, the problem of evaluation of interventions in community-based arts for health activities and the need for a more solid evidence base remain (Madden and Bloom 2004; South 2004). For Stickley and Duncan (2010, p. 105), the problem lies in the fact that '[s]pecific research into the arts, creativity and its benefits for physical and mental health is in its infancy, being in a hypothesising/generating stage'. As Mike White (2009, p. 201) pithily puts it:

'There is a lot we do not and cannot empirically know that is nevertheless an integral yet immeasurable part of the wellbeing experienced by the participants. The benefits of participation in arts community health are to date only partly substantiated and so are also partly unknown.'

The question of the availability and reliability of evidence for the effectiveness of the arts in the context of health interventions is central to the financial sustainability of this strand of arts practice. The importance of this connection is clearly articulated in the evaluation of 'Time Being 2', a participatory arts on prescription project piloted and delivered between 2002 and 2012 by the Isle of Wight National Health Service (NHS) primary care trust, and targeted at patients with depression:

'Existing qualitative evidence overwhelmingly suggests that the benefits of participatory arts programmes are in the areas of self-esteem, social participation, and mental wellbeing for those participating. However, there have been few quantitative studies and those that have been undertaken are of questionable rigour; the need for more definitive evidence is frequently rehearsed in the research and policy literature. Without rigorous evidence of the specific contribution made by participatory arts programmes to (mental) health outcomes and their cost-effectiveness, it is unlikely that existing or future governments will see fit to encourage local health commissioners to invest in them.'
Baumann and MatrixInsights (2010, p. 28)

The problem of the reliability of the evidence base for the claims made on behalf of arts participation within public policy is a wider one in relation to cultural policies (Belfiore 2009; Belfiore and Bennett 2010), and the issue of evidence is not limited to the field of arts and health. In fact, the work of Katherine Smith (2013) shows how, despite the centrality that the principle of evidence-based policy holds in the sphere of public health, research consistently demonstrates that public health policies are not, in reality, evidence based, and that it is fairly easy to identify a fair few policies that actual run *counter* to the available scientific evidence.

## Arts and health: the public's view

The general impression that emerges from a consideration of the literature is that of a field in which the gathering of scientific evidence is trying to catch up with the rapid expansion of arts practice (and this is, often, publicly funded practice): 'The race to capture an evidence base to support the ascendancy of practice in arts and community health can sometimes seem like a treadmill' (White 2009, p. 204).

It is interesting to note that within modern cultural life there is an evident widespread belief in the power of the arts to deeply affect both the psyche and the body, which does not seem to be predicated on the availability of supporting scientific evidence but rather relies on the strength of a common sense belief. The popular author and television presenter Alain de Botton has recently teamed up with the philosopher John Armstrong to co-author a book entitled *Art as Therapy*, whose self-professed ambitious aim is to introduce a new method of interpreting art, whereby art is to be seen as a form of therapy (de Botton and Armstrong 2013). Writing in the *Guardian* newspaper about his new book, de Botton (2014) explicitly draws upon this deeply held commonsensical belief in the therapeutic powers of the arts, suggesting that thinking of the arts as therapeutic 'comes naturally to us', and that, indeed, this almost instinctive search for healing drives our creative consumption, as demonstrated, for instance, by our everyday attempts to lift our mood via our choice of music or TV viewing.

De Botton's observation on the *naturalness* of our belief in the therapeutic powers of music is worth further consideration. At the more eccentric end of the spectrum the continuing popularity of ideas such as the so-called 'Mozart effect' is further proof of the public's belief in the profound effects that the arts (most notably music) can have on minds and bodies. According to its proponents, the Mozart effect is allegedly based, albeit very loosely, on scientific research. The general idea of the Mozart effect has been creatively extrapolated from a piece of research conducted in 1993 at the University of California, Irvine which showed that college students exposed to Mozart displayed temporarily improved spatio-temporal abilities (that is, the ability to visualize something in space which unfolds over time, such as reading a map). However, the legitimacy and robustness of the 'evidence base' used to prop up the lucrative Mozart effect merchandise, including the classical music CDs that purport to make children smarter, has been hotly contested by scientific experts. In an interview for a feature on the CNN website, Frances Rauscher, co-author of the original study said: 'I'm horrified—and very surprised—over what has happened. It's a very giant leap to think that if music has a short-term effect on college students that it will produce smarter children. When we published the study results, we didn't think anyone would care. The whole thing has really gotten out of hand' (in Jones 1999).

Thus, the enduring popularity of the Mozart effect (which is now, interestingly, a registered trademark) is best explained in relation to its appeal to a pre-existing conviction in 'the power of music to heal the body, strengthen the mind and unlock the creative spirit', as the subtitle of Don Campbell's best-selling book, *The Mozart Effect* (2001) argues. Campbell's book offers a range of examples that testify, in his view, to the fact that, in recent years, the 'enhanced effects of music—and especially Mozart's—on health and healing have become more widely acknowledged and appreciated'. Some of them are, frankly, bemusing, including as they do the (unsubstantiated) claim that monasteries in Brittany have found that listening to Mozart made cows produce more milk, and that sake brewed in Japan by a company that plays Mozart in the background managed to increase tenfold the quality of the yeast sake is made from (Campbell 2001, p. 14). Alongside these more bizarre statements are others that argue, more plausibly, that listening to music might reduce the need for pain relief in hospitalized patients, reduce hypertension, and have other mild beneficial health effects.

It would be very easy to simply discredit and dismiss much of Campbell's book as nonsense misleadingly purporting to be based on science, as has indeed been done by several members of the scientific community. What I think is more interesting for the purposes of our discussion is to observe and take stock of the popularity of Campbell's arguments, which have now given rise to a whole industry (and a very profitable one at that), and to acknowledge that there might be something more powerful at work here than merely the gullibility of naïve consumers.

How can we explain, then, the flourishing—ahead of the scientific evidence—of a form of arts practice and a body of public health initiatives predicated on the belief that the arts can improve health, help address illness, and generally promote good health and desirable wellbeing outcomes for participants in arts and health interventions? Furthermore, how can we explain the fact that, as we have seen, this seems to be a view that is also held within popular culture and by the general public? If we accept its veracity, how can we explain the often-made claim that '[m]ost people tacitly understand how dancing, making music, writing poetry, and other forms of creative expression relieve tension and provide feelings of fulfilment' (McNiff 2004, p. 290)?

This chapter aims to address these questions by embracing an 'ideational' approach to understanding how public policy works that emphasizes the key role that ideas, values, and beliefs play in shaping policy alongside (and often in competition with) evidence from research (Belfiore and Bennett 2010; Smith 2013). The argument that will be developed is that it can be helpful to consider the growing popularity of (and policymakers' commitment to) arts and health work in the light of the long history of the belief in the healing powers of the arts. The persisting influence of such history on our culture might go some way towards making sense of the continued engagement of people and institutions in arts participation for health gains, even in the face of the scarcity of the kind of evidence base, rooted in large-scale randomized controlled trials (RCTs), which represents the 'gold standard' in medical research.

## Arts and healing: a long history

Madden and Bloom (2004, p. 140) helpfully distinguish between two different approaches to understanding the ways in which the power of the arts to impact on health and wellbeing can be harnessed: the 'art *as* therapy' approach, according to which artistic creation is inherently healing and cathartic, and the 'art *in* therapy' approach, according to which artistic creation is one of the tools clinicians have at their disposal for the purposes of diagnosis, prognosis, and treatment. Both approaches are predicated on the belief that the arts can have healing powers, especially of a psychological nature (in line with the particular popularity of participatory arts interventions in relation to minor mental health conditions). As Malchiodi (2002) puts it:

'Art therapy, the use of the creative process for emotional restoration and healing, grew out of the idea that images are symbolic communications and that art making helps us to express and transform difficult life experiences. It has expanded our understanding of how image making and imagination help during the dark night of the soul, carrying forward the ancient knowledge of art's healing powers

as well as the work of Freud and Jung. Artistic expression is one of our elemental tools for achieving psychological integration, a universal creative urge that helps us strive for emotional wellbeing.'

Malchiodi (2002, p. 11)

Malchiodi's reference to 'the ancient knowledge of art's healing powers' is echoed by Gilroy and Skaife's (1997, p. 58) classification of this view as part of a 'shamanic, spiritual and soul-making, studio-based tradition' that sees the value of making art in the cathartic release it offers. It is a common trope of the literature on the beneficial impact of the arts on health (especially that produced by arts and health practitioners and art therapists) to trace the historical origins of a practice back to shamanic practices of healing and creative expression that might date as far back as the Palaeolithic, and which are still alive and practised in a number of cultures.

The figure of the shaman fulfilled a number of roles within early societies: priest, medicine man, sorcerer, political leader, and artist. His *modus operandi* involved dance, music, acting, image making, and the induction in his patients of altered states of consciousness promoting psychological self-healing. The shaman accomplished this therapeutic task in the context of ritual practices that often encompassed the achievement of a state of ecstasy (Achterberg 2002, p. 6). The healing and transformative powers of the shaman were therefore linked to the capacity attributed to him to connect mind, body, and soul, in a time that preceded the distinction that would eventually characterize Western thought between mind and body (and therefore between bodily and mental disease) which was established by Plato (Szasz 1988, p. 12). It is quite common in some quarters of the arts therapy profession to claim a direct link between the practice of the shaman and modern practices of arts and health. For instance, Shaun McNiff (2004) has argued:

'The struggle of the shaman to find meaning and order within the flux of experience is akin to the artistic process. Like the dramatist of later cultures, the shaman attempts to attach spiritual significance to unsettling and tragic circumstances. [. . .] Rather than attempting to tranquilize eruptions of psychological tension by external means, the artist and the shaman go to the heart of the inner storm and enact its furies in a way that benefits the individual and the community. The end result is not just emotional catharsis but deepened insight into the nature of human emotion.'

McNiff (2004, pp. 185–6)

As we will see, the concept of catharsis, and particularly the version that emerged from the interpretation of Aristotle's writing on tragedy, holds a pivotal place in the set of ideas and beliefs about the healing power of the arts that are under consideration here. However, it is interesting to note that ideas about purification and healing through the creative expression of intense and troubling emotions were already in circulation long before their influential formulation in Aristotle's *Poetics* in Athens in the fourth century BC. In other words, such beliefs in the therapeutic possibilities offered by dance, music, and words have a history that not only stretches way back into the past but also extends beyond the western intellectual tradition. For example, incantation, poetry and other remedies reliant on the belief in 'the magical instrumentality of the voice' were important healing and ritual practices in Native American cultures, as emerges from the fascinating account offered by Rafael Campo (2003, pp. 31–2). He refers to the Navajo 'night chant', a poem transmitted orally through the generations, in which the poetic appeal to the moon, the sky, the sun, the land, and other elements in the sufferer's surroundings was believed to have therapeutic effects on the ill. The Iroquois 'condolence ritual', a ceremonial incantation usually performed by a shaman, worked in a similar way to bring relief to the depression of those who struggled to cope with bereavement (Campo 2003). The Egyptians showed a similar reliance on the healing power of words in the era of the Pharaohs (whose Early Dynasty dates back to 3000 BC): according to the Greek historian Diodorus Siculus, the famous library at Thebes in Egypt bore the inscription 'The healing place of the soul' (McCulliss 2012, p. 24). Campo (2003, p. 34) further draws parallels with the Judeo-Christian tradition, which also displays a faith in the connection between poetry and healing, as shown by poetry found in the Bible, and especially in the Psalms and the Song of Solomon.

This historical account cannot hope to be exhaustive, but rather aims to be illustrative and to offer some intellectual and historical context for current arts and health policy debates such as those discussed in the rest of this volume. There is a moment in intellectual history, however, that played a key role in the development of western ideas around the therapeutic potential of the dramatic arts (although the argument was later extended beyond them) and which is worthy of more detailed exploration. The Greek poets and philosophers, and particularly Aristotle's concept of tragic catharsis, have had a marked influence on how in the west we conceive of the connection between artistic expression and representation, emotions, and psychological wellbeing, and the next section explores their legacy.

## Aristotle, dramatic catharsis, and the origins of 'arts and health'

For the Ancient Greeks poetry had always been connected to the process of healing and the restoration of health. The work of Stephen Rojcewicz (2004, 2009) paints a fascinating picture of the epic poems of Homer as a celebration of poetry therapy, and the first powerful statement of the belief in the healing powers of words in western culture. Both the *Iliad* and the *Odyssey* contain references to the use of story-telling as part of the cure of wounds acquired in battle. The famous scene in the *Iliad* that sees Patroclus bringing succour and aid to his friend Eyryplus, who had been wounded in battle, might indeed be seen as prefiguring the modern practice of integrating psychotherapy, or even art therapies, with pharmacological treatment. In the poem, Patroclus sat by his injured friend's side 'Trying to lift the soldier's heart with stories/ Applying soothing drugs to his dreadful wound/As he sought to calm the black waves of pain' (Rojcewicz 2004). Rojcewicz (2004) discusses a number of similar examples within Greek poetry, theatre, and philosophical writing, including Plato's dialogue *Ion*, which, he argues, 'refers to the madness of poets, and the possibility of creativity flourishing in individuals with mental illness' (Rojcewicz 2004, p. 211).

There is therefore abundant evidence of the longstanding connection in Ancient Greek culture between poetry (a term which in classical Greece indicated an individual or group performance of verses with the accompaniment of a musical instrument in front of an audience) and therapy which even found embodiment in religious imagery: Apollo, one of the main gods of the Greek pantheon was both the god of poetry and of healing. His symbols were the lyre (an instrument that in Greece was played as accompaniment to the recital of poetry) and the staff, which is still an emblem of medicine in popular iconography which Apollo shared, together with the epithet of 'healer', with his son Asclepius, himself a god of medicine and healing (Hart 1965). It is, however, with the writings of the philosopher Aristotle, in fourth-century BC Athens, that this connection between poetry and healing finds its single most influential articulation in the concept of dramatic catharsis.

Aristotle presents the idea of catharsis as the effect upon the audience of the performance of tragic theatre in a later work of his, *Poetics*, which has only partially been preserved. Despite the loss of large sections of it, critics agree that the *Poetics* was an essay that Aristotle had written in response to the writing of his master, Plato, who famously had suggested that poets ought to be evicted from the ideal polity, and literature and the theatre—alongside other mimetic, or in other words, representative art—ought to be the object of careful censorship by the state. The fundamental aim of the *Poetics*, then, was to rehabilitate poetry and the theatre from Platonic censure, and to advance a positive articulation of their cultural value in terms of the potential they offer for education, ethical development, and catharsis (Belfiore and Bennett 2008).

Aristotle's *Poetics* effectively represents the first recorded example of literary theory in western culture. The work explores the nature and characteristics of poetry, a definition that in Greek culture extended to dramatic tragedy, comedy, and poetry. Not much is known about the detailed contents of the *Poetics*, which were structured in two books, because only part of the first one has survived and secondary sources give only a general indication of what could be found in the remaining sections. It is remarkable that the concept of dramatic catharsis, which has proved remarkably and unfailingly influential over the centuries, is only briefly mentioned once in the whole *Poetics* (or at least the surviving portion). Aristotle's own work does not advance a fully developed definition of catharsis or a detailed explanation of how it might be achieved via tragic performances. And yet a short and cryptic passage in the *Poetics* has given impetus to centuries—indeed over two millennia—of enquiry, intellectual development, and empirical research aiming to pin down how 'purification' from troubling emotions might be achieved as a result of engagement with theatrical performances. Interestingly, the English literature scholar Baxter Hathaway (1962) has suggested that the vagueness and ambiguity of the definition of catharsis as offered by Aristotle in his *Poetics* might in fact be one of the reasons for its longstanding popularity with critics through the ages. According to this view, it is precisely the combined brevity and ambiguity of the Aristotelian original that might have encouraged different people in different times to develop distinctive interpretations of the concept of catharsis for their own intellectual purposes.

The idea of catharsis appears, in all its mysteriousness, in the context of a definition of the stylistic properties of tragic drama:

'serious, complete in itself, and of a certain magnitude; in language embellished with each kind of artistic ornament, the several kinds being found in several parts of the play; in the form of action, not of narrative; *through pity and fear effecting the proper purgation of these emotions* [emphasis added].'

Butcher (1951, p. 23)

The bone of contention among critics is how 'purgation'—that is, the Greek word κάθαρσιν—is to be translated and interpreted in the passage above: indeed different (and equally influential) theories of the effects of engagement with theatre and the arts more generally can be seen to have derived from different interpretations of this one word. I have offered elsewhere a full discussion of the different ways in which catharsis has been translated and the phenomenon adumbrated in the definition of tragedy has been explained (Belfiore and Bennett 2008). Here, it is sufficient to consider the three principal possible interpretations that have been put forward: catharsis as a process of intellectual, moral, or emotional purification, the latter being the interpretation most relevant to the discussion in hand, and therefore the principal focus of the following. The idea of 'intellectual catharsis' conceives the purification Aristotle refers to as a process of elimination of intellectual confusion, that is, as a process in which something that was initially intellectually murky is made clear and intelligible. An illustrious proponent of this line of interpretation is Martha Nussbaum, who in *The Fragility of Goodness* (1986, p. 389) suggests that '[k]*atharsis* is the clearing up of the vision of the soul by the removal of these obstacles; thus the *katharon* becomes associated with the true or truly knowable, the being who has achieved *catharsis* with the truly or correctly knowing'. An alternative interpretation attributes a moral and didactic nature to the process of catharsis: in this view tragedies, by means of the example offered by the vicissitudes of the tragic heroes as portrayed on the dramatic scene, teach audiences to restrain their own emotions and passions, thus avoiding the consequences that would befall them should those feelings be left unfettered. This interpretation proved especially popular in the Renaissance, and eventually fed into ideas of the civilizing and moralizing powers of the arts (Belfiore and Bennett 2008).

Finally, the interpretation that is more relevant to understanding the history of the belief in a deep connection between the arts and psychological health is the one that interprets catharsis as a process of emotional release. According to this reading of Aristotle's definition of catharsis, theatrical performances offer audiences an outlet for pent-up emotions and an opportunity for a beneficial (even if the audience is unaware of this) 'psychic discharge' (Nuttall 1996, p. 39). According to this interpretation, by witnessing the unfolding of difficult and emotionally intense dramatic action on the scene, spectators are able to confront those same troubling emotions and troubling feelings, gaining some relief from the process.

The eminent mid-nineteenth-century German philologist Jacob Bernays was a staunch proponent of this interpretive hypothesis, and a scathing critic of the moral and didactic interpretation of catharsis that was then the received one. Bernays (2004, p. 325) arrived at what he refers to as 'the *pathological point of view*' by bringing references to catharsis in other works by Aristotle, namely *Rhetoric* (a treatise on the art of persuasion) and *Politics* (a treatise on political philosophy), to bear on the interpretation of the definition of tragedy in *Poetics*. Bernays (2004) started from the observation that in those other texts, Aristotle referred to catharsis as a 'pharmakon', to mean 'a lifting or alleviation of illness brought about by means of medical relief'. Referring in particular to the discussion, in *Politics*, of dance- and music-based rituals that entailed participants

achieving a state of temporary rapture followed by a feeling of calm and serenity, Bernays explains that the pathological one is the kind of catharsis that can be identified in early Greek writing and which is likely to have offered the philosopher a model and a metaphor for phenomena occurring in the human mind (as opposed to the human body):

'The Phrygian songs derived from the mythical singer Olympus [. . .] transport otherwise calm people into rapture. Conversely, those possessed by rapture undergo, *after* they have heard or sung those intoxicating songs, a calming down.'

Bernays (2004, pp. 325–6)

Bernays justifies the 'medical interpretation' mostly on philological grounds, but he also notes that Aristotle was the son of a royal physician and himself practised the art of medicine in his youth, and therefore was naturally attuned to the complexity of the workings of the body, so much so that 'an unflagging alert consideration and awareness of the corporeal' runs through both his scientific and philosophical writings. Hence Bernays' claim that, for Aristotle, catharsis is a label that is transferred from the somatic to the mental level in order to refer to the kind of treatment that addresses the disturbance to be healed not by suppressing it but rather by aiming to 'arouse and drive it into the open, and thereby to bring about the relief of the oppressed person' (Bernays 2004, p. 329).

This understanding of catharsis is echoed in modern versions of the 'medical interpretation' of catharsis in connection with the theatrical experience and arts engagement more generally. Here too the potential for personal and social transformation is attributed to the emotional outlet offered by the arts. The definition proffered by Dani Snyder-Young (2013) is a good example:

'Catharsis is a product of empathy. Audience members identify with elements of a character they recognize in themselves, and, as a result, may take a vicarious emotional journey leading to an organic, extreme emotional release.'

Snyder-Young (2013, p. 91)

Indeed, whilst Bernays lamented, in the mid 1800s, the lasting influence of the moral interpretation of the process of catharsis, largely due to the Renaissance Humanists' endorsement, the 'pathological view' he championed has proved quite fruitful in the modern age and a powerful influence in ensuring the endurance of the belief in the connection between creative arts and psychological healing. A key moment in this unfolding tradition of thinking of catharsis as emotional release is represented by the early writings of Freud and Bauer. Whilst they both eventually moved away from it, their concept of 'abreaction' clearly bears the imprint of the Aristotelian notion of catharsis. With the term abreaction, Freud and Bauer indicated the procedure through which the analyst can facilitate emotional release in his or her patients by leading them to relive past traumatic experiences through talking or creative expression exercises (Belfiore and Bennett 2008, p. 86). Psychotherapeutic theatre, psychodrama, the psychodynamic acting method devised by Stanislavski, as well as other theorizations of theatre as vehicle of transformation can all be seen to stem from Aristotelian catharsis, and are equally predicated on the therapeutic potential that performances hold. Fintan Walsh (2013) offers a compelling modern articulation of this potential in his *Theatre and Therapy*, offering further proof that catharsis is still an active driver of thinking and practice in this area:

> 'Theatre, like therapy, can prompt us to reflect upon our own thoughts, feelings and behaviours in the presence of others, within a specific time frame. As we observe lives play out before us as spectators, or actively collaborate in the process as performers, practitioners and participants, theatre can illuminate and stimulate mental and emotional activity, those primary targets of therapeutic intervention. In the arousal of emotion, theatre can coax us to emphatically identify with others. By stepping into another person's shoes, we might increase our sensitivity to others, and learn more about ourselves. Encounters with performance can deepen our awareness of behavioural patterns in a way that might even spur change. Theatre, like therapy, can lead us into a richer understanding of ourselves and our worldly relationships.'
>
> Walsh (2013, p. 1)

A cathartic process with beneficial health impacts such as we have just considered in relation to theatre has also been posited and documented for other arts forms. For example, modern bibliotherapy has been defined as 'the guided use of reading, usually as an adjunct to psychotherapy in mental health care settings, for learning about and developing insights into illness, and for stimulating catharsis, to aid in the healing process' (Katz and Watt, cited in Campo 2003, p. 35). Similarly, in her very personal account, the writer and academic Louise DeSalvo (1999, pp. 25ff.) explains how for writing to have positive health effects, a description of past traumatic events is not sufficient—it needs to be accompanied by the description of the concurrent feelings, in both the past and present. Reliving and acknowledging the feelings that are linked to past traumas are therefore, in her view, key to achieving catharsis and healing through writing.

## Conclusion

This chapter started with an acknowledgment of the growing support among policy makers, within both the arts and health sectors, for the therapeutic potential of participation in the arts and creative activities, resulting in the flourishing over the past 30 years of the 'arts and health' movement. The persisting problem of evidence was also discussed, and it was noted how research documenting, testing, and verifying the wellbeing and therapeutic claims made on behalf of arts engagement has not yet provided the kind of indisputable scientific evidence that can 'prove' the effectiveness of the diverse arts and health interventions that are part of current practice. This is problematic, of course, especially because if we hypothesize that the arts can be harnessed for their powers to effect deep psychological and social transformations, then it is necessary to acknowledge that such power may be abused, or provoke undesirable and harmful as well as beneficial impacts (Belfiore and Bennett 2008). A much better understanding of the psychological mechanisms at play and of the workings of arts-based interventions is therefore important to ensure that the risk of harm to participants is minimized.

The question of evidence also poses obvious problems of justification and legitimacy, especially where arts and health practice is publicly funded. Particularly during times of austerity and contracting budgets for the provision of public services, developing robust evidence of the kind that scientists consider reliable and credible will remain a priority for the arts and health community. This poses many challenges, especially as there is, as Clift (2012, p. 123) observes, a well-known 'hierarchy of evidence' in the field of medicine, in which RCTs and systematic reviews constitute the gold standard in the development of evidence-based medical practice. This poses several challenges for arts and health practitioners and funders: these approaches are costly and arts interventions often involve numbers of participants that are too small to lend themselves to RCTs (Smith 2012). But there are other observations of a methodological nature to make here: there are important aspects of arts and health practice that are central to understanding the experience of participants and that would be best captured by qualitative methodologies and not necessarily by RCTs. Hence Clift's (2012) call for the acceptance of a range of qualitative approaches (such as observations, interview, focus group discussions, and narrative and content analysis) as equally important sources of legitimate and credible scientific evidence in assessing the health impacts of arts participation. As Clift (2012) observes:

> 'In discussing evidence in relation to arts and health, it is important to recognise that the growth, scope, and variety of practical initiatives in this field should, in itself, be regarded as important evidence of the feasibility, acceptability, flexibility and vitality of working through the creative arts in supporting health care and promoting health. Such activities would not happen and certainly would not continue to happen, if their value was not recognised and if the experiences of such initiatives on the part of artists, health professionals and participants did not point to tangible effects.'

The aim of this chapter has been to offer a necessarily brief and illustrative (rather than exhaustive) history of the belief that the arts have a therapeutic dimension that can be seized upon for health benefits. This is a history that goes back to the earliest written records of western culture, as in the case of Homer's poems and the writings of the Greek philosophers, and indeed further back to even more ancient shamanic rituals. If the progress of arts and health practice ought to be seen as a valid indication of their widely recognized therapeutic value, then this chapter argues that so does the long history of the idea of the healing power of the arts, and the way it has survived through the ages. This is of course not to suggest that this powerful intellectual history can or should suffice as a substitute for solid and rigorous scientific evidence. Indeed, the case of the enormous profits that a blind trust in the so-called 'Mozart effect' has brought its creator, despite having no real foundation in science, is a perfect illustration of the perils of detaching the promotion of therapeutic arts activities from rigorous research. And yet there is an argument to be made for historical research to join qualitative research methodologies in the attempt to broaden the research approach to arts and health, and my ambition in this chapter was to begin to construct precisely that argument.

# References

ACE (2007). *A Prospectus for Arts and Health*. London: Arts Council England.

ACE (2014). *The Value of Arts and Culture to People and Society*. London: Arts Council England.

Achterberg, J. (2002). *Imagery in Healing: Shamanism and Modern Medicine*. Boston: Shambala.

Baumann, M. and MatrixInsights (2010). *Evaluation of 'Time Being 2': A Participatory Arts Programme for Patients With Depression (and Low Levels of Personal Social Capital)*. Newport, Isle of White: Healing Arts, Isle of Wight NHS PCT.

Belfiore, E. (2009). On bullshit in cultural policy practice and research: notes from the British case. *International Journal of Cultural Policy*, **15**, 343–359.

Belfiore, E. and Bennett, O. (2008). *The Social Impact of the Arts: An Intellectual History*. Basingstoke: Palgrave.

Belfiore, E. and Bennett, O. (2010). Beyond the 'toolkit approach': arts impact evaluation research and the realities of cultural policy-making. *Journal of Cultural Research*, **14**, 121–142.

Bernays, J. (2004). On catharsis. From *Fundamentals of Aristotle's Lost Essays on the 'Effects of Tragedy' (1857)*. *American Imago*, **61**, 319–341.

de Botton, A. (2014). Alain de Botton's guide to art as therapy. *Guardian*, 2 January 2014. Available at: <http://www.theguardian.com/artand-design/2014/jan/02/alain-de-botton-guide-art-therapy> (accessed 10 March 2014).

de Botton, A. and Armstrong, J. (2013). *Art as Therapy*. London: Phaidon Press.

Butcher, S.H. (1951). *Aristotle's Theory of Poetry and Fine Art*. Translated and with critical notes by S. H. Butcher, New York: Dover Publications.

Campbell, D. (2001). *The Mozart Effect: Tapping the Power of Music to Heal the Body, Strengthen the Mind, and Unlock the Creative Spirit* [reprint of 1997 edition]. New York: Quill.

Campo, R. (2003). *The Healing Art: A Doctor's Black Bag of Poetry*. New York: W.W. Norton.

Clift, S. (2012). Creative arts as a public health resource: moving from practice-based research to evidence-based practice. *Perspectives in Public Health*, **132**, 120–127.

DeSalvo, L. (1999). *Writing as a Way of Healing: How Telling Our Stories Transforms Our Lives*. London: The Women's Press.

Gilroy, A. and Skaife, S. (1997). Taking the pulse of American art therapy: a report on the 27th annual conference of the American Arts Therapy Association, November 13th–17th, 1996, Philadelphia. *Inscape*, **2**, 57–64.

Hart, G.D. (1965). Men and books: Asclepius god of medicine. *Canadian Medical Association Journal*, **92**, 232–236.

Hathaway, B. (1962). *The Age of Criticism: The Late Renaissance in Italy*. New York: Cornell University Press.

Jones, R. (1999). Mozart's nice but doesn't increase IQs. *CNN website*. Available at: <http://edition.cnn.com/health/9908/25/mozart.iq/> (accessed 10 March 2014).

London Health Commission (2002). *Culture and Health: Making the Link*. London: London Health Commission.

McCullis, D. (2012). Bibliotherapy: historical and research perspectives. *Journal of Poetry Therapy*, **25**, 23–38.

McNiff, S. (2004). *Art Heals: How Creativity Cures the Soul*. Boston: Shambala.

Madden, C. and Bloom, T. (2004). Creativity, health and arts advocacy. *International Journal of Cultural Policy*, **10**, 133–156.

Malchiodi, C.A. (2002). *The Soul's Palette: Drawing on Art's Transformative Powers for Health and Wellbeing*. Boston: Shambala.

Nussbaum, M.C. (1986). *The Fragility of Goodness: Luck and Ethics in Greek Tragedy and Philosophy*. Cambridge: Cambridge University Press.

Nuttall, A.D. (1996). *Why Does Tragedy Give Pleasure?* Oxford: Clarendon Press.

Rojcewicz, S. (2004). Poetry therapy in ancient Greek literature. *Journal of Poetry Therapy*, **17**, 209–213.

Rojcewicz, S. (2009). Psychotherapy in the *Odyssey*. *Journal of Poetry Therapy*, **22**, 99–103.

Secker, J., Hacking, S., Spandler, H., Kent, L., and Shenton, J. (2007). *Mental Health, Social Inclusion and Arts: Developing the Evidence Base*. London: National Social Inclusion Programme, Care Service Improvement Partnership.

Smith, J. (2012). *Can the Arts Really Make You Happy? A Study of the Methods Used for Evaluating the Impact of Arts Projects on Mental Health and Wellbeing*. Unpublished MA dissertation. Coventry: Centre for Cultural Policy Studies.

Smith, K. (2013). *Beyond Evidence-Based Policy in Public Health: The interplay of ideas*. Basingstoke: Palgrave.

Smith, R. (2002). Spend (slightly) less on health and more on the arts—health would probably be improved. *British Medical Journal*, **325**, 1432–1433.

Snyder-Young, D. (2013). *Theatre of Good Intentions: Challenges and Hopes for Theatre and Social Change*. Basingstoke: Palgrave.

South, J. (2004). *Community-based Arts for Health: A Literature Review*. Leeds: Leeds Metropolitan University. Available at: <http://www.leedsmet.ac.uk/hss/docs/Literature_Review.pdf> (accessed 10 March 2014).

Stickley, T. and Duncan, K. (2010). Learning about community arts. In: V. Tischler (ed.), *Mental Health, Psychiatry and the Arts: A Teaching Handbook*, pp. 101–110. Oxford: Radcliffe Publishing.

Szasz, T. (1988). *Myth of Psychotherapy: Mental Healing as Religion, Rhetoric and Repression*. Syracuse, NY: Syracuse University Press.

Walsh, F. (2013). *Theatre and Therapy*. Basingstoke: Palgrave.

White, M. (2009). *Arts Development in Community Health: A Social Tonic*. Oxford: Radcliffe Publishing.

# CHAPTER 3

# The fifth wave of public health and the contributions of culture and the arts

Phil Hanlon and Sandra Carlisle

## Introduction to the fifth wave of public health

The Faculty of Public Health of the Royal College of Physicians of the United Kingdom (Faculty of Public Health 2013) defines public health as the art and science of improving health. Yet within the profession of public health much is written about the science and little about the art of public health, and still less about the arts. This chapter is a modest attempt to redress this balance.

## How modernity improved health

Many of the health problems which cause the greatest concern today are of a different nature from those we have successfully overcome in the past. They are an emergent manifestation of our late modern culture rather than manifestations of diseases caused by known pathogens (Harrison 1993; Hanlon and Carlisle 2008). Problems like obesity, loss of wellbeing, greater inequality, and problematic drug and alcohol use reflect our culture (Hanlon and Carlisle 2010; Hanlon et al. 2010). With these problems public health faces a series of challenges that do not seem to be amenable to the approaches that have worked so well in the past (Homer-Dixon 2000). This, of course, begs the following questions: how has public health succeeded in the past and how and why has health improved in the modern era?

To help answer these questions we can consider four phases (we will call them waves) of health improvement in the United Kingdom since the Industrial Revolution. We call them waves because their dynamic takes the form of a wave. Each emerged from major shifts in thinking about the nature of society and health itself to achieve maximum impact. However, once a peak of effectiveness was achieved, new problems came into focus that required a new wave of intervention. The old wave remained important and ran on as a trough of activity—but never with the same impact it enjoyed when first implemented (Lyon 2003; Hanlon et al. 2011a).

The first wave of public health (roughly 1830–1900) arose in direct response to the Industrial Revolution. Overcrowding, lack of clean water and sanitation, poor nutrition, and a dire built environment created the ideal milieu for infectious diseases and a range of social problems (Fukuyama 1999). The imperative was to create order out of disorder. Human faeces had to be removed from the water supply. Factories had to be made safe. Violence on the street cried out for control (Wohl 1983). The senses were assailed by squalor and this created an aesthetic motivation, as well as practical and ethical reasons, for improvement. The public health response was led by early pioneers in the field of social medicine (Hamlin 1988) and politicians like Edwin Chadwick (Chadwick 1842). Great public works (in particular clean water and sewerage), improvements in housing, and enhanced living and working conditions were the key interventions (Hardy 2001). In time, these improvements caused a reduction in water-borne diseases and, later, respiratory diseases. Importantly, this happened before their causes were discovered: science was rudimentary in this wave. It was social institutions like local government, cooperative societies, modern police forces, health visitors, orphanages, and much else that brought the first wave of improvements in health (Lyon 2003; Hanlon et al. 2011a) (Table 3.1).

The second wave of public health, roughly spanning the decades 1890–1950, saw scientific rationalism allied to technological change and institutional development applied to manufacturing, medicine, engineering, transport, and many other fields. It brought improved living standards (in particular better nutrition, housing, and employment) and it is this, above all, that improved health (McKeown and Record 1962). Scientific discovery suggested new approaches based, for example, on the shift from miasmic to germ-based theories of disease. So if social reformers were key figures in the first wave, scientists like Koch and Pasteur were integral to the second. The second wave of public health might be best thought of as the appliance of science allied to continuing economic development.

A third wave proved to be needed because the so-called giants that William Beveridge described (want, disease, ignorance, squalor, and idleness) had palpably not been slain by the material progress of the Industrial Revolution or the previous two waves of public health response (Beveridge 1942). The fruits of the Industrial Revolution and the prosperity it brought were unevenly distributed (Williams 2005). The key determinants of health were

**Table 3.1** Four waves of public health improvement

| First wave | Second wave | Third wave | Fourth wave |
|---|---|---|---|
| Approximately 1830–1900. Order needed to be established in rapidly industrializing cities. Classical public health interventions, such as clean water and sanitation reduced deaths | Approximately 1890–1950. Greater prosperity brought better nutrition, housing, and working conditions. Scientific rationalism provided breakthroughs in many fields | Approximately 1940–1980. Emergence of the welfare state and the post-war consensus: the National Health Service, social security, social housing, and universal education extended the benefits of a modern state | Approximately 1960–2000. Effective healthcare interventions helped to prolong life. Risk factors and lifestyle issues became of central concern to public health. Life expectancy rose but with high levels of morbidity in older age |

now seen as inadequate education, lack of social security, substandard housing, and poor healthcare. The policy objective of the welfare state was therefore to use the power of government legislation and a set of new programmes to bring the benefits of a modern industrial economy to the whole population. The pioneers of the welfare state believed that a transformation in the material circumstances of the population, allied to the provision of high-quality healthcare, would increase the health of the people of Britain to such an extent that the need for the National Health Service (NHS) would diminish over time.

This, as we now know, did not happen and the fourth wave (approximately 1960–2000) arose as a partial response to this realization. By the 1960s the results of the first three waves were clear (Bell 1976). Each had built upon its predecessor(s) and death rates continued to decline throughout the twentieth century (McKeown and Record 1962). In the first two waves, public health action and economic improvements benefited the young more than the old. During the third wave, chronic diseases like ischaemic heart disease, stroke, chronic obstructive pulmonary disease, and cancer replaced infection as the central concern of public health and the NHS. This was the era in which epidemiologists like Sir Richard Doll established the health hazards of smoking and long-term cohort studies were set up. This was also the era where public health experts came to the fore and a wider range of specialties began to contribute to the increasingly professionalized area of public health (Bonita and Beaglehole 2004).

By the 1980s, and for the first time in history, death was being delayed by the expansion of medical technology (e.g. treatments for cardiovascular disease including bypass surgery, angioplasty, drug therapy, and coronary care units and their combined effects increased survival for ischaemic heart disease). Social and economic interventions were the drivers of improved health in the first three waves but, while these remain important, medical interventions have been responsible for much of the decline in mortality in the last quarter of the twentieth century. However, medical advances provided few solutions to emergent social pathologies. In such a complex context the fourth wave became partly characterized by a concern for risky behaviours in relation to major disease patterns. Issues such as diet, exercise, tobacco, alcohol, and

consumption of illegal drugs took centre stage in concerns about public health (Rollnick 1999)

The argument, therefore, is that each wave arose as a response to historically, geographically, and culturally defined needs, drawing upon emerging ideas in science and society (Szreter 1997). Each wave's power, however, diminished in the face of new challenges that needed new responses.

## The dis-eases of modernity

What new challenges do we now face? Three important examples—obesity, inequality, and loss of wellbeing—will be discussed briefly. What seems to be important is that these problems are emergent manifestation of modernity itself and cannot be 'fixed' by technical interventions. The four waves already described do not seem to work for this category of problems.

In industrialized countries obesity is now a population-wide problem: the weight distribution of almost the entire population is shifting upwards (Foresight 2007). There have always been a few obese individuals in most (but not all) societies, but the emergence of obesity as a population-wide phenomenon is unprecedented: in 2006, the number of obese and overweight people in the world overtook the number who were malnourished and underweight (Booth et al. 2005). The key point is that obesity is not the result of a pathogen (like cholera) or an identifiable social problem (like poor housing). It is, therefore, not a problem for which we will be able to easily develop a technically driven intervention. The best analyses suggest that we humans are obesogenic organisms: that is, we have a propensity to consume calorie-dense food and preserve energy when we can. This is a survival strategy developed in our evolutionary past which has served us well for all of our previous history. The problem is that for the first time we find ourselves in an obesogenic environment—that is, a society where calorie-dense food is so inexpensive and ubiquitous and the opportunities for reducing energy expenditure so pervasive that weight gain is now widespread (Stanton 2007). For these reasons, the obesity epidemic has developed rapidly since the 1980s and is not automatically self-limiting.

If left unchecked, it may bring other unforeseeable changes and difficulties. If it is to be reversed, we will probably have to change our whole food economy, the balance of what we eat, and our whole pattern of physical activity. This is only likely to happen if we change the way we organize our lives and our society. However, we have yet to achieve anything like the change that will be needed. We are, for example, adapting to and normalizing a much larger body shape. For some this may be a positive and anti-discriminatory development. However, it remains problematic for the public health community because of the implications of unhealthy weight gain for health outcomes and quality of life over the longer term. Our choice is clear. We can either continue as we are (choosing only to treat the exponential rise in secondary clinical consequences of obesity) or we can choose to reverse the social and commercial changes which have conspired to make overweight/obesity more 'normal'. The latter is the only plausible solution but its implementation seems improbable because it would require an entirely new mindset in modern society.

Inequalities in health constitute another challenge for which we need a new approach (Marmot and Wilkinson 2000). Global economic activity has quintupled in the last 40 years (Brown 2007).

Yet, by 2004, the income of the richest 10% of the world's population was around the same as the income of the bottom 50% (Kattan 2006). In the United Kingdom a series of reports on inequalities in health (e.g. Black et al. 1980; Department of Health 1998; Marmot Review 2010) have provided conclusive evidence for the harm caused by inequalities. These reports have each made a raft of policy recommendations to combat the problem, yet inequalities in health in the United Kingdom continue to widen. Wilkinson and Pickett (2009), in their popular and influential book *The Spirit Level: Why More Equal Societies Almost Always Do Better*, have shown that the whole population benefits when a wealthy county adopts a more egalitarian distribution of income and wealth. Mostly, this advocacy falls on deaf ears. There is one further, and indeed more profound, problem. Historically, public health advocates have suggested that inequalities will be combated by levelling up the circumstances of the poor to those of the rich. What is now clear is that such a strategy, if it were to succeed globally, would require a level of resource consumption that is not available (Simms et al. 2006). Today, if everyone consumed as much as the average UK citizen, we would need more than three Earth-like planets to support them. In short, inequalities in health are profound and widening and current public health interventions are not solving the problem (Wilkinson and Pickett 2006). Worse, even if they were to succeed on their own terms, they are ecologically unsustainable.

After the Second World War, the industrial economies of the west saw reconstruction, a rise in average incomes, and reductions in inequalities. These positive changes were accompanied by improved wellbeing. However, since the mid 1970s, increased economic growth in the United States, Europe, and Australasia has not been accompanied by commensurate improvements in wellbeing (Lane 2000; Layard 2005). In short, becoming even wealthier has not made us happier (Easterbrook 2003). In addition, there has been an increase in depression and anxiety: the World Health Organization predicts that depression will soon be one of the leading global causes of disability (WHO 2001). These rises in levels of depression and anxiety and the associated loss of mental and emotional wellbeing provide strong evidence of the degree to which modern populations are feeling overwhelmed. There are various hypotheses linking this stasis or decline in wellbeing to the effects of economic growth and the underlying consumerist society. One theory is that of the 'hedonic treadmill' where, no matter how much one owns, the persistent visibility and marketing of goods provokes a constant feeling of being without, which gives rise to a diminished sense of wellbeing. Another is termed 'choice anxiety', where the multitude of decisions (often trivial) that are made every day give rise to unhappiness. The loss of meaning and purpose as the practice of consumption replaces identity and deeper motivations and meanings in life has also been cited as a causal pathway (Eckersley 2004). Linked to this is the phenomenon of satisfied expectations, where achievement of material wealth leaves an emptiness of hope (Ransome 2005). A further feature of the globalized capitalist world has been uncertainty and insecurity in areas such as employment and pensions (New Economics Foundation 2004): this 'footloose' existence has stretched social ties and made interpersonal relations shallower (Putnam 2000).

Importantly, the four waves of public health interventions are helpless in the face of these trends. Antidepressants are being prescribed in unprecedented numbers but fail to address root causes: talking therapies like cognitive behavioural therapy provide modest benefit but only work at an individual level and fail to address the cultural and structural underpinnings of the problem. Improved material circumstances or welfare provision can help some dimensions of mental health, but the rise of these problems in the face of widely increasing affluence suggests that we need different solutions.

We might be better to call problems like obesity, inequalities, and loss of wellbeing 'dis-eases' rather than diseases, because they reflect an 'inner world'—the realm of our individual consciousness, beliefs, and motivations—that is struggling to cope with modern life. These dis-eases are a product of late modernity. That is, they are an emergent consequence of the very nature of the lives we have created for ourselves. Modernity (i.e. what has emerged since the Enlightenment) has been characterized by a distinctive and integrated inner and outer world. The inner world of modernity has taught us to think of ourselves as complex biological machines that are the product of chance and time. We understand ourselves as individuals, subject to biological competition (survival of the fittest) and social competition (the market). The outer world of modernity is dominated by materialism, individualism, consumerism, and economism (i.e. economics is regarded as more important than any other discipline in understanding society) (Eckersley 2004). We understand the world both as a resource to be used and a complex machine that needs managing. We accept that the task of an organized society is to satisfy the inexorable, growing needs of the human population. If it is true that the dis-eases of modernity reflect the inner and outer worlds of modernity, then problems like obesity, inequality, or loss of wellbeing cannot be fixed by conventional policy interventions. More profound, more integral and embodied change will be needed (Wilber 2001).

## Modernity is in crisis

Will our societies change radically to combat obesity, inequality, or loss of wellbeing? Whilst evidence to date suggests not, a series of influences make change inevitable, and if change is inevitable it opens up the possibility that we might create new inner and outer worlds that confront these dis-eases. Change is inevitable, because modernity is built on economic growth and growth cannot continue indefinitely in a finite system, but several parameters are currently growing exponentially. For example, the human population has risen from around a billion in about 1830 to approximately 7 billion in 2015, and projections suggest that there will be around 9 to 10 billion people by 2050. When combined with several other aspects of human-related systems and their interaction with each other and the biosphere, population growth becomes a significant challenge. Two further systems currently in a period of exponential increase are energy use and money. For energy (oil, gas, uranium, etc.), the problem comes when production peaks: the remaining resource is more difficult and thus more expensive to extract (Hanlon and McCartney 2008) and if we burn all the fossil fuel that is in the Earth's crust we will simply exacerbate climate change (McCartney and Hanlon 2008). The link between the exponential growth of money and health is less well recognized. Money is created by debt, and continuing growth of money is built into the current system. In the years leading up to the credit crunch we experienced an exponential growth in credit. As long as the supply of credit keeps growing, loans (with their attendant interest) can be paid off: but, if there is a major default, the whole system collapses. In short, our current phase of development is fuelled by exponential rises which are not sustainable: the current pattern of growth will have to come to an end sooner or later. The question is whether we can make a transition to a more stable state without undergoing a major collapse.

If we embark on a radical programme of transformational change we could experience a (relatively) smooth adaptation of the human footprint to the carrying capacity of the globe. What is not possible is for the current growth in many systems to continue uninterrupted. This is why change is inevitable. However, the good news is that if change is inevitable we have an opportunity to create transformational change which could give rise to a society and a world that is sustainable, equitable, and healthy. Such a prize lies within our grasp. However, the mindset that created the problem—the mindset of modernity—will not create the transformation we need.

## The Afternow project

This hypothesis—that health and wellbeing in modern, western-type societies is threatened by particular aspects of modern culture—has been investigated in a research study called the Afternow project (<http://www.afternow.co.uk/>). The study has been distinctive in drawing together and integrating knowledge from a wide range of literatures and disciplines, including public health, psychology, economics, philosophy, neuroscience, sociology, and anthropology (Carlisle et al. 2012). This approach led to an appreciation that a new approach—a 'fifth wave' of public health—is needed (Hanlon et al. 2011). Although our analysis began with our own discipline of public health, we also reached the broader conclusion that many spheres of modern life are now subject to diminishing returns, which means that it is not just public health but the whole modern project that is involved in this transition (Homer-Dixon 2000). As yet, however, there is little evidence that the majority of people are embracing a new wave of change. Instead, we observe denial, resistance, or, at best, passive adaptation.

### Three common objections

When we and others have spoken about the urgent need to move beyond the inner and outer worlds of modernity and create a 'fifth wave', three objections are commonly voiced. An obvious objection is that the majority find the fruits of modernity beneficial. That is true. Modernity has brought diverse benefits to many, not least through the insights of science and technology. Therefore, one of our greatest challenges as we create a fifth wave will be to preserve these benefits while acknowledging that modernity is not sustainable and, therefore, change is inevitable. The crucial question then becomes, can we create change that preserves the best of modernity while enhancing wellbeing, sustainability, and equity? Others ask: is the current age so different? Have people not always worried about the future? It does seem to be true that human beings have some predilection for apocalyptic thinking and have always worried about the future. While conceding this point, there are two further arguments to consider. First, some ages in human history have been characterized by a confidence in the future and a belief in 'progress'. Indeed, this was the case earlier in the modern period.

However, two world wars, the Great Depression, the atomic bomb, and the ecological crisis are among the factors that have altered this mindset. More importantly, the ecological crisis we face over the whole globe is unprecedented (Roberts 2005; Rifkin 2009). Just because we are prone to apocalyptic thinking does not alter the nature of this threat. Human consciousness is slowly being changed by an awareness of the degree to which human beings are growing in numbers while already overshooting the ecological constraints of the globe (Rifkin 2009). Importantly, the 'Afternow' analysis is not at all apocalyptic: it is profoundly optimistic. It simply starts by concluding from available trends that change is inevitable, and that the thinking that has created the problem will not provide the solution. A third common objection is that these are concerns confined to a privileged, liberal elite. This is only true in part. Climate change is already affecting some of the poorest people on Earth. Consumerism has some of its most damaging impacts on the poorest and most excluded in the United Kingdom. Our fieldwork has heard accounts of the malign effects of modernity from groups like prisoners, recovering addicts, those suffering from mental health problems, and residents of some of our most troubled housing estates. Many in the most disadvantaged sections of society are concerned about these problems.

### Creating a fifth wave of public health

The Afternow project has argued that to create the fifth wave we will need to learn to integrate three perspectives: science (the true), ethics (the good), and aesthetics (the beautiful) (Hanlon et al. 2011a) (see Fig. 3.1). 'The true, the good, and the beautiful' is derived from Platonic thinking—so it is old (O'Hear 2007). However, the new model that might inform a fifth wave in a future public health has yet to be created—it is emergent.

We can be optimistic about the prospects for this model because it is intrinsic to our humanity—we naturally integrate the true, the good, and the beautiful. Consider the example of food. We care about the safety and nutritional quality of our diet: scientific insights from nutrition and hygiene matter. Food also has an ethical dimension. In the United Kingdom it is estimated that we waste between a third and a half of all food that is produced. This fact pricks our consciences as well as our wallets. We are becoming

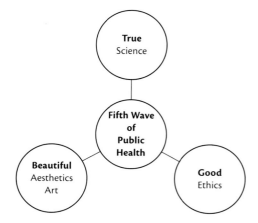

**Fig. 3.1** A model that might inform the fifth wave of public health.
Reproduced with permission from Hanlon P, Carlisle S, Hannah M, Lyon A, and Reilly D. Learning our way into the future public health: a proposition. *Journal of Public Health* 3(3): 335–342. Copyright © 2011 Oxford University Press, UK: Oxford.

more conscious that we are all citizens of the world and need to find an approach to food security that is universal and equitable. However, we do not eat with either science or ethics as our most prominent motivations. We eat because we get hungry—but eating is not empty of social meaning. We eat to share fellowship with friends and family. We prepare food to show love and care for others. We express our creativity when we prepare food and our appreciation when we receive food. We use food to create our identities (vegetarian, gourmet, 'locavore', always rushing and eating on the run . . . and so on). In truth, we eat out of an integrated mixture of all these factors.

Any public health approach to food in the fifth wave will need to build on this awareness because integration and emergence extend very widely. Everything we have said about food could be expanded to create an approach that is also more sustainable and more equitable. In short, our conversation about food cannot be confined to nutrition, ethics, hunger, fellowship—or any single factor. It needs to integrate them all and consider them all not just in the context of food but in the wider contexts of sustainability, health, and equity.

Compare such a holistic approach with current public health sciences which are overly reliant on reductionist approaches. Reductionism has helped us to understand a great deal about the natural world, yet a complex system is always more than the sum of its parts and the social world has intra- and interpersonal dimensions which are missing from the objective world view. Different and more diverse types of thinking are needed to help explain reality and to help us understand the nature of the health challenges that we face (Hanlon et al. 2012).

Public health ethics has its roots in the four foundational principles of medical ethics (i.e. autonomy, beneficence, non-maleficence, justice) but has also attempted to create a distinctive set of principles that apply to population health interventions rather than individually applied treatments (Nuffield Council on Bioethics 2007). Whilst they are helpful, current ethics fail to address some of the truly difficult ethical questions with which public health of the future will have to grapple. The great achievement of current ethics, built on a long tradition, is that it encourages us to place a high value on each human life and has invested each person (irrespective of status or circumstance) with fundamental human rights. When we speak of an emergent ethics for a fifth wave of public health it is vital that this does not weaken or dilute the achievements of current ethics. Nevertheless, the current approach to ethics in public health does not adequately address the two major and linked issues of social justice and ecological public health. At present we lack a true ethic of connectedness. A move in this direction implies a very real change in values and mindset, and many think that this unlikely. Yet consider the fact that there was a time when our circle of empathy was confined to the tribe: this became expanded to the nation (Rifkin 2009). If our understanding of who we are as people and those to whom we relate with care and inclusion has changed in the past, can we change again? Can we develop a truly global consciousness?

However, the idea of a changing human consciousness takes us into the territory of the final component of the model, 'the beautiful'—which includes art, aesthetics, and creativity. Since *Homo sapiens* emerged we have been engaged in creating: making tools, painting the walls of caves, crafting personal decorations, and much more, as part of the in-built human impulse to create meaning. Without creativity, our work can become commonplace and without meaning. Yet in modern culture even this aspect of our humanity has been commandeered for instrumental purposes and commodified within the consumer marketplace. So, art becomes of value to public health if it is part of regeneration or therapy but not for its own sake or for its capacity to inspire.

If we are to create widespread change, we will need new art, stories, myths, symbols, and much else to help us make the inner and outer transformations that will be needed. We may also need to reclaim old stories or reinvent old myths for new purposes. The term 'emergent' applies here because, while we are sure change is coming, the manner in which we will respond in our individual and collective imaginations will need to emerge from a continuing and dynamic process of discovery and creativity. Activities in this dimension of the model will centre on being fully human: being creative, being playful, developing consciousness, fostering empathy, and much else. Creativity is important because it is part of our nature and, as positive psychology has shown, we are often at our happiest and most fulfilled when lost in the flow and challenge of being creative (Huppert 2005). It is also from our creative selves that solutions to our most profound problems often arise. Creativity is also important because it balances some of the more instrumental modes of being that tend to dominate our working lives.

The point we are making here is that the role of 'the arts' in the fifth wave is central. However, the manner in which the arts currently interact with health is often problematic. We have felt a degree of unease when reading of reductionist studies that seek to show biomedical benefits from interventions that involve art or music. These are valuable in themselves but they run the risk of distracting us from the much larger challenge of discovering a shared act of creation—nothing less than the reimagining of what it is to be fully human and live together in a healthy, sustainable, just, but also beautiful, world.

What the Afternow project has argued is that we need to develop a practice that is first of all *integrative*—bringing together science, ethics, and aesthetics. It must also be *ecological*—recognizing limits to growth and engaging with other complex adaptive systems that influence human health. It should also be *ethical*—respecting individual human rights and raising human consciousness globally. To achieve some of this we will have to be more *creative*—envisioning a better future and unblocking the forces that impede creativity. To inspire us, the future for which we work should be *beautiful*—a future that raises our spirits and fires our imagination. We should encourage and support each other to *embody* the change we want to see in the world and to become more *reflexive* and more self-aware of our own mindset and practice (Hanlon et al. 2012). Our current 'maps' of the world (paradigms and worldviews) are not working. If we are to successfully navigate the transition in which we find ourselves we need to be able to imagine a future that is profoundly different. The good news is that this type of imagination and creativity is widely evident: we have seen many examples on our learning journeys (Carlisle et al. 2012). We have also learned that the arts and creative communities have much to teach those of us on the 'scientific' side of the house. We urgently need to find ways to better fire our imaginations and live with greater creativity: to this end we might consider the need to make more time for fun and adventure in our lives—as a vital necessity not a luxury. We could make more time for reflection and the cultivation of 'flow'—that state where one is completely absorbed in something, such that a sense of time passing disappears. It is from these experiences that new 'maps' will emerge. The challenge of sustainability means that we all have to learn to 'use less stuff'. However, we should remember that less can often be more. It is not trite to say that we would plausibly improve our wellbeing if we had less advertising, less pornography, less consumerism, and less waste. Also, many would like less busy-ness, less mindless choice, fewer targets, and less bureaucracy.

There are reasons for hope. It must have been tough for our earliest ancestors in the African forests when the climate changed. Yet that hardship forced our ancestors to learn how to survive on grassland and led to the 'out of Africa' migration and subsequent population of the rest of the world by early humans. Equally, it must have been difficult to develop agricultural techniques and domesticate animals for the first time. How traumatizing it must have been for crofters to be pulled off the land and into factories when the Industrial Revolution started. Yet each of these transitions represented an important chapter in human history. Human beings have made great transitions before and we can do so again.

## Acknowledgement

We are grateful to all who have contributed to and supported the Afternow project but particular thanks goes to our main collaborators—Dr Andrew Lyon, Dr David Reilly, and Dr Margaret Hannah.

# References

Bell, D. (1976). *The Coming of Post-Industrial Society: A Venture in Social Forecasting*. New York: Basic Books.

Beveridge, W. (1942). *Social Insurance and Allied Services*, CMD 6404 [the Beveridge Report]. London: HMSO.

Black, N., Morris, J.N., Smith, C., and Townsend, P. (1980). *Inequalities in Health*. Harmondsworth: Penguin.

Bonita, R. and Beaglehole, R. (2004). *Public Health at the Crossroads: Achievements and Prospects*. Cambridge: Cambridge University Press.

Booth, K.M., Pinkston, M.M., and Walker, S.C.P. (2005). Obesity and the built environment. *Journal of the American Dietetic Association*, **105**(Suppl. 1), S110–S117.

Brown, E.H. (2007). *The Web of Debt: The Shocking Truth About Our Monetary System and How We Can Break Free*. Louisiana: Third Millennium Press.

Carlisle, S., Hanlon, P., Reilly, D., Lyon, A., and Henderson, G. (2012). Is 'modern culture' bad for our wellbeing? Views from 'elite' and 'excluded' Scotland. In: S. Atkinson, S. Fuller, and J. Painter (eds), *Wellbeing and Place*, pp. 123–140. Aldershot: Ashgate.

Chadwick, E. (1842). *The Sanitary Conditions of the Labouring Population of Great Britain*. London: Poor Law Commission.

Department of Health (1998). *Independent Inquiry into Inequalities in Health. Report.* Chairman: Sir Donald Acheson. London: The Stationery Office.

Easterbrook, G. (2003). *The Progress Paradox. How Life Gets Better While People Feel Worse*. Toronto: Random House.

Eckersley, R. (2004). *Well and Good: How We Feel and Why it Matters*. Melbourne: Text Publishing.

Faculty of Public Health (2013). *What is Public Health?* Available at: <http://www.fph.org.uk/what_is_public_health> (accessed 4 July 2013).

Foresight (2007). *Tackling Obesities—Future Choices*. Project Report. London: Government Office for Science.

Fukuyama, F. (1999). *The Great Disruption: Human Nature and the Reconstitution of Social Order*. New York: Free Press.

Hamlin, C. (1988). *Public Health and Social Justice in the Age of Chadwick. Britain, 1800–1854*. Cambridge: Cambridge University Press.

Hanlon, P. and Carlisle, S. (2008). Do we face a third revolution in human history? If so, how will Public Health respond? *Journal of Public Health*, **30**, 355–361.

Hanlon, P. and Carlisle, S. (2010). Re-orienting public health: rhetoric, challenges and possibilities for sustainability. *Critical Public Health*, **20**, 299–309.

Hanlon, P. and McCartney, G. (2008). Peak oil: will it be public health's greatest challenge? *Public Health*, **122**, 647–652.

Hanlon, P., Carlisle, S., Reilly, D., Lyon, A., and Hannah, M. (2010). Enabling wellbeing in a time of radical change: Integrative public health for the 21st century. *Public Health*, **124**, 305–312.

Hanlon, P., Carlisle, S., Hannah, M., Reilly, D., and Lyon, A. (2011a). Making the case for a fifth wave in public health. *Public Health*, **125**, 30–36.

Hanlon, P., Carlisle, S., Hannah, M., Lyon, A., and Reilly, D. (2011b) Learning our way into the future public health: a proposition. *Journal of Public Health*, **33**, 335–342.

Hanlon, P., Carlisle, S., Hannah, M., Lyon, A., and Reilly, D. (2012). A perspective on the future public health: an integrative and ecological framework. *Perspectives in Public Health*, **132**, 313–319.

Hardy, A. (2001). *Health and Medicine in Britain Since 1860*. London: Palgrave.

Harrison, P. (1993). *The Third Revolution: Population, Environment and a Sustainable World*. London: Penguin.

Homer-Dixon, T. (2000). *The Ingenuity Gap: Facing the Economic, Environmental, and Other Challenges of an Increasingly Complex and Unpredictable Future*. New York: Vintage.

Huppert, F.A. (2005). Positive mental health in individuals and populations. In: F.A. Huppert, N. Bayliss, and B. Keverne (eds), *The Science of Wellbeing*, pp. 307–340. Oxford: Oxford University Press.

Kattan, E. (2006). *Annual Report: Global Partnership for Development*. New York: United Nations Development Programme.

Lane, R.E. (2000). *The Loss of Happiness in Market Democracies*. London: Yale University Press.

Layard, R. (2005). *Happiness: Lessons From a New Science*. London: Penguin.

Lyon, A. (2003). *The Fifth Wave*. Edinburgh: Scottish Council Foundation.

McCartney, G. and Hanlon, P. (2008) Climate change and rising energy costs: a threat but also an opportunity for a healthier future? *Public Health*, **122**, 653–656.

McKeown, T. and Record, R.G. (1962). Reasons for the decline of mortality in England and Wales during the nineteenth century. *Population Studies*, **16**, 94–122.

Marmot, M.G. and Wilkinson, R.G. (2000). *The Social Determinants of Health*. Oxford: Oxford University Press.

Marmot Review (2010). *Fair Society, Health Lives. Strategic Review of Inequalities in Health England Post-2010*. Chair: Sir Michael Marmot. London: University College London.

New Economics Foundation (2004). *A Wellbeing Manifesto for a Flourishing Society*. London, New Economics Foundation.

Nuffield Council on Bioethics (2007). *Public Health: Ethical Issues*. London: Nuffield Council on Bioethics.

O'Hear, A. (ed.) (2007). Philosophy: the good, the true and the beautiful. *Royal Institute of Philosophy Supplement*, **47**.

Putnam, R.D. (2000). *Bowling Alone: The Collapse and Revival of American Community*. New York: Simon & Schuster.

Ransome, P. (2005). *Work, Consumption and Culture: Affluence and Social Change in the 21st Century*. London: Sage.

Rifkin, J. (2009). *The Empathic Civilization: the Race to Global Consciousness in a World in Crisis*. Cambridge: Polity Press.

Roberts, B. (2005). *The End of Oil*. London: Bloomsbury.

Rollnick, S. (1999). *Health Behaviour Change: A Guide for Practitioners*. Edinburgh: Churchill Livingstone.

Simms, A., Moran, D., and Chowler, P. (2006). *The UK Interdependence Report: How the World Sustains the Nation's Lifestyles and the Price it Pays*. London: New Economics Foundation.

Stanton, R. (2007). Nutrition problems in an obesogenic environment. *Medical Journal of Australia*, **184**, 76–79.

Szreter, S. (1997). Economic growth, disruption, deprivation, disease and death: on the importance of the politics of public health for development. *Population Development Review*, **23**, 693–728.

WHO (2001). *Mental Health: New Understanding, New Hope*. Geneva: World Health Organization.

Wilkinson, R.G. and Pickett, K.E. (2006). Income inequality and population health: a review and explanation of the evidence. *Social Science and Medicine*, **62**, 1768–1784.

Wilkinson, R. and Pickett, K. (2009). *The Spirit Level: Why More Equal Societies Almost Always Do Better*. London: Allen Lane.

Williams, B. (2005). *Victorian Britain*. London: Jarrold Publishing.

Wilber, K. (2001). *A Theory of Everything: An Integral Vision for Business, Politics, Science and Spirituality*. Dublin: Gateway.

Wohl, A.S. (1983). *Endangered Lives: Public Health in Victorian Britain*. London: JM Dent.

# CHAPTER 4

# The social determinants of health, empowerment, and participation

Jessica Allen and Matilda Allen

## Health inequalities and the social determinants of health

Length of life and levels of health vary significantly between countries across the world. In Japan, on average, people live to 83, whereas in Sierra Leone the life expectancy is 47 (World Health Organization 2011). These startling differences are not confined to different countries at very different levels of development—they exist also within countries. In England, those who live in the most deprived areas spend 17 years longer with a disabling illness than those who live in the richest areas, and they live on average 7 years less (The Marmot Review Team 2010). Even in smaller areas and regions there are significant and persistent health inequalities. For example in the borough of Westminster in London, one of the richest areas in England, there is a difference of 22 years in male life expectancy between the richest and the poorest wards (City of Westminster 2014).

These differences in health outcomes are not inevitable, and they cannot be explained away by reference to chance or genetics. They are the result of the social, economic, environmental, and political conditions in which people live. These are summarized as the 'social determinants of health', and include (but are not limited to) early years experiences, education, income, employment and quality of work, and the physical and social environment.

Health inequalities are largely avoidable, and therefore profoundly unjust. Taking action on health inequalities is, first and foremost, a demand of social justice, and tackling health inequalities should be a priority for all governments. Taking action on health inequalities through action on the social determinants on health also means taking action on the many ways in which circumstances affect a range of outcomes for people throughout their lives—early years, education, income, and quality of work for instance. There are multiple social and economic benefits arising from activities to improve the social determinants of health. Reducing health inequalities is also economically advantageous. Preventing illnesses before they occur tends to be more cost-effective than dealing with them once they are manifest (Wanless 2002). Economic analysis of the English context suggests that inequality in illness accounts for losses of £31–33 billion in productivity per year, welfare payments that are £20–32 billion higher, and well over £5.5 billion a year in extra NHS costs (The Marmot Review Team 2010).

## Previous work on the social determinants of health

The Commission on the Social Determinants of Health (CSDH) gathered global evidence on the ways in which social determinants affect health, and concluded that the unequal distribution of power, money, and resources determines people's life chances and mental and physical health outcomes. It studied the impact of the conditions in which people are born, grow, live, work, and age, and concluded that 'social injustice is killing on a grand scale'. (Commission on the Social Determinants of Health 2008). It also proposed a wide range of areas for action and made recommendations which were organized under three over-arching recommendations:

1. Improve daily living conditions

2. Tackle the inequitable distribution of power, money, and resources

3. Measure and understand the problem and assess the impact of action

The Marmot Review which followed (The Marmot Review Team 2010) built on the global evidence from the CSDH and applied it to an English context. It proposed six areas for action, designed to improve health and reduce inequalities:

1. Give every child the best start in life

2. Enable all children, young people, and adults to maximize their capabilities and have control over their lives

3. Create fair employment and good work for all

4. Ensure a healthy standard of living for all

5. Create and develop healthy and sustainable places and communities

6. Strengthen the role and impact of ill health prevention

The Marmot Review provided detailed recommendations, evidence, and examples for each of these six areas and also proposed a monitoring and measurement framework.

Subsequently the Review of Social Determinants and the Health Divide in the WHO European Region (UCL Institute of Health Equity and WHO Regional Office for Europe 2014) assessed and analysed evidence from across Europe, and concluded with the following recommendations:

1a. Ensure that the conditions needed for good-quality parenting and family-building exist, promote gender equity, and provide adequate social and health protection

1b. Provide universal, high-quality, and affordable early years, education and childcare systems

1c. Eradicate exposure to unhealthy, unsafe work and strengthen measures to secure healthy workplaces and access to employment and good-quality work

1d. Introduce coherent, effective, intersectoral action to tackle inequities at older ages to prevent and manage the development of chronic morbidity and improve survival and wellbeing across the social gradient

2a. Improve the level and distribution of social protection according to needs to improve health and address health inequities

2b. Ensure concerted efforts are made to reduce inequities in the local determinants of health through co-creation and partnership with those affected, civil society, and a range of civic partners

2c. Take action to develop systems and processes within societies that are more sustainable, cohesive, and inclusive, focusing

particularly on those groups most severely affected by exclusionary processes

3a. Promote equity through the effective use of taxes and transfers. In particular, the proportion of the budget spent on health and social protection programmes should be sustained in all countries and increased for countries below the current European average

3b. Plan for the long term and safeguard the interests of future generations by identifying links between environmental, social, and economic factors and their centrality to all policies and practice

4a. Improve governance for the social determinants of health and health equity. This requires greater coherence of action at all levels of government—transnational, national, regional, and local—and across all sectors and stakeholders—public, private, and voluntary

4b. Develop a comprehensive, intersectoral response to the long-term nature of preventing and treating ill-health equitably to achieve a sustained and equitable change in the prevention and treatment of ill-health and the promotion of health equity

4c. Undertake regular reporting and public scrutiny of inequities in health and its social determinants at all governance levels, including transnational, country, and local

The recommendations of each of these reviews were based on the analysis of evidence across the social determinants of health, some of which will be referred to later in this chapter.

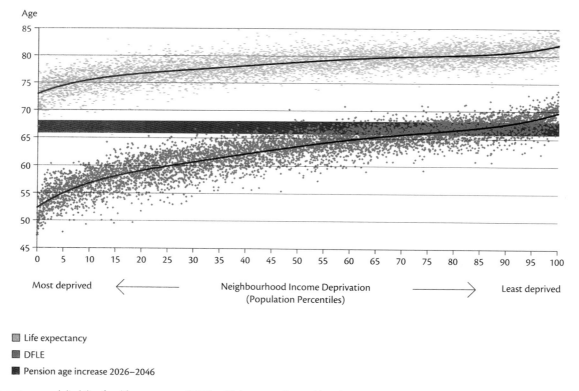

**Fig. 4.1** Life expectancy and disability-free life expectancy (DFLE) at birth, persons by neighbourhood income level, England, 1999–2003.
Source: data from Office for National Statistics (2014) Health Expectancies at birth and age 65 in the United Kingdom, <http://www.ons.gov.uk/ons/rel/disability-and-health-measurement/health-expectancies-at-birth-and-age-65-in-the-united-kingdom/index.html>, accessed Oct.2014.

# The social gradient

Each of the reviews mentioned showed that health outcomes are not just a case of a simple difference between the richest and the poorest. Instead, health is so closely related to a number of social factors that the relationship between social class and health is graded.

For example, Fig. 4.1 shows that life expectancy (the upper line) and disability-free life expectancy—the number of years someone can expect to live in good health (the lower line)—are related to neighbourhood-level deprivation. We can see a finely graded distribution, which we call 'the social gradient'. For this reason, although essential, it is not sufficient just to tackle chronic disadvantage (i.e. those at the very bottom of the social gradient). Actions to improve the conditions in which people are born, grow, live, work, and age should be universal, but implemented with increasing intensity according to position on the social gradient. We call this 'proportionate universalism'. Those who are the worst off should receive the greatest focus of action, those in a slightly higher position, slightly less focus, and so on. To effectively reduce health inequalities, the gradient in health outcomes should 'level up', so that everyone's outcomes move towards those of the most well off (Fig. 4.2).

# The life course approach and intergenerational equity

The recommendations in the reports described in 'Previous work on the social determinants of health' were developed in accordance with a life course approach which sees advantage and disadvantage as accumulating throughout life, beginning at the very earliest (prenatal) stages and manifesting as a shortened life and worse health in later life for those who are most disadvantaged. Those who are born into disadvantage or poverty are less likely to have the social and economic advantages which lead to success in education, good-quality employment, and a sufficient income to achieve a healthy standard of living (The Marmot Review Team 2010; UCL Institute of Health Equity and WHO Regional Office for Europe 2014), while those who are born into wealthier, less deprived environments will have a greater range of opportunities and advantages available to them and are more likely to have a range of better outcomes, live longer, and be healthier.

Actions taken early on in life are particularly important: here actions can have the greatest impact because this is the stage at which later-life advantage or disadvantage begins to build. However, action is necessary across every stage of life, from prenatal, through early childhood and education, to living and working conditions and family-building for adults, and experiences of ageing. Actions and intervention should be adapted according to the stage in the life course, because those at different ages and stages of their life will have different needs and be affected in different ways.

The European Review of Social Determinants of Health (UCL Institute of Health Equity and WHO Regional Office for Europe 2014) conceptualized this life course approach, and the range of structural and environmental factors that impact on health, in a diagram (see Fig. 4.3). The arrow labelled 'perpetuation of inequities' refers to the process whereby advantage and disadvantage may be transmitted through generations. For example, children of mothers with depression are more likely to have a low birth weight (Surkan et al. 2011), which then has an impact on later health outcomes (Barker 2004), including increasing their likelihood of depression (Surkan et al. 2011). Children of mothers with mental ill-health are five times more likely to have mental health disorders themselves (Melzer et al. 2003). Analysis from the United Kingdom shows that there is a gradient of socio-economic difficulties in children according to their family income (Kelly et al. 2011), and the transmission of ill-health and disadvantage relates mainly to the

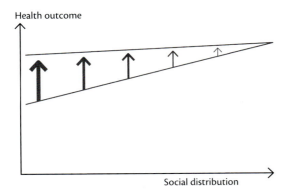

**Fig. 4.2** Levelling-up the social gradient in health.
Reproduced from UCL Institute of Health Equity and WHO Regional Office for Europe, *Review of Social Determinants and the Health Divide in the WHO European Region.* (Copenhagen: WHO, 2013, updated reprint 2014), http://www.euro.who.int/__data/assets/pdf_file/0004/251878/review-of-social-determinants-and-the-health-divide-in-the-who-european-region-final-report.pdf, accessed Oct. 2014. Copyright WHO © 2013 (updated reprint 2014), with permission from the World Health Organization.

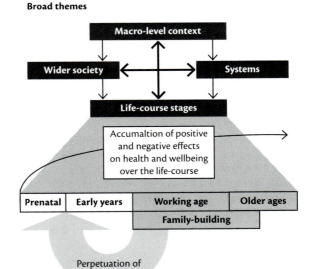

**Fig. 4.3** Broad themes of the review of social determinants and the health divide in the WHO European Region.
Reproduced from UCL Institute of Health Equity and WHO Regional Office for Europe, *Review of Social Determinants and the Health Divide in the WHO European Region.* (Copenhagen: WHO, 2013, updated reprint 2014), http://www.euro.who.int/__data/assets/pdf_file/0004/251878/review-of-social-determinants-and-the-health-divide-in-the-who-european-region-final-report.pdf, accessed Oct. 2014. Copyright WHO © 2013 (updated reprint 2014), with permission from the World Health Organization.

transmission of disadvantage (or, conversely, advantage) via social and economic factors, rather than by genetic transmission.

Maternal education is particularly important in overcoming the intergenerational transmission of disadvantage. A lower level of maternal education is related to increased infant mortality, stunting and malnutrition, overweight in children, lower scores on vocabulary tests, conduct problems, emotional problems, lower cognitive scores, mental health problems, and infections (Bicego and Boerma 1993; Case et al. 2005; Gleason et al. 2011; Schady 2011; Allen et al. 2014). Therefore activities which improve the education of girls and women will have an impact on the current generation of women, reduce inequalities, and help reduce the intergenerational transmission of disadvantage.

In sustainable development, the principle of 'intergenerational equity' is often cited: this states that the actions of one generation should not compromise the environment for the next. The same principle should be applied to health. For example, current responses to the economic crisis are likely to have effects on future generations and may well have a negative effect on health (Stuckler and Basu 2013). Polices should therefore be assessed for their likely future impact on health equity as well as their impact on health equity for the current generation.

## Control, stress, and empowerment

Income has an effect on health as it (in part) determines what individuals and families can afford to buy and which services they have access to. Health-promoting factors such as good-quality housing, good education, and healthy food can all be purchased by adults who earn sufficient amounts. However, income is only one factor affecting health. For example, in 2011 men in Russia had a life expectancy 1 year lower than men in India (World Health Organization 2011), despite the fact that Russia's gross domestic product (GDP; measured here as purchasing power parity per capita) is over five times that of India (The World Bank 2013).

Sufficient income, or a minimum income for healthy living, is important to provide individuals with some control over their lives as well as to facilitate access to goods, services, and other prerequisites for a healthy life. However, income is not the only means of providing control over one's life. This is reflected in the capabilities approach, most famously espoused by Amartya Sen (1992). Sen argues that poverty, and other conditions of life, are important because they shape the extent to which people are able to do and to be that which they have reason to value. The capacity to have control over one's life is an essential component of being a free, respected, and successful citizen, all of which in turn affects an individual's capacity for good health and wellbeing.

### Children and young people

While the early years may offer little opportunity for control, stress is an important factor because later experiences of stress vary according to experiences in early childhood. Stressors experienced in early childhood affect biological stress regulatory systems—the neural processes by which stress responses are regulated in the brain (Taylor 2010). Later in the life course, experiences of stress may be shaped by these early experiences and the formation of neural pathways. However, early years experiences should not be seen as definitive predictors of later

levels of stress and control. Conditions at any point can positively or negatively modify an individual's experiences. For example, later on in life, the amount of control that young adults have over their lives, which is partly dependent on the opportunities and support offered to them through their education and training, can have a positive or negative impact on their health and wellbeing.

### People of working age

The Whitehall studies led by Professor Sir Michael Marmot showed the impact of control and stress within the context of employment. The Whitehall studies took cohort data gathered from staff in the UK Civil Service and measured health outcomes in relation to status within the organization. Those in the most junior positions had a mortality rate three times higher than those in the most senior positions, even controlling for income, access to medical care, lifestyle choices, genetic predisposition, and upbringing (Marmot 2004). Part of the reason for this is due to the increased stress involved in being in a junior or low-status position, positions which are often characterized by a lack of control, minimal rewards, and repetitive tasks. When the body is under stress, it releases cortisol. This is a natural response, but too much cortisol can increase the chances of disease (Steptoe et al. 2003; Chandola et al. 2006). Increased stress can also have a negative effect on unhealthy behaviours (Marmot et al. 1991). Conversely, job security and control at work have been shown to be protective of good mental health (Anderson et al. 2011).

A lack of control is also experienced by those who have poor-quality housing, a low income, or who experience discrimination based on their race, gender, ethnicity, sexual orientation, or some other characteristic. For example, being in debt (which involves a lack of control as well as stress) has a clear relationship with mental disorder, even after controlling for income and socio-demographic variables (Jenkins et al. 2008). Similarly, low educational attainment, material disadvantage, and unemployment are also associated with higher frequencies of depression and anxiety (Fryers et al. 2005), which may relate to levels of stress.

### Summary

Social determinants affect health in many ways. They may have a direct impact—for example poor-quality housing may be damp, which increases respiratory problems and the risk of cardiovascular disease (University College London Institute of Health Equity 2011). However, a lack of control, and the resulting stress this causes, can also have an effect on physical and mental health. For example, as well as having a direct impact on morbidity, living in poor-quality damp or cold housing creates stress which then has a negative effect on physical and mental health and affects productivity at work, educational development, children's outcomes, and older people's wellbeing and levels of social contact. On the other hand, situations of control, resulting in empowerment, can be protective of health.

## Social contact, social capital, and participation

One particularly important way to improve health and potentially reduce health inequalities is by fostering strong, good-quality

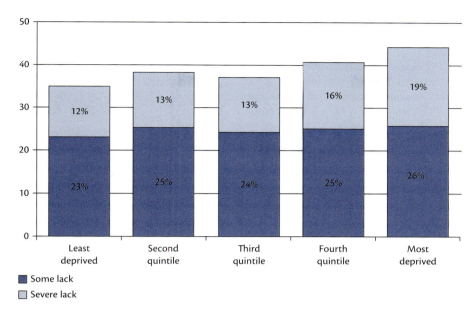

**Fig. 4.4** Percentage of those lacking social support, by deprivation of residential area, 2005.
Source: data from *Health Survey for England 2005: The health of older people, Summary of key findings* , The Information Centre, http://www.hscic.gov.uk/catalogue/PUB01184/heal-surv-heal-old-peo-eng-2005-rep-v5.pdf. Copyright © 2007 The Information Centre.

social contacts and high levels of participation in society. Public arts institutions and voluntary arts organizations can be important in these respects, as contributions to this volume demonstrate. It has been shown that low levels of social contact increase mortality (Bennett 2002) and depression (Morgan and Swann 2004). Individuals who are socially isolated are two to five times more likely to die prematurely than those who have good social ties and contact (The Marmot Review Team 2010). While those with high levels of social contact don't fall ill less than others, the support they receive from their social networks enables them to recover more quickly and successfully (Halpern 2004). Social capital is more specifically defined than social contact, as it refers to the quality of relationships. These relationships can include 'community networks, civic engagement, sense of belonging and norms of cooperation and trust' (Almedom 2005).

Participation can refer to a range of social contacts, but tends to involve an active role for the individual, particularly in their community. Social contact, capital, and participation follow a social class gradient. Figure 4.4 shows the gradient in social support by deprivation in England. However, some people are particularly deprived of social capital and participation. These are often people who have been severely affected by exclusionary processes, such as irregular migrants, Roma, people with disabilities, and the very old (UCL Institute of Health Equity and WHO Regional Office for Europe 2014). Exclusionary processes can include exclusion from good-quality education or work, exclusion from wider participation in the community, and poor living conditions and can create vulnerability, undermine social cohesion, and have a negative effect on health (UCL Institute of Health Equity and WHO Regional Office for Europe 2014).

### Children and young people

Analyses of the role of social capital and participation in fostering good health don't often focus on the early years; however,

they have an important role in fostering social interaction and the development of social skills in the early years. There is evidence that for the primary carers of very young children the level of social support and capital can be significant in helping to foster loving, stable, secure, and stimulating relationships which are crucial for the health of both the child and caregiver (UCL Institute of Health Equity and WHO Regional Office for Europe 2014). Family support, good child care and education, and reduction of child poverty, can, , act as protective factors against intergenerational transmission of isolation, deprivation, and ill-health and improve equity of outcomes amongst children (UCL Institute of Health Equity and WHO Regional Office for Europe 2014).

### People of working age

Social capital improves people's resilience and capacity to deal with challenging times because social support and connections help to build psychosocial wellbeing and provide connections that help people access formal and informal support, which are also protective of health (The Marmot Review Team 2010). Good-quality work is also a good source of social capital and empowerment, partly because it fosters strong social status and social identity (Siegrist et al. 2012). While social contact is important across the working age population, for some parents with young children a lack of social networks is particularly significant (Wilkinson and Pickett 2009), and this group may require particular support, as may older people.

### Older age

Many older people (over 65) experience poor mental and physical health as a result of social isolation. Loneliness in older people is linked to depressive symptoms, poor mental health and cognition, alcoholism, suicidal ideation, and mortality (Cacioppo et al. 2006; Hawkley et al. 2008), and one study suggested that nearly 20% of older people in the United Kingdom felt lonely or isolated

(Actor et al. 2002). On the other hand, higher levels of social support (e.g. regular contact with friends) tend to reduce the risk of depression amongst the older population, even amongst those with poor physical health (Prince et al. 1998). Social networks and social participation have also been shown to act as protective factors against dementia or cognitive decline over the age of 65 (Fabrigoule et al. 1995; Bassuk et al. 1999). Volunteering and participation in communities can give the opportunity to improve social contact and capital and therefore reduce the likelihood of depression, increase satisfaction, and improve morale and self-esteem (Surr et al. 2005).

## Summary

It is important to recognize and build capabilities for individuals and communities in order to improve health. One way to do this is by strengthening social networks, control, and inclusion at a community level, which can enhance and protect health. Volunteering, which was mentioned in reference to the older population, also has benefits at other stages of the life course. A study conducted by Volunteering England found that volunteers experience positive effects in the areas of self-rated health status, mortality, adoption of healthier lifestyles, quality of life, depression, psychological distress, and self-esteem (Casiday 2008). There is also evidence that volunteering created a stronger immune system and reduced blood pressure (Neuberger 2008). Those who receive support from community programmes also experience improved outcomes. For example, there is evidence that community health workers or volunteers tend to increase their knowledge, improve access to and uptake of services, promote changes in health behaviour, and improve health status amongst those they work with (World Health Organization 2007; South et al. 2010).

The Marmot Review states that in order to reduce social isolation, we must 'develop social capital by enhancing community empowerment. This helps to develop relationships of trust, reciprocity and exchange within communities, strengthening social capital . . . increasing control and community empowerment may (also) result in communities acting to change their social, material and political environments' (The Marmot Review Team 2010).

The European Review builds on this idea, summarizing the importance of social relationships, control, social capital, and resilience as follows:

'How people experience social relationships influences health inequities. Critical factors include how much control people have over resources and decision-making and how much access people have to social resources, including social networks, and communal capabilities and resilience. Social capital has been identified as a catalyst for coordination and cooperation, serving as an essential means to achieve better social and economic outcomes.'

UCL Institute of Health Equity and WHO Regional Office for Europe (2014)

As the contributions to this volume show, engagement in participative creative arts activities in communities can help to build social capital, address loneliness and social isolation, and build personal confidence and a sense of empowerment. In all of these respects, the creative arts have a role to play in

addressing the social determinants of health and wellbeing so powerfully documented through the work of the Institute of Health Equity.

## Conclusion

There is a significant and growing body of evidence demonstrating that inequalities in power, money, and resources affect levels of population health and wellbeing. The circumstances in which people are born, grow, live, work, and age shape their chances and opportunities for good health. These factors, called the 'social determinants of health', include early years experiences, education, income, employment and quality of work, and the physical and social environment. The social determinants of health contribute to unacceptable differences in length and quality of life both within and between countries. Differences are not just a result of the wealth or level of development in a country or area, but the extent to which people have the opportunity to live lives that they have reason to value.

There are some key concepts which have been outlined in this chapter in order to help understand health inequalities. First, there is the understanding that health inequalities are a result of unfair and unequal social determinants. Secondly, we have described the social class gradient in health outcomes, the finely graded distribution of health outcomes according to wealth or other social determinants of health. The best response to the social gradient is to adopt policies of proportionate universalism, in order to 'level up' the slope. The third area of importance is the life course approach, which recognizes that approaches must be targeted and adapted according to the stage of life of the individual. The life course approach demonstrates the cumulative effect of advantage and disadvantage over the life span, from prenatal and early years to old age. Furthermore, there is intergenerational transmission of inequity, whereby the opportunities of future generations for good health are in part determined by conditions and events occurring long before they are born.

The second half of this chapter applied these key concepts to important impacts of social determinants—control, stress, and empowerment. People who are able to make decisions about how they want to live their lives tend to have better health as a result. This is partly because a lack of control (through, for example, poverty or a low-quality job), heightens the risk of stress, which has a negative impact on health. Across the life course, the distribution and level of control relate to levels of health and inequalities between groups or populations.

Amongst the wide range of approaches that can be used to reduce health inequalities, one important strategy is to reduce social isolation and thereby increase people's levels of control and reduce stress. In this way, social contact, social capital, and participation in the community are important ways of fostering control, empowerment, and better health. There are various ways to reduce social isolation and increase participation within communities and community organizations, including participation in creative arts activities. Those who support and foster strong communities have significant impacts on health equity.

## References

Actor, C., Bowling, A., Bond, J., and Scambler, S. (2002). *Loneliness, Social Isolation and Living Alone in Later Life*. Swindon: ESRC.

Allen, J., Balfour, R., Bell, R., and Marmot, M. (2014). Social determinants of mental health. *International Review of Psychiatry*, **26**, 392–407.

Almedom, A.M. (2005). Social capital and mental health: an interdisciplinary review of primary evidence. *Social Science and Medicine*, **61**, 943–964.

Anderson, P., McDaid, D., Basu, S., and Stuckler, D. (2011). *Impact of Economic Crises on Mental Health*. Copenhagen: World Health Organization European Office.

Barker, D.J. (2004). The developmental origins of adult disease. *Journal of the American College of Nutrition*, **23**(6 Suppl.), 588S–595S.

Bassuk, S.S., Glass, T.A., and Berkman, L.F. (1999). Social disengagement and incident cognitive decline in community-dwelling elderly persons. *Annals of Internal Medicine*, **131**, 165–173.

Bennett, K.M. (2002). Low level social engagement as a precursor of mortality among people in later life. *Age and Ageing*, **31**, 165–168.

Bicego, G.T. and Boerma, J. (1993). Maternal education and child survival: a comparative study of survey data from 17 countries. *Social Science and Medicine*, **36**, 1207–1227.

Cacioppo, J.T., Hughes, M.E., Waite, L.J., Hawkley, L.C., and Thisted, R.A. (2006). Loneliness as a specific risk factor for depressive symptoms: cross-sectional and longitudinal analyses. *Psychology and Aging*, **21**, 140–151.

Case, A., Fertig, A., and Paxson, C. (2005). The lasting impact of childhood health and circumstance. *Journal of Health Economics*, **24**, 365–389.

Casiday, R. (2008). *Volunteering and Health: What Impact Does it Really Have?* London: Volunteering England.

Chandola, T., Brunner, E., and Marmot, M. (2006). Chronic stress at work and the metabolic syndrome: prospective study. *British Medical Journal*, **332**, 521–525.

City of Westminster (2014). Area profiles. URL: <https://www.westminster.gov.uk/ward-profiles> (accessed 5 March 2015).

Commission on the Social Determinants of Health (2008). *Closing the Gap in a Generation: Health Equity Through Action on the Social Determinants of Health. Final Report of the Commission on Social Determinants of Health*. Geneva: World Health Organization.

Fabrigoule, C., Letenneur, L., Dartigues, J.F., Zarrouk, M., Commenges, D., and Barbergergateau, P. (1995). Social and leisure activities and risk of dementia—a prospective longitudinal-study. *Journal of the American Geriatrics Society*, **43**, 485–490.

Fryers, T., Melzer, D., Jenkins, R., and Brugha, T. (2005). The distribution of the common mental disorders: social inequalities in Europe. *Clinical Practice and Epidemiology of Mental Health*, **1**, 14.

Gleason, M.M., Zamfirescu, A., Egger, H.L., Nelson, C.A. 3rd, Fox, N.A., and Zeanah, C.H. (2011). Epidemiology of psychiatric disorders in very young children in a Romanian pediatric setting. *European Child and Adolescent Psychiatry*, **20**, 527–535.

Halpern, D. (2004). *Social Capital*. Cambridge : Polity.

Hawkley, L.C., Hughes, M.E., Waite, L.J., Masi, C.M., Thisted, R.A., and Cacioppo, J.T. (2008). From social structural factors to perceptions of relationship quality and loneliness: the Chicago Health, Aging, and Social Relations Study. *Journal of Gerontology Series B: Psychological Sciences and Social Sciences*, **63**, S375–S384.

Jenkins, R., Bhugra, D., Bebbington, P., et al. (2008). Debt, income and mental disorder in the general population. *Psychological Medicine*, **38**, 1485–1493.

Kelly, Y., Sacker, A., Del Bono, E., Francesconi, M., and Marmot, M. (2011). What role for the home learning environment and parenting in reducing the socioeconomic gradient in child development? Findings from the Millennium Cohort Study. *Archives of Disease in Childhood*, **96**, 832–837.

Marmot, M. (2004). *Status Syndrome: How Your Social Standing Directly Affects Your Health and Life Expectancy*. London: Bloomsbury.

Marmot, M., Smith, G.D., Stansfeld, S., et al. (1991). Health inequalities among British civil servants: the Whitehall II Study. *Lancet*, **337**, 1387–1393.

Melzer, D., Fryers, T., Jenkins, R., Bhugra, T., and McWilliams, B. (2003). Social position and the common mental disorders with disability: estimates from the National Psychiatric Survey of Great Britain. *Social Psychiatry and Psychiatric Epidemiology*, **38**, 238–243.

Morgan, A. and Swann, C. (eds) (2004). *Social Capital for Health: Issues of Definition, Measurement and Links to Health*. London : Health Development Agency.

Neuberger, J. (2008). *Volunteering in the Public Services: Health and Social Care. Baroness Neuberger's Review as the Government's Volunteering Champion*. London: Cabinet Office/Office of the Third Sector.

Office for National Statistics (2014). *Health Expectancies at Birth and Age 65 in the United Kingdom*. Available at: <http://www.ons.gov.uk/ons/rel/disability-and-health-measurement/health-expectancies-at-birth-and-age-65-in-the-united-kingdom/index.html> (accessed October 2014).

Prince, M.J., Harwood, R.H., Thomas, A., and Mann, A.H. (1998). A prospective population-based cohort study of the effects of disablement and social milieu on the onset and maintenance of late-life depression. The Gospel Oak Project VII. *Psychological Medicine*, **28**, 337–350.

Schady, N. (2011). Parents' education, mothers' vocabulary, and cognitive development in early childhood: longitudinal evidence from Ecuador. *American Journal of Public Health*, **101**, 2299–2307.

Sen, A. (1992). *Inequality Reexamined*. Oxford: Clarendon Press.

Siegrist, J., Rosskam, E., and Leka, S. (2012). Report of Task Group 2: Employment and Working Conditions Including Occupation, Unemployment and Migrant Workers. Available at: <https://www.instituteofhealthequity.org/members/workplans-and-draft-reports>

South, J., Raine, G., and White, J. (2010). *Community Health Champions: Evidence Review*. Leeds: Centre for Health Promotion, Leeds Metropolitan University.

Steptoe, A., Kunz-Ebrecht, S., Owen, N., et al. (2003). Socioeconomic status and stress-related biological responses over the working day. *Psychosomatic Medicine*, **65**, 461–470.

Stuckler, D. and Basu, S. (2013). *The Body Economic: Why Austerity Kills*. New York: Basic Books.

Surkan, P.J., Kennedy, C.E., Hurley, K.M., and Black, M.M. (2011). Maternal depression and early childhood growth in developing countries: systematic review and meta-analysis. *Bulletin of the World Health Organization*, **89**, 608–615.

Surr, C., Boyle, G., Brooker, D., Godfrey, M., and Townsend, J. (2005). *Prevention and Service Provision: Mental Health Problems in Later Life*. Leeds: Centre for Health and Social Care, University of Leeds/Division of Dementia Studies, University of Bradford.

Taylor, S.E. (2010). Mechanisms linking early life stress to adult health outcomes. *Proceedings of the National Academy of Sciences of the United States of America*, **107**, 8507–8512.

The Marmot Review Team (2010). *Fair Society, Healthy Lives: Strategic Review of Health Inequalities in England post-2010*. London: Marmot Review Team.

The World Bank (2013). *GDP per capita, PPP (Current International $)*. Available at: <http://data.worldbank.org/indicator/NY.GDP.PCAP.PP.CD?order=wbapi_data_value_2012+wbapi_data_value+wbapi_data_value-last&sort=desc> (accessed 15 September 2013).

UCL Institute of Health Equity and WHO Regional Office for Europe (2014). *Review of the Social Determinants of Health and the Health Divide in the WHO European Region* [updated reprint].

Copenhagen: WHO. Available at: <http://www.euro.
who.int/__data/assets/pdf_file/0004/251878/Review-of
-social-determinants-and-the-health-divide-in-the-WHO-
European-Region-FINAL-REPORT.pdf> (accessed October 2014).

University College London Institute of Health Equity (2011). *The
Health Impacts of Cold Homes and Fuel Poverty*. Available
at: <http://www.instituteofhealthequity.org/projects/
the-health-impacts-of-cold-homes-and-fuel-poverty>

Wanless, D. (2002). *Securing Our Future Health: Taking a Long-term
View. Final Report* [known as the Wanless Report]. London: HM
Treasury. Available at: <http://webarchive.nationalarchives.gov.
uk/20130129110402/http://www.hm-treasury.gov.uk/consult_
wanless_final.htm>

Wilkinson, R.G. and Pickett, K. (2009). *The Spirit Level: Why More Equal
Societies Almost Always Do Better*. London: Allen Lane.

World Health Organization (2007). *Community Health Workers: What Do
We Know About Them?* Geneva: WHO.

World Health Organization (2011). *Life Expectancy Data by Country*.
Available at: <http://apps.who.int/gho/data/node.main.688?lang=en>
(accessed 12 September 2013).

# CHAPTER 5

# Case Study: Southbank Centre London and the social utility of the arts

Shân Maclennan

## The social utility of the arts

Depending on who you are talking to, those who know it may describe London's Southbank Centre as an arts centre, an education centre, a social space, a concert hall gallery, or a found space for street arts. They may describe it as a place where something significant happened to them, or where they witnessed an engagement, a political announcement, a birthday, an awakening, a reunion, a wedding, a meeting, a great performance, a change of heart, a memorable exhibition, a farewell, or the setting for a transformative experience. They may describe it as a good place for a day out near to the river. Southbank Centre is all of these things.

The idea of social utility is rooted both in the way people choose to use this highly visible site on the southern bank of the Thames in London—the range of experiences they describe and the often deep emotional responses they elicit—and in the site's heritage as the place where the centrepiece of the 1951 Festival of Britain, the South Bank Exhibition, took place.

In this chapter I am going to suggest that Southbank Centre's history and its present-day practice make its work intrinsically useful to society. I will explain how an experience of the arts on this festival site can be life-enhancing for both individuals and groups. It can make things better. Apart from the obvious pleasure which the arts can provide, an experience here can offer a route to identity, better health, collective purpose, and a feeling of belonging as well as increased knowledge and confidence. Rather than running special programmes which attend to social and educational agendas, Southbank Centre believes that social usefulness is essential to its identity as a modern festival site. It examines and then produces all its work by asking the questions how can this be useful to society and how is Southbank Centre part of society? I am going to give examples of where these questions have been most clearly articulated and answered.

## A tonic to the nation

To understand the particular ideological and social DNA which runs through all of Southbank Centre's work, we need to start at the beginning, in 1951, when the 28-acre site on the southern banks of the Thames was chosen by the British government as the place to stage the South Bank Exhibition at the heart of the Festival of Britain. The festival, developed by the Labour politician Herbert Morrison, deputy prime minister and leader of the House of Commons, had been generated by the same post-war radical idealism which had created the National Health Service, passed the Education Act and founded the Arts Council: health, welfare, education, and culture for all.

There had been a lot of discussion about where the South Bank Exhibition would happen, but in the end the riverside location (consciously the unfashionable and undeveloped southern side where even the London Underground barely reached), almost directly opposite the Houses of Parliament, was settled upon.

Morrison's 'tonic to the nation' as it became known was at once an unforgettable festival to celebrate the end of the Second World War and to imagine the future many had believed would never come and an accelerated regeneration plan to attend to the southern bank of the Thames. Morrison was inspired by the Great Exhibition of 1851, but this was to be a new kind of festival for a new age.

Gerald Barry was appointed as the festival organizer, and after just over 3 years of planning his grand festival engaged everyone's imagination the length and breadth of the country. Some 17,000 towns and villages staged an event: every summer fair, Women's Institute cake sale, Brownie camp, school orchestra, amateur drama club, gardening show, and astronomy society joined in, and new local amenities were honoured with a festival tag—pubs, theatres, and parks. From Aberdeen to Llangollen, from York to Inverness, from Bath to Perth, every existing festival was rebranded as part of the Festival of Britain (Fig. 5.1).

The South Bank Exhibition was the epicentre of the festival, where the Royal Festival Hall, the Dome of Discovery, the Skylon (a sculptural structure which astonished visitors with its scale and beauty and the ingenuity of its construction), pop-up buildings and pavilions, open-air cafés, flags, fountains, art installations, and soundscapes delighted the eight and a half million people who were able to purchase a ticket. It was a completely new format, neither an arts festival nor a science expo, including masses of information about the achievements and potential of the British people (to the extent that at least one famous visitor, the Welsh poet Dylan Thomas, was exhausted if exhilarated!) but also making sure that there was light and joy, gaiety and playfulness: in short, that everyone could have a very good time. The Architect

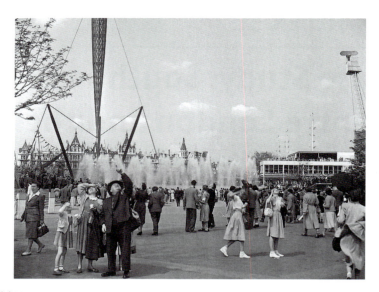

**Fig. 5.1** Visitors to the South Bank Exhibition 1951.
Reproduced from *Southbank Centre Celebrates Festival of Britain Souvenir Guide*, The Southbank Centre. Copyright © 2011, with kind permission of the Southbank Centre.

H. T. Cadbury Brown who worked on fountain design, remarked, 'There was a real sense in which the Festival marked an upturn in people's lives . . . it was an event for a new dawn, for enjoying life on modern terms, with modern technology.'

Under the head of architecture, Hugh Casson, a team of young architects and designers conceived of the site as 'a pattern book for a new urban landscape'. Casson planned the site as if it were a small town and his implausibly young team (some were still students) demonstrated how this new world could look different and promoted alternative ways of living. Furniture and textiles were also integral to this presentation of modern life, and designers like Robin and Lucienne Day who created chairs and fabrics went on to be recognized as among the most influential figures of the time.

Art was central to the exhibition, and many artists—both known and unknown—were commissioned to make paintings, murals, sculptures, flags, and fountains. Likewise science and scientific development were part of the backbone of the experience both as exhibition content and in design. Britain was a world leader in crystallography and the Festival Pattern Group, including pioneering scientists like Dorothy Hodgson, used crystallography diagrams to inspire the design of wallpaper, fabrics, graphics, and restaurant menu cards.

The Festival of Britain made tremendous gestures depicting how culture and the arts could bring about a change in society complete with dozens of tiny blueprints suggesting how to do it. Schoolchildren were as important to the festival as professional people: dancing in your overcoat makes you happy; artists can be part of everyday life; colour cheers you up; seriousness and fun—'serious fun'—can go hand in hand. These gestures stood out in a post-war society which was visibly changed, more progressive and more receptive to new ideas than that which preceded it. The benefits and privileges of universal education and healthcare were soon to be tangibly felt. But there was still food rationing in London in 1951, and although the South Bank Exhibition was always intended to be temporary there was something in the almost violent and brisk dismantling of the site by the new Conservative government that seemed to want to quash the

utopian dreams which had been allowed to flourish and to resist the 'propaganda of the imagination' which had been unleashed.

When the festival ended, the progressive arts and education agenda it had laid out went underground. The fragile territory where the practice of the arts is discussed in relation to the 'everyday reality' of individuals, communities, and neighbourhoods fully consumed by the business of simply living risked being confined to a 'very minor footnote in the margin of our cultural history' (Lane 1978). Even on the festival site itself, the Royal Festival Hall, left lonely in a landscape which had been packed with activity and ideas, swiftly became a more traditional kind of concert hall, presenting great concerts and events of many kinds but rarely stopping to ask what purpose such presentations had in the political reality of the day. There were exceptions to this—for example, Guitar-in, a benefit concert organized by Liberal International's Fighting Racialism Appeal Fund in September 1967 and featuring a young Jimi Hendrix, addressed a growing modern problem—but this was the exception rather than the rule.

## This sacred site

It was not until the early part of the twenty-first century, under the leadership of Jude Kelly who joined the organization as artistic director in 2005, that Southbank Centre (as the site was constituted in the mid 1980s and registered as a charity) fully reclaimed its history as a festival site. She set about a conscious, collective act of 'remembering the history of this sacred site' in order to establish a pathway for the future.

Jude's vision is fundamentally based on a reclamation of the entire site (now technically 21 acres rather than 28) with art, fountains, gardens, flags, pop-ups, shops, and cafés (all echoes of the site in 1951) and the re-establishment of it in the public imagination as an engine where the arts and culture are agents of change in a global society.

Her vision places great art alongside the discussion of the important issues of the day. It values the truly international and deep cultural exchange and gives the young child, the teenager, and in fact anyone who feels excluded, equal rights with the experienced art-lover and the expert. Her emphasis on human rights and on the central importance of creative education give urgency and radical intention to the day-to-day programming of the site both inside the buildings and outdoors. A tremendous shift since 1951 has been that the site is now completely free to visit, and over half of its entire artistic programme is free for audiences and participants.

If you visit Southbank Centre today you will find practical demonstrations of this vision all around you. It might be the annual exhibition of art by offenders, secure patients, and detainees from the Koestler Awards (see the case study by Tim Robertson in Chapter 35). It could be a rehearsal by a group drawn from the 400 young musicians who make up In Harmony Lambeth, a social project inspired by the Venezuelan Sistema method of music education which brings hope and aspiration to children through the learning of a musical instrument (see the case study by Andrea Creech and colleagues in Chapter 24). You might be consulting The Book Doctor hoping to be prescribed a book to help you with a particular problem. (Since 2013, there has been a National Books on Prescription Scheme created by The Reading Agency working with the Society of Chief Librarians and health partners aimed at addressing mild to moderate mental health problems.) You might find professional artists working alongside others in a performance or at an exhibition presented as part of the mainstream programme. You may be joining with many other people to enjoy a Big Sing or a Big Busk in one of the public spaces. The effect of people singing and playing instruments together in a public place creates feelings of infectious joy for those taking part which very quickly transmits to those who are observing or who are nearby. Or you might simply want to be there—to meet a friend, or have a business meeting, or simply watch the world go by in a refreshingly open and unregulated environment.

The sense of being part of society is particularly present in the garden on the roof of the Queen Elizabeth Hall. This garden in the sky was created by Southbank Centre in association with the Eden Project in Cornwall, and it is grown, maintained, and developed by gardeners from Grounded Ecotherapy, part of the housing association Providence Row.

The idea to green the roof had existed in the minds of the original architects of the Queen Elizabeth Hall but only became a reality as part of the celebrations for the 60th anniversary of the Festival of Britain. The garden has wonderful river views and features a lush lawn sprinkled with daisies, a wildflower garden which has over 90 varieties of plant and fruit and olive trees as well as a café. It is a very popular place for people to come and relax (Fig. 5.2). For Grounded Ecotherapy the garden at Southbank Centre has a very particular purpose. In making a beautiful amenity for the public to enjoy, Grounded Ecotherapy have established a place where the vulnerable, excluded people whom they support can rebuild their sense of themselves; one gardener talks of reprogramming himself to be 'a gardener, not a fighter.'

This change begins by making the journey to Southbank Centre in the first place. Kelvin Barton, the Grounded mental health and wellbeing coordinator says, 'It's a place they probably would never have come; they'd have thought it was for other, middle-class people. If they had had a diagnosis of schizophrenia or depression, they might have felt that they didn't deserve to be spoken to by "normal" people. They might have been ignored by people who walked past them when they were sleeping rough in a shop doorway'. Once they are here, the work in the garden and the pleasure it brings to others allows the gardeners to see themselves as 'valid human beings'. People ask for advice on how to grow runner beans and how to make a wild flower area in their own garden. They admire the trees and marvel at what can be achieved in such a small space. This authentic communication with the public allows the gardeners to 'leave their diagnosis at the gate' and to re-reference their sense of themselves and their perception of how they are seen by others.

The public come to the garden because they love it not because they are curious about the gardeners. Kelvin says, 'People like it because it's good. It has to be the best it can be. It's a nice addition that it helps individuals.'

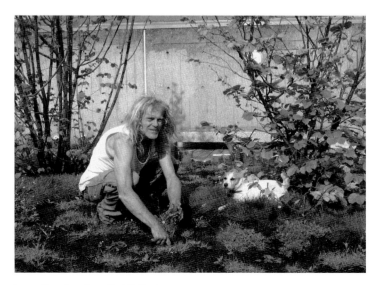

**Fig. 5.2** The Southbank Centre roof garden and head gardener Paul Pulford.
Reproduced by kind permission of the Southbank Centre. Copyright © 2015 The Southbank Centre.

## The story of festivals

Inevitably, however, Southbank Centre's central purpose is most present in its year-round programme of festivals. Like the Festival of Britain, modern-day Southbank Centre festivals grow from our times—from ideas and issues that are in the public imagination, in the *zeitgeist,* which require urgent attention at this moment. The work of creative people is at the heart of every festival, and although there are countless moments of inexplicable pleasure and pain, knowing, and understanding brought about by an encounter with great art, this is not an 'arts for arts' sake' agenda. The festivals are designed to re-imagine the arts and culture as supporting practical enquiry and human need. This applies as much to communities as to the individual, and festivals tend to be characterized by moments of congregation (from the traditional audience to the joiners-in) as well as by those seeking a solitary experience or one shared by friends and family. There are up to 20 festivals each year. Some last for a weekend, others for several months. Some are aimed at a particular audience—Imagine, every February, is for the under 12s—whereas others, like Festival of Love, are for everyone.

The making of festivals at Southbank Centre is codified in an internal working document known as the 'festival methodology'. This is a kind of checklist against which the curators, programmers, and delivery teams measure the initiation and development of festivals against specific principles.

As stated in the festival methodology, it is a given that a Southbank Centre festival is 'a platform for high-quality international art (free and ticketed)' in support of 'artistic experiment and innovation' and that it should aim to attract intergenerational and diverse audiences. It is also a given that Southbank Centre's work should have rich local and regional community engagement and use both indoor and outdoor space. The more radical elements of the methodology, which require that learning and participation shape and lead the artistic programme from the beginning and that demand cultural activism to challenge the curators and programmers to consider communities and influences beyond their own professional sphere, allow the festival to emerge as a collective effort with unexpected voices and actions often taking centre stage. Evaluation of the festivals against precise social objectives is considered, and we have recently begun to experiment with the social return on investment instrument as a method. We commissioned a report from Mandy Barnett Associates to consider the participation of children in Southbank Centre's 2013 Imagine Festival.

The Festival of Death happened over a long weekend in January 2012. Styled as Southbank Centre's Festival for the Living, the festival determined not only to confront the taboos surrounding the discussion of death in many societies including ours but to reclaim, according to Jude Kelly, 'the greatest and most challenging of all certainties' (Southbank Centre 2012) and examine it with delight and humour as well as dignity and seriousness.

Far from presenting artistic events for their own sake, it placed them inside a meticulously designed philosophical framework. The festival included learned talks (the artistry of cemeteries, death in the Hindu tradition, a discussion of suicide) alongside personal testimony (a father on the agonizing decision of who to save when he and his twins were drowning, surviving breast cancer, surviving land-mines); there were debates (assisted dying considered

by an expert panel chaired by news journalist Jon Snow), there were exhibitions (Boxed: Fabulous Coffins From Ghana and the UK, Before I Die, Sam Winston's Birthday); there was theatre for children (Goodbye Mr Muffin) and theatre for adults (An Instinct for Kindness); there was comedy (The Sandi Toksvig Memorial Lecture, Marcus Birdman); and then, of course, music and poetry of many kinds.

Perhaps unsurprisingly, Festival of Death brought a very wide variety of people of different ages and backgrounds to Southbank Centre. They came for all kinds of reasons, ranging from a very particular desire to hear a talk on a specific subject to a generalized curiosity. Some people found the festival by accident, whereas for others it provided an overdue opportunity to discuss urgent and unresolved matters.

Other festivals have similarly layered programmes to different effect. The 4-month long Festival of Neighbourhood in summer 2013 brought allotments, wheelbarrows groaning with fruit and vegetables, and giant topiary figures (one duo made to honour those neighbours who began the great clear-up in the aftermath of the London riots in 2011) to the outdoor spaces. Alongside an exhibition of outsider art in the Hayward Gallery, The Alternative Guide to the Universe, and an impressive programme of performing arts events including a Meltdown season curated by Yoko Ono and a family of lumberjacks from Canada presenting a show for everyone called Timber, there were weekends featuring the South London communities of Deptford, Brixton, and Vauxhall and the neighbourhood of Pelourinho in the Brazilian city of Salvador, all programmed by and for the communities allowing them to profile and discuss their current ideas and concerns.

The Rest is Noise told the story of music in the twentieth century by relating it to the politics and science of the time in the dramatization of the eponymous book by the American music critic Alex Ross (2007). Over 150 concerts carried the musical story while 12 themed weekends of talks, debates, and seminars (a staggering 600 in total)—among them, The Rise of Nationalism, Berlin in the 1920s and 1930s, Art of Fear, Superpower, and New World Order—allowed participants to relate music directly to the stories of politics, history, and science. It gave audiences, and those wishing to learn, a new way to approach modern music, which is often thought of as difficult, to understand the political and social circumstances in which it was made, and to consider their own relationship to these.

WOW, Women of the World, which started in 2011, has become an international festival with programmes in Australia, the United States, and Ireland and further ones planned in other parts of the world. A co-designed programming model has enabled both women and men from all walks of life to come together to discuss a barely imaginable range of topics from art, comedy, women in the military, rocket science, motherhood, sex, cosmetic surgery, and dozens of others. At the heart of the festival, the Southbank Centre version features an all-woman symphony orchestra—even more staggering to witness than to contemplate—and a night of comedy, stories, and music inspired by great women.

## A new kind of art-making

A profound consequence of attending to the arts and culture in this way, allowing the work of artists to directly serve individuals and communities in their search for understanding and identity, is that the arts themselves change. The restless and ongoing making of Southbank Centre, like the creation of the South Bank Exhibition in 1951, continuously produces new styles of artistic presentation which in themselves make it more possible for more people to think of the arts as useful in their everyday life and relevant to their own concerns. It is unthinkable now that people would come here just to 'listen to music in a soundproof box' (Mullins 2007); the question is always about how to place music and the arts in society where it can not only inspire us but give us permission to act differently.

The arc of inclusion which reaches from 'ordinary people', from all of us, to people who are leading and defining the world is very clear: the symbolism was unmistakable when the leader of the Labour Party, Tony Blair, chose the balcony of the Royal Festival Hall from which to address his supporters following his historic election victory in spring 1997. Equally, Malala Yousafzai, the young campaigner for girls' education who was shot by the Taliban in 2012, chose Southbank Centre to give her first UK public speech knowing that her visit underscored our Day of the Girl which brings hundreds of young women here to discuss the challenges that girls face in reaching their potential.

Now, it seems very obvious that someone is as likely to come to Southbank Centre to be close to great art and artists as to meditate on universal or personal questions. Social utility, usefulness to society at large, sits harmoniously with the striving for new forms of expression and exceptional art. These actions are all part of each other and they create the unique conditions which allow Southbank Centre—a social space in the true sense—to have potency for the many, to be truly a caring place, a 'peoples' place.'

## References

Lane, J. (1978). *Arts Centres: Every Town Should Have One.*
    London: Paul Elek.
Mullins, C. (2007). *A Festival on the River: The Story of Southbank Centre.*
    London: Penguin Books.
Ross, A. (2007). *The Rest Is Noise—Listening to the Twentieth Century.*
    New York: Farrar, Straus and Giroux.
Southbank Centre (2012) *Festival of Death Brochure: January 2012.*
    London: Southbank Centre.

## Websites

Southbank Centre: <http://www.southbankcentre.co.uk/>
The Eden Project: <http://www.edenproject.com>
Grounded Ecotherapy: <http://groundedproject.org/>
Books on Prescription: <http://www.booksonprescription.org.uk/
    about-the-scheme>

# CHAPTER 6

# The means to flourish: arts in community health and education

Mike White

## The emergence of arts in community health

Arts in community health projects first appeared in the United Kingdom in the late 1980s, placing local arts development in health promotion and primary-care contexts. I have previously defined this work as 'a distinct area of activity operating mainly outside of acute healthcare settings and characterised by the use of participatory arts to promote health' (White 2009, p. 3). In communities and schools in disadvantaged areas participatory arts have combined creative activities with health education and amassed testimony from participants as to its value. In recent years, community-based projects using arts to address local health issues have proliferated and have become, through their increasing presence in the international field of arts in health, a small-scale global phenomenon in imaginative health promotion. For example, Ireland has a thriving national festival of arts for older people, Bealtaine, which takes place through the month of May and is inspiring similar developments in several other countries (Ni Leime and O'Shea 2008). Furthermore, reality TV programmes like the BBC's *The Choir* and ABC Australia's *Choir of Hard Knocks* have demonstrated the potential of communal singing for social bonding, health improvement, and wellbeing. A growing interest in the social wellbeing that can be achieved through participatory arts, particularly with regard to mental health across the life course and the care needs of an ageing population, has begun to characterize the community outreach programmes of major cultural institutions such as New York's Museum of Modern Art (MOMA) (Rosenberg 2009), Tate Modern (Independent 2009), the National Gallery of Australia (Artworks ABC Radio 2009), and Sage Gateshead (Sing Up 2012).

There have even been stadium-scale representations of arts in health for global audiences. As an example, the centrepiece of the closing ceremony for the Commonwealth Games in Manchester in 2002 was a gigantic illuminated figure assembled from lantern tableaux created with local communities to express a theme of social integration and wellbeing. This image was orchestrated by Walk the Plank Theatre, an offshoot of the Welfare State Arts Company which pioneered sculptural lantern parades through the 1980s and with which I worked on my first arts in health projects. Ten years on from those Commonwealth Games, one of the most resonant images from the post-modernist jamboree of the opening ceremony of the 2012 Olympics in London was that of hundreds of children bouncing on beds to the choreographed attendance of health workers from National Health Service (NHS) hospitals. Daring to epitomize our national values at a global sporting event in a concern for the health and imagination of children produced a populist tableau. There was a lot of sentiment in it, even some of the proud socialism in which the NHS was conceived. It was a massive declaration for arts in health as the bedrock of healthcare, expressed with a sweeping confidence that the viewing public would understand such an association.

Whilst the field of arts in health is now primed to make statements on the world stage, we should not forget that the practice is essentially about relationship-based working, whether it is in acute care settings or a community health context (White 2010). In looking for impact, we also should not underestimate the inherent strength of the arts to shape people's world views and influence lifestyle choice, autonomy, perception of human worth, and social engagement—factors which the United Kingdom's 'new public health' movement claims have significant effects on health (Wilson 1975; Ashton and Seymour 1988; Marmot 2004). The central importance of creativity to public health is highlighted in the declaration of health philosopher David Seedhouse (2001, p. 121) that 'The major theme of health education has been prevention. However, since a person's health is inextricably linked to the quality of life, the primary aim of health education and promotion should be to create.'

## Arts in community health and education

I want to share some lessons learned from my own management and research of arts in community health and set it in a broader context of health education in schools, social inclusion, and the emphasis on creativity in the new public health. The big challenge for me and my artist colleagues has been to sustain our projects for long enough to consolidate an emergent practice and to undertake longitudinal research that can utilize and analyse participants' testimony in a more rigorous ethnographic framework. At the core of the work that we have been doing in this field has been support for schools and the communities they serve to develop new traditions that celebrate health awareness and occasions of transition through resonant imagery and the reflective practice that comes from relationship-based working (White and Robson 2011).

Given the longitudinal nature of this work, with some projects running for over 10 years, there is an accumulated wealth of data from them demonstrating how arts-led approaches can contribute to mental health and wellbeing (Raw 2006; Loca 2009; Atkinson and Robson 2012). The arts in health practice has helped to shape educational practice on different levels, and the links developed between both arts and health professionals as well as academics and participants are now many and varied. These sustained relationships make for a rather complex network of practitioners, participants, and academics all seeking a reciprocal understanding about the work that can help to originate participatory research with mentoring from various departments within Durham University, where I am based in the Centre for Medical Humanities (CMH). The arts in health programme is guided by the CMH's over-arching and interdisciplinary theme of 'human flourishing', and in long-term fieldwork it interprets this theme as a more dynamic and socially connected form of wellbeing.

In recent years, my work in community-based arts in health has attempted to apply the policy directives for both child and community health practice that were established in the United Kingdom, first in *Every Child Matters* (Department for Education and Skills 2005) and later in the Marmot Review *Fair Society, Healthy Lives* (Marmot Review 2010) which attracted interest and support across the political spectrum. The previous UK Labour government's Every Child Matters strategy introduced and identified five national outcomes that all professionals working with children and young people needed to be working towards; these are being healthy, staying safe, enjoying and achieving, making a positive contribution, and socio-economic wellbeing. They provided a context through which to have joint conversations, joint planning, and joint working by statutory and voluntary agencies, with clear processes to achieve those outcomes for children and young people; but crucially they have had to involve children and young people in learning to take responsibility for achieving those outcomes for themselves. The National Children's Bureau came to see those five outcomes as integrated rather than separate (Worthy 2005), and identified characteristics of good practice residing particularly in projects that foster creativity and emotional and social development. Such projects can help to ameliorate the process of transition, not only as it occurs in the school system but also possibly when a child undergoes difficult changes and loss in their personal life.

The Marmot Review's key policy objectives to reduce health inequalities included 'Enable all children, young people and adults to maximise their capabilities and have control over their lives', with a priority to 'ensure that schools, families and communities work in partnership to reduce the gradient in health, wellbeing and resilience' and 'create and develop healthy and sustainable places and communities'. On the social determinants of health it concluded that 'All these influences are affected by the socio-political and cultural and social context in which they sit' (Marmot Review 2010, p. 10). It encouraged extension of the role of schools into communities and developing the education workforce to address social and emotional wellbeing in school, family, and community life. Furthermore, it called for support for communities to find their own whole-system solutions so that top-down approaches are reduced and 'avoid drift into small-scale projects focused on individual behaviours and lifestyle' (Marmot Review 2010, p. 18). It needs to be noted, however, that neither this Marmot Review nor the World Health Organization's committee report on global health inequalities *Closing the Gap* (World Health Organization 2008) on which Marmot was the chair, called specifically for arts interventions to address these issues; an omission which subsequently prompted an advocacy campaign editorial in the international journal *Arts & Health* (Clift et al. 2010).

## The Roots and Wings project

One UK community arts in health and education project connected to the research portfolio of the CMH that attempted to give substance to the Marmot recommendations through the example of participatory arts addressing children's emotional health was Roots and Wings. This was based in a primary school in Chickenley, West Yorkshire, and ran for 10 years from 2003. Chickenley is a socio-economically deprived area on the outskirts of Dewsbury. Its primary school had a troubled history, and in 2001 it was taken into 'special measures' on the recommendation of the inspectorate. A newly installed headteacher saw potential in having artists in residence in the school to help address its difficulties, funded initially through the Children's Trust Fund and later from the local healthcare trust responsible for primary-care provision. The project's artists, led by CMH's associate artist Mary Robson, worked year-round with pupils, their families, school staff, and the wider community to foster social and emotional development and encourage cultural change through new traditions that mark significant moments in the life of the community. They applied the 'positive regard' theory of Carl Rogers (1959) to their work and adapted child development theories about curiosity from US psychologist Bruce Perry (2008).

The project's title 'Roots and Wings' expresses its ethos and approach. Central to the project has been the art room, a space run by the children at break and lunchtimes with artist support. Encouragement to reflect on feelings led to the children creating greetings cards, initially for friends and family but later also sold into craft outlets in the town, with the proceeds providing charitable donations that the children were able to determine. Sometimes there could be as many as 40 children in the art room but order somehow emerged in this bedlam as children assisted each other in realizing their art from concept to appraisal. The children devised their own ground rules for behaviour in the art room and, guided by the artists, their activities focused on self, emotions, expression of emotions, and different ways to depict complex messages through a range of art forms. Roots and Wings gave children the responsibility to help change some aspects of school culture, prevent mental ill-health, and set the scene for a more nurtured generation. A deeply held belief that an emphasis on unconditional positive regard would lead to children gaining a perceptive understanding of alternative ways of behaving and enhance their ability to learn pervaded the project. It was more than just an activity room, but rather a space to foster empathy, and to model and analyse relationships in a child-friendly way. Every aspect of the project came to involve reflective practice, whether between the professional practitioners or the pupils.

Within 3 years, the Roots and Wings programme had a significant impacted on Chickenley Primary's performance at all levels. The Office for Standards in Education (Ofsted) inspection report stated:

'One child wrote about her marvellous work of art, 'I think I am a painter now. I could work in a fast food restaurant, but being a painter is better'. Pupils are cherished as individuals. Education for personal and social health and citizenship is well organised to promote healthy and safe lifestyles. The initiative entitled 'Roots and Wings' is an outstanding element which has raised the school's profile locally. Pupils' artistic skills, writing and personal development, for example, are enhanced by its many superb activities. Pupils who are talented in sports or the arts thrive on a curriculum which offers many worthwhile opportunities in these areas. This is reflected in their trusting attitudes and confident bearing.'

Ofsted (2006, pp. 3–4)

In addition to the art room sessions, other activities included projects to raise aspirations, encourage effective thinking, and increase self-esteem—and how to apply these qualities and skills to other areas of life. In particular, from 2004, two annual carnival-style parades were developed that celebrated transition (Fig. 6.1). One was for the youngest children moving up to 'big school' and the other with the oldest, as they prepared to begin life at the high school. The significance of these transition parades was grasped by the then headteacher Lesley Finnegan, who saw them as key to raising the self-esteem and attainment of the children:

'We wanted anything that would engage them in learning, in activity and enjoyment; to put smiles on their faces and give them some confidence. We wanted to engage their curiosity and develop belonging. These children needed to feel like they belonged somewhere. A big part of it is friendship, respect for individuality. We are still working on that day by day. We came across enormous challenges around friendship and transition because I was aware that our children were anxious about transition to high school. It didn't feel right so we needed to do some work around that. I passionately believe that we needed to break cycles, break habits. In breaking cycles of deprivation we had to get in there somewhere. This is a long-term piece of work because Chickenly doesn't have a huge movement of its population; families stay. And so our children will become our parents. If

we can create a different attitude in our schools with our children, when they come back as our parents we are on to a winner.'

Finnegan and Robson (2005)

The 'transition' parade became an annual tradition whereby the Year 6 class, just before the end of the summer term, would walk from their familiar school gates up the long hill to the rather foreboding high school carrying large, team-designed sculptures that represented their aspirations and apprehensions for their future learning environment. Over the years, a growing number of parents followed in their wake, locals came out of their homes to watch, and the younger children cheered them on from the playground. The sculptures were given morale-boosting titles like 'The rocky mountains of strength', 'The fearless flames of destiny' and 'The waterfall of wishes'. Ex-pupils of Chickenley would line the drive of the secondary school to applaud the children's entrance, guiding them to the hall for a ritualistic exchange between the headteachers in which the Year 6 pupils are commended and entrusted to the bigger school with the words 'Take care of our children, they are special and talented'. The occasion became customarily commemorated with the presentation to the secondary headteacher of a garland of paper birds, on each of which is written a child's hopes and fears for their continuing education. Then the sculptures would be arranged for exhibition in the hall and the audience invited back to Chickenley Primary to view the self-portraits that each child had painstakingly worked on in their last term in a guided exploration of the meaning of inspiration and reflexive creativity. As one child declared to me 'a self-portrait isn't just drawing your face, you know, it's showing what's inside you, your feelings.'

The significance of transition for children's wellbeing is identified in the end report on the major arts in schools initiative Creative Partnerships, *The Impact of Creative Partnerships on the Wellbeing of Children and Young People*, (University of Cambridge 2012) which concludes that children's wellbeing diminishes over time as they progress through school, with positive feelings peaking around Year 6 (aged 10–11), and with girls losing their sense of wellbeing more than boys later on. For pupils at this time of transition, art was cited as the most motivating subject and literacy the least. This is not only a crucial phase in childhood development (Worthy 2005) but also an important time for

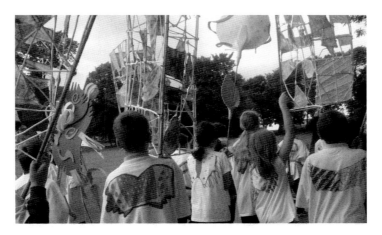

**Fig. 6.1** The Chickenley transition parade.
Reproduced by kind permission of M. Robson, Copyright © 2015 M. Robson.

determining health prospects in later life, with literacy—both emotional literacy and reading and writing—being, as the World Health Organization (2008) asserted, the single most important social determinant of health. Roots and Wings created a seedbed of reflection for participatory arts practice that proved a nurturing environment for both professionals and pupils as they aimed together to stimulate emotional literacy. It placed at the heart of the practice a belief that curiosity is the fuel of development. While some professional talk might be of attainment, resilience, attendance, and expectations, the real quality of Roots and Wings lay in the relationships it fostered, and in the creation of a fund of memories, both individual and collective, that helped to redefine perceptions of the community.

Despite the reflective environment developed by Roots and Wings over several years, it came as something of a deflating disappointment to realize in 2010 that all was not well. A new senior management team had brought changes to the school, but there appeared to be a shortfall in their understanding of the project and what its committed practice brought to the learning environment. Other staff changes inevitably added to the misunderstanding as they were not inducted as to the role of Roots and Wings' much beyond that it produced fantastic art work. The overall relationship between project staff and school staff was amiable yet somewhat diminished. Without adequate attention, relationships began to falter. Project staff felt the problem to be an ethical one because it seemed impossible for the work to develop without a mutually understood communal will. The way forward initially was to talk to senior management and explain that the project would not seek further funding and why. It required a frank, honest yet sensitive approach. Senior management had no idea that the problem existed but found it impossible to imagine the school without Roots and Wings. The new headteacher declared that the nurturing environment provided by the project was crucial for the children and their ability to learn. Both sides were able to admit responsibility and to move on to a new phase of development; the project continued as a result and to everyone's credit. The problem of maintaining the communal will for the project, however, resurfaced 2 years later, exacerbated further by funding difficulties and the changed priorities in education introduced by the government, such as the downgrading of arts in schools and the de-prioritization, coupled with removal of national control, of the healthy schools programme. (Lancet 2011)

In summer 2013, with great regret, the project closed after the 10th annual transition parade for Year 6 pupils. Shortly afterwards, at a final day of celebration and positive reflection in the art room base of Roots and Wings, there were dozens and dozens of communal journals, photo files, 'artist statements', and scrapbooks, dating back 10 years, laid open for all to see. Old friends of the project, parents, and former pupils turned up to offer congenial support and condolences. Display boards and art works, especially the self-portraits that came to characterize Roots and Wings, spoke volumes and sparked conversations, and visitors were invited to contribute memories of the project to a timeline on the wall. The Year 6 children, fresh from their transition parade and sporting the winged T-shirts they designed, had set up an impromptu café to offer visitors drinks and an all-cake buffet on arrival. The confidence and good humour of Chickenley children are always remarkable, and are so evidently at odds with their estate's reputation in the media as a sink of under-achievement and social dysfunction. While visitors leafed through the journals with mixed emotions, they were periodically entertained with raps and songs the children had composed.

It was a sad and unsought demise, but the legacy of the Chickenley project is considerable. It influenced and generated a lot of research-guided arts in health practice in schools in Yorkshire, initiated with the help of Loca, Kirklees Council's arts and regeneration agency. Inspired by the successes of Roots and Wings the agency was keen to take some of the working practices that were proving so successful in Chickenley and extend similar work to other schools. Loca successfully bid for funding in 2006 to develop 'Inside Me', a programme which for its first 3 years involved artists working in a cohort of six primary schools to deliver a series of 18 short projects with a particular focus on emotional literacy and emotional health. This in turn led to Kirklees Primary Care Trust commissioning Loca to be a delivery partner in its TaMHS (Targeted Mental Heath in Schools) initiative. Loca's creative input involved some of the most experienced artists from Inside Me and Roots and Wings working alongside other specialists (primary mental health workers, educational psychologists, and social and emotional aspects of learning specialists) to find innovative, creative, interdisciplinary ways of delivering interventions and training with children and staff in 15 participating schools (only one of which had been previously been involved with Inside Me).

As news got out that the Chickenley project was closing, the artists were immediately invited and resourced to establish another Roots and Wings project in a primary school in a neighbouring district. In a very palpable sense, the artists too have had their time of transition, and in a manner akin to the observation of Emerson that 'everything teaches transition, transference, metamorphosis: therein is human power, in transference, not in creation; and therein is human destiny, not in longevity but in removal. We dive and reappear in new places' (Emerson, 2001).

## Developing an international dimension

Artists from Roots and Wings have together modelled their practice to a higher level of interpersonal skills, innovation, and influence. In the project's final year they were able to share their learning in an international context. In 2011, CMH created an opportunity for leading practitioners and researchers from the United Kingdom, United States, South Africa, Australia, Ireland, and Mexico to come together at Durham in what was termed a 'critical mass' meeting. Participants explored community-based arts in health in a global context, identified key issues for international collaboration in both practice and research, and envisioned what success would look like in 5 years' time, with a detailed timeline to get there.

In preparation for this international 'critical mass' at Durham, the 20 or so participants (an equal number of practitioners and researchers) were invited to explain what were the principles and values that informed their interest in community-based arts in health and their current lines of enquiry. Their responses were collated and summarized as follows:

◆ We have a sense of crossing professional boundaries—in hybrid and unconventional roles—with a tendency to generalism and/or interdisciplinary collaboration rather than specialism.

◆ We have a commitment to social justice—addressing health inequalities through a nexus of collective creativity, health education, and citizenship.

◆ We seek transformational change more than instrumental effects.

◆ Some of us thrive on complex connections; others strive to disentangle complexity—either way, we try to turn complexity into revelation.

◆ We focus on relationship-building through shared reflective practice.

◆ We are interested to connect the diversity of global practice of arts in health through a better understanding of process and context.

One of the practical initiatives that arose from that 'critical mass' meeting was a pilot exchange in community-based work for two artists from Yorkshire and two from Western Australia providing placements in each other's jobs, networks, and communities for 8 weeks guided by reflective practice and research. The exchange put young and emerging artists at the heart of complex communities and practices at an international level. The host projects provided avenues for production and critical reflection through which the participating artists could develop new approaches to their practice and inform the recommendations and frameworks to guide future investments in the next generation of outstanding artists working in a participatory community context. The artist exchange took place through the autumn of 2012. The placements offered in Western Australia to the two visual artists from Yorkshire, who had previously been working on Roots and Wings, were in fieldwork projects run by the Australian arts in health agency DADAA (<http://www.dadaa.org.au/>). Reciprocally, the UK placements for DADAA's artists were based mostly at Chickenley Primary School. Within a framework of supervised reflective practice, all the artists worked with their host communities and explored similarities and differences in approaches to community-based arts in health.

The culmination of the exchange was when the four artists came together at an international arts and health conference in Fremantle, Western Australia, to share their learning, firstly in a reflection seminar with their mentors and then in a keynote presentation and open forum. The artists' feedback on the exchange indicated that despite working with very different people in very different environments, there was a realization by all that there were shared values in the work that provided a basis for ethical practice. All four artists aimed to develop meaningful connections with health population groups through arts and health processes at the grass roots level, and it was an opportunity to understand the significant characteristics of their practice.

Further annual exchanges are planned and will be more closely integrated into ongoing research programmes. The UK placements will be in the successor project to Chickenley at Knowleswood Primary on the Holme Wood estate in Bradford, West Yorkshire, continuing the Roots and Wings approach, and at Tilery Primary in Stockton-on-Tees, a rapidly developing project with a multicultural focus which has overlapped with the later years of work at Chickenley. The arts development at Tilery is envisaged as another long-term project to test a hypothesis that exploring the local history of a neighbourhood and its social and economic relations

outwards can build temporal, or vertical, community connectedness. This will complement how, through an annual lantern parade, the building of a local cultural tradition can formulate and promote through narratives a spatial, or horizontal, community connectedness. This next phase of our research-guided practice draws on a range of art forms and interventions to connect the history of the area, of indigenous families and of newcomers.

## The Tilery lanterns project

Tilery Primary is the latest addition to a cluster of schools-based arts in heath programmes in areas of social disadvantage in northern England that CMH has assisted and/or investigated. The school's roll is drawn from the St Ann's and Portrack estates which in the last decade have seen a significant increase in the number of refugees and asylum seekers. The headteacher, John Repton, estimates there are now over 20 languages spoken on the local estates, and the growing ethnic diversity is both reflected and addressed in the school. Historically, there has been some hostility between the two estates, and those tensions have been further raised by the influx of 'newcomers' perceived as having arrived from afar as either migrant workers from eastern Europe or refugees from sub-Saharan Africa, the Middle East, and Sri Lanka. The common ground between the communities on the estates, however, is literally a footpath across a strip of common land that connects St Ann's to Portrack, and over which a now-annual lantern parade passes in both directions each year, giving the participants the opportunity to view the full span of the procession before it weaves through each estate. From the comments of participants, this seems to provide a potent image of a joined together community that resonates long after the event.

The Tilery project began in October 2008 when a group of school staff and parents attended a well-established annual lanterns parade at Southwick School in Sunderland. That parade is another project that CMH has been involved with for over 10 years and the neighbourly connection that was developed between Southwick and Tilery shows how arts in health projects,

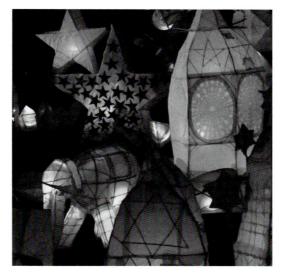

**Fig. 6.2** Tilery lanterns.
Reproduced by kind permission of M. Robson. Copyright © 2015 M. Robson.

and the participating communities, can motivate and influence one another. A group of Southwick parents and staff made a gift of a special star-shaped lantern to lead the first Tilery procession in the hope it would provide a tangible and powerfully symbolic message of passing on community knowledge. The first Tilery lanterns event took place in March 2009, and the annual parades since then have seen an exponential growth in participants and spectators and firmly established the event as an annual 'tradition' (Fig. 6.2).

Due to the proximity of Tilery Primary to Durham University's Stockton campus, it has been possible to draw in the support of the School of Medicine through the regular placement of medical students in Tilery to develop their understanding of community health and primary care in a region of England with the worst population health profile. The students usually take part in the lantern-making, and are taught how to do it by the children. Other regular contributors to the event include staff from the local library, from the supermarket and local radio station, and from most of the voluntary agencies that work in the area. The event becomes a means of gathering and displaying the community's assets within a health promotion model. As the headteacher John Repton observed in an interview in 2012:

'I wanted our school to make a difference in our community and improve wellbeing in an area with a poor health profile. I always felt intervention would need to be long-term, aiming to reach the 'softer' bits that connect to the kids' feelings. The arts channel emotional responses to situations. They are a vehicle to promote equality, whatever race or background. There's something special about this event for the community. It has rejuvenated it and it's welcomed by different generations. Many children say 'this is the best day of my life'. We want to transform the school for the development of learning by all the family. The university could help us to become more reflective.'

Crucial to the success of the event each year is the atmosphere generated in the lanterns workshop space. At the 2012 Tilery lantern workshops some semi-structured interviews were conducted with a small group of parent volunteers and staff, revealing that the most valued outcomes of the parades were that they assisted remembrances, empathic insight, capacity building, and improvements in mental and emotional health.

On the subject of remembrances, and specifically the large star lantern which has been transformed into an armature on which to record lost or absent relatives, one volunteer said:

'I liked the Remembrance Star we made this year for who's here and who's not. The idea came naturally from us.'

Another reported:

'I took our lanterns to the cemetery for a memory thing for the kids. It's important and that's why we've got more remembrances this year. It's not just sticks and paper, there's deep meanings.'

Members of a focus group that was convened to review the 2012 procession also commented that:

'The Star of Remembrance worked well. The commemoration made it all the more challenging to do it right. We were surprised by how many remembrances there were. We want to continue this. The community reflects on what has happened and children respond well to it. People were putting poems and their own writing on the stars. Kids connect the light with the remembrance, as though it were enabling the dead person to 'see' the event. There aren't usually opportunities in community and cultural life to do this.'

As regards the empathic insight developed through the event, one volunteer said:

'It's about bringing the community together and seeing it. I feel safer because I know people. There was a feeling of strangeness about being with other races at first, but now I'm fascinated by other cultures and the opportunity to be involved through the school. Lanterns show people as they really are and you get an insight into their lives.'

Another added:

'It's good to meet all these new people too and have more conversation at the school gates. You get different impressions of people from a lantern workshop and you change your opinion of them.'

Arising from the growing perception of a connected community created through the event there is a keenness to share the experience with others, establish a network hub for community development, and build capacity. As one volunteer noted:

'We need to keep addressing multicultural issues and get more of other cultures into the workshops. We should go to other communities and the campus and involve other schools and make it bigger as a town event.'

The school's community liaison worker said:

'I want to see us pass this tradition to somewhere else. We shouldn't keep it to ourselves. Lantern 'twinning' would be great. It would be fabulous to link with a community in another part of the world, for example.'

The impact on mental and emotional health was expressed by one volunteer as follows:

'When you get your child with you making something, you have a different kind of conversation and make a bond. There's no stress and it's good for your health. You can spend time with your child and not worry, you're both engaged and it eases the burden on yourself. All in all you're in a better mood. It helps you to understand and deal with your feelings. It gives you time to reflect and get your worries out and not take them home. I can be easier on myself.'

Together these comments suggest that staff and parent volunteers at Tilery have come to see the event as providing a space for transformation with a guiding ethos that is most clearly articulated in the lantern workshops. At the heart of the workshops is the making of the candle-lit lanterns, from willow sticks, masking tape, tissue paper and glue. Most lanterns are small and house-shaped, to represent home and community. Makers frequently include a star shape somewhere in their lantern as a common connecting image. Staff and volunteers from local organizations and teams of Year 6 pupils make large lanterns. As CMH's artist Mary Robson has observed:

'There is now significant expertise in lantern making in the community. Some Tilery residents have become proficient makers and construct complex sculptural lanterns that demand a lot of commitment and a whole range of decisions in their making. Participants work together to consciously create a shared history. There is a purposeful, collaborative atmosphere that builds in the last couple of days. The shaping of a communal memory of the lanterns event appears crucial to the solidarity that sustains the repetition of the event in the social calendar.'

White and Robson (2015)

Through a wider programme of work entitled 'The Tilery Chronicles' the project now aims to build on the momentum of recent activities and introduce new ones, looking particularly at how nurtured conversation around these activities may generate communal memories and shared meanings, interpreted across the diversity of the community. It will support the intergenerational collection of personal stories and communal journals, create 'suitcase stories' for children in transition from primary to secondary school, support family events in the school, and build historical aspects into the community's awareness of its changing identity.

## Next steps and lessons learned

The inspiration and content of The Tilery Chronicles is to be drawn from the local history of the area and from the heritage of local people and their widely differing cultural backgrounds. We aim to provoke new and alternative narratives of a socially included self within a more connected neighbourhood and community through sharing the individual and collective experiences of a cultural event and by assisting the rediscovery of personal, intergenerational, and neighbourhood histories. As a case study, Tilery affords a highly innovative approach to contemporary place-shaping through building connected communities in which health and wellbeing can thrive. The relationships between individual and collective narratives, social connectedness, and individual and collective health and wellbeing are highly complex but are possibly amenable to interpretation, with permission of the participants, through the nuanced detail and depth of ethnographic research. Thus to elaborate the pathways through which creative and collective arts projects enable the renegotiation of narratives and the role of such narratives in social connectedness, health, and wellbeing, we are documenting the processes of project implementation and the historical and current everyday life of the area.

The key lesson that we take from Chickenley and now apply to Tilery is that although individual arts in community health projects may eventually come to an end there is rarely a final outcome from this relationship-based way of working because it is always ongoing. This is why the narrative of a project becomes so important because, as the 'new public health' pioneer Michael Wilson asserted (Wilson 1975, p. 61), health requires 'the languages of story, myth and poetry [to] also disclose its truth'. The development of projects like those described here is informed by the individual and collective narratives of the participants and their perception of producing new traditions for their community through the event.

Commitment to a long-term relationship with a community-based arts in health project means that both the quantity and quality of documentation and dissemination is improved. Such work lends itself readily to interdisciplinary analysis as well as generating a richly detailed evocation of the process of the work, so that participants' tales become vital testimony. As the World Health Organization (2008, p. 33) has observed, 'evidence is only one part of what swings policy decisions—political will and institutional capacity are important too. But more than simply academic exercises, research is needed to generate new understanding in practical, accessible ways, recognising and utilising a range of types of evidence, and recognising the added value of globally expanded Knowledge Networks and communities.'

Effective health promotion is more than addressing topical health issues and priorities, but rather it is also about issues of identity, meaning and place. These are essential issues in arts in community health, and the development of this field is now poised to provide concrete examples in both practice and research of what those 'globally expanded Knowledge Networks and communities' might look like.

## References

Artworks ABC Radio. *Art and Alzheimers*. ABC Radio, Canberra, audio recording 15 November 2009. Available at: <http://www.abc.net.au/radionational/programs/artworks/art-and-alzheimers/3086220> (accessed 8 August 2013).

Ashton, J. and Seymour, H. (1988). *The New Public Health*. Milton Keynes: Open University.

Atkinson, S. and Robson, M. (2012). Arts and health as a practice of liminality: managing the spaces of transformation for social and emotional wellbeing with primary school children. *Health & Place*, **8**, 1348–1355.

Clift, S., Camic, P.M., and Daykin, N. (2010) The arts and global health inequities. *Arts & Health: An International Journal for Research, Policy and Practice*, **2**, 3–7.

Department for Education and Skills (2005). *Every Child Matters: An Overview of Cross-Government Guidance*. London: DfES.

Emerson, R.W. (2001) *Journals of Ralph Waldo Emerson, 1820–1824*. Bridgewater, NJ: Replica Books.

Finnegan, L. and Robson, R. (2005). *Audio recording of the proceedings of the Children's Fund Conference at Dewsbury Minster on 9 November 2005*. Durham: Centre for Medical Humanities.

Independent (2009). Arts and minds at the Tate. *The Independent*, 10 May 2009. Available at: <http://www.independent.co.uk/.../news/arts-and-minds-at-the-tate-1682307.html> (accessed 8 August 2013).

Lancet (2011). National healthy schools programme. *The Lancet UK Policy Matters*, 6 May 2011. Available at <http://ukpolicymatters.thelancet.com/policy-summary-national-healthy-schools-programme/> (accessed 30 October 2013).

Loca (2009). '*Inside Me' Evaluation Report April 2008 to March 2009*. Dewsbury: Loca.

Marmot, M. (2004). *Status Syndrome: How Your Social Standing Directly Affects Your Health and Life Expectancy*. London: Bloomsbury.

Marmot Review (2010). *Fair Society, Health Lives. Strategic Review of Inequalities in Health England Post-2010*. Chair: Sir Michael Marmot. London: University College London.

Ni Leime, A. and O'Shea, E. (2008). *The Bealtaine Festival: An Evaluation*. Dublin: Age & Opportunity.

Ofsted (2006). Chickenley Community Junior Infant and Nursery School. Ofsted Inspection 282150, Kirklees Education Authority, Huddersfield. Available at: <http://www.chickenleycommunityschool.com/kgfl/primary/chickenleypri/arenas/websitecommunity/web/ofstedreportmay2006.pdf> (accessed 7 August 2013).

Perry, B. (2008). *Curiosity: The Fuel of Development*. Available at: <http//www.teacher.scholastic.com/professional/bruceperry/curiosity.htm> (accessed 7 August 2013).

Raw, A. (2006). *Chickenley Creative Kids Project: Independent Evaluation For Year 3*. Dewsbury: The Children's Fund.

Rogers, C. (1959). A theory of therapy, personality and interpersonal relationships as developed in the client-centered framework. In: Koch, S. (ed.), *Psychology: A Study of a Science. Vol. 3: Formulations of the Person and the Social Context*, pp. 184–256. New York: McGraw Hill.

Rosenberg, F. (2009). The MOMA Alzheimer's project: programming and resources for making art accessible to people with Alzheimer's disease and their caregivers. *Arts & Health: An International Journal for Research, Policy and Practice*, **1**, 93–97.

Seedhouse, D. (2001). *Health: The Foundations For Achievement*, 2nd edn. Chichester: Wiley and Sons.

Sing Up (2012). *Synthesis Report*. Available at: <http://www.singup.org/fileadmin/singupfiles/previous_uploads/Sing_Up_Evaluation_synthesis_report.pdf> (accessed 8 August 2013).

University of Cambridge Education Department (2012). *The Impact of Creative Partnerships on the Wellbeing of Children and Young People*. London: Creative Partnerships.

White, M. (2009). *Arts Development in Community Health: A Social Tonic*. Oxford: Radcliffe.

White, M. (2010). Developing guidelines for good practice in participatory arts-in-health-care contexts. *Journal of Applied Arts and Health*, **1**, 139–155.

White, M. and Robson, R. (2011). Finding sustainability: university-community collaborations focused on arts in health. *Gateways International Journal of Community Research and Engagement*, **4**, 48–64.

White, M. and Robson, R. (2015). Lantern parades in the development of arts in community health. *Medical Humanities*, **36**, 59–69.

Wilson, M. (1975). *Health is For People*. London: Darton, Longman and Todd.

World Health Organization (2008). *Closing the Gap in a Generation: Health Equity Through Action on the Social Determinants Of Health*. Geneva: World Health Organization.

Worthy, A. (2005). *Supporting Children and Young People Through Transition*. London: National Children's Bureau.

# CHAPTER 7

# Community cultural development for health and wellbeing

## Paul M. Camic

## Introduction to community cultural development

Community cultural development (CCD) is a broad-based term to describe the philosophy, practices, intentions, and outcomes of community-based cultural and artistic practices. Within the context of public health and healthcare, the aim of CCD is to improve the health and wellbeing of those individuals who participate in such activities but also to benefit, perhaps more indirectly, those who live or work in—or even visit—a particular community (Minkler 1999). It is also important to consider that CCD is not only an 'intervention' but also 'a phenomenon that communities engage in, at various levels of intensity, as an ordinary part of being, or becoming, communities' (Hawkes 2003, p. 1).

Hence, CCD can be seen as a formally organized plan for intervention as part of government policy, such as the 'colourful condom' campaign seen on London Transport in the 1970s to reduce unplanned pregnancies and sexually transmitted infections, but also as a part of everyday life in a community that is not policy or intervention driven but developed from local interests and needs, such as the annual village art fair or a town's music festival.

Community cultural development has also been described as 'the work of artist-organizers and other community members collaborating to express identity, concerns and aspirations through the arts and communication media. It is a process that builds individual mastery and collective cultural capacity while contributing to positive social change' (Goldbard 2006, p. 20). Social change in the context of cultural development has meant a range of activities, such as increasing positive attitudes towards older people, helping to make a community more accessible for those with physical disabilities, bringing awareness to the problem of unemployed youth, and harnessing the creative capacity of children to help clean up a neighbourhood, to give just a few examples. The programmes discussed in this chapter focus on arts-based contexts, which draw on a diversity of cultural development initiatives related to public health planning, policy, and intervention at international, national, and local levels.

The colourful condom campaign involved artists' depictions on bus and train posters of different coloured condoms looking happy and friendly while dancing condoms greeted people on Friday and Saturday nights in various locations across the city. The campaign sought not to moralize or warn about the dangers of unprotected sex but to encourage people to laugh and talk about and ultimately use aesthetically interesting protective devices. On a smaller scale, local art fairs and other cultural events can be enjoyable in and of themselves but they can also seek to raise support for health-related charities by bringing awareness of public health issues while also creating opportunities for social engagement and encouraging the use of cultural activities to develop local communities. Fringe festivals, for example, have been gaining popularity worldwide in a variety of communities from small villages to large cities like Edinburgh as a way for local inhabitants to create on-going cultural events that reflect the cultural creativity of a local area (see the World Festival Network, <http://www.worldfestivalnet.com/>). These home-grown creative activities are rarely policy or evidence driven, yet they are often very successful in bringing a community together for a set period of time to participate in socially and culturally enjoyable activities (Fig. 7.1).

Adams and Goldbard (2001) in their well-received *Creative Community* report for the US-based Rockefeller Foundation, advanced the term 'community cultural development' for community-engaged cultural practice, describing this type of practice as a cultural response to social conditions that transcends ethnicity, socio-economic status, gender, and age. As an example of local CCD practice, Yung (2007) received federal funding to work with low-income immigrant Korean and Japanese older adults in Seattle, communities that have often had longstanding historical animosity towards each other. She describes CCD as an approach that can help to loosen cultural entrenchments and act as bridge between and within communities. In particular, Yung sees community-based cultural development as a way to use art as an essential asset and as a connection between arts practice, practitioners, and community members.

## Community + culture + development

*Community* can refer to a geographical location such as a neighbourhood, village, town, or city; a group of people with shared interests or values; but also, increasingly, to a virtual community based on shared interests, problems, or activities. The term also refers to a participatory process, which encourages collaboration between community members, artists, and others. One of the best and most comprehensive descriptions of *culture* that I have seen comes from Bill Flood (1998), then at the Oregon Arts

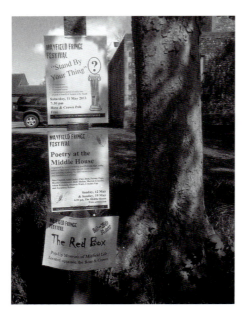

**Fig. 7.1**  Advertising the local village fringe festival.
Reproduced by kind permission of Paul Camic, Copyright © 2015 Paul Camic.

Commission in the United States: 'It gives us identity and meaning. It takes many forms, including how we adapt our natural environment; the institutions we create to express our social and political beliefs; the performing arts, visual arts, literature, crafts, and handwork; our history; and language and communication forms through which we express our beliefs. Culture is both what we create and the societal glue that holds us together—or tears us apart.'

Development, not unlike the terms community and culture, is likely to mean a range of things to different people and can include improving and enhancing the social, health, economic, policy, and commercial components (Todaro and Smith: 2011) of a given community. CCD is being practised when people in a community, often together with local organizations (e.g. arts, sports, and leisure organizations—including both popular culture and more traditionally considered cultural activities), are actively engaged in social action by building, enhancing, supporting, connecting, and enlivening their communities, through creativity, problem-solving and compassion (Flood 1998; Camic 2008). In the context of CCD, 'development suggests the dynamic nature of cultural action . . . including empowerment . . . and incorporating principles of self-development rather that development imposed from above' (Goldbard 2006, p. 22). CCD takes many forms and does not involve a unitary approach; depending on where you live in the world it may also be referred to by different names including community arts, participatory arts, community-based arts, cultural work, and participatory arts projects.

Historically, delivering public health promotion and prevention programmes has most often been undertaken at regional or national levels, yet many arts and health practitioners, artists, and researchers, with notable exceptions, have tended to target individuals or small groups and not community-wide populations (e.g. Clift et al. 2009; Sonke et al. 2009; Wreford 2010; Cox et al. 2010; Cuypers et al. 2011). CCD offers an opportunity to consider systemic 'interventions' such as changes in policy, enhancing the built environment, delivering new community cultural initiatives, and considering alternative management and funding models that affect a community's cultural experiences, all of which in turn have the possibility to impact on health and wellbeing.

One possible impediment, however, to cultural development, and particularly the arts within cultural development, is often the lack of well-formulated policy at national or regional levels. The California-based James Irvine Foundation (2006) has drawn attention to this deficit by highlighting that arts and cultural policy 'lack the essential policy arguments available to many other sectors, including: broad-based consensus over public value, acceptance of the legitimacy of public support due to market failures in making it broadly and equitably available, a solid causal model of the effects of investments, and standardized evaluative measures for measuring success' (James Irvine Foundation 2006, p. 12). Within many European and Asian countries further attention has been directed toward developing arts and cultural policy (e.g. the European Union (EU), Australia, China, and Japan) than has generally occurred in the United States, for example, at both federal and state levels. This is probably due to many factors including a closer shared understanding about the public value of culture that is often expressed across the political spectrum and the acceptance that the state has a role to play in fostering cultural value (Arts and Humanities Research Council 2013).

The remaining sections of this chapter will describe illustrative examples of international, national, and local CCD initiatives.

## International initiatives

### UNESCO Creative Cities

Launched in 2004, and involving cities from across the world, the UNESCO Creative Cities Network is a platform for partnership, for sharing experience, and for joint action in order to make the most of culture for empowerment, social inclusion, and sustainable development (UNESCO 2013) through both policy and programme activities. Although health and wellbeing aims are not explicitly stated, several aims of the network can be linked to local wellbeing agendas (UNESCO 2013, p. 1):

- Strengthen the creation, production, distribution, and enjoyment of cultural goods and services at the local level
- Promote creativity and creative expressions especially among vulnerable groups, including women and youth
- Enhance access to and participation in cultural life as well as enjoyment of cultural goods
- Integrate cultural and creative industries into local development plans

The Creative Cities Network has identified seven thematic areas and cities must choose only one theme to develop as part of their application: cinema, crafts and folk art, design, literature, media arts, music, and gastronomy. Each city is required to complete an annual self-evaluation report while they remain a member; reports are available from the Creative Cities Network website (<http://www.unesco.org/new/en/culture/themes/creativity/creative-cities-network/>) and offer a detailed explanation of activities and how they are evaluated, which in turn feeds into the overall evaluation process across all current and future city members. Member cities range from small to large, with new cities joining each year. A mentorship process is part of the network and has been developed to help cities work together in clusters to support and learn from each other and to promote international engagement.

## European Action Plan/World Health Organization (WHO)

The purpose of the European Action Plan, a regional international initiative, is to ensure that public health services continue to develop and evolve in order to respond to the public health challenges facing the WHO European Region at present and in the future (WHO 2012a). Together with Health 2020 (WHO 2012b), these two Europe-wide initiatives provide a policy framework and flexible action plan to address regional health and wellbeing issues. While neither initiative provides a template or roadmap for cultural involvement in health, they do provide opportunities for involvement of the community cultural sector in public health through two essential public health operations:

♦ tackling the social determinants of health and inequities in health experience (WHO 2012a, p. 3) and

♦ advocacy, communication, and social mobilization for health (WHO 2012a, p. 21)

Addressing these issues through a community cultural development approach would involve transcending well-established professional and sectoral boundaries. Doing so, however, would allow public health and healthcare agencies to engage with local and regional cultural organizations with the aim of broadening social inclusion and enhancing communication (European Commission 2005; Alcock et al. 2011) and addressing specific healthcare problems through community-based initiatives (e.g. Angus 2002; Nyonator et al. 2005; Camic and Chatterjee 2013). This possibility was reinforced by the European Commission's 7-year approval of funding for Creative Europe (European Commission 2013), a new programme which seeks to enhance creative development and cross-border cultural engagement across the EU. One such result of Europe-wide cultural development has been 'One Land, Many Faces', an EU-sponsored programme that seeks to explore European identity through commissioning visual and performing artists across Europe to address various components of what it means to be European. Issues such as displacement, loss, isolation, connectedness, separation, and cohesion, which are also public health concerns, are some of the experiences being addressed.

While not necessarily an easy or straightforward task, the mechanisms and structures are beginning to be put in place within the EU for more linked up arts, public health, and wellbeing development.

## National programmes

### Cultural Development Network/Australia

Based in Melbourne, the Cultural Development Network (CDN) is a unique organization in several ways. It is both independent and not-for-profit but also serves to link 'local government, communities, artists, researchers and related agencies [by] advocating for the importance of arts and cultural expression in the development of creative, healthy, engaged and sustainable communities' (Cultural Development Network 2013). In addition, the network supports local government and local communities by providing

evidence-based resources virtually and through conferences, workshops, and publications. They are managed through a voluntary board that includes representation from local government, academia, cultural organizations, and the community.

A sample of CDN projects includes:

1. A research project that examined how participation can be increased at cultural events for both audience members and artists who have physical disabilities, with recommendations being made for both government and the cultural community for ways to widen access.

2. The 'HomeLands' project, which worked with young people from refugee backgrounds to help them develop a positive cultural identity as settlers in a new country. Supporting young people to develop audiovisual materials that they shared over the Internet with local and overseas friends and family, the project allowed participants to experiment with different forms of expression by producing short films, recording music videos, and writing lyrics to new songs.

3. The 'Generations' project, which sought to build civic engagement through the arts in five communities across Australia by assessing how community art practices can enrich the practice of local government (see Mulligan and Smith 2010). This extensive project sought to answer the following research questions: how to increase the strategic importance of community art; how are partnerships built and sustained; and what are the best ways to engage community members? The results from this 3-year project are relevant to many communities around the world seeking to engage in community cultural development.

Mulligan and Smith's report provides evidence of good practice for 'socially engaged art' (Mulligan and Smith 2010, p. 108) that is well documented and links local government practice to community art practice across a range of different communities.

### Animating Democracy

Animating Democracy is a programme sponsored by Americans for the Arts, a national not-for-profit US-based organization. It seeks to 'cultivate a landscape for positive social change' by inspiring, promoting, informing, and connecting 'arts and culture as potent contributors to community, civic and social change' (Animating Democracy 2013). Its website (<http://animatingdemocracy.org/>)is a treasure trove of resources, available to anyone who registers, and includes valuable information about the arts and social change, planning projects, obtaining funding, measuring impact, collaborating with others, and disseminating results. The website provides links to many current and previous projects, one for example, is a virtual community project, '100 Faces of War Experience: Portraits and Words of Americans who Served in Iraq and Afghanistan' (<http://www.100facesofwarexperience.org/>) that gives us a glimpse into the lives of 100 servicemen and -women through their painted portraits, poems, stories, and diaries. The project provides a voice for 'people who have gone from America into these wars or posthumously by their families', who are rarely seen or heard.

Another project example is 'A Day at Stateville' developed by the Illinois Institute for Community Law and Affairs, which is a play detailing a newcomer's first day at Stateville

Correctional Facility in Joliet, Illinois (<http://illinoisinstitute.net/idea-exchange/a-day-at-stateville/>). The play was developed and written by inmates, all of whom are serving life sentences without parole. These inmates sought to inform members of the community about the importance of helping to support at-risk youth in order to reduce their chances of entering prison. Inmates had taken the prison's course on transformation and communication, which inspired them to write and perform the play. The play continues to be performed in the Chicago area by former prisoners in the form of a theatrical reading (see the Animating Democracy website for additional information: http://animatingdemocracy.org/).

This project has implications for prisons across the United States as well as the rest of the world through its involvement of people who have no parole options and those who have been released from prison as a way to help young people at high risk but who are not yet in the prison system. Taken within a public health context, this can be seen as both a health promotion and a violence prevention initiative, which allows those convicted of serious crimes to give back something positive and help to support others.

### ArtPlace America

In 2011 an unprecedented, large-scale private–public collaboration was announced bringing together 11 of the United States' leading philanthropic foundations together with the federal government's National Endowment for the Arts and seven other federal agencies to establish ArtPlace, a national initiative to drive revitalization in cities and towns with a new investment model that put the arts at the centre of economic development (see <http://www.artplaceamerica.org/>). Although not specifically identified as a public health programme, the implications of improving economic development in areas needing revitalization have a direct relationship to important public health goals such as reducing unemployment, providing opportunities for enhancing social cohesion, and increasing social inclusion. The ArtPlace initiative seeks to use the arts as vital economic drivers to help improve the wellbeing of local communities following an economic model that supports public–private partnership development to shape social, physical, and economic futures (Landesman 2011). The approach underlying the development of ArtPlace is that of 'creative placemaking' (Markusen and Gadwa 2010), an evolving field of practice, initially developed in the 1980s

> 'that intentionally leverages the power of the arts, culture and creativity to serve a community's interest while driving a broader agenda for change, growth and transformation in a way that also builds character and quality of place.'
>
> ArtScape Toronto (2014)

A strength of ArtPlace is the extensive support it has received across several US federal agencies and its close partnership links to private organizations and companies, thus forming for the first time in the United States a mechanism for active involvement of the national government and private sector in CCD. Rather than depending solely on state resources, which have a host of limitations including political concerns, restricted financial support, and lack of a climate of entrepreneurial development, a large-scale partnership with private companies provides additional financial capital, creative resources, and an environment that values experimentation and innovation.

## Local communities: large and small

### European Capitals of Culture

Although the yearly European Capitals of Culture cites are designated and supported by European Commission funding, the events themselves and the cultural development resulting from these events are decidedly local. Since the programme began in 1985, dozens of cities have been awarded this coveted title, with commissioned research indicating significant cultural development and economic benefits as two of the many results (Palmer et al. 2011). The process of developing an application to this scheme brings together various local government agencies, cultural organizations, artists, and community planners and encourages cities to think about their identity, cultural capital, links to other European cities, and their own cultural futures. A report on the experience of Liverpool as a European Capital of Culture in 2008 (Garcia et al. 2010) cited the significant economic gain to the local economy through tourism (£130 million), the inclusivity of cultural access and participation, enhanced cultural vibrancy and sustainability, and a change in media image and perceptions as the major impacts.

### The local village fête

Scaling down a notch or two from nationally and internationally funded cultural events, there is probably nothing as quintessentially small town and local than the annual village fête, county fair, autumn festival, or travelling carnival (Fig. 7.2). Occurring in many countries across the globe, these annual, local events bring people together through planning and organizing, fundraising, advertising, setting up stalls, selling goods, and probably best of all being collectively engaged in enjoyable, socially inclusive activities, very often at low cost or without charge. Often overlooked

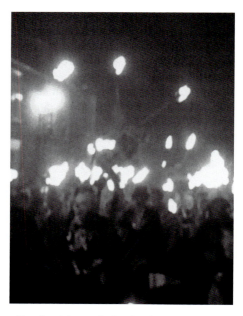

**Fig. 7.2** Annual bonfire night parade, Rye, East Sussex, UK.
Reproduced by kind permission of Paul Camic, Copyright © 2015 Paul Camic.

or possibly dismissed by government planners whose attentions are on large-scale urban cultural development, these local community cultural activities help to culturally enrich the villages and towns that host them. As Mulligan and Smith (2010) demonstrated in their study of five small Australian towns, CCD in small towns and rural communities can creatively engage people and help to build more inclusive societies, which enhances wellbeing and quality of life (European Commission 2011).

## Concluding comments

The brevity of this chapter has meant that only a glimpse of community cultural development and its possible links to health and wellbeing from a public health perspective could be presented. These links are not always straightforward and may require a great deal of negotiating and planning, as was the case for the projects described in this chapter. Like many public health programmes, the focus of community-based cultural development, within a culture and health framework (Camic and Chatterjee 2013), seeks to foster attention on populations or communities rather than on individuals. This approach to health promotion and illness prevention initiatives has the possibility of engaging an ever-widening audience through evocative, stimulating, enjoyable, and participatory cultural activities.

## References

Adams, D. and Goldbard, A. (2001). *Creative Community: The Art of Cultural Development*. New York: Rockefeller Foundation.

Alcock, C., Camic, P.M., Barker, C., Haridi, C., and Raven, R. (2011). Intergenerational practice in the community: an applied ethnographic evaluation. *Journal of Community and Applied Social Psychology*, **21**, 419–432.

Angus, J. (2002). *A Review of Evaluation in Community-based Arts and Health Activity in the UK*. London: Health Development Agency.

Animating Democracy (2013). *A program of Americans for the Arts*. Available at: <http://animatingdemocracy.org/

Arts and Humanities Research Council (2013). *Cultural Value Project*. Available at: <http://www.ahrc.ac.uk/funded-research/funded-themes-and-programmes/cultural-value-project/pages/default.aspx>

ArtScape Toronto (2014). *DIY Creative Placemaking*. Available at: http://www.artscapediy.org/creative-placemaking/approaches-to-creative-placemaking.aspx>

Camic, P.M. (2008). Playing in the mud: health psychology, the arts, and creative approaches to health care. *Journal of Health Psychology*, **13**, 287–298.

Camic, P.M. and Chatterjee, H.J. (2013). Museums and art galleries as partners in public health interventions. *Perspectives in Public Health*, **133**, 66–73.

Clift, S., Camic, P.M., Chapman, B., et al. (2009). The state of arts and health in England. *Arts & Health: An International Journal of Research, Policy and Practice*, **1**, 6–35.

Cox, S., Lafrenière, D., Brett-MacLean, P., et al. (2010). Tipping the iceberg? The state of arts and health in Canada. *Arts & Health: An International Journal for Research, Policy and Practice*, **2**, 109–124.

Cultural Development Network (2013). *Cultural Development Network*. URL: <http://www.culturaldevelopment.net.au/>

Cuypers, K.F., Knudtsen, M.S., Sandgren, M., Krokstad, S., Wikström, B.M., and Theorell, T. (2011). Cultural activities and public health: research in Norway and Sweden. *Arts & Health: An International Journal for Research, Policy and Practice*, **3**, 6–26.

European Commission (2005). *The Role of Culture in Preventing and Reducing Poverty and Social Exclusion*. Available at: <http://ec.europa.eu/employment_social/social_inclusion/docs/studyculture_leaflet_en.pdf>

European Commission (2011). *Mental Wellbeing for a Smart, Sustainable and Inclusive Europe*. Available at: <http://ec.europa.eu/health/mental_health/docs/outcomes_pact_en.pdf>

European Commission (2013). *Creative Europe: Support Programme for Europe's Cultural and Creative Sectors from 2014*. Available at: http://ec.europa.eu/culture/creative-europe/index_en.htm)

Flood, B. (1998). What is community cultural development and how do we practice it? *Culture Work*, **2**(4). Available at: <http://pages.uoregon.edu/culturwk/culturework7.html>

Garcia, B., Melville, R., and Cox, T. (2010). *Creating an Impact: Liverpool's Experience a European Capital of Culture*. Liverpool: University of Liverpool. Available at: <http://www.liv.ac.uk/impacts08/>

Goldbard, A. (2006). *New Creative Community: The Art of Cultural Development*. Oakland, CA: New Village Press.

Hawkes, J. (2003). Community cultural development according to Adams & Goldbard, *Artworks*, 56, 1–7.

James Irvine Foundation (2006). *Critical Issues Facing the Arts in California*. San Francisco: James Irvine Foundation.

Landesman, R. (2011). A powerful new collaboration of foundations and federal agencies puts arts at the center of the revitalization of cities and towns across the U.S. *The Rockefeller Foundation News & Media*. Available at: <http://www.rockefeller foundation.org/newsroom/powerful-new-collaboration-foundations>

Markusen, A. and Gadwa, A. (2010). *Creative Placemaking*. Washington, DC: National Endowment for the Arts.

Minkler, M. (1999). *Community Organizing and Community Building for Health*. New Brunswick, NJ: Rutgers University Press.

Mulligan, M. and Smith, P. (2010). *Art, Governance and the Turn to Community: Putting Art at the Heart of Local Government*. Melbourne: Globalism Research Centre, RMIT University.

Nyonator, F.K., Awoonor-Williams, J.K., Phillips, J.F., Jones, T.C., and Miller, R.A. (2005). The Ghana community-based health and planning services initiative for scaling up service delivery innovation. *Health Policy and Planning*, **20**, 25–34.

Palmer, R., Richards, G., and Dodd, D. (2011). *European Cultural Capital Report 3*. Arnhem: Atlas.

Sonke, J., Rollins, J., Brandman, R., and Graham-Pole, J. (2009). The state of the arts in healthcare in the United States. *Arts & Health: An International Journal for Research, Policy and Practice*, **1**, 107–135.

Todaro, M. and Smith, S.C. (2011). *Economic Development*, 11th edn. Boston, MA: Pearson Education.

UNESCO (2013). *Creative Cities Network: Applicant's Handbook*. Paris: UNESCO.

WHO (2012a). *European Action Plan for Strengthening Public Health Capacities and Services*. Copenhagen: WHO Regional Office for Europe.

WHO (2012b). *Health 2020: A European Policy Framework and Strategy for the 21st Century*. Copenhagen: WHO Regional Office for Europe.

Wreford, G. (2010). The state of the arts and health in Australia. *Arts & Health: An International Journal for Research, Policy and Practice*, **2**, 8–22.

Yung, R. (2007). Community cultural development: the next generation. *GIA Reader*, **18**(1). Available at: <http://www.giarts.org/article/community-cultural-development>

# CHAPTER 8

# Epidemiological studies of the relationship between cultural experiences and public health

Töres Theorell and Fredrik Ullén

## Issues and concepts

Cultural participation can be defined in several ways: in the present chapter it is defined as participation in any cultural activity—music, dance, theatre, painting, drawing, sculpture, photography, or writing. The authors, however, make no judgement with regard to genre. For instance, classical music is not considered to be more relevant than folk music or heavy metal and ballet no more relevant than jazz dance or folk dance. Although there is a clear difference between active participation (e.g. performing music, playing theatre roles, making photographs) and passive consumption of culture (e.g. reading, going to concerts or exhibitions) we will discuss both kinds of participation—the borderline between them is not so clear as one might think!

Participation in cultural activities such as those mentioned shows enormous variation between different national populations around the world and also varies strongly between different areas and different groups within populations. Therefore, participation in cultural activities has often been analysed within a broader context, as part of social capital and social networks. From that perspective cultural participation could include participation in sports clubs, unions, and social networks in general. We do not intend to cover these broad topics, although it is sometimes impossible to define a border between participation in cultural activities and wider social participation.

Clift et al. (2012) have discussed various kinds of evidence in the field of culture and health science, emphasizing that there is a hierarchy of evidence. The studies that are based upon observations in populations provide necessary evidence of relevance for policy makers, but controlled intervention studies occupy a higher position in the hierarchy since they may provide evidence not only showing 'what works' but also 'what does not work'. In epidemiology it is possible to combine these approaches, but so far there have been very few such studies.

Do cultural activities such as singing, playing a musical instrument, writing poetry, or going to the theatre somehow influence standard epidemiological outcome measures such as longevity, mortality, or morbidity? To start with we will discuss conceptual issues from different disciplinary perspectives.

## The evolutionary perspective

Music, dance, and painting could be regarded as 'social tools' that may have been used throughout the history of humankind in order to fulfil functions that have been proposed to be of survival value, for example increasing group cohesion. On the basis of findings of flutes made from bones in remnants from Neanderthals who may have lived 200,000 years ago, Mithen (2005) has speculated that these people were performing music and perhaps dancing. Paintings on cave walls estimated to be between 10,000 and 30,000 years old (for instance in Altamira, Chauvet, and Lascaut) indicate that painting has been important for a very long time in human history. There is a long-running scientific debate regarding the role of art in early human history. Some authors (e.g. Lewis-Williams 2002) argue that the cave paintings indicate that modern humans had arrived and that the Neanderthals were unable to produce that kind of art. Aiken (1998) has emphasized that early on art became a powerful tool for social and political manipulation. It became 'conditional to fear leaders, nations, gods and ideas'. Dissanayake (1988) has discussed culture as behaviour as well as the fact that science has a difficulty when it approaches the arts and similarly that the producers of art hesitate to accept scientific explanations of art. Benzon (2001) believes that music evolved as a means of 'brain coupling', i.e. a technique to increase the likelihood of cooperation between individuals. Promotion of musical communication may have been enhanced due to evolutionary pressures when human beings were living in small groups in a threatening environment. It was necessary to create tight groups, the members of which would help one another in crisis situations, for instance at night when one of several members had to stay awake and promise to wake the group when dangers were approaching. This may even have been important to evolution in a Darwinian sense: those who were unable to relate to dance and music may have had poorer survival chances than others. An illustration of this—albeit speculative—is that only 4% of normal populations could be regarded as 'tone deaf' (Peretz et al. 2007). Tone deafness means a consistent inability to differentiate the high note from the low note when notes are played randomly in pairs.

### Adverse effects of cultural activities

It must be kept in mind that not all stereotypical concomitants of cultural behaviours are unequivocally deemed to be 'good' or 'healthy' practices. On the contrary, for example, histories of some styles of music, poetry, and theatre in western cultures seem associated with the use of narcotic drugs, cigarette smoking, and other health-damaging behaviours. Such concomitant practices may create adverse relationships between some types of music experiences and public health (e.g. Bellis et al. 2007; Zhao et al. 2010).

One word of caution: participants in most choirs or dance groups will stop participating when they develop illnesses that interfere with their participation, such as lung, voice, and muscle disorders, as well as illnesses that reduce energy, such as psychiatric, cardiovascular, and metabolic disorders. Therefore, in cross-sectional studies, choir singers or people participating actively in folk dance groups may be healthier than the general population as a result of a 'healthy singer/dancer effect'. Therefore, other strategies including longitudinal assessments of musical interventions are mandatory to establish their effects on wellbeing and health.

## Cultural consumption in the general population

In some countries there is epidemiologically based information concerning the extent to which citizens participate in cultural activities. Sweden is a stable and relatively secularized society with a high level of education in the population. Statistics Sweden performed interviews about cultural activities (Survey of Living Conditions; Kulturrådet 2008) with randomly selected men and women (aged 16–74) from the general population. Statistics have been published showing the development of the prevalence of various cultural activities between 1976 and 2006 (with data from the years 1976, 1982–83, 1990–91, 1998–99, and 2006). In 2006 some interviews were performed by telephone whereas during the preceding waves all interviews had been face to face and this created some methodological difficulties; the differences between face to face and telephone interviews are small but in the few cases where there are differences we have presented the average. Taking some examples from the surveys these statistics (Kulturrådet 2008) show that:

◆ In 1976, 37% of Swedes had attended a concert or a theatre performance at least once during the past year. In 2006, the figure had increased to 65%; 6% had done so at least five times during the year preceding the interview in 1976 and in 2006 this had increased to 8%.

◆ In 1976, 51% had visited a museum (art or other) at least once during the past year. In 2006 this had increased to 53%. However, the corresponding percentages for visits to a museum at least five times during the past year had decreased from 12% in 1976 to 6% in 2006.

◆ In 1976, 44% had visited a library at least once during the past year. In 2006 the corresponding figure was 65%. Visits to a library at least five times during the past year were reported by 24 and 25% in 1976 and 2006, respectively;

◆ In 1976, 46% had been to the cinema at least once during the past year and in 2006 it was 66%. In 1976, 16% had visited the cinema at least five during the past year, and in 2006 15% had done so.

◆ In 1976, 77% reported that they had been reading a book at least once during the past year; the figure for 2006 was 79%. The corresponding percentages for having read a book at least five times during the past year were 39% (1976) and 38% (2006), respectively.

These numbers show that the consumption of fine arts is extensive in Swedish society. Some activities have increased. During the 20 years when these statistics were being produced the level of education of Swedes increased considerably and it was also a period of relative affluence. This development was interrupted in the first years of the 1990s, but the financial crisis with increased unemployment did not markedly influence the patterns of culture consumption.

Technological developments were dramatic during the period from 1976 to 2006. This has influenced patterns of cultural consumption in many ways. One of the modes of consumption that has not been included in the surveys performed by Statistics Sweden is listening to music by means of portable equipment. A recent study in Uppsala, Sweden (Västfjäll et al. 2012) showed that among students (aged 20–31) music listening took place on 37% of the randomly scattered occasions during their waking hours (over a period of 14 days) when a palmtop computer told them to report what they were doing. If this finding is representative of young adults in general it would mean that men and women in this age group in Sweden spend a third of their waking hours listening to music! This is probably much more than in previous generations. Similarly it could be argued that exposure to movies, video games, photos, and other kinds of visual culture has increased dramatically in our population due to technological advances.

There are also pronounced differences between the consumption of various kinds of culture in different socio-economic strata. From the Swedish surveys it is possible to calculate the ratio between the reported prevalence of various cultural activities in higher-level white collar workers and lower-level blue collar workers. For visits to theatre and concert performances (at least once a year) this ratio was 2.91 in 1976, decreasing progressively to 1.53 in 2006. This means that this type of cultural activity became less socio-economically divided during the 30 years' follow-up of the study. Visiting libraries followed a similar development, the corresponding ratio decreasing from 2.15 in 1976 to 1.32 in 2006. In 1976 going to the cinema was been approximately 50% more frequent among high-level white collar workers than among low-level blue collar workers. This has not changed during the 30 years of follow-up. Visits to museums have been consistently more frequent among high-level white collar workers than among low-level blue collar workers, the ratio varying between 2.09 and 2.26 with no time trend.

There are also other differences between subgroups in the population. In general women report a greater consumption of culture than men, at least with regard to going to the theatre or concerts, going to libraries, and reading books. In addition, the general pattern is that the consumption of culture decreases with increasing age.

### Active participation in arts and culture

Data regarding active participation (e.g. playing a musical instrument, dancing, performing theatre) from the Swedish surveys are available for a shorter period than the data regarding passive consumption, namely from 1982–83 until 2006. In addition this information is based upon a wider age range, 16–84.

In 1982–83, 17% of Swedes reported that they had played a music instrument during leisure at least once during the past year and 8% that they had played an instrument every week. In 2006 these numbers had decreased to 14% (at least once) and 6% (every week). The corresponding numbers for singing in a choir during leisure were between 5 and 6% (at least once) and around 4% (every week). There are opposing trends among the youngest and oldest in the population. Active music training has decreased between 1982–83 and 2006 in the youngest age group (16–19), from 33% at least once during the past year and 20% every week to 20% at least once and 11% every week, respectively. The corresponding percentage decrease in the prevalence of singing in a choir in this age group was 12% (once) and 9% (every week) to 10% (once) and 7% (every week). In contrast playing an instrument and singing in a choir have become more prevalent in the oldest age group (75–84). In general music training has been much more common in younger age groups and there is also a gender difference: whereas men more often play an instrument than women do, women more often sing in a choir.

Painting and drawing or making sculptures during leisure was reported by 18% (at least once during the past year) in 1990–91 (no data for 1980–81). This had decreased to 14% in 2006. This kind of activity was reportedly engaged in weekly by 5% with no obvious change during the observed period. Writing diaries, poetry, letters, and articles during leisure was an activity that was reported by 36% (once during the past year) in 1981–82. This had decreased to 29% in 2006. Between 11 and 13% reported that they had been doing this every week—with no change during the period studied. For both these activities, particularly for writing, there was a pronounced difference between men and women—women had much more activity than men. Painting and drawing were more frequent activities in young subjects than in old. An interesting phenomenon was observed with regard to writing: in 1981–82 this activity was much more common in the younger than in the older age groups. However, writing then decreased in the young and increased in older Swedes. This resulted in a reversed pattern in 2006, at least with regard to writing weekly—13% in the 16–19 age group and 23% in the 75–84 age group. There was a decreasing tendency among younger subjects with regard to both production of visual arts and in writing during the studied period.

A conclusion from these Swedish surveys is that there is a high level of consumption of culture and that the patterns are changing. In general, participation in active cultural production during leisure is much less common. In addition, for some of these activities there seems to be a downward trend in the youngest age group. This may be surprising in view of the fact that technology makes it easier to draw, to write, and to produce music. It could be described as a trend towards more passive consumption and less active production during leisure time.

Although the socio-economic differences have decreased during later years there are still clear differences between social groups, with more active and passive activities related to culture among high-level white collar workers than among low-level blue collar workers.

## Empirical population studies and findings

Epidemiological studies of the effects of cultural experiences on public health are rare, but there are some published studies of

relevance. For example, Hyyppä and Mäki (2001a) used longevity and disability-free life expectancy as dependent measures to compare two groups of people living on the north-eastern part of the Finnish Baltic coast. One group belonged to a minority speaking both Swedish and Finnish (Swedish speaking Ostro-Bothnians) and the other group spoke only Finnish. The authors observed that the former group had significantly higher values with regard to both longevity and disability-free life expectancy. Detailed examination revealed that neither genetics nor accepted risk factors were likely to explain this difference. However, 'social capital' independently and significantly differentiated the two language groups from one another. Social capital is related to a community's cohesiveness. In fact, the authors subsequently showed that factors to do with social capital were strongly related to self-rated health (Hyyppä and Mäki 2001b). These findings suggest that certain cultural activities, for instance singing in a choir, make a significant contribution to building social capital, which has direct implications for improved health and longevity.

Bygren et al. (1996) and later Konlaan et al. (2000) conducted a cohort study based upon 10,609 Swedish men and women aged 25–74. The participants were interviewed in 1982 and 1983 about their living conditions including attendance at cultural activities and health status. Participants were followed up with regard to survival (regardless of diagnosis at death) until the end of 1996. After adjustment for age, sex, financial security, education, long-term disease, smoking, and physical exercise at baseline, it was shown that there was a higher mortality risk for those people who rarely (less than once a week) visited the cinema, concerts, museums, or art exhibitions compared with those visiting them more often. Among the strengths of this study was the inclusion of a large, representative cohort, high compliance at baseline (75%), and perfect coverage in public registers, facilitating follow-up assessments. Moreover, several important health factors were controlled for in this study. For example, one of the adjustment factors was health at the start of the follow-up. This means that associations between cultural activities and lower health risks could not be explained by the fact that participants who were ill were also less likely to attend cultural activities—and also more prone to die early. In addition, the observed association remained stable even when variables related to individual socio-economic background were included in the analysis. Therefore, explanations other than socio-economic status are needed for why cultural participation may be advantageous for public health in general, and mortality risk in particular. A later study of a similar cohort (Bygren et al. 2009) of 9011 Swedish men and women showed that the beneficial effect on longevity was confined to cancer mortality.

In Finland, Väänänen et al. (2009) performed a similar study of 7922 industrial workers who were followed between 1986 and 2004. High cultural engagement was shown to be associated with age-specific all-cause mortality and external causes of death (e.g. suicide, accidents), even after adjustment for socio-demographic factors, socio-economic status, work stress, social characteristics, diabetes, and hypertension. In the Finnish study, activities other than those related to creative pursuits were added to the cultural activities, such as activity in associations, societal action, and studying.

A large cross-sectional Norwegian study (Cuypers et al. 2012) of 50,797 randomly selected citizens of Nord-Trøndelag examined the relationship between cultural activities—both receptive (consumption) and creative (performing)—and perceived health, anxiety, depression, and satisfaction with life. Analyses showed that participation in receptive and creative cultural activities was significantly associated with good health, good satisfaction with life, and low anxiety and depression scores in both genders. In men in particular, attending receptive, rather than creative, cultural activities was more strongly associated with all health-related outcomes. Statistically significant associations between several single receptive, creative cultural activities and health-related outcome variables were revealed. As in the Swedish and Finnish studies, all analyses were adjusted for possible confounders such as age, gender, education, and health. This study is the largest such detailed epidemiological study published so far. It should be cautioned, however, that the findings are cross-sectional. This means that some of the associations may be due to reverse causality: subjects who are healthy and have good social circumstances will be more active in general.

## Cultural participation and health across the life span

Community actions aimed at introducing or increasing cultural participation will have to use different methodologies in different age groups. A crude division of ages is between growing up, working age, and old age. These will be discussed separately.

### Growing up

Musical experiences differ in their significance for people of different ages and across different cultures. It has often been claimed that early musical training stimulates general cognitive development. There is certainly extensive cross-sectional data showing positive associations between musical training in childhood and performance on a wide range of both musical and non-musical tasks (for a recent review see Schellenberg and Weiss 2013). Such associations have been reported, for example, for various auditory discrimination tasks, including speech perception (Pantev and Herholz 2011; Schellenberg and Weiss 2013), verbal, auditory, and visual memory (Chan et al. 1998; Degé et al. 2011), vocabulary (Moreno et al. 2011), reading ability (Moreno et al. 2009; Degé and Schwartzer 2011), visuo-spatial abilities (Rauscher and Zupan 2000; Costa-Giomi et al. 2001), and general IQ (Schellenberg 2006). However, it appears likely that these associations, at least in part, are driven by selection effects, i.e. that the children who choose to engage actively in music and remain in training are supported in this by their family and tend to have higher cognitive abilities to begin with so perform well on non-musical tasks for that reason. More studies addressing possible causal effects of music would clearly be useful. Behavioural genetics studies can provide important information on genetic and non-genetic components of associations between musical activity and various outcomes in cross-sectional data. Longitudinal studies in which both psychological functions and brain development can be followed in comparable groups of children with/without early training would be informative, although randomized experimental designs would be ideal. Another issue to keep in mind is that voluntary musical training in the general population, which is typically what is studied in cross-sectional designs, and imposed and monitored training in randomized intervention studies, may differ fundamentally in various important ways. The former, but not the latter, is, for

example, presumably dependent on personality traits, motivation, and interests that in part have a genetic basis. Conceivably, voluntary and imposed training could also differ in their effects on outcome variables such as cognitive and emotional ability.

Two published studies (Costa-Giomi 1999; Schellenberg 2004) have shown effects of musical training on IQ in a randomized experimental design. They both started with 6-year-old children in ordinary living conditions. The children were randomized into a group with early music training and a group without such training and cognitive development was followed by means of standardized methods. Both studies showed that the children in the music training group did have a small but significant advantage in IQ development compared with the comparison group. In Costa-Giomi's study this advantage decreased as the follow-up continued. It thus appears possible that musical training can have small, positive causal effects on general cognition. One should also mention that another randomized experimental study only found a non-significant trend for a larger increase in IQ in a group that received musical training (6 months) than in a control group that received training in painting (Moreno et al. 2009). Limited statistical power may have been an issue in that study, since the studied sample was relatively small ($n = 32$).

A very recent study (Mehr et al. 2013) was based upon two randomized experiments with 4-year-old children, some of whom were randomly assigned to music sessions. The results were diverging with regard to the effects of music on cognitive ability. While the first smaller experiment showed significant results in favour of the non-music intervention the second experiment did not show any difference. However, it could be argued that both the experiments also had relatively small samples (23 and 22, respectively) and that the music intervention was of short duration (6 weeks). Such a short intervention period could certainly be insufficient for effects on cognition. One should finally consider the possibility that datasets with null effects have remained unpublished. Clearly, however, these are interesting and important clues to be followed up in future research. The development of cognitive functions in environments that stimulate learning during childhood has been shown, in epidemiological research, to be important to the health of adults (Power et al. 2006).

From the perspective of child development, helping children to progress intellectually through music lessons may be just one factor that could be relevant to long-term health. Development of social and emotional skills appears to be of no less importance. A famous and scientifically robust study—large enough and with study groups sufficiently representative of the population to be labelled epidemiological—to illustrate this point has been conducted by Spychiger and co-workers in Switzerland (Spychiger 2002). Fifty-two ordinary school classes distributed across Switzerland were randomly allocated to 'extra music' or 'no extra music' education with an equal number of classes and pupils in both groups. They were followed for 3 years with repeated observations regarding achievements and behaviour at school. The fact that the pupils in the music classes had slightly less time for language and mathematics was of particular importance in the evaluation. When the results were collated after 3 years it became evident that the children in the music group developed better social cohesiveness in the classroom than the controls. Moreover, students in both groups still performed similarly in language and mathematics assessments. This example suggests that in competitive environments such as schools, music can be a medium to enhance cooperation in children to counterbalance competitiveness (see also Chapter 35).

Lindblad et al. (2007) have illustrated a mechanism that could possibly underlie the effect of extra music lessons in the school environment in their small-scale study of fifth and sixth graders in a Stockholm school. Three comparable groups of children in these grades were assigned to 'music intervention', 'extra computer education', and 'ordinary curriculum' groups, respectively, with 17 children in each group. The music intervention was very similar to the one used by Spychiger and colleagues. The goal was to use enjoyable music exercises requiring collaboration of all children in the classroom to achieve increased cohesiveness and a calm social climate. These exercises lasted for an hour and took place once a week. The ultimate goal was to improve the learning environment—not only during the extra music lessons but during the school week as a whole. The children in the three groups were followed for a year with assessments at the start of the school year, at Christmas time, and just before the end of the school year in June. Salivary cortisol was measured on four occasions during the day but the most important occasion was 1 hour after lunch when the climate in the classroom tends to be at its worst. This afternoon salivary cortisol concentration decreased significantly in the music intervention group after a year but did not change in the other groups during the school year; this was possibly an illustration of a stress-reducing effect of the extra music intervention. This study was not conclusive due to its small size but may illustrate the potential cohesive power of added 'social' music exercises.

### Working age

People in full-time employment spend half of their waking hours at work. Work is considered an important arena for health promotion. Possible health effects of cultural activities in the workplace could arise because (1) such activities may strengthen cohesion between employees and between management and employees, resulting in an improved psychosocial environment or (2) because of direct effects of the cultural activities themselves. Our group (Theorell et al. 2013) followed 6214 randomly selected Swedes for 2 years between 2008 and 2010 with regard to depressive symptoms and emotional exhaustion, assessed by means of standardized questionnaires before and after follow-up. At the start of the project participants answered questions about cultural activities (movies, theatre performances, concerts, exhibitions) organized for employees during the year preceding the survey. They also answered questions regarding their working environment and their mental health. Half of the participants reported that no cultural activities had been organized by the workplace. Forty per cent reported that such activities had taken place at least once during the past year. Accordingly, cultural activities were uncommon. However, the findings indicated that the more cultural activity there had been in the workplace, the lower was the likelihood that the employees would experience worsened emotional exhaustion during follow-up.

In our population study of cultural activity at work a very superficial question about 'culture' was used. Of course different activities give rise to different effects. Some activities could even have adverse effects on health. Our group (Hartzell and Theorell 2007) performed a study of the immediate psychological effects of 'passive' attendance at cultural activities in a work situation during working hours. For these studies we used a visual analogue scale (VAS) for the assessment of 'tiredness/vitality' before and after the activity. Most of the participants were naïve with regard to participation in fine culture and represented lower as well as higher social classes. The county arranged for a 'culture producer' to come to the worksite and organize a performance once a week for 3 months. Producers could be theatre groups, music ensembles, art lotteries, and movie shows. Averages were calculated for each participant with regard to 'increase in vitality.'

The activities with the highest mean VAS change were activities with a high degree of interaction between the actors/musicians and the audience. The theatre performances used the audience as active parts in their plays. In the interactive music performances the listeners were clapping hands and moving with the music. At the opposite end, those who watched a movie in many cases became even more tired during the performance. Accordingly more 'active' experiences have stronger immediate effects on vitality. This does not mean, however, that the more interactive experiences are more effective in the longer term in promoting health than the more passive ones. This will be an important theme for future research.

In general, participants who had experienced the highest average increase in vitality and joy during the cultural activities were those who had had the most favourable development over time compared with other participants with regard to sleep disturbance and the biological stress marker plasma fibrinogen (Theorell et al. 2009). On the other hand it was also observed that these participants experienced worsened social support at work. This may be due to the fact that the participants only comprised a very small part of the total number of employees in these worksites. An important conclusion from this is that cultural activities at work should be organized in such a way that the majority of workers should have the opportunity to participate and that possible effects of 'jealousy' are avoided.

A study of the importance of cultural activity in healthcare professionals in Finland involved 336 subjects. The association of creative leisure activities (art-making or creative expression) and receptive cultural activities (consuming culture) with wellbeing at work was analysed. Wellbeing was looked at from three points of view: creative working mode, personal achievement, and work engagement. The authors found that a high frequency of cultural leisure activities was associated with wellbeing at work. Both types of cultural activities were associated with a sense of personal achievement at work, but only creative leisure activities were associated with the creative working mode. In contrast, only receptive cultural activities were associated with work engagement.

There is a socio-economic perspective in cultural activities at work. Subjects with a high level of education are more likely in general to be involved in cultural activities, and this was also observed in the Swedish study of cultural activities at work—the correlation between education and frequency of cultural activities at work being highly significant (0.23). However, this depends to a great extent on which cultural activity is offered. A recent Norwegian study (Vaag et al. 2013) of a choir singing experiment showed that it is possible to obtain good participation among staff having lower levels of education. All employees in two county hospitals were offered the opportunity to participate in rock music choral singing led by professional musicians with rehearsals and a final concert. Three hundred employees completed questionnaires both before and after the intervention. Middle-aged female employees with a lower level of education were more likely to participate in this cultural work-based activity than others. A change was observed in the choir participants after the choir period since there was more engagement and organizational commitment as well as more self-reported positive change with regard to the psychosocial work environment and global health in participants compared with non-participants. These results point at concrete possibilities for using the workplace for health-promoting cultural activities.

A study by Romanowska et al. (2011, 2013) has indicated that cultural participation may be a tool for improving manager competence resulting in improved employee health. The underlying idea has been that *laissez-faire* managers who lack engagement, in particular social and emotional, with their employees give rise to poor mental health in their staff. For instance, a tendency among managers to formalize difficult social problems in the work environment may cause unnecessary delay in problem solving, with resulting emotional suffering among employees. A programme named 'Schibbolet' was created as an 'art tool' in order to generate increased engagement among managers. The programme is a collage of poetry pieces read to the participants by professional actors. The participating managers in both groups were examined before the start, after 1 year, and after 18 months. Four subordinates per manager were also examined on the same occasions. There were 136 subjects in total in the study. The results after 18 months indicated that the subordinates of the Schibbolet managers had a significant improvement in mental health (sleep problems, depressive symptoms, emotional exhaustion) and also in their ability to actively deal with problems at work (decreasing scores for covert coping) than the subordinates of the managers in the comparison group. This experiment points at a possible use for arts in improving managers and that the changes in the managers may favourably influence the health of subordinates.

According to results published by Bygren et al. (2009), a programme including self-selected cultural activities once a week for 8 weeks for workers in a municipality had favourable effects on various self-reported aspects of health. However, the authors are not aware of published studies of health effects on whole workplaces with a longer follow-up period.

## Old age

It is frequently stated that old people can increase their vitality and promote their health by participating in cultural activities. Indirect support for this was found in observational epidemiological studies by Konlaan et al. (2000) and Bygren et al. (2009). Our own research group performed an experimental study including participants with a minimum age of 65 years (mean age 74) living in an apartment building for elderly people in Stockholm. Participants were exposed to cultural activities having biographical relevance to each of them. Measurement instruments included questionnaires, staff ratings, and blood concentrations of a number of biomarkers. These observations were made at baseline prior to the intervention as well as at 3 and 6 months later (Arnetz et al. 1983). Another part of the apartment building (with different staff) was selected under strict conditions for comparison to construct a matched control group. Analyses of

the biomarkers showed that participants on the experimental floor had a more favourable development during the experimental period than those in the control group—with decreased stress (mirrored in improved blood sugar) and improved cell regeneration (mirrored in the concentration of 'positive' hormones stimulating regeneration).

Later, a study was performed concerning the effects of pictures of fine art on the health of older women. The older women living in a service home were randomly allocated to a 'art group' or a 'talk group' (20 women in each group). The interventions lasted for 4 months. The investigator met the participants once a week over the 4 months. In the art group a series of pictures of fine art were used to introduce talks, while in the other group talks were regular conversations without art introductions (Wikström 1994). Observations (questionnaires and blood pressure assessments) were made before the start as well as 4 (end of interventions) and 8 months later (4 months following the intervention). In general there were significantly more favourable effects in the art group than in the other group, and these effects lasted longer than the 4 months of the intervention. For instance, there were significantly improved coping, blood pressure control, and improvement in physical health (indicated also by a decreased usage of laxatives) in the art group compared with controls. Figures 8.1 and 8.2 show two examples of results (Wikström et al. 1993; Wikström 1994). Figure 8.1 shows the development of group means for 'emotional balance' assessed by using a 'coping wheel'. Whereas a lasting improvement in emotional balance is reported in the art group no change is observed in the talk group. Figure 8.2 shows the corresponding

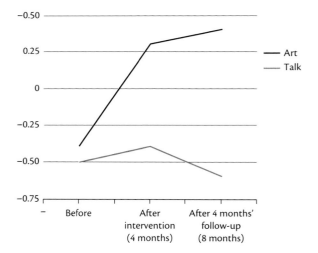

**Fig. 8.1** Means for emotional balance in two groups of elderly women randomly allocated to either the art group or the talk group (*n* = 20). The means are presented before intervention, immediately after the intervention (4 months after the start) and again after a follow-up period of 4 months (8 months after the start). Two-way analysis of variance showed significant difference in development over time. In both groups the participants met the experimenter for an hour once a week for 4 months. In the art group the session was initiated by specially selected pictures of fine art upon which a conversation followed. In the talk group there was no art introduction to the conversation, just talking.
Source: data from Wikström, B.-M., *Pleasant guided mental walks via pictures of works of art*, Academic Thesis, Karolinska Institute, Stockholm, Copyright © 1994; and Wikström B.-M. et al., Medical health and emotional effects of art stimulation in old age, *Psychotherapy and Psychosomatics*, Volume 60, pp. 195–206. Copyright © 2010 Karger Publishers, Basel, Switzerland.

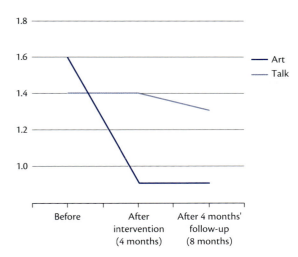

**Fig. 8.2** Means for self-reported laxative pill consumption in two groups of elderly women randomly allocated to either the art group or the talk group (n = 20). The means are presented before intervention, immediately after the intervention (4 months after the start) and again after a follow-up period of 4 months (8 months after th estart). Two-way analysis of variance showed significant difference in development over time. In both groups the participants met the experimenter for an hour once a week for 4 months. In the art group the session was initiated by specially selected pictures of fine art upon which a conversation followed. In the talk group there was no art introduction to the conversation, just talking.

Source: data from Wikström, B.-M., *Pleasant guided mental walks via pictures of works of art*, Academic Thesis, Karolinska Institute, Stockholm, Copyright © 1994; and Wikström B.-M. et al., Medical health and emotional effects of art stimulation in old age, *Psychotherapy and Psychosomatics*, Volume 60, pp. 195–206. Copyright © 2010 Karger Publishers, Basel, Switzerland.

means for consumption of laxative pills. Whereas the consumption of laxative pills decreased in the art group no change was observed in the talk group. In both these examples there are significant differences between the groups (two-way analysis of variance). These experiments with elderly people were not epidemiological in the sense that the participants were drawn randomly from the population, but the study samples were typical of the elderly population with normal health living in homes for the elderly in Sweden.

Several studies have indicated that singing in a choir may be of particular importance for health promotion in old age. The most extensive study published so far is that by Cohen (2009) whose research group studied 166 older people living in Washington, New York City, and San Francisco. Those who were willing to participate in singing were randomly assigned to either cultural activity or a control group. In New York City and San Francisco other forms of cultural activity took place, but in Washington all three participating centres had choral weekly singing groups which in the end formed a big choir. This continued for 2 years and the participants were followed by means of standard questionnaires. In assessments performed at baseline as well as after 1 and 2 years there were 61 participants in the choral group and 57 in the control group. Several health indicators showed the same pattern, with significantly improved scores (for instance number of health problems) in the choral group and deteriorated scores in the control group. The main difference was particularly pronounced after 2 years. From this study of a representative group of institutionalized elderly people it was concluded that organized choir singing could have a particular health-promoting value in old age, at least among those who want to sing and have no opportunity to do so without organized help. A large cross-national interview study of older adult choir singers in Australia, England, and Germany (Clift et al. 2007, 2008) has explored the potential benefits of active involvement in choral singing. At least six mechanisms were identified as potential explanations for a health-promoting effect of choir singing in this age group, among which are positive affect, focused attention, deep breathing, and social support.

## Conclusion

Although epidemiological research throwing light on the health effects of cultural activities has been relatively limited it is a rapidly growing field. There are several indications from epidemiological research that cultural activities may promote health. Researchers are facing many challenges. For instance, a significant positive relationship between a cultural activity and an indicator of health may not necessarily be causal. Therefore, carefully designed large-scale controlled interventions with follow-up of long-lasting effects on defined aspects of health and physiological parameters are needed.

# References

Aiken, N.E. (1998). *The Biological Origins of Art*. Westport, CT: Praegen/Greenwood.

Arnetz, B., Theorell, T., Levi., L., Kallner, A., and Eneroth, P. (1983). An experimental study of social isolation of elderly people: psychoendocrine and metabolic effects. *Psychosomatic Medicine*, **45**, 395–406.

Bellis, M.A., Hennell, T., Lushey, C., Hughes, K., Tocque, K., and Ashton, J.R. (2007). Elvis to Eminem: quantifying the price of fame through early mortality of European and North American rock and pop stars. *Journal of Epidemiology and Community Health*, **61**, 896–901.

Benzon, W. (2001). *Beethoven's Anvil: Music in Mind and Culture*. New York: Basic Books.

Bygren, L.O., Konlaan, B.B., and Johansson, S.E. (1996) Attendance at cultural events, reading books or periodicals, and making music or singing in a choir as determinants for survival: Swedish interview survey of living conditions. *British Medical Journal*, **313**, 1577–1580.

Bygren, L.O., Johansson, S.-E., Konlaan, B.B., Grjibovski, A.M., Wilkinson, A.V., and Sjöström, M. (2009). Attending cultural events and cancer mortality: a Swedish cohort study. *Arts & Health: An International Journal for Research, Policy and Practice*, **1**, 64–73.

Bygren, L.O., Weissglas, G., Wikström, B.M., et al. (2009). Cultural participation and health: a randomized controlled trial among medical care staff. *Psychosomatic Medicine*, **71**, 469–473.

Chan, A.S., Ho, Y.C., and Cheung, M.C. (1998). Music training improves verbal memory. *Nature*, **396**, 128.

Clift, S. (2012). Creative arts as a public health resource: moving from practice-based research to evidence-based practice. *Perspectives in Public Health*, **132**, 120–127.

Clift, S., Hancox, G., Morrison, I., Hess, B., Kreutz, G., and Stewart, D. (2007). Choral singing and psychological wellbeing: findings from English choirs in a cross-national survey using the WHOGOL-BREF. In: A. Williamon and D. Coimbra (eds), *Proceedings of the International Symposium on Performance Science, Porto. Portugal, 25–27 October*.

Clift, S., Hancox, G., Morrison, I., Hess, B., Kreutz, G., and Stewart, D. (2008). *Findings from a Cross-National Survey on Choral Singing, Wellbeing and Health. Canterbury: Canterbury Christ Church University*. Available at: <http://www.canterbury.ac.uk/centres/sidney-de-haan-research/> (accessed 3 February 2010).

Cohen, G. (2009). New theories and research findings on the positive influence of music and art on health with ageing. *Arts & Health: An International Journal for Research, Policy and Practice*, **1**, 48–63.

Costa-Giomi, E. (1999). The effects of three years of piano instruction on children's cognitive development. *Journal of Research In Music Education*, **47**, 198–212.

Costa-Giomi, E., Gilmour, R., Siddell, J., and Lefebvre, E. (2001). Absolute pitch, early musical instruction, and spatial abilities. *Annals of the New York Academy of Sciences*, **930**, 394–396.

Cuypers, K., Krokstad, S., Lingaas Holmen, T., Skjei Knudtsen, M., Bygren, L.O., and Holmen, J. (2012). Patterns of receptive and creative cultural activities and their association with perceived health, anxiety, depression and satisfaction with life among adults: the HUNT study. *Norway Journal of Epidemiology and Community Health*, **66**, 698–703.

Degé, F. and Schwartzer, G. (2011). The effect of a music program on phonological awareness in preschoolers. *Frontiers of Psychology*, **2**, 124, doi: 10.3389/fpsyg.2011.00124

Degé, F., Wehrum, S., Stark, R., and Schwarzer, G. (2011). The influence of two years of school music training in secondary school on visual and auditory memory. *European Journal of Developmental Psychology*, **8**, 608–623.

Dissanayake, E. (1988). *What is Art For?* Seattle, WA: University of Washington Press.

Hartzell, M. and Theorell, T. (2007). *Regelbundet Återkommande Kulturella Aktiviteter på Arbetsplatsen*. [Regularly Occurring Cultural Activities in the Workplace]. Stockholm: National Institute for Psychosocial Factors and Health.

Hartzell, M. and Theorell, T. (2009). A note on designing evaluations of health effects of cultural activities at work. *Arts & Health: An International Journal for Research, Policy and Practice*, **1**, 89–92.

Hyyppä, M.T. and Mäki, J. (2001a). Why do Swedish-speaking Finns have longer active life? An area for social capital research. *Health Promotion International*, **16**, 55–64.

Hyyppä, M.T. and Mäki, J. (2001b). Individual-level relationships between social capital and self-rated health in a bilingual community. *Preventive Medicine*, **32**, 148–155.

Konlaan, B.B, Bygren, L.O., and Johansson, S.E. (2000). Visiting the cinema, concerts, museums or art exhibitions as determinant of survival: a Swedish fourteen-year cohort follow-up. *Scandinavian Journal of Public Health*, **28**, 174–178.

Kulturrådet [Swedish National Arts Council] (2008). Svenska Kulturvanor i Ett 30-Årsperspektiv: 1976–2006. *Kulturen i Siffror*, no. 6 [Swedish Cultural Habits in a 30 Years Perspective: 1976–2006. *Culture in Numbers*, no. 6]. Stockholm: Kulturrådet.

Lewis-Williams, D. (2002). *Consciousness and the Origins of Art*. London: Thames and Hudson.

Lindblad, F., Hogmark, Å., and Theorell, T. (2007). Music intervention for 5th and 6th graders—effects on development and cortisol secretion. *Stress and Health*, **23**, 9–14.

Mehr, S.A., Schachner, A., Katz, R.C., and Spelke, E.S. (2013). Two randomized trials provide no consistent evidence for nonmusical cognitive benefits of brief preschool music enrichment. *PLoS ONE*, **8**(12): e82007. doi:10.1371/journal.pone.0082007

Moreno, S., Marques, C., Santos, A., Santos, M., Castro, S.L., and Besson, M. (2009). Musical training influences linguistic abilities in 8-year-old children: more evidence for brain plasticity. *Cerebrum and Cortex*, **19**, 712–723.

Moreno, S., Bialystok, E., Barac, R., Schellenberg, E.G., Cepeda, N.J., and Chau, T. (2011). Short-term music training enhances verbal intelligence and executive function. *Psychological Science*, **22**,1425–1433.

Mithen, S. (2005). *The Singing Neanderthals. The Origins of Music, Mind and Body*. London: Weidenfeld and Nicholson

Pantev, C. and Herholz, S.C. (2011). Plasticity of the human auditory cortex related to musical training. *Neuroscience and Biobehavioral Review*, **35**, 2140–2145.

Peretz, I., Cummings, S., and Dubé, M.P. (2007). The genetics of congenital amusia (tone deafness): a family-aggregation study. *American Journal of Human Genetics*, **81**, 582–588.

Power, C., Jefferis, B.J., Manor, O., and Hertzman, C. (2006). The influence of birth weight and socioeconomic position on cognitive development: does the early home and learning environment modify their effects? *Journal of Pediatrics*, **148**, 54–61.

Rauscher, F.H. and Zupan, M.A. (2000). Classroom keyboard instruction improves kindergarten children's spatial-temporal performance: a field experiment. *Early Childhood Research Quarterly*, **15**, 215–228.

Romanowska, J., Larsson, G., Eriksson, M., Wikström, B.-M., Westerlund, H., and Theorell, T. (2011). Health effects on leaders and co-workers of an art-based leadership development program. *Psychotherapy and. Psychosomatics*, **80**, 78–87.

Romanowska, J., Larsson, G., and Theorell, T. (2013). Effects on leaders of an art-based leadership intervention. *Leadership and Organization Development Journal*, **32**, 1004–1022.

Schellenberg, E.G. (2004). Music lessons enhance IQ. *Psychological Science*, **15**, 511–514.

Schellenberg, E.G. (2006). Long-term positive associations between music lessons and IQ. *Journal of Educational Psychology*, **98**, 457–468.

Schellenberg, E.G. and Weiss, M.W. (2013). Music and cognitive abilities. In: D. Deutsch (ed.), *The Psychology of Music*, pp. 499–550. London: Academic Press.

Spychiger, M. (2002). Music education is important—why? In: G. Matell and T. Theorell (eds), *Barn och Musik [Children and Music]*. Stockholm: Stress Research Institute, Stockholm University.

Theorell, T., Hartzell, M., and Näslund, S. (2009). A note on designing evaluations of health effects of cultural activities at work. *Arts & Health: An International Journal for Research, Policy and Practice*, **1**, 89–92.

Theorell, T., Osika, W., Leineweber, C., Magnusson Hanson, L.L., Bojner Horwitz, E., and Westerlund, H. (2013). Is cultural activity at work related to mental health in employees? *International Archives of Occupational and Environmental Health*, **86**, 281–288.

Vaag, J., Saksvik, P.Ø., Theorell, T., Skillingstad, T., and Bjerkestad, O. (2013). Sound of wellbeing—choir singing as an intervention to improve wellbeing among employees in two Norwegian county hospitals. *Arts & Health: An International Journal for Research, Policy and Practice*, **5**, 93–102.

Wikström, B.-M. (1994). Pleasant guided mental walks via pictures of works of art. Academic Thesis. Stockholm: Karolinska Institute.

Wikström, B.-M, Theorell, T., and Sandström, S. (1993). Medical health and emotional effects of art stimulation in old age. *Psychotherapy and Psychosomatics*, **60**, 195–206.

Västfjäll, D., Juslin, P.N., and Hartig, T. (2012). Music, subjective wellbeing, and health: the role of everyday emotions. In: R. MacDonald, G. Kreutz, and L. Mitchell (eds), *Music, Health, and Wellbeing*, pp. 405–423. Oxford: Oxford University Press.

Väänänen, A., Murray, M., Koskinen, A., Vahtera, J., Kouvonen, A., and Kivimäki, M. (2009). Engagement in cultural activities and cause-specific mortality: prospective cohort study. *Preventive Medicine*, **49**, 142–147.

Zhao, F., Manchaiah, V.K.C., French, D., and Price, S. (2010). Music exposure and hearing disorders: an overview. *International Journal of Audiology*, **49**, 54–64.

# CHAPTER 9

# Psychophysiological links between cultural activities and public health

Töres Theorell

## Introduction

In this chapter the physiological mechanisms that could mediate the health effects of cultural activities are reviewed. Neurobiological research indicates that cultural activities during childhood may influence the development not only of cognitive but also of emotional skills. Both active and passive cultural experiences influence the activity of the brain, and a number of hormonal, cardiovascular, and immunological influences have been described. Both beneficial and adverse effects of cultural participation can arise. Long-term beneficial health effects have not yet been studied extensively using physiological assessments. Combined effects of different modalities of cultural participation (for instance visual and auditory experiences) have been shown.

## Neurobiological background

Joseph Le Doux (1998) and colleagues made the discovery that emotionally charged stimuli are transmitted to the brain via two different routes that they labelled the 'upper' and the 'lower' routes. The same routes could also be labelled the 'slower' and the 'faster' routes, respectively. The sound or light impulse first reaches a relay station in the thalamus located in the midbrain. A musical tune or a specific picture may be associated with anxiety. If this is the case, the faster lower route transmits the impulse to the amygdala. This brain structure has an important role in stress and anxiety reactions. The amygdala—part of the emotional brain—rapidly triggers a stress response in the brain and the rest of the body. The emotional brain could be regarded as a primitive part of the human brain (see Fig. 9.1).

The impulse is transmitted via the higher route up to the brain cortex, which processes the cognitive interpretation (e.g. Which piece of music or picture? Where did I hear or see this before? Does it mean danger?). If the cognitive analysis leads to the conclusion that the situation associated with the music is dangerous, an impulse is sent to the amygdala from the cortex as well. Since this transmission is relatively slow, the amygdala has already reacted, but the cortical reaction can now modify the primitive stress reaction. If the sound or picture impulse lasts for a very short time (less than 40 ms; e.g. a dissonant chord or a picture of a monster

in a movie that disappears rapidly) the cognitive cortex may never become aware of the phenomenon and may therefore not be able to process the information on a conscious level. In such a case it is only the lower route that has been activated, and the brain may never become aware of the source of the anxiety reaction. This has been clearly shown in brain research on picture perception. If simplified pictures of neutral, sad, happy, and angry faces are shown in random order very rapidly, the subject will not be able to know cognitively which faces he or she has seen. But functional magnetic brain imaging (a method for studying the activation of different parts of the brain during stimulation) shows that the amygdala is activated every time the angry face is shown but not when the other faces are shown—despite the fact that the subject is unable to say when the angry face is being shown. There are similar routes (with other combinations of brain structures in the emotional brain) for other emotions, such as joy, anger, and sadness (Morris et al. 1998).

An important concept in the psychophysiological understanding of possible beneficial health effects of cultural experiences is 'emotional competence' (e.g. Morris and Dolan 2013) This refers to the fact that emotional impulses and rational understanding are handled differently by different parts of the brain and that the cooperation of these is vital to health.

## Emotional and social competence

In psychosomatic medicine the concept of *alexithymia* is important. Alexithymia means a lack of the ability to differentiate feelings (Sifneos 1996). Someone with a good ability to identify, describe, differentiate, and deal with different emotions has a great advantage. By contrast those who are lacking in this skill could suffer from alexithymia. Our emotions serve as a driving force and a compass in many situations. Biologically speaking we show anger because we want others to be afraid of us. Sadness, particularly when accompanied by tears, shows that we are in need of help (Hendriks et al. 2008). We show pride because we expect those around us to give us praise. This feeling can also amplify a positive collective feeling. All our emotions serve as signals to the environment and at the same time they are driving

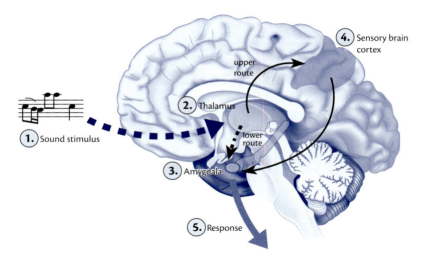

**Fig. 9.1**  Musical impulses (1) are first transmitted to the thalamus in the mid brain (2) and then along two different routes when they reach the brain. The lower (and faster) route (from 2 to 3) is from the thalamus to the emotional brain, in the diagram represented by amygdala which is important in the regulation of anxiety. The upper (and slower) route (from 2 to 4) is from the thalamus to the sensory (cognitive) brain cortex.
Reproduced by kind permission of Annika Röhl. Copyright © 2015 Annika Röhl, Töres Theorell.

forces in our own acts. Every emotion has both bodily and psychological expressions. Someone who is good at differentiating his or her feelings is also likely to be able to differentiate feelings in relatives, friends, and family members (see Baughman et al. 2013). Accordingly, emotional competence relates to social competence. In accordance with the development of other kinds of skills it is likely that training in emotional skills should start as early as possible in life. Alexithymia is associated with an increased risk of illness; the most well-documented example being hypertension (high blood pressure) which arises more often in people with alexithymia than in others (Grabe et al. 2010).

So how early should we start? Probably already by the foetal stage! In the third trimester of pregnancy the foetus already has fairly good hearing and it is able to differentiate sounds (Granier et al. 2011). It has also been shown that the foetus can learn to differentiate vowels that are audible to it during this part of the pregnancy: newborn babies show physiological signs (sucking behaviour) indicating that they recognize the mother's speech sounds from the foetal period (Moon et al. 2013). A newborn American baby recognizes typical American speech sounds while a Swedish baby recognizes typical Swedish speech sounds. Speech melody—so-called prosody—is close to music for the baby!

It could be assumed that the emotional experiences of the foetus *in utero* are primitive. It is likely to recognize some aspects of its mother's movements, ranging from no movement at all to slow and fast and from chaotic to rhythmic. The chemical environment may also change in association with these components of sensory input. It is a fact that some stress hormones, for instance cortisol, pass the placental barrier. In other words, when the mother is stressed, joyful, or sad the chemical situation for the foetus will correspond to those maternal conditions (e.g. Harris and Seckl 2011). Other kinds of auditory stimuli may also play a role in this. For instance, the mother's heart sounds are audible to the foetus. In some way the foetus may perhaps be able to differentiate between a fast maternal heart rate associated with fast bodily movements on one hand and maternal tachycardia without bodily movements on the other.

After birth, interaction with the environment becomes more intensive. The social anthropologist Dissanayake (2000) has performed detailed studies of mother–infant interaction before the age of 6 months. Mimics, gestures, speech sounds, and singing become important components of emotional communication, particularly frequently with the mother.

During the first years after birth the child develops an increasing ability to recognize different emotions and to differentiate between more and more fine-grained emotional states. That children's social competence can benefit from cultural training has been shown in Schellenberg's study (2004) of randomly selected 6-year-olds who were assigned to music training (two groups), theatre training, and a control condition. One of the significant observations was that children in the theatre training group developed better social competence than children in the other groups. Accordingly we can assume that cultural experiences can help children in their emotional development.

In addition, a study by Romanowska et al. (2013) with managers and business leaders showed increased emotional engagement after participation in a cultural programme with sessions once a month for a period of 9 months. Each session contained a mix of poetry interspersed with specially selected pieces of music. The selected pieces of poetry had ethically provocative themes. Each session was followed by diary writing and group discussions. This was a randomized controlled study and the managers in the cultural programme were compared with managers who went through a programme aimed at improved social competence using structured lectures and discussions. One year after the start, managers in the cultural training programme had improved their 'agreeableness' and 'sense of coherence' scores significantly more than the managers in the comparison group.

These observations on both children and adults give support to the idea that cultural interventions can benefit the development of emotional and social competence.

Multimodality (several modes at the same time) is important in such emotional education. For instance, if one reads a story to a child, a musical and pictorial accompaniment may amplify the emotional context of the text. This will help the child to identify the 'correct' emotions and also to differentiate between sadness, anger, and anxiety for instance. Rhythmic dance movements may further amplify emotional expressions.

A large ongoing study by Theorell et al. (2014) involving 8000 participants aged 27–54 from the Swedish twin registry has shown that there is an association between musical ability (rhythmic as well as melodic capacity objectively assessed) on the one hand and emotional competence on the other (assessed by means of a widely used internationally standardized alexithymia questionnaire, TAS 20). There is also a significant (but weak) relationship between the amount of musical training and emotional competence; the more musical training a participant reported throughout life the better his or her emotional competence. Musical ability, the amount of music training, and general intelligence are all intercorrelated.

'Mirror neurons' are instrumental when a person looks passively at someone doing something, activating the cells in his or her brain that correspond exactly to that act. For instance, if a movement is performed by the active person's hands, the brain cells corresponding to those hand movements are also activated in the passive observer. This does not just pertain to movements (motor neurons) but is also applicable to emotions, and is the basis of human empathy. The existence of such processes for 'internal simulation' of what other people do, think, and feel may explain part of the power of music (Vickhoff 2008).

## Psychophysiology of music

In a large-scale project, Gabrielsson (2011) recruited more than 900 participants for an interview study. He asked people to describe in their own words the most profound musical experience that they had had in their lives and then went on to categorize those experiences with regard to content, context, and consequences. Gabrielsson stated that it was very difficult to do such a categorization since the experiences covered a very large area, and asserted that music seems to comprise the 'whole psychological reality'. Many of these situations were seen as being turning points in people's lives. Gabrielsson provided examples of people who reported being in deep depression 'discovering' a kind of music that they had never been interested in before, but in that situation they become passionately engaged in listening to it and they believe that it had helped them out of the depression.

Krumhansl (1997) described how a group of individuals reacted physiologically to three different kinds of musical pieces which were assumed to induce sadness (Albinoni's *Adagio* and Barber's *Adagio for Strings*), fear (Mussorgsky's *Night on Bald Mountain* and 'Mars' from *The Planets* by Holst) and joy (Vivaldi's 'Spring' from *The Four Seasons* and Alfvén's *Midsummer Wake*), respectively. First of all it was shown that the music really did induce the expected feelings in most experimental subjects. Secondly, it turned out that physiological reactions were indeed different in these induced emotional states. During the sad music the subjects had a lower heart rate, higher blood pressure, and sweated more (galvanic skin response). When the fearful music was played there was an increased respiratory rate (number of breaths per minute) and decreased blood flow in the periphery (finger tips). The joyful music was associated mainly with an increased respiratory rate.

In an experiment performed on a group of 37 young adults, the participants were asked to select two of their own favourite pieces

of music (Lingham and Theorell 2009), one piece that according to their own assessment was 'stimulating' and one that they considered 'relaxing'. While sitting quietly they listened in random order to these pieces. Their heart rate, breathing frequency, and emotional state were recorded, and recordings made when listening to their favourite pieces were compared with the preceding restful silence. During the stimulating piece the average increase in heart rate was seven beats per minute compared with the quiet condition. However, in some individuals the relaxing music did not produce the expected reduction in heart rate. Quite the contrary, in 11 cases it was even associated with a small increase in heart rate. There were similar observations with regard to breathing. During the stimulating music breathing frequency increased significantly, the average increase being four breathing cycles per minute. During the relaxing music, on the other hand, there was no significant change. Emotional self-recordings verified this in the psychological domain, whereas the stimulating music quite clearly induced feelings of arousal, the relaxing piece triggered both relaxed and aroused feelings. The conclusion to be drawn from this seems to be that these highly educated people were skilful in selecting their own stimulating music but were not as successful with regard to relaxing music—it frequently did not have the expected calming effect on heart rate and breathing.

Listening to music influences biochemical bodily processes as well. One example is the secretion of immunoglobulin A in saliva which is influenced by music experiences (Rider et al. 1990). This could have significance for resistance to infections. In many activities typical of the modern world music is used in ways that may seem new but are in fact very old. A striking example is the playing of music in gyms—indeed special kinds of music have been developed for this. One is reminded of all the music that has been used in human history in order to facilitate physical work, for example pulling boat songs, sailors' songs for rowing or managing large sails, and marching music to facilitate long troop marches.

A modern line of research has shown that specially adapted music may decrease both the subjective experience of physical effort and the physiological reactions to it. Szmedra and Bacharach (1998), for example, performed an experiment on this several years ago. Young men were asked to do exactly the same physical work on the treadmill during two different conditions. One condition was in silence and the other was while listening to special gym music. The two conditions were randomly ordered. The blood concentration of lactic acid was assessed. Heart rate and blood pressure were recorded and the subjects were asked to make a self-rating of effort. Despite the fact that the physical work was fixed and exactly the same in the two conditions, elevation of blood pressure and heart rate were lower during the exercise performed to music and the same observation was made for subjective effort and lactic acid concentration.

Other research in this field has shown that in long-distance cycling (10 km), when the cyclists choose their own tempo, listening to fast dance music ('trance' with a tempo of 142 beats per minute) is likely to induce an elevated cycling pace, with the work being perceived as harder without music (Atkinson et al. 2004). In another study the effects of different types of music on heart rate, rating of perceived exertion, and time to exhaustion were studied. The subjects performed their physical work on a treadmill and the conditions were randomly allocated to 'soft music', 'loud, fast and exciting music', and silence. The results showed that the soft music reduced physiological and psychological arousal during submaximal exercise and also increased endurance (Copeland and Franks 1991)

## Psychophysiology of music performance

The physiological effects of performing music have also been studied. The performance of music requires physical effort and hundreds of muscles are engaged during singing and also when playing an instrument. Singing in groups frequently entails bodily movement and dance. Even listening can induce strong physical activity, for instance when moving to dance music or attending a rock concert. Therefore, enhancement of aerobic skills and fitness may be inherent to large parts of musical experience. Vice versa, while performing aerobic exercises music can act as a motivating stimulus. Some of these effects appear to be exploited in commercial dance and gymnastics studios. In another vein, empirical studies of professional and amateur singers suggest that learning to sing in a controlled way can be associated with systematic training of breathing techniques. Professional singers differ from amateurs with regard to heart rate variability (HRV) during singing (Grape et al 2003), with professionals showing much greater HRV than amateurs. Most of the HRV is determined by activity in the parasympathetic nervous system that in many ways counterbalances the sympathetic nervous 'stress' system. During singing the professionals manage to activate a high degree of HRV. This may be due to a trained breathing technique with emphasis on diaphragmatic breathing, which stimulates the vagus nerve—the most important component in the parasympathetic nervous system. Breathing techniques acquired through musical practice could be used in situations outside the music room as well, producing a 'transfer' effect—from music performance to everyday life.

Stage performers can sometimes experience 'flow' (often referred to as 'effortless attention'; see Czikszentmihalyi 1990; Ullén et al. 2010). The state of flow typically arises when someone is performing a difficult task and has a sufficient skill level to match the challenge of the task. Characteristic components of the flow experience are high but include subjectively effortless attention, a sense of control, low self-awareness, a distorted sense of time, and positive affect (Csikszentmihalyi and Nakamura, 2010). This state may arise in many activities and is in no way confined to stage performances. Flow experiences can elevate quality of life. An online study by De Manzano et al. (2010) of physiological states in professional pianists when they played a difficult piece (which they liked and had selected) on five different occasions with varying degrees of flow (according to a standardized questionnaire-based assessment) showed that the flow state was characterized by a high state of arousal (with high heart rate), increased activity in the 'smile muscle', and increased depth of breathing. The increased depth of breathing is likely to have increased the parasympathetic activity mediated by the vagus nerve. One possibility, therefore, is that flow, in physiological terms, is a state of high arousal which is counterbalanced by high activation of the vagus nerve. Clearly, however, more research is needed on the physiological underpinnings of flow in various activities.

What are the possible mechanisms mediating the health-promoting effects of music in adult participants? Immediate effects of singing have been shown in several studies. For instance,

choral singers have been reported to have increased salivary immunoglobulin after a rehearsal compared with before the rehearsal (Beck et al. 2000; Kreutz et al. 2004). A study of the immediate effects of an individual singing lesson (Grape et al. 2003) showed that singing—in both amateurs and professionals—was associated with an increased plasma concentration of oxytocin. This may be a non-specific reaction to a situation with a strong social interaction component (between the singing teacher and their pupil). It could be speculated that the frequent repetition of active singing with all its hormonal effects could give rise to a cumulative wellbeing effect, but the significance in the long term of this kind of effect on health is unknown.

In a randomized small-scale study of patients with irritable bowel syndrome (IBS), a bowel disease with symptoms that are aggravated by worsened life conditions, the excretion of testosterone in the saliva was assessed (Grape et al 2010). None of the participants had been participating in choral singing, but half of the patients selected at a random were offered the possibility of singing in a choir once a week for a year. Those randomly allocated to the control group had IBS-related group activities without singing once a week for a year. Assessments were made on all participants before the start of the intervention and then 6, 9, and 12 months later. Among the variables studied was salivary testosterone. This was assessed on six occasions during waking hours on the four measurement days. Testosterone is important in both men and women for the regeneration of cells and for protecting the body against stress-related disorders. Variations in the concentration of testosterone in the saliva reflect variations in blood concentration and hence in regenerative activity. In studies of testosterone excretion in normal populations it has been shown that concentration of this hormone in both blood and saliva is related to the general psychosocial situation. When this improves testosterone excretion increases, and vice versa.

The findings in the choir study showed that after 6 months there was a pronounced increase in the excretion of testosterone in the choir group but not in the comparison group. After a year the differences were no longer statistically significant. Blood samples were collected before the start of the intervention and 1 year later. Plasma fibrinogen concentration, an indicator of long-lasting arousal, was assessed in these samples—the findings indicating a favourable 1-year effect on the choir group relative to the other group (Grape et al. 2009). These results indicate that singing in a group may stimulate regeneration and reduce long-term stress but also that these effects may depend on context. These findings illustrate physiological mechanisms that may explain the perceived health-promoting effects of group singing, but much larger studies of representative samples are required for sound conclusions.

## Cognitive effects of music training?

Whether or not early training in music performance might influence the development of children's brains has been an important topic in neurobiology. Effects of musical training have been found in both the grey and the white matter of the brain.

In the grey matter, the primary motor cortex (M1) of musicians is larger in both hemispheres than in non-musicians (Amunts et al., 1997; Gaser and Schlaug, 2003; Han et al., 2009). This effect has been found to be associated with the age at which training started (Amunts et al., 1997) and 'musician status' (professional > amateur > non-musician) (Gaser and Schlaug 2003). Strikingly, Bangert and Schlaug (2006) have shown that M1 morphology varies with instrument played, with pianists and string players showing a left- and right-side advantage, respectively. Such instrument-specific effects naturally suggest causal influences of training on brain anatomy. Conclusive evidence for a causal effect was found by Hyde and colleagues, who demonstrated increases in volume of the motor cortex after 15 months of musical training in children (Hyde et al. 2009). Plastic changes in the anatomy of the motor system also include premotor and parietal areas (Bermudez et al. 2009). Gaser and Schlaug (2003) found increases in regional volume in bilateral clusters in the cortex, extending from M1 to premotor areas and the parietal cortex. Broca's area, which is important for speech, music, and sequential organization of behaviour in general, likewise shows an increased volume in musicians (Sluming et al. 2002; Gaser and Schlaug 2003; Abdul-Kareem et al. 2011a), and this effect is associated with the age at which training started (Sluming et al. 2002) and musician status (Gaser and Schlaug 2003).

Differences in grey matter between musicians and non-musicians are also found in other parts of the cortex. The auditory cortex in the bilateral superior temporal gyrus shows a larger regional volume (Gaser and Schlaug, 2003; Bermudez et al., 2009) and cortical thickness (Bermudez et al., 2009) in musicians. Hyde et al. (2009), using a longitudinal design, demonstrated increases in volume of the auditory cortex after 15 months of training. Finally, Groussard et al. (2010) showed a larger regional volume of the left hippocampal head in musicians than in non-musician controls, an effect that may reflect the processing of musical memories.

The most well-replicated finding in the white matter of the brain of musicians is that the cross-sectional area of the corpus callosum (CC) is larger (Schlaug et al. 1995; Öztürk et al. 2002; Lee et al. 2003; Hyde et al. 2009; Steele et al. 2013). This is of particular relevance to this chapter because the CC is the bridge between the right and left hemispheres of the brain and has been shown to be very important for emotional competence. As a dramatic illustration of this, Paul et al. (2003) have shown that subjects who lack this structure in the brain can be perfectly normal with regard to cognitive functioning (verbal understanding) but have serious deficits in emotional and social skills. As already mentioned, there is a correlation between musicality and emotional competence. Studies using the magnetic resonance technique of diffusion tensor imaging to study the organization of white matter in musicians have found a positive association between musical training in childhood and adolescence and fractional anisotropy (FA) of the CC in pianists (Bengtsson et al. 2005). FA is a commonly used index of white matter integrity that may reflect a number of microstructural variables such as myelination, axonal size, and the spatial organization of axons in a fibre tract (Le Bihan 2003). Interestingly, recent studies have reported stronger effects on CC anatomy in musicians who started their training at an early rather than a later age (Steele et al. 2013). Diffusion imaging studies have also demonstrated higher FA in the pyramidal tract of musicians than in non-musicians (Bengtsson et al. 2005; Han et al. 2009; Halwani et al. 2011), and that practice in childhood and pyramidal tract FA in pianists are positively associated (Bengtsson et al. 2005). The pyramidal tract is essential for the cortical control of finger movements (Armand et al. 1996). Associations between musical training and more well-organized white matter structure

have also been found for other white matter tracts, including the arcuate fasciculus (Bengtsson et al. 2005; Halwani et al. 2011) and superior and inferior frontal tracts (Bengtsson et al. 2005). The regional pattern of white matter structure may differ between categories of musicians, and interesting differences have been reported between instrumentalists and singers—the latter group was found to have a larger arcuate fasciculus on the left than on the right side (Halwani et al. 2011). Longitudinal evidence for causal effects of musical training on white matter structure were obtained by Hyde et al. (2009), who found an increase in CC volume after 15 months of musical practice.

Finally, two studies have reported that the volume of the cerebellum is greater in musicians than in non-musicians (Hutchinson et al. 2003; Abdul-Kareem et al. 2011b). The size of this effect was related to intensity of long-term musical practice.

In summary, there is a fairly large neurobiological literature on brain anatomy in musicians. Taken together, these studies support the idea that musical training stimulates development of the brain, and that the effects of such training are widespread and involve many regions in both the grey and white matter. Interestingly, several of the studies also suggest that training in early childhood may be particularly effective.

## Dance and music

In his research Krantz (2006) has shown that lay people in Sweden react in a predictable way when diatonic ascending chords (two notes at the same time) are being played. Minor seconds (two notes as close as possible to one another on a 12-tone scale, for instance C and C♯) and major sevenths (two notes that are as almost and as close as possible to an octave, for instance A and A ♭) are the most disharmonic diatonic chords. When these chords are being played the experimental subjects tend to report disharmonic emotions, such as worry, irritation, and sadness. Chords in the middle range tend to trigger soft or agreeable feelings. The major sixth was associated with the most pronounced joy whereas the fifth was associated with wholeness, the major third with embracing, and the major seventh with uncoordinated jittery movements. These kinds of observations indicate that dance and music may be programmed together in our brains and that this may have phylogenetic meaning.

In a small randomized trial study of 36 patients, Bojner Horwitz et al. (2003) evaluated the effects of dance therapy for patients with fibromyalgia. A novel procedure in that research was film recording of movement patterns in standardized situations. Such recordings were performed before the dance therapy started as well as 14 months later. After 14 months standardized ratings of the patients' movements showed that the movement patterns had improved in the dance group compared with the control group. Self-ratings and assessments of hormones did not show significant improvements. Patients in the dance group, however, tended to have higher concentration of cortisol in their plasma and saliva after therapy compared with before—a possible indicator of activation of the hypothalamic–pituitary–adrenocortical (HPA) axis. The HPA axis is instrumental in the mobilization of energy in stressful situations, so increased activity of the HPA in healthy subjects is an indicator of increased energy mobilization, i.e. stress. However, inability to activate the HPA axis is a frequent component in long-lasting physiological exhaustion. An increased level of cortisol in patients who have shown clinical symptoms of exhaustion (as patients with fibromyalgia do) could be interpreted positively because of this known association between chronic stress conditions and passivity in the HPA axis. This study illustrates some of the methodological difficulties encountered in quantitative scientific studies of the effects of dance. Patients are often unaware of their own improved movement patterns and several effects may be associated with activation of hormonal systems rather than soothing of hyperactive patterns.

Dancing may also activate anabolic/regenerative hormones. A study by Quiroga et al. (2009) of the hormonal effects of dancing the Argentinean tango showed that during tango dancing, with a partner and when music is being played, testosterone excretion was stimulated both in women and men. A randomized study has been published by Kattenstroth et al. (2013) of the effects of a dance class once a week for 6 months on elderly women and men (aged 60–94), with 25 subjects in the intervention and 10 in the control group. Significant improvements in lifestyle index and tests of cognition, reaction time, posture, hand/motor function, and tactile ability were found after the intervention period in the experimental group but not in the control group. These promising results show that dance classes may be a very beneficial activity for elderly.

It has been known for a long time in physiotherapy that a thorough analysis of patients' body language reveals a lot about their emotional state. This has been used extensively in dance therapy.

## Art psychotherapy in rehabilitation

Sometimes several forms of cultural experience may interact in generating forceful effects (e.g. dance and music, visual arts and music, music and words). For instance, there is controversy over the existence of music modules in the brain (i.e. regions of the brain that are specific to processing music). Very briefly, many neural structures and functions that are activated during musical experiences are shared or overlap with other domains, such as emotion, movement (corresponding to correlates of finger or limb movements during listening to music, for example), and speech and language. There is initial evidence showing that music can enhance the activation of brain regions that are relevant in one type of activity, and vice versa. For instance, Baumgartner et al. (2006) investigated the responses of the brains of healthy participants to unimodal and bimodal presentations of images and music. Unimodal presentations led to differential activations depending on the visual or auditory modality. These activations were combined and further enhanced in the bimodal condition. The point to be made here is that contextual factors can significantly modulate the responses to musical activities in the brain.

The conclusion is that musical experiences may amplify concomitant experiences in other modalities, which can be significant in a health context.

Theorell et al. (1998) performed a study on 24 patients who suffered from chronic pain and other psychosomatic conditions. They were all on sick leave and had been so for at least a year. These patients were followed for 2 years with blood samples and standardized questionnaires illuminating their mental state every fourth to sixth month. Each patient was informed that she or he would be treated over a 2-year period. In the art psychotherapy programme patients were treated once a week. Patients were assigned according to anticipated needs and preferences to one of the programmes: visual art, music, dance, or psychodrama. However, the group of therapists met once a month and the patients' therapy courses were reviewed by the therapists together. Sometimes painting or drawing was used for patients who did not participate in the visual art group. Similarly movement (dance), theatre experiences, and music were used in the groups not specializing in these activities. Because of the longitudinal nature of the data collection it was possible to follow typical time courses in these treatments. When the patients started they were mostly in a state of low energy (mirrored by a low serum concentration of uric acid). When the therapist and patient began to get to know one another, crucial art experiences during the therapy sessions could evoke memories of traumatic experiences. During this phase—mostly after about 6 months—the energy levels (serum uric acid as well as self-reported) were rising. At the end of the first year most patients had calmed down and their energy levels were intermediate. During this phase the levels of anxiety and depression had decreased. However, it was 2 years after the start of the course before somatic symptoms tended to decrease.

## Conclusion

Research on the psychophysiological links between cultural activity and health is increasing rapidly. The research efforts firstly deal with detailed descriptions of immediate physiological reactions to passive (listening) and active (performing) music situations—as for instance during 'chills' when listening and 'flow' when performing. Secondly researchers are beginning to follow more long-lasting effects of continuous repeated cultural experiences, for instance effects on regenerative hormones after 6 months of dancing once a week or choral singing. The effects of cultural activities on brain development in children are being increasingly studied—with possible consequences for cognition and emotional competence. This field of research should be regarded as a difficult one: it is often tricky to draw firm conclusions regarding causality, and great attention must be paid to research design.

## References

Abdul-Kareem, I.A., Stancak, A., Parkes, L.M., and Sluming, V. (2011a). Increased gray matter volume of left pars opercularis in male orchestral musicians correlate positively with years of musical performance. *Journal of Magnetic Resonance Imaging*, 33, 24–32.

Abdul-Kareem, I.A., Stancak, A., Parkes, L.M., et al. (2011b). Plasticity of the superior and middle cerebellar peduncles in musicians revealed by quantitative analysis of volume and number of streamlines based on diffusion tensor tractography. *Cerebellum*, 10, 611–623.

Amunts, K., Schlaug, G., Jäncke, L., et al. (1997). Motor cortex and hand motor skills: structural compliance in the brain. *Human Brain Mapping*, 5, 206–215.

Armand, J., Olivier, E., Edgley, S.A., and Lemon, R.N. (1996). The structure and function of the developing corticospinal tract: some key issues. In: A.M. Wing, P. Haggard, and J.R. Flanagan (eds), *Hand and Brain*, pp 125–146. San Diego: Academic Press.

Atkinson, G., Wilson, D., and Eubank, M. (2004). Effects of music on work-rate distribution during a cycling time trial. *International Journal of Sports Medicine*, 25, 611–615.

Bangert, M. and Schlaug, G. (2006). Specialization of the specialized in features of external human brain morphology. *European Journal of Neuroscience*, 24, 1832–1834.

Baughman, H.M., Schermer, J.A., Veselka, L., Harris, J., and Vernon, P.A. (2013). A behavior genetic analysis of trait emotional intelligence and alexithymia: a replication. *Twin Research and Human Genetics*, 16, 554–559.

Baumgartner, T., Lutz, K., Schmidt, C.F., and Jäncke, L. (2006). The emotional power of music: how music enhances the feeling of affective pictures. *Brain Research*, 1075, 151–164.

Bengtsson, S.L., Nagy, Z., Skare, S., Forsman, L., Forssberg, H., and Ullén, F. (2005). Extensive piano practicing has regionally specific effects on white matter development. *Nature Neuroscience*, 9, 1148–1150.

Bermudez, P., Lerch, J.P., Evans, A.C., and Zatorre, R.J. (2009). Neuroanatomical correlates of musicianship as revealed by cortical thickness and voxel-based morphometry. *Cerebral Cortex*, 19, 1583–1596.

Bojner Horwitz, E., Theorell, T., and Anderberg, U. (2003). Dance/movement therapy and changes in stress-related hormones: a study of fibromyalgia patients with video-interpretation. *The Arts in Psychotherapy*, 30, 255–264.

Copeland, B.L. and Franks, B.D. (1991). Effects of types and intensities of background music on treadmill endurance. *Journal of Sports Medicine and Physical Fitness*, 31, 100–103.

Czikszentmihalyi, M. (1990). *Flow: The Psychology of Optimal Experience*. New York: Harper and Row.

Csikszentmihalyi, M. and Nakamura, J. (2010). Effortless attention in everyday life: a systematic phenomenology. In: B. Bruya (ed.), *Effortless Attention: A New Perspective in the Cognitive Science of Attention and Action*, pp. 179–190. Cambridge, MA: MIT Press.

De Manzano, Ö., Harmat, L., Theorell, T., And Ullén, F (2010). The psychophysiology of flow during piano playing. *Emotion*, 10, 301–311.

Dissanayake. E. (2000). Antecedents of the temporal arts in early mother–infant interaction. In: N.L. Wallin, B. Merker, and S. Brown (eds), *The Origins of Music*, pp. 389–410. Cambridge, MA: MIT Press.

Gabrielsson, A. (2011). *Strong Experiences With Music: Music is Much More Than Just Music*. Oxford: Oxford University Press.

Gaser, C. and Schlaug, G. (2003). Brain structures differ between musicians and non-musicians. *Journal of Neuroscience*, 23, 9240–9245.

Grabe, H.J., Schwahn, C., Barnow, S., et al. (2010). Alexithymia, hypertension, and subclinical atherosclerosis in the general population. *Journal of Psychosomatic Research*, 68, 139–147.

Granier-Deferre, C., Ribeiro, A., Jacquet, A.Y., and Bassereau, S. (2011). Near-term fetuses process temporal features of speech. *Developmental Science*, 14, 336–352.

Grape, C., Sandgren, M., Hansson, L.-O., Ericson, M., and Theorell, T. (2003). Does singing promote wellbeing? An empirical study of professional and amateur singers during a singing lesson. *Integrative Physiological and Behavioral Science*, 38, 65–74.

Grape, C., Theorell, T., Wikström, B.M., and Ekman, R. (2009). Choir singing and fibrinogen, VEGF, cholecystokinin and motilin in IBS patients. *Medical Hypotheses*, 72, 223–225.

Grape, C., Wikström, B.M., Hasson, D., Ekman, R., and Theorell, T. (2010). Saliva testosterone increases in choir singer beginners. *Psychotherapy and Psychosomatics*, 79, 196–198.

Groussard, M., La Joie, R., Rauchs, G., et al. (2010). When music and long-term memory interact: effects of musical expertise on functional and structural plasticity in the hippocampus. *PLoS ONE*, 5, e13225, doi: 10.1371/journal.pone.0013225.

Halwani, G.F., Loui, P., Rüber, T., and Schlaug, G. (2011). Effects of practice and experience on the arcuate fasciculus: comparing singers, instrumentalists, and non-musicians. *Frontiers in Psychology*, 2, 156.

Han, Y., Yang, H., Lv, Y.-T., et al. (2009). Gray matter density and white matter integrity in pianists' brain: a combined structural and diffusion tensor MRI study. *Neuroscience Letters*, 459, 3–6.

Harris, A. and Seckl, J.(2011). Glucocorticoids, prenatal stress and the programming of disease. *Hormones and Behavior*, 59, 279–289.

Hendriks, M.C., Croon, M.A., and Vingerhoets, A.J. (2008). Social reactions to adult crying: the help-soliciting function of tears. *Journal of Social Psychology*, 148, 22–41.

Hutchinson, S., Lee, L.H., Gaab, N., and Schlaug, G. (2003). Cerebellar volume of musicians. *Cerebral Cortex*, 13, 943–949.

Hyde, K.L., Lerch, J., Norton, A., et al. (2009). Musical training shapes structural brain development. *Journal of Neuroscience*, 29, 3019–3025.

Kattenstroth, J.-C., Kalisch, T., Holt, S., Tegenthoff, M., and Dinse, H.R. (2013). Six months of dance intervention enhances postural, sensorimotor and cognitive performance in elderly without affecting cardio-respiratory functions. *Frontiers in Aging Neuroscience*, 5, doi: 10.3389/fnagi.2013.00005.

Krantz, G., Madison, G., and Merker, B. (2006). Melodic intervals as reflected in body movement. In: M. Baroni, A.R. Addessi, R. Caterina, and M. Costa (eds), *Proceedings of the Ninth International Conference on Music Perception and Cognition, Bologna August 22–26*. Available at: <http://www.marcocosta.it/icmpc2006/pdfs/149.pdf>

Krantz, G., Kreutz, G., Ericson, M., and Theorell, T. (2010). Bodily movements influence heart rate variability (HRV) responses to isolated melodic intervals. *Music and Medicine*, 3, 108–113.

Kreutz, G., Bongard, S., Rohrmann, S., Hodapp, V., and Grebe, D. (2004). Effects of choir singing or listening on secretory immunoglobulin A, cortisol, and emotional state. *Journal of Behavioral Medicine*, 27, 623–635.

Krumhansl, C.L. (1997). An exploratory study of musical emotions and psychophysiology. *Canadian Journal of Experimental Psychology*, 51, 336–352.

Le Bihan, D. (2003). Looking into the functional architecture of the brain with diffusion MRI. *Nature Reviews Neuroscience*, 4, 469–480.

Le Doux, J. (1998). *The Emotional Brain*. New York: Weidenfeld and Nicolson.

Lee, D.J., Chen, Y., and Schlaug, G. (2003). Corpus callosum: musician and gender effects. *NeuroReport*, 14, 205–209.

Lingham, J. and Theorell, T. (2009). Self-selected 'favourite' stimulative and sedative music listening—how does familiar and preferred music listening affect the body? *Nordic Journal of Music Therapy*, 18, 150–166.

Moon, C., Lagercrantz, H., and Kuhl, P.K.(2013). Language experienced in utero affects vowel perception after birth: a two-country study. *Acta Paediatrica*, 102, 156–160.

Morris, C.A., Denham, S.A., Bassett, H.H., and Curby, T.W. (2013). Relations among teachers' emotion socialization beliefs and practices, and preschoolers' emotional competence. *Early Education and Development*, **24**, 979–999.

Morris, J.S., Öhman, A., and Dolan, R.J. (1998). Conscious and unconscious emotional learning in the human amygdala. *Nature*, **393**, 467–470.

Öztürk, A.H., Tasçioglu, B., Aktekin, M., Kurtoglu, Z., and Erden, I. (2002). Morphometric comparison of the human corpus callosum in professional musicians and non-musicians by using in vivo magnetic resonance imaging. Journal of Neuroradiology, **29**, 29–34.

Paul, L.K., Van Lancker-Sidtis, D., Schieffer, B., Dietrich, R., and Brown, W.S. (2003). Communicative deficits in agenesis of the corpus callosum: nonliteral language and affective prosody. *Brain and Language*, **85**, 313–324.

Quiroga, M.C., Bongard, S., and Kreutz, G. (2009). Emotional and neurohumoral responses to dancing tango Argentino: the effects of music and partner. *Music and Medicine*, **1**, 14–21.

Rider, M.S., Achterberg, J., Lawlis, J.F., Goven, A., Toledo, R., and Butler, J.R. (1990). Effect of immune system imagery on secretory IgA. *Biofeedback and Self-Regulation*, **15**, 317–333.

Romanowska, J., Larsson, G., and Theorell, T. (2013). Effects on leaders of an art-based leadership intervention. *Journal of Management Development*, **32**, 1004–1022.

Schellenberg, E.G. (2004). Music lessons enhance IQ. *Psychological Science*, **15**, 511–514.

Schlaug, G., Jäncke, L., Huang, Y., Staiger, J.F., and Steinmetz, H. (1995). Increased corpus callosum size in musicians. *Neuropsychologia*, **33**, 1047–1055.

Sifneos, P.E. (1996). Alexithymia: past and present. *American Journal of Psychiatry*, **153**(7 Suppl.), 137–142.

Sluming, V., Barrick, T., Howard, M., Cezayirli, E., Mayes, A., and Roberts, N. (2002). Voxel-based morphometry reveals increased gray matter density in Broca's area in male symphony orchestra musicians. *NeuroImage*, **17**, 1613–1622.

Steele, C.J., Bailey, J.A., Zatorre, R.J., and Penhune, V.B. (2013). Early musical training and white-matter plasticity in the corpus callosum: evidence for a sensitive period. *Journal of Neuroscience*, **33**, 1282–1290.

Szmedra, L. and Bacharach, D.W. (1998). Effects of music on perceived exertion, plasma lactate, norepinephrine and cardiovascular hemodynamics during treadmill running. *International Journal of Sports Medicine*, **19**, 32–37.

Theorell, T., Konarski, K., Westerlund, H., et al. (1998). Treatment of patients with chronic somatic symptoms by means of art psychotherapy: a process description. *Psychotherapy and Psychosomatics*, **67**, 50–56.

Theorell, T.P., Lennartsson, A.K., Mosing, M.A., and Ullén, F. (2014). Musical activity and emotional competence - a twin study. *Frontiers in Psychology*. **16**, 774.

Ullén, F., de Manzano, Ö., Harmat, L., and Theorell, T. (2010). The physiology of effortless attention: correlates of state flow and flow proneness. In: B. Bruya (ed.), *Effortless Attention. A New Perspective in the Cognitive Science of Attention and Action*, pp. 205–217. Cambridge, MA: MIT Press.

Vickhoff, B. (2008). A perspective theory of music perception and emotion. *Skrifter från Musikvetenskap*, no. 90. Gothenberg: Institutionen för Kulturvetenskaper, University of Gothenberg.

# CHAPTER 10

# The role of qualitative research in arts and health

## Norma Daykin and Theo Stickley

## Qualitative research in arts and health: state of the art

Qualitative research designs are adopted in many arts and health contexts. Interest in qualitative methods has burgeoned in recent years, and multiple qualitative approaches are available to researchers and practitioners seeking to explore arts and health. Common approaches in arts and health research include ethnography and grounded theory, while other approaches include narrative research, discourse analysis, participatory action research, and arts-based methods. The choice of methodologies can seem baffling to new researchers or practitioners seeking to understand the impact of their work. The present authors both have many years' experience of applying qualitative approaches to a wide range of research topics, as well as teaching qualitative methodologies to students and practitioners. In this chapter we draw on recent experience of researching arts and health issues in order to discuss challenges and highlight some issues of best practice. We aim to help novice researchers to avoid some of the pitfalls, and support practitioners in their attempts to negotiate the minefield of qualitative research and evaluation.

In recent years there has been an increased focus on the need for evaluation of arts and health programmes. This focus on evaluation derives from our experience of applied health research, where qualitative approaches are often used in the context of evaluation studies, most commonly within mixed-methods designs. In these contexts, qualitative methods are usually used to illuminate or add to findings from quantitative data analysis, or as a foundation for further studies involving quantification where appropriate. They can provide insights into participants' experiences of the arts as well as revealing processes involved in project delivery. However, the potential for qualitative methods is broader than this, since they also lend themselves to the investigation of a wide range of questions not directly connected with project evaluation. While reviewing methodologies and reflecting on our experience, we hope not to lose sight of these broader questions.

The use of qualitative methods to support evaluation of arts and health interventions is sometimes poorly understood, with a lack of clear differentiation between the aims of qualitative and quantitative approaches. Recent evidence reviews have found that qualitative researchers and evaluators sometimes fail to report procedures for selection and recruitment of participants, data collection and analysis, and addressing ethical issues (Daykin et al. 2008b, 2011, 2013). The purpose of this chapter is to provide an overview of some of the different approaches used in qualitative research as well as to explain some of the philosophy and theory that lie behind them. This is needed in order to clarify the different purposes and applications of different methods. In short, we seek to examine what qualitative methods can achieve and, importantly, what they should not seek to achieve, in the study of arts and health. We also discuss the topic of ethics in relation to this work.

## The purpose of qualitative research

It is helpful to begin by considering the aims of qualitative research. Quantitative experimental research can investigate whether an arts intervention is capable of producing a desired change in the health status of participants. However, qualitative research is not well suited to measuring effects. Hence qualitative researchers do not tend to talk about outcomes or variables but rather phenomena in specific contexts. Qualitative research is useful for exploring experience and perspectives. This can include examining apparent associations and generating theory. However, while quantitative research is generally used to test theories that are established before data collection begins, qualitative research is better suited to more open-ended questions, allowing theories and models to be developed iteratively as the research proceeds. Such theories and models could potentially be tested in further quantitative research if appropriate.

Quantitative and qualitative methods are often combined in evaluation research. Mixed-methods research programmes are increasingly guided by the Medical Research Council (MRC) framework for evaluating complex interventions (Craig et al. 2008). Within this framework, qualitative methods can strengthen quantitative research in a number of ways. They can guide feasibility studies that precede and inform quantitative data collection. They can explore participants' experiences of arts activities, helping to establish whether particular interventions are acceptable to stakeholders, They can also help to clarify how observed effects are produced, revealing the processes or generative mechanisms involved.

However, some qualitative research approaches do not fit easily into this framework. Traditionally, quantitative research has derived from the standpoint of positivism, which focuses on what is observable and measurable. Researchers seeking to explore deeper questions of meaning, particularly those using 'extended epistemologies' to capture symbolic, expressive, and experiential ways of knowing (Heron and Reason 1997), may generate data that are difficult to combine with traditional quantitative research.

Research in the social sciences has also been influenced by realism, which assumes an objective reality that scientific research is increasingly coming to know. More recently, this view has softened as researchers acknowledge that the limitations of the research process mean that the truth can only be imperfectly and incrementally understood (Fox et al. 2007). While qualitative research can derive from a realist standpoint, it is also common for qualitative research to reflect a constructionist view of the world. In this, objective reality is elusive or even unknowable, since phenomena such as health and wellbeing are shaped by language and interaction in particular social contexts.

This discussion demonstrates the limitations of reducing qualitative data collection and analysis to questions of feasibility, acceptability, or modelling as suggested by the complex interventions evaluation framework. It should be borne in mind that while the framework is a useful model for evaluation research, it is not intended to encompass all research, and there are many arts-based research questions that fall outside of it.

## Sampling in qualitative research

Consideration of sampling is important in both quantitative and qualitative research. Poor attention to sampling in programme evaluation can lead to bias, since it is important to sample a wide variety of experiences and not just select participants who successfully complete projects and report positive experiences. A number of sampling approaches can be used in qualitative research. A common technique is purposive sampling, where participants or cases are selected in accordance with pre-defined criteria. In more advanced qualitative research, theoretical sampling, where participants or cases are selected as the research progresses in response to emergent theory, or until data saturation is reached, can also be used. Since the aim of sampling in qualitative research is not to ensure representativeness or eliminate bias, it is not necessary to use techniques of randomization or include control groups. However, it is important to understand the backgrounds of participants since the ability to make limited generalizations from qualitative findings depends upon a detailed knowledge of the characteristics of study participants, or cases, in relation to those of the wider study population.

## Qualitative data collection

Qualitative research is usually associated with interviews and focus groups. However, other data can be generated, for example art works, music, film, photographs, and even dance and song. We are unable to explore all of these approaches in this chapter, but we will address some of the issues around using interviews and focus groups in arts and health settings.

Qualitative data collection is usually guided by an overarching research framework. For example, interviews and focus groups undertaken as part of a grounded theory study will be different from those undertaken as part of narrative research. These two

research approaches are discussed in more detail later. The point here is that before collecting any qualitative data it is important to consider the type of analytical procedure that is likely to be undertaken.

## Interviews and focus groups

Researchers thinking about conducting one-to-one interviews need to be very clear about why they are doing them. Although research and evaluation are closely related, and indeed share similar methods, they are not the same. For example, when thinking about interviews, evaluators seek to elicit people's views about a project or programme, while researchers may wish to explore more broadly the meaning people ascribe to their experiences. Questions like these help to differentiate between evaluation and research. It is right and proper to build evaluation into every programme, but it is important not to stray from what an evaluation should be aiming to achieve. An evaluation should aim to establish whether the programme is meeting its aims. It should ask questions about the processes involved in delivering the programme and it should also ask questions about whether the aims of the programme have been met. This is why care needs to be taken when defining aims for any arts and health programme and associated evaluation. If they are ambitious (e.g. a 6-week hourly group to generate clinical outcomes such as reduced anxiety and depression, or produce outcomes related to wellbeing such as increased self-esteem) it may be extremely difficult to evaluate them qualitatively. An interview that is for evaluation will not usually try to measure outcomes but will seek qualitative feedback about participants' experiences and views about the programme. This can encompass questions about what participants gained and what they enjoyed as well as whether they believe the intended outcomes were realized. It is therefore usual to use an interview schedule asking specific questions when a service is being evaluated through interviews or focus groups.

An interview for research purposes is much more exploratory and seeks deeper revelations and stories from participants. Research interviews can follow a topic guide, but they rarely follow a detailed schedule: it is more common for them to be semi-structured or open-ended. Because qualitative research interviews often deal with sensitive issues, there is the potential for them to cause anxiety and distress for participants and researchers. This is something that arts and health researchers need to be aware of, particularly as they are likely to be working with vulnerable and disadvantaged people. In such situations the inexperienced interviewer may quickly become out of their depth. Hence it is important to think carefully about the management of qualitative interviews. Ethics committees increasingly demand that qualitative researchers consider the potential risks and have in place appropriate support systems and resources for participants and researchers should they be needed.

For evaluation purposes, it is best, wherever possible, to think about using an external evaluator,—somebody from outside the organization brought in to conduct the evaluation. This helps to bring more objectivity to the process. Participants may also be more frank or honest if it is not someone from the host organization asking the questions. It is imperative that research interviews are conducted by someone who has had research training.

For both interviews and focus groups it is usual to audio-record the meeting and, wherever possible, to transcribe the discussion verbatim. The subsequent transcripts are usually referred to as data.

Before any data are collected, it is essential to secure informed consent from the participants. This is usually done by providing people with all the information they need to decide for themselves if they wish to take part and then for them to read and sign a consent form. In the case of evaluation, it is important that any data collection complies with policies and procedures for data protection and ethical good practice. In the case of research, projects must undergo formal ethics review before they can proceed.

Although qualitative research is not guided by hypotheses, it is still important prior to data collection to have considered the type of analysis that will be used. In evaluation, descriptive reporting and thematic analysis of participants' responses is often sufficient, but this will depend on the goals and aims of the project. In qualitative research, analytical techniques can be more complicated. We now go on to discuss approaches to data analysis.

## Qualitative data analysis: common approaches in arts and health research

### Thematic analysis

While there are numerous methods of analysis available to qualitative researchers, a large number of qualitative research studies use some form of thematic analysis (Braun and Clarke 2006). In general, this proceeds through a series of stages, organizing data into initial codes from which broader themes are generated and refined. Many procedures in thematic analysis are influenced by the overarching research approach of grounded theory. This draws on the work of Corbin and Strauss (2008) and others and usually involves detailed initial coding followed by an iterative process of analysis which proceeds through stages of refinement until nothing new can be identified in the data. The aim of grounded theory is the formation of overarching categories and, ultimately, the generation of an explanatory framework. A useful example of an arts and health project that has adopted grounded theory methods is the study by Roberts et al. (2011) of the role of art-viewing as a community intervention for family carers of people with mental health problems. The constructivist grounded theory approach recognizes the existence of multiple interpretations rather than trying to determine essential truths (Charmaz 2000). An example of a study that follows a constructivist grounded theory approach is the study by Barker et al. (2009) of occupational strain affecting professional artists.

The techniques of thematic analysis are used in a wide range of research approaches, not just in grounded theory. While the generation of themes in qualitative research is sometimes characterized as an inductive process, i.e. coding proceeds in a bottom-up fashion without the imposition of prior theories or hypotheses, qualitative thematic analysis can also be led by theory, if not by specific hypotheses. Indeed, it is difficult to imagine a scenario in which the researcher starts with a completely blank slate. In reality, the generation of themes needs to be guided by the overarching research question, which tends to be broken down into a series of sub-questions as the analysis proceeds. As Braun and Clarke (2006) caution, the generation of questions for analysis requires reasonable skills of interpretation: researchers are advised against reproducing 'results' that simply reflect the headings of the topic guide that was used for interviews.

Braun and Clarke (2006) also advise researchers to consider the extent to which the generation of themes relies on semantic or latent meaning. In the former, meaning is projected from participants' accounts and is limited to the words they use. In weaker qualitative studies, participants' accounts are reproduced as 'truth' without filtering or exploration: in other words, they are not interpreted at all. Methodologies that explore latent meaning usually interpret participants' accounts in relation to wider questions, such as the influence of power relationships or the broader social context in which these accounts are generated. These approaches use thematic analysis but they tend to be considered as more advanced qualitative methods. They include constructionist approaches such as discourse analysis as well as more commonly used approaches such as narrative analysis. We will discuss examples of these later.

In summary, the popularity of thematic analysis arises from its flexibility. It can suit the underlying purposes of a wide range of approaches, including realist and constructionist approaches. It can be applied to different data sets, including primary data (information collected for the purposes of the research), secondary data (information that already exists), interviews, and focus groups as well as documentary data. It is also an approach that is accessible to novice researchers and fits relatively easily within multidisciplinary and mixed-methods research, including much arts and health evaluation. For those seeking to engage with qualitative research for the first time, Braun and Clarke (2006) provide a useful six-point guide as well as a discussion of the pitfalls of thematic analysis.

### Case study: discourse analysis

This case study discusses discourse analysis (DA) both in relation to sources of information and the choice of analytical approach. The most common forms of data in qualitative research are interviews and focus groups; however, there are many more potentially useful data sources including naturally occurring conversation, interaction, documents, images, and sounds, to name a few. This case study focuses on a piece of research in which DA was found to be particularly useful in analysing documentary data. These data were not primary data, i.e. they was not generated by the research processes but were secondary data that already existed at the start of the project and had been collected for different purposes. Doing DA is a bit like doing content analysis, but DA differs is that it can go beyond a 'face value' reading of the text. Hence it can be useful where there is a need to explore latent as well as semantic meaning (Braun and Clarke 2006). As well as identifying key themes, DA explores tensions, absences, and silences within the data.

Here we discuss a research project that included DA undertaken by Norma Daykin and Ellie Byrne as part of mixed-methods study of an arts and mental health project (Daykin et al. 2010). In a modernization project, new hospital environments included 36 integrated commissions by leading artists, along with participatory arts designed to enhance the wellbeing of patients and staff (Figs 10.1 and 10.2). We draw on the report of the documentary analysis undertaken Byrne and Daykin (Daykin et al. 2008a) which adopted DA for the analysis of 442 project documents including business, strategy and finance documents, meeting notes,

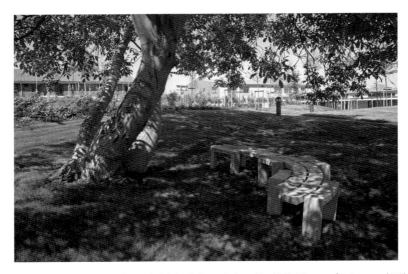

**Fig. 10.1** Walnut tree seating by Angus Ross at Callington Road Hospital, Bristol. Commissioned by Willis Newson for Avon and Wiltshire Mental Health Partnership NHS Trust.

minutes, and feedback from stakeholders following consultation events.

There are many challenges and limitations that need to be recognized in the analysis of documentary data. For example, informal meeting notes and minutes cannot always provide a complete record of all the discussions and views expressed. Similarly, data taken from comment and feedback forms may be influenced by a range of factors including group dynamics, confidentiality, and emotional or mental wellbeing. In complex projects there are likely to be conflicting views, as well as claims that some views, particularly negative ones, are not adequately recorded. In this project we addressed these concerns by combining analysis from different data sources, including interviews and focus groups, and by using Foucauldian discourse analysis (FDA), a form of DA

which emphasizes contextual issues rather than focusing solely on the meanings generated from specific texts. FDA is undertaken with reference to the wider social and political context from which documents draw meaning.

An overview of procedures used in FDA is provided by Carabine (2001). Within FDA, the word 'discourse' has two meanings. As well as a piece of text or an image, a discourse is a set of words, thoughts, and actions surrounding a particular topic. Hence discourses impact on our collective values and assumptions, helping to maintain the status of social institutions such as medicine or the law. A central premise of FDA is that knowledge and power are intimately bound; so much so that they cannot be divorced from each other in any analysis. FDA therefore looks at the way that knowledge and power are discursively incorporated our ways

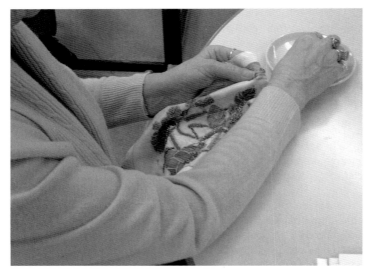

**Fig. 10.2** Older adult textile workshops led by June Heap at Callington Road Hospital, Bristol. Commissioned by Willis Newson for Avon and Wiltshire Mental Health Partnership NHS Trust.

of thinking and speaking through the ways they are textually represented. It helps to unmask how dominant groups in society promote their own interests by constructing a fitting version of reality through texts and images. It also reveals ways in which dominant versions of reality are challenged.

In this project, a structured sampling frame was used to select a sample of 10 core documents and 275 operational documents for analysis. We began by identifying broader contextual discourses that shaped the project, including 'evidence-based design' and 'patient and public involvement'. We then went on to explore specific project discourses, including: 'appropriate art', 'service user participation', and 'stigma'. This analysis strengthened the thematic analysis that we undertook from qualitative interviews with patients and staff, giving context and meaning to participants' accounts. Together, these data highlighted the value of participatory arts in providing meaningful activity, reinforcing non-stigmatized identities, and encouraging engagement (Daykin et al. 2010).

This example illustrates some of the insights that DA can provide that would not be easily gained from thematic analysis. The FDA analysis allowed us to go beyond what was represented in the texts to explore significant tensions, absences, and silences. In terms of tensions, the project seemed to be marked by an underlying conflict between notions of 'prestige', used to suggest that artworks by 'high calibre' artists were needed in order to enhance the environments and reduce stigma, and, on the other hand, 'authenticity', used to demand that artworks within mental healthcare settings should reflect the identities of those within and provide opportunities for service users to be considered as 'artists' and not just 'patients'. The FDA allowed us to trace these issues through the development of the project, mapping shifts in power and influence as stakeholders grappled with evolving definitions of 'art', 'artist', 'service user', and 'therapy'. The FDA enabled us to understand the standpoints of key stakeholders, including occupational therapists, arts therapists, and clinicians, and the influences shaping collaboration between these groups.

In terms of absences, we noted that powerful voices, such as those of finance and business partners, were relatively silent in the documents. Their perspectives did not seem to be strongly articulated as the project developed. On the other hand, the voices and views of service users were frequently recorded. However, the volume of reporting was not a true reflection of the influence that each of these groups was able to wield. A simple content analysis with no reference to contextual issues of power and stakeholding would have failed to understand the mechanisms driving the project.

A further opportunity in documentary analysis is the incorporation of diverse data sources including images and sounds. In this project, the body of data included 291 photographs taken by service users and staff depicting 'love' and 'hate' images within the mental healthcare environment. As the photographs did not include narrative, their interpretation was not straightforward. A very basic content analysis revealed that 'love' images often included scenes of nature, including open space, trees, grass, and sky. In contrast, 'hate' images often depicted concrete and urban built environments, including roads, walls, and car parks. Many of the 'hate' photographs show areas of the hospital in a poor state of cleanliness or in need of maintenance. These include dirty carpets and sink areas, broken garden furniture, and overflowing ashtrays. Service users also used the cameras to reflect on the experience of being in hospital. However, the ambiguity of these images made it difficult to know the intended meaning and we decided to undertake a further study to explore the extent to which interpretation of visual data is possible without access to accompanying text or narrative (Byrne 2013).

## Narrative research in arts and health

The word 'narrative' is widely used in arts circles. It simply means 'a story'. The way the word is used, though, implies something more than a story; it also implies that the story has meaning and purpose. In some way when we use the word 'narrative' it implies something more serious than a story. We refer to a play or book having a 'strong' or 'fragmented' narrative; we innately expect cohesion in the story, for example we like to be satisfactorily introduced to a plot and see the resolution of that plot in a conclusion to the narrative. It is argued that creating narratives (story-telling) has been fundamental to the development of human history and culture and individual identity (Benwell and Stokoe 2006), and storytelling provides meaning to events and enables people to make sense of their world. The study of narrative is the study of the ways in which human beings experience the world, that is, through the recounting and retelling of that experience. Narrative is seen as universal and intrinsic to life. 'Narrative is present in every age, in every place, in every society; it begins with the very history of mankind and there nowhere is, nor has been a people without narrative. All classes, all human groups, have their narratives ... narrative is international, transhistorical, transcultural: it is simply there, like life itself' (Barthes 1977, p. 79).

Narrative has been shown to be very important in experiences of illness. In narrative analysis (NA) the assumption that individuals seek to impose order on experience is brought to bear in the interpretation of disrupted biographies that people face when they are confronted with a threat to their wellbeing, identity, or beliefs about the life course (Bury 1982, 2001). Procedures for NA differ, but they focus on identifying stories that are not just personal, since they draw on shared linguistic and cultural resources and therefore illuminate broader questions and themes (Riessman 1993). This is illustrated in a study by Daykin (2005) which explored the stories of a small sample of musicians who experienced ill-health or other circumstances that threatened their identities as creative professionals. The research explored the way that these stories reflect and challenge received ideas about creativity. It showed some of the negative aspects of these ideas, including the idea that creativity is innate and individual, requiring significant personal sacrifice. These ideas can be used to justify poor working conditions and economic insecurity for professional musicians and artists as well as reinforce their isolation within society. The research showed that these ideas are unsustainable in the longer term. When faced with crises of vulnerability, musicians reworked their stories to embrace a more 'therapeutic' creativity; some used this as a springboard to engage with arts and health practice.

Because narrative is also central to artistic expression, it is only to be expected that narrative research has been used extensively in arts and health research. A narrative approach in research focuses upon the stories related by people; this might be through qualitative interviews or through creative expression. Once data collection is completed, the data are subjected to a NA process. There is no standard format for this, unlike with other data analysis methods; a NA might depend on one's understanding of narrative theory. A researcher may choose to interpret the data through certain theoretical or analytical lenses (see Chase 2005).

As the researcher completes his or her analysis, which inevitably involves some form of interpretation, the researcher may write up his or her findings from the analytic process. In a way, because the process involves interpretation, the researcher is regarded as co-constructing the narrative. The researcher brings to the narrative his or her own ideas, beliefs, and values. Developing a reflexive awareness of these is an important issue for researchers.

An example of an arts and health study that used the narrative approach is that by Stickley and Hui (2012). That research explored the experiences of people who have engaged with an Arts On Prescription programme in a UK city. It explored how people experience the social, psychological, and occupational impacts of arts participation. It showed that, by feeling accepted and amongst people of similar experiences, people also gain a sense of social belonging from arts participation. It also indicated that longer-term changes in identity may be stimulated by participation, with several participants going on to find new opportunities for creative activity beyond the life of the project.

A narrative approach can elicit greater depth than can be achieved through a more usual interview with a list of questions and a subsequent thematic analysis. In narrative interviewing we deliberately ask for the person's story. Through the story-telling, people may speak more openly and personally and are often highly motivated to give their story, needing little in the way of prompts from the researcher.

This is of course only a brief introduction to narrative research related to arts and health practice (for a detailed overview of the different types of NA see Murray (2003)). One important point to remember, though, is that while many people are happy to tell their stories, some people may find this painful and difficult. It is essential to provide safe and supportive environments where people do not feel pressurized in any way to contribute to research if they do not feel or think they want to, especially for those who work with vulnerable people.

## Participatory action research and participatory arts—a good fit with arts practice

Those of us who have led or taken part in arts activities will know intuitively whether or not they have been genuinely participatory. This kind of art-making invariably involves people being creative together and there exists a sense of harmony. Every ancient civilization records community-based rituals that usually involved singing, dancing, craft making, story-telling and poetry, and so on. Sometimes, because these kinds of activities involve communities of people, this approach has been referred to as *community arts*. This is in contrast to art-making that it conducted as a solitary experience or art-making that is overtly therapeutic, such as arts psychotherapy. In participatory art-making, participants become the artists, the authors, the performers. Participatory arts, when implemented well, leave participants feeling they have achieved something good. People often feel uplifted and proud

of what they have done. Participatory arts can also be politically engaged and aim to bring about change in society, as powerfully illustrated by the work of Augusto Boal (1931–2009) in his *Theatre of the Oppressed* (Boal 1979).

Participatory action research (PAR) assumes a similar philosophy; people become co-authors of the research in the same way people become artists in participatory arts activities. This is in contrast to traditional academic research where people are the subjects (or objects) of the research. In traditional research, the academics design the research and implement it in a research site; people are studied and the results of the research are published in academic journals. The academics benefit from the research, but often the people involved hear very little if anything from the researcher again. Unlike traditional research practices, PAR can also seek to bring about political change, by giving power to people to design and implement their own research. A good example in the literature is the work of Murray and Crummett (2010) which describes a participatory arts project with a group of older people, how they represented their community, and how they experienced the community arts intervention.

If PAR is done well, again, people feel an ownership of the process and may also feel valued. The approach aims to incorporate the fundamental differences in the varied stakeholder's perspectives and acknowledges that the academic or clinical researcher may have different motives from the participant.

The process of PAR is similar to action research, but places greater emphasis upon the role of the participant in the design, implementation, and dissemination of the research. Similar to action research, the process of implementation may be described as a spiral of self-reflective cycles of planning change, acting, and observing the process and consequences of the change, reflecting on these processes and consequences, re-planning, acting, and observing again, reflecting again, and so on. In reality the stages will overlap, and initial plans may become obsolete in the light of learning from experience. Each of the steps outlined in the spiral of self-reflection is undertaken collaboratively by all the stakeholders in the research process (Chevalier and Buckles 2013).

PAR demands a very different role for the researcher compared with more traditional methods. Instead of being unbiased and impartial they are expected to act from an explicit value-base and to be committed to change. This is due to PAR having the capacity to act as a basis for change. By combining research with action it has the potential to close the gap between research and practice.

## Arts-based methods

While there is a general move within research communities towards more formal and controlled methods, there is at the same time a move in the opposite direction towards methods that are flexible and diverse, including arts-based methods. The impetus for this has come from growing critiques of conventional forms of knowledge and representation. Heron and Reason (1997) outlined an 'extended epistemology' that included alternatives to 'propositional' or conceptual ways of knowing derived from the natural and social sciences. These alternatives value symbolic, expressive, experiential, and practical knowledge. This notion of extended epistemology has greatly stimulated the development of qualitative and arts-based methodologies.

The topic of arts-based methods is vast and there are too many methodologies to be reviewed here. They include creative story-telling, painting and drawing, photographic methods, film, dance, performance, and music. For those interested in exploring the subject further, there are some useful texts available, including collections by Liamptuttong and Rumbold (2008); Knowles and Cole (2008), and Leavy (2009). Here, we consider in general terms how arts-based approaches might be applied at different stages of the research process, what they might add to research and evaluation, and some of the challenges we ourselves have encountered when incorporating arts into research.

A systematic review by Fraser and al Sayah (2011) examined arts-based methods used in 30 health research studies. They found that visual arts were the most common, followed by performance arts, and literary arts. The purposes of using arts in health research were primarily for knowledge production and knowledge translation. This is borne out by our own experience. Processes of data collection can be greatly enhanced by techniques such as photo elicitation or other techniques that use arts to encourage reflection, stimulate discussion, or trigger memories. These techniques can be easily incorporated into conventional research methods such as interviews and focus groups. Similarly, the use of arts can greatly enhance the dissemination of research, whose findings can be made much more interesting and accessible to a wide audience when represented in many formats including film, imagery, and music as well as traditional reports.

The use of arts-based methods is less well developed in relation to questions of interpretation. Arts-based approaches can enhance the interpretive process by bringing in new sensory experiences, enhancing perception, engendering empathy, and evoking emotions (Eisner 2008). However, arts are by virtue ambiguous, and when it comes to art forms like music there are complex debates about whether and how meaning can be derived from them (Daykin 2008, see also Byrne 2013).

There are also a number of pitfalls in using arts-based approaches. McNiff (2008) warns that arts-based researchers can become lost when their enquiries become overly personal or over ambitious. There are times when artistic values may clash with research credibility. For example, the artist may be driven to generate a powerful narrative whereas the researcher may wish to treat data comprehensively, as advised by Silverman (2011) in order to strengthen credibility and fully explore emergent theories. There may be ethical conflicts. For example, artistic conventions value ownership and authorship but when it comes to artworks made by study participants, research conventions value confidentiality and anonymity. These issues need to be carefully navigated when using arts-based methods. However, it is our experience that the use of arts-based approaches can bring projects to life, creating enjoyable experiences for participants, enhancing collaboration, and adding both value and meaning to the research process.

## Ethics in qualitative research

Naturally, all participatory arts practitioners endeavour to work in an ethical way. At the heart of any kind of arts for health initiative would be a desire to do good and to do no harm. It is easy, though, to make assumptions about the people with whom one works. For example, a client or patient may have once agreed to have their photograph taken for a leaflet, but might be surprised 6 months later to see that photograph on a website. Of course, good practice in this situation would require the artist to get written consent to cover such use of a photograph, both at the time and, if possible, later on as well if it is used for more than one purpose. This may not be always possible, but nevertheless one should always get some kind of written consent for such use. Another example of when consent should be sought might be when photographing someone's artwork and using it for your own publicity or (as we have done) used people's artworks in books or journals or conference presentations. It could be argued that academics and practitioners can exploit artworks made by research participants for their own gain. Working ethically in practice is complex and we may not always think in advance about potential ethical dilemmas.

In arts and health research there are also many potential ethical minefields. We would emphasize the point that any kind of research that is conducted in practice should have previously been granted ethical approval from an ethics committee. But we need to be clear about how research is defined. Some people may refer to research in a casual way such as: 'I'm going to do some research on singing with people with dementia'. This kind of research may involve Internet searches, reading books and journal articles, etc. Of course, this kind of documentary research does not require ethical approval. Other practitioners may be conducting an evaluation and they mistakenly refer to it as 'research'. Evaluating an arts and health project would not normally be referred to as research because evaluation, such as measuring outcomes against objectives does not normally need ethical approval. However, if a practitioner (or academic) conducts an evaluation and then seeks to get it published as research, then they should have acquired ethical approval from an ethics committee.

## Acquiring ethical approval from an ethics committee

Any research that involves human participants, whether or not they are healthcare clients, requires approval by an appropriate ethics committee or institutional review board. In this way, the researcher is not only ensuring that their data collection method is ethical but is also acquiring some kind of endorsement for their study and providing an additional safeguard for participants. Ethics committees are made up of individuals with wide-ranging experiences and they can offer useful insights and raise awareness of issues that researchers may not have considered. In most countries individual hospitals or local health and social care authorities have an ethics review procedure. These are often found on the Internet or by contacting the hospital directly. Similarly, most health faculties of universities also have ethics committees that can be approached.

In the United Kingdom any research conducted on National Health Service (NHS) patients requires NHS ethics approval. Research in the social care sector is subject to ethics review. The UK Health Research Authority (<http://www.hra.nhs.uk>) is a useful source of information about the principles and procedures that underpin ethical research.

In community-based studies it is important to establish whether or not participants are healthy volunteers. In other words, are the people we wish to study patients in some kind of health service or are they 'well' members of the public? It is a grey area, because although researchers may access the participants of the study through community resources the participants may also be users of health services. The message is, if in doubt ask! The chairperson of an ethics committee is usually very approachable and can advise at an early stage whether or not a research project might need to acquire ethical approval.

In summary, research processes can be complicated, including the decision whether or not ethical approval is required from an ethics committee. On occasions ethical approval may not be 'needed' but it may be helpful to acquire it as the process can clarify issues and strengthen research design. One final note is that if in the future you wish to get your work published most journals will expect a comment on ethics and usually only publish studies that have acquired ethical approval from an ethics committee.

## Concluding thoughts

This chapter has reviewed key issues and methodologies for qualitative research, identifying the strengths and challenges of these in arts and health contexts, including evaluation research. We have sought to clarify the distinct purposes of qualitative as opposed to quantitative methods. While we have been unable to cover the entire range of qualitative methods, we have drawn attention to some common issues and highlighted the need for rigorous procedures and clear reporting of sampling, data collection, data analysis, and ethical issues.

While qualitative research is not subjected to the same procedures for testing validity and reliability as those used in quantitative research, the claims made by qualitative researchers need to be credible, and transparent research procedures can enhance credibility. Silverman (2011) argues that if rigorous procedures are applied, including close attention to sampling, comprehensive data treatment, and deviant case analysis, qualitative research can be generalized within defined parameters and can therefore produce meaningful results to inform policy and practice. Beyond this there is no clear agreement about the specific procedures to be adopted, and different qualitative methods may require different procedures. Those embarking on a qualitative study may wish to consult with one of a number of available guidelines and checklists covering areas such as research design, sampling, data collection, data analysis, reporting, reflexivity, ethics, auditability, relevance to policy, and practice. Examples include structured tools by the Critical Appraisal Skills Programme (CASP) (2014) and the Quality Framework (Spencer et al. 2003).

This chapter has demonstrated the breadth and richness of qualitative methods, which can make a strong contribution to the development of the evidence base surrounding arts and health as well as addressing broader questions about the meaning and experience of arts, health, and society.

# References

Barker, K.K., Soklaridis, S., Waters, I., Herr, G., and Cassidy, J.D. (2009). Occupational strain and professional artists: a qualitative study of an underemployed group. *Arts & Health: An International Journal for Research, Policy and Practice*, **1**, 136–150.

Barthes, R (1977) Introduction to the structural analysis of narratives. In: *Roland Barthes, Image-Music-Text* (transl. S. Heath), pp. 79–124. Glasgow: Collins.

Boal, A (1979). *Theatre of the Oppressed*. London: Pluto Press.

Benwell, B. and Stokoe, E. (2006). *Discourse and Identity*. Edinburgh: Edinburgh University Press.

Braun, V. and Clarke, V. (2006). Using thematic analysis in psychology. *Qualitative Research in Psychology*, **3**, 77–101.

Bury, M. (1982). Chronic illness as biographical disruption. *Sociology of Health and Illness*, **4**, 167–182.

Bury, M. (2001). Illness narratives: fact or fiction? *Sociology of Health and Illness*, **23**, 263–285.

Byrne, E. (2013). Visual data in qualitative research: the use of photography to evaluate mental health hospital environments. Unpublished PhD Thesis. University of the West of England, Bristol.

Carabine, J. (2001). Unmarried motherhood 1830–1990: a genealogical analysis. In M. Wetherell, S. Taylor, and S. Yates (eds), *Discourse as Data: A Guide for Analysis.*, pp. 267–307. London: Sage.

Critical Appraisal Skills Programme (CASP) (2013). *10 Questions to Help You Make Sense of Qualitative Research*. Available from: <http://media.wix.com/ugd/dded87_951541699e9edc71ce66c9bac4734c69.pdf> (accessed 19 March 2014).

Charmaz, K. (2000). Grounded theory: objectivist and constructivist methods. In: N.K. Denzin and Y.S. Lincoln (eds), *Handbook of Qualitative Research*, 2nd edn, pp. 509–535. Thousand Oaks, CA: Sage.

Chase, S.E. (2005). Narrative inquiry: multiple lenses, approaches, voices. In: N.K. Denzin and Y.S. Lincoln (eds), *The Sage Handbook of Qualitative Research*, 3rd edn, pp. 651–679. London: Sage.

Chevalier, J.M. and Buckles, D.J. (2013). *Participatory Action Research: Theory and Methods for Engaged Inquiry*. London: Routledge.

Corbin, J. and Strauss, A. (2008). *Basics of Qualitative Research: Techniques and Procedures for Developing Grounded Theory*. London: Sage.

Craig, P., Dieppe, P., Macintyre, S., Michie, S., Nazareth, I., and Petticrew, M. (2008). *Developing and Evaluating Complex Interventions: New Guidance*. Medical Research Council. Available at: <http://www.mrc.ac.uk/documents/pdf/complex-interventions-guidance/> (accessed 27 September 2013).

Daykin, N. (2005). Disruption, dissonance and embodiment: creativity, health and risk in music narratives. *Health: An Interdisciplinary Journal for the Social Study of Health, Illness and Medicine*, **9**, 67–87.

Daykin, N. (2008). Knowing through music. In: P. Liamputtong and J. Rumbold (eds), *Knowing Differently. Arts-Based and Collaborative Research Methods*, pp. 229–244. New York: Nova Science Publishers.

Daykin, N., Byrne, E., Soteriou, T., and O'Connor, S. (2008a). *Building on the Evidence: Qualitative Research on the Impact of Arts in Mental Health Care*. Final Report. Department of Health Pathfinder Project Report P (05) 07. Bristol: University of the West of England. Available at: <http://hsc.uwe.ac.uk/net/research/data/sites/1/movingoneval%20jan08.pdf> (accessed 19 March 2014).

Daykin, N., Orme, J., Evans, D., and Salmon, D. [with McEachran, M. and Brain, S.] (2008b). The impact of participation in performing arts on adolescent health and behaviour: a systematic review of the literature. *Journal of Health Psychology*, **13**, 251–264.

Daykin, N., Byrne, E., Soteriou, T., and O'Connor, S. (2010). Using arts to enhance mental healthcare environments: findings from qualitative research. *Arts and Health: An International Journal of Research, Policy and Practice*, **2**, 33–46.

Daykin, N., Moriarty, Y., de Viggiani, N., and Pilkington, P. (2011). *Evidence Review: Music Making with Young Offenders and Young People at Risk of Offending. Report for Youth Music*. Bristol: University of the West of England. Available at: <http://www.youthmusic.org.uk/assets/files/Research/YM_YoungOffenders_web.pdf> (accessed 12 March 2015).

Daykin, N., Moriarty, Y., de Viggiani, N., and Pilkington, P. (2013). Music making for health, wellbeing and behaviour change in youth justice settings: a systematic review. *Health Promotion International*, **28**, 197–210.

Eisner, E. (2008). Art and knowledge. In: J.G. Knowles and A.L. Cole (eds), *Handbook of the Arts in Qualitative Research*, pp. 3–12. London: Sage.

Fox, M., Martin, P., and Green, G. (2007). *Doing Practitioner Research*. London: Sage.

Fraser, K.D. and al Sayah, F. (2011). Arts based methods in health: a systematic review of the literature. *Arts and Health: an International Journal of Research, Policy and Practice*, **3**, 110–145.

Heron, J. and Reason, P. (1997). A participatory inquiry paradigm. *Qualitative Inquiry*, **3**, 274–294.

Knowles, J.G. and Cole, A.L. (eds) (2008). *Handbook of the Arts in Qualitative Research*. London: Sage.

Leavy, P. (ed.) (2009). *Method Meets Art: Arts-Based Research Practice*. London: Guildford Press.

Liamptuttong, P. and Rumbold, J. (eds) (2008). *Knowing Differently. Arts-Based and Collaborative Research Methods*. New York: Nova Science Publishers.

McNiff, S. (2008). Arts-based research. In: J.G. Knowles and A.L. Cole (eds), *Handbook of the Arts in Qualitative Research*, pp. 29–40. London, Sage.

Murray, M. (2003). Narrative psychology and narrative analysis. In: P.M. Camic, J.E. Rhodes and L. Yardley (eds), *Qualitative Research in Psychology: Expanding Perspectives in Methodology and Design*, pp. 95–112. Washington, DC: American Psychological Association.

Murray, M. and Crummett, A. (2010). 'I don't think they knew we could do these sorts of things': social representations of community and participation in community arts by older people. *Journal of Health Psychology*, **15**, 777–785.

Riessman, C.K. (1993). *Narrative Analysis*. London: Sage.

Roberts, S., Camic, P.M., and Springham, N. (2011). New roles for art galleries: art-viewing as a community intervention for family carers of people with mental health problems, *Arts & Health: An International Journal for Research, Policy and Practice*, **3**, 146–159.

Silverman, D. (2011). *Interpreting Qualitative Data*. London: Sage.

Spencer. L., Ritchie, J., Lewis, J., and Dillon, L. (2003). *Quality in Qualitative Evaluation: A Framework for Assessing Research Evidence* [online monograph]. London: Cabinet Office. Available at: <http://dera.ioe.ac.uk/21069/2/a-quality-framework-tcm6-38740.pdf> (accessed 12 March 2015).

Stickley, T. and Hui, A. (2012). Social prescribing through arts on prescription in a UK city: participants' perspectives (Part one). *Public Health*, **126**, 574–579.

# CHAPTER 11

# Ethical issues in arts-based health research

Susan M. Cox and Katherine M. Boydell

## Overview of ethical issues in arts-based health research

The arts are powerful mediators in our understanding and experience of health and wellbeing. Increasingly, the arts are also employed as an innovative method of doing research and disseminating the findings of studies employing more traditional methods (Cox et al. 2010). Some benefits of using the arts in research include greater attention to the meaning and experience of health, illness, and the body and increased ability to convey research findings in a way that captivates target audiences and facilitates change in healthcare practice.

The use of the arts in research—arts-based health research (ABHR)—is a positive development but it also raises new ethical challenges for researchers, artists, patients, and other participants (Boydell et al. 2012b). For example, in research employing theatre, research participants may feel uncomfortable with the interpretations that actors give to their words unless they are meaningfully involved in co-creation of the play (Lafrenière et al. 2013). Playwrights, on the other hand, may wish to dramatize specific elements in order to effectively convey their insights and create an aesthetically powerful piece. Another example comes from the use of photography and visual arts. Research participants taking photos or creating artwork as part of their participation in a project may wish to identify themselves by name as artists, yet the images may reveal potentially sensitive or even stigmatizing information about them that research ethics boards (REBs) would argue should remain confidential (Boydell et al. 2012a).

There are currently few guidelines that address such challenges arising in ABHR (Lafrenière et al. 2012) and there is a poor fit between existing ethical guidelines and the needs of health researchers using ABHR. One obstacle to creating appropriate guidelines is that ABHR can involve a broader and very different range of participants from more traditional research. This requires the rethinking of typical research roles as it may no longer be appropriate for researchers to maintain control over collaboratively generated data or for research participants to provide consent in advance of actually experiencing what is involved in using the arts to document their health and/or illness experience.

This chapter identifies a range of ethical challenges arising throughout the life cycle of ABHR, from research design through to dissemination of the findings. Key issues are illustrated through examples drawn from the authors' and others' research and possible responses to these challenges are identified. Questions for discussion highlight useful topics for teaching and for deepening understanding between research collaborators.

## Arts-based health research

Arts-based research refers to the use of any art form (or combinations thereof) at any point in the research process in generating, interpreting, and/or communicating knowledge (Knowles and Cole 2008). Within health research, ABHR refers to the use of any art form(s) to identify and describe, understand and interpret, represent and communicate social and individual experiences of health and illness across the life span.

### Benefits of ABHR

ABHR initiatives continue to emerge as insightful approaches to social inquiry and represent innovation in qualitative research (Cox et al. 2010; Boydell et al. 2012a). Artistic forms of expression offer different ways of thinking about research processes, alternative ways of working with colleagues and research participants, and a variety of forms for representing and sharing research findings. Thus there are many reasons why health researchers are making creative use of the arts, both in doing research and in disseminating research findings.

There has been a recent steady increase in the number and variety of health research projects adopting arts-based approaches to conducting research and/or disseminating research findings (Sonke et al. 2009; Cox et al. 2010; Wreford 2010). One important reason for this growth is that ABHR offers a means of expanding our understanding of health and social care, obtaining new insights about experiences of illness, such as how it feels to live with heart disease (Guillemin and Drew 2010) or how life changes as we age and the body declines (Pauwels 2010). Arts-based methods also highlight the human aspects of medicine and healthcare that help to reduce interdisciplinary barriers and improve our understanding of health and medicine. ABHR can also open up opportunities for those voices that are not heard as a result of culture, language, disability, or other forms of marginalization.

The arts reach out and speak to people about health, illness, and the body in powerful ways and hence have great potential to capture public interest in a range of health-related topics

(Lafrenière and Cox 2010, 2012, 2013). They offer alternative ways of producing and communicating research findings and best practices in healthcare (Keen and Todres 2007; Parsons and Boydell 2012) and expanding representational opportunities as a more fully embodied response is invited from research participants and audiences of the work (Boydell et al. 2012c). Thus research becomes more accessible to a wider range of stakeholders (Colantonio et al. 2008). ABHR shows great promise in health research translation: it has been shown to increase knowledge about the illness (Piko and Bak 2006; Fleming et al. 2009), raise awareness (Streng et al. 2004; Frith and Harcourt 2007), offer therapeutic benefit (Wang and Pies 2004; Thompson et al. 2008), and encourage participant empowerment (Frith and Harcourt 2007; Catalani and Minkler 2010). In the dissemination of research, arts-based approaches stimulate public engagement (Nisker et al. 2006; Cox et al. 2009), increase knowledge about health issues (Roberts et al. 2007), mobilize research to the scientific (Lafrenière et al. 2012) and broader community (Wang and Pies 2004; Levin et al. 2007; Vaughn et al. 2008), and change attitudes (Herman and Larkey 2006) and behaviour (Bosompra 2007).

Research-based collaborations between artists and health researchers can offer stimulating potential for crossing interdisciplinary boundaries, moving beyond traditional research dissemination, and developing innovative types of research (e.g. Kontos and Naglie 2006; Mitchell et al. 2006; Belliveau 2007; Boydell and Jackson 2010; Boydell 2011a,b; Parsons and Lavery 2012). This work opens up the way to explore creative forms of research that reflect the richness and complexity of health data and invite multiple levels of engagement that are cognitive, sensory, emotional, and aesthetic.

### Challenges of ABHR

We are at a crossroads in the use of ABHR. Despite its many benefits, there remain a great many challenges for researchers as well as artists, policy-makers, and members of REBs. The arts are not a panacea, and ABHR ought not to be embraced uncritically. Unfortunately, however, there is little critical inquiry into, reflection on, or debate about the use of arts in research (Fraser and al Sayah 2011; Boydell et al. 2012a). For example, the methodological, aesthetic, collaborative, funding, and other challenges inherent in doing this work need to be reflected on critically. Arts-based research is currently under-theorized and the methodological challenges and benefits have rarely been addressed (Knowles and Cole 2008; Boydell et al. 2012a). Pauwels (2010, p. 548) comments that, 'few authors have ventured to provide an analytical and integrated approach' to arts-based research, focusing instead on specific modes or techniques (e.g. photo-elicitation) or presentational forms (e.g. film). There is a significant need to address issues of knowledge creation, knowledge dissemination, and impact, while also focusing on the theoretical and methodological challenges of engaging in ABHR. A more refined analytical and synthetic approach is required in order to contribute to conceptual and methodological grounding of the field and provide an evidence base for this work. There is also a need to identify appropriate methods of evaluating the validity of research in light of the differing norms and values of the artistic and scholarly world (Knowles and Cole 2008). These differing norms and values also give rise to tensions in how research and /or artistic

practice ought to be conducted; hence there is also an urgent need to examine the ethical challenges introduced by ABHR (Boydell et al. 2012b).

### Ethical issues arising in ABHR

Mounting evidence indicates that greater attention needs to be devoted to the ethical aspects of ABHR. Three recent articles reviewing the scope and significance of ABHR conclude that knowledge about the methodologies of ABHR is increasing rapidly; however, many ethical challenges remain to be addressed (Cox et al. 2010; Fraser and al Sayah 2011; Boydell et al. 2012a). There are few existing ethical guidelines for ABHR, and those that do exist are not as explicit as they need to be to provide solid guidance. Some key ethical issues warranting renewed attention include ownership of the products of artistic collaboration and the risks associated with the identifiability of participants. There is also a need to focus on related methodological and aesthetic issues of appropriate methods for analysing artistically generated data and criteria for assessing the trustworthiness and/or quality of ABHR.

REBs and funding agencies are also identifying the need for study and guidance in this area. For instance in Canada during the last round of revisions to the policy document governing the ethics of research (the Tri-Council Policy Statement or TCPS2), a special chapter on the arts was recommended by a committee chaired by Mary Blackstone et al. (2008) in recognition of the numbers of researchers from a wide range of disciplines—not just traditional Fine Arts disciplines—currently using creative practices in their research.

## Procedural ethics and ethics in practice

It is helpful here to make a distinction between procedural ethics and research ethics in practice. *Procedural ethics* involves obtaining approval from a relevant ethics committee to undertake research with human subjects. This process of ethical approval typically includes consideration of the potential risks to research participants and balancing research benefits against those risks, the strategies required to safeguard confidentiality of data, and the inclusion of consent forms and plain language statements in the material provided to participants to ensure that their consent is both meaningful and voluntary.

Not all issues that have ethical significance in research can or should be subject to procedural ethics. *Research ethics in practice (microethics)* refers to the day-to-day ethical issues that arise in the practice doing of research—difficult, often subtle, and usually unpredictable situations. These issues are typically not addressed in applications to research ethics committees and represent events that are not easily anticipated when applying for approval. Guillemin and Gillam (2004) note that procedural ethics cannot alone provide all that is required for addressing *ethically important moments* in qualitative research. Likewise, White and Belliveau (2010) suggest that the ethical implications of arts-based work should not be regarded as potential distractions or obstructions, or as a responsibility that is solely addressed prior to the actual undertaking of research. Ethically important moments arise throughout the research process and, thus, researchers must maintain a critical awareness of emergent ethical dilemmas and explicitly raise these issues with participants as an integral part of the research.

## Ethical challenges and creative solutions

We now illustrate some of the challenges encountered in our work and the work of others using different art genres both to conduct research and to disseminate research findings. We also identify possible strategies to address these issues. Table 11.1 summarizes these examples and identifies key ethical concerns.

### Co-creation of a mural by young people with psychosis

Boydell (2013) used mural art to provide young people with psychosis with an opportunity to visually depict their help-seeking experience (Fig. 11.1). Young people worked with an artist facilitator over 8 days. The REB for the institution required that the anonymity of the young people be preserved. However, the research team was faced with a dilemma. On the one hand they had concerns that to remain invisible was to perpetuate the stigma of

mental illness. They noted that several participants wanted to have their names in the public domain as they were proud of their work and felt that it was one way to create awareness and understanding of the experience of psychosis and, hopefully, decrease stigma. Conversely, several members of the research team had concerns about identifiability with some of the very intimate and personal experience stories in the public sphere. They worried about the possibility of this resulting in harm. They wanted to ensure that participants were fully aware of the possible ramifications of being identified as a young person with psychosis. Would young people feel the same way about being identified in 10 years' time? Might this affect future job opportunities? If REBs view research participants as vulnerable, does that mean that confidentiality should be required? What if the key research purpose is to empower individuals and allow a space for sharing their personal stories?

### Photovoice study with women experiencing partner violence

Ponic and Jategaonkar's (2012) photovoice study with women experiencing partner violence represents an example of a feminist participatory action research project that used arts-based methods. It aimed to document and take action to address barriers to housing faced by women who have left abusive relationships. Forty-five women in four rural communities were provided with cameras and asked to take photos as data. Meanings were ascribed to these photos during photo-elicitation interviews in which the women engaged in group discussions as a form of knowledge generation and consciousness raising. The authors identified four major barriers to housing for these women, including unsafe housing, the health effects of violence, poverty, and persistent patterns of revictimization. They acknowledge the complex ethical tensions inherent when involving vulnerable groups in research that aims to use the data in local knowledge exchange and action activities that may place them at increased risk in their communities.

A variety of ethical challenges are particular to the use of photographs as data in the case of women who have left abusive relationships. For example, when the photos are shown in public venues they may uncover identities and experiences that could evoke negative reactions from ex-partners, families, friends, and other community members. In this study, such concerns were heightened because the research took place in small towns in which individuals had an increased chance of knowing one another and recognizing a place or person depicted in a photo. The researchers worried that this could negatively affect a research participant's access to resources in the community.

Consequently, participant training was incorporated in the research and included presentations and discussion on the study context and goals, an overview of photovoice research, the confidentiality and safety implications of taking photos for research, procedures for providing ongoing consent, and legal and privacy guidelines for taking photos of individuals and public places. Women were encouraged to think carefully about the safety and confidentiality implications of their decisions. They collectively explored alternative ways to depict their ideas with less risk—this resulted in use of metaphor to convey the barriers encountered with respect to their housing situation. Instead of having the women take pictures of the rundown building they lived in—which might place them at risk if they lived in a small town and their landlord saw the pictures—they used metaphoric photos. For example, one

**Table 11.1** Key ethical concerns arising from recent research

| Research study | Artistic genre | Stage of research | Ethical issues |
|---|---|---|---|
| Mural co-creation by young people with psychosis (Boydell 2011b; Boydell et al. 2012) | Visual arts; mural | Knowledge dissemination | Confidentiality <br> Anonymity <br> Stigma and other potential harm |
| Photovoice study with women experiencing partner violence (Boydell 2013) | Visual arts; photographs | Knowledge creation and dissemination | Consent <br> Confidentiality <br> Anonymity <br> Risk of violence and other harm |
| Dance representing pathways to care for youth with psychosis (Ponic and Jategaokar 2011) | Performative arts; dance | Knowledge dissemination | Aesthetic qualities versus research validity <br> Audience misinterpretation and potential harm |
| Found poetry about experiences of being a human subject in health research (Lafrenière et al. 2013) | Literary arts; found poetry | Knowledge creation and dissemination | Informed consent <br> Authorship and ownership of artistic works <br> Validity of research representations |
| Poetry and photography installation about patient narratives of heart disease (Lapum et al. 2012a) | Literary and visual arts; photos, poems | Knowledge dissemination | Dangerous emotional terrain and risk <br> Audience vulnerability |
| Risky moments in applied theatre with children experiencing dialysis (Walsh and Ledgard 2013) | Performative, literary and visual arts; poems, paintings, monologues | Knowledge creation and dissemination | Participant safety <br> Risk and empowerment <br> Trust and professional judgment |

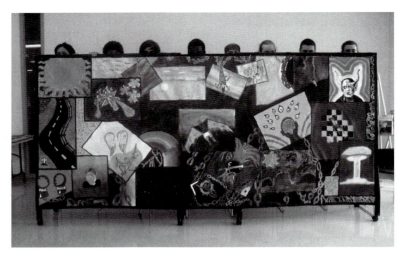

**Fig. 11.1**  A mural installation.
Reproduced by kind permission of Katherine Boydell. Copyright © 2015 Katherine Boydell.

metaphoric photo depicting discrimination as a barrier to housing included an image of a hand reaching for a house key and a large boot stepping on the hand that was reaching out and another depicting poverty as a barrier included an image of an old pair of ripped jeans. Consent was conceptualized as an ongoing process that helped to keep awareness of the possible risks and rewards of involvement at the forefront. (See Clark et al. (2010) for a further discussion about ethical issues in image-based research.)

### Dance representing pathways to mental healthcare for young people experiencing psychosis

Concerns regarding the potential for (mis)interpretation surfaced in a research-based dance project (Boydell 2011a) created as a research dissemination strategy based on an in-depth examination of pathways to mental healthcare for young people experiencing psychosis. It included 60 qualitative interviews with young people and their significant others (including parents, general practitioners, friends, psychiatrists, teachers, and case managers) involved in the pathway. Findings highlighted the complexity and connectedness of the family, school, community, and treatment system in the lives of young people.

The experience of creating the dance emphasized ongoing adjustments made as the choreography was scripted. The struggle between the content and the aesthetic qualities of the dance was paramount in this process—the issue of balancing didactic and aesthetic claims. What may have been sacrificed for the sake of performance and what may have been sacrificed for the sake of the research were questioned by the members of the research and creative teams. For example, would leaving the performance open to a greater level of interpretation result in a product that was less true to the research? We arrived at a mutual agreement that it was essential to maintain the integrity of key features of the experience; however, the ways in which to do this were frequently ambiguous. When the dance was performed at an international symposium on early psychosis one audience member stated 'But I think psychosis is more isolating and lonely than portrayed—patients would love to be able to have that sense of contact with one another'. This example highlights the dangers of misinterpretation—it indicates

that psychosis is an isolating experience and the audience member questioned the interaction that occurs among dancers throughout the performance. The research team emphasized to the creative team that lots of interaction was needed because we wanted to depict the fact that the pathway to care is *not* an individual decision-making process, that there are many 'others' involved, whether they represent a help or hindrance to the help-seeking process.

Misguided assumptions by audience members regarding the association between violence and mental illness were also uncovered as one audience member noted the performance was 'Moving, excellent, wonderful for cross-cultural work reaching public and high school students. I am a little concerned that the first image was a violent one with markers depicted as knives'. The dancers begin the performance by using large markers to write the key concepts/themes from the research on each other's white T-shirts. Some of these themes reflecting the help-seeking process included 'stigma', 'hope', 'holding back', and 'reaching out'. Unfortunately one audience member mistook the markers for knives. Upon reading this comment, the research team was concerned that the dance had the potential to perpetuate stigma rather than reduce it, but they have since come to believe that it is an important function of the dance performance to open up the space to have these types of dialogue with the audience (Boydell 2011b). Should audience members be made aware in advance of the emotional or other effects an artistic work could have for them, specifically, the potential for distress?

### Found poetry about experiences of being a participant in health research

The experiences of people who volunteer to participate in health research have, despite the attention given to research ethics, been largely neglected. A pilot project using several artistic genres to represent the experiences of research participants illustrates several emerging ethical challenges in the use of ABHR, both for knowledge creation and dissemination. The project was part of a 5-year study entitled 'Centring the Human Subject in Health Research: Understanding the Meaning and Experience

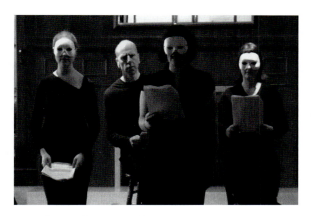

**Fig. 11.2** Performing *The Human Subject*.
Reproduced by kind permission of Susan M. Cox. Copyright © 2015 Susan M. Cox.

of Research Participation'. Two researchers (Cox and Lafrenière) coordinated an interdisiplinary group of scholars and professional artists in creating works in one of four artistic forms—'found' poetry, drama, song, or visual arts. These creative works were based on selected portions of the verbatim transcripts arising from previously conducted in-depth interviews with research participants, all of whom consented to have their interview material used in this way. The project involved more than 50 artist collaborators who worked over an 18-month period. The works were integrated to create a 40-minute performance piece that was performed for participants in the research and the wider community (Fig. 11.2). Assessment of audience responses was carried out through survey methods and short open-ended interviews conducted after each performance (Lafrenière and Cox 2012). All stages of the research and artistic creation were approved by the relevant REB.

A number of ethical challenges can be identified with the use of 'found' poetry. With found poetry 'the researcher uses only the words of the participant(s) to create a poetic rendition of a story or phenomenon' (Butler-Kisber 2002, p. 232). The technique is therefore appropriate where researchers want to give voice to neglected experiences. It can also be easily deployed with participants who have little experience in writing more conventional poetry. As Lafrenière and Cox (2013, p. 328) explain:

> 'We decided . . . to write found poetry as opposed to other genres because we thought it would, on the one hand, be less intimidating if they were using the existing words of the human subjects, and on the other hand, it would ensure that the voices of initial research participants were 'heard'.'

Found poetry workshops were held with scientists, philosophers, and graduate and undergraduate students. Participation was voluntary and required no prior knowledge of research ethics or experience with writing poetry. Consent was obtained from participants in these workshops and permission was sought to display/perform and/or publish, totally or in part, any poems created during the workshop.

The 39 poems arising from the workshops were the co-creations of the people who participated in the research interviews, the researchers who conducted the interviews, and the poetry workshop participants who 'found' the poems within the transcript excerpts provided to them. The process of creative collaboration

leading to the generation of found poetry therefore raises a whole set of questions relating to authorship and ownership of the work, consent to use the work, and the truthfulness or adequacy of the poem as a representation of participants' experiences. Who is/are the author(s) of 'found' poems such as these? Must all parties consent to have the poem displayed or performed? Should research participants have an opportunity to review and/or approve the poems before they are displayed, performed, or published? If the found poems deviate from the intended emphasis of research participants, are they still valid research representations? Who ought to make such determinations?

## Poetry and photography installation about patient narratives of heart surgery

The work of Lapum et al. (2012a,b) provides an example of the use of poetry and photography in the dissemination of patient narratives of heart surgery and recovery. Based on study results, they engaged in an arts-informed secondary analysis to design a product to highlight the experiential and subjective qualities of illness. The authors translated participants' stories into poetry and photographic imagery, displayed as a three-dimensional sculptural installation. As they aimed to physically and emotionally engage the audience, stories were aesthetically translated into an installation of poetry and photography designed as a winding path. Sixteen participants undergoing heart surgery were recruited via a hospital pre-operative clinic. Two semi-structured interviews were conducted with each participant between 48 and 96 hours after surgery and 4 to 6 weeks following discharge.

Results were based on analysis of the 32 interview transcripts and 94 journal entries; based on this analysis, composite poetry was composed based on words taken directly from participants' interviews and journals. Following team discussion, concepts for the photographic imagery were developed, drawn from recurring themes and motifs generated from research data and the poetic text. The imagery provided metaphorical representations of emotional and embodied patient experiences. Subjects in the photographs were volunteer models, rather than original research participants. The final product included 13 poems and 35 photographic images, combined in textile compositions and housed within seven sections of a 1739 square-foot installation. (The installation can be viewed online at <https://www.youtube.com/watch?v=pYcSmsRW21g>.)

With the intention of immersing the audience in the emotions, fears, and trauma of heart transplant patients there arise the ethical challenges associated with the danger of encountering difficult, emotionally charged, risky, and traumatic issues which have the potential to lead to crisis. In arts-informed work, the goal is often to push viewers beyond their typical comfort zones and expose them to varied perspectives and experiences in a meaningful manner. Although audience response is generally positive and the experience of sharing research results via art genres has an informative, liberating, and empowering effect (Sinding et al. 2005), the dangers of dramatizing certain topics to vulnerable audiences must be considered (Mienczakowski 2003). Should ethics protocols attempt to constrain artists by ensuring that they avoid so-called dangerous emotional grounds or are the provocative aspects of such work simply part and parcel of what art ought to do?

## Risky moments in applied theatre with children

Walsh and Ledgard's (2013) insightful exploration of 'risky moments' emerging from the use of applied theatre with young people illustrates some of the risks as well as the powerful impact the arts can have for all participants. 'For the Best', a site-specific performance created by Mark Storor and Anna Ledgard, involved the delivery of one-to-one and group activities for children undergoing dialysis in a renal unit at a London hospital. This stage of the work resulted in creation of paintings, poetry, and monologues that were then translated into participatory activities for workshops with 60 children in two London primary schools. The aim was to engage the young people who could not attend school with their at-school peers. The final phase of the project involved development of a performance with actors at the Unicorn Theatre, the premiere venue for children's theatre in London, about the effects of long-term critical illness for a fictionalized family. Maintaining the integrity of the original stories and images created by the children, this performance allowed the materials to appear in 'a multilayered and exaggerated form in the performance—often strikingly—in the voices of the children themselves' (Walsh and Ledgard 2013, p. 217).

What is perhaps most unusual about this project is Storor's method of reframing the traumatic elements of the children's experiences through the use of metaphor and imagery. He is not attempting to represent trauma or tell the story of one participant, but rather to incorporate the many contributions of participants into a learning space wherein participants encounter themselves experiencing precarious situations. In one workshop, the at-school children encounter a ferocious tiger that they must attempt to get past and into a safe space. Many children attempt to placate the tiger but cannot get past. A brave young girl talks to the tiger and then attempts to climb up the climbing frame to reach the safe space, the tiger nipping at her heels. The child is, according to Walsh and Ledgard (2013, p. 223), 'clearly genuinely frightened and at the same time absolutely determined'. This raises many questions for those responsible for the production and for the safety of the children in the school. The child is a performer in this unfolding drama and she is highly motivated to overcome the obstacle and get to a safe space. As Walsh and Ledgard (2013, p. 223) ask, 'What are the risks? Who is really taking a risk? How important to the learning of the children is the risk? How important to the artistic process?' The apparent risks are, however, managed through the close attention given to monitoring and communication amongst the actor performing the tiger, the producer, and the deputy head of the school. They have evolved a kind of split-second responsiveness around how the performance can be modified to allow the risk, uphold the child's agency, and encourage learning in a safe way. In this example, the tiger responds to the brave girl's whistling and becomes docile, causing the class to shout out that the tiger is listening. This moment of learning 'highlights the fragility of arts processes within schools and the need to trust split-second judgments by professionals' (Walsh and Ledgard 2013, p. 223).

## Discussion

The ethical challenges encountered in using mural art, photography, dance, found poetry, and a multimedia installation highlight both procedural ethics and ethics in practice issues. The latter are the day-to-day ethical issues that surface when engaged in the 'doing' of the research, issues that are typically unaddressed in REB applications and not always anticipated when applying for approval.

The examples include projects where the focus is on generating data (as in the case of the mural) as well as projects whose aim is dissemination (in the case of the multimedia installation) of empirical research findings. They demonstrate difficulties in determining ownership of the work, ensuring whether representation and interpretation is 'true', how and whether to maintain confidentiality and anonymity, the potential for negative emotional responses or upset, and the aesthetic value of the work (Boydell et al. 2012b). These examples also highlight the need to rethink traditional research roles as it is no longer appropriate for researchers to maintain control over data that are collaboratively generated or for research participants to provide consent in advance of actually experiencing what is involved in using the arts to document their health and/or illness experience.

Standard approaches to confidentiality and anonymity are also problematic in the context of ABHR. As seen with the mural art example, many artist participants feel strongly about claiming authorship of the work created, despite the possibility of long-term implications associated with stigma arising from being identifiable as someone who has experienced psychosis. On the other hand, the photovoice study example on partner violence illustrates that there may be other times when it is important for researchers to devise appropriate methods to protect the identity of participants. Clearly, these are matters that must be determined within the context of each study and with the active involvement of study participants.

With respect to the challenges inherent in considering representation and audience interpretation, the notion of relational art or 'relational aesthetics' may help to frame the work as an on ongoing opportunity for dialogue and continued co-construction of data. Relational aesthetics, a term coined by French art critic Nicolas Bourriaud (2002), refers to the notion of artistic practices viewed as a shared social and interactive encounter, rather than an independent and private space.

The power of the arts to inspire, engage, and stimulate also raises the potential for a dangerous emotional terrain. As the example of the poetry and photo installation reveals, there may be a fine line between depicting the raw experience of heart surgery and opening up viewers to possible crisis. The example of the applied theatre project with children on dialysis points to similarly risky moments, as participants in the workshops are encouraged to learn from their engagement with potentially terrifying material.

These ethical issues are not completely separable from questions of aesthetics. As the example of found poetry about the experiences of research subjects suggests, there is a tension between the need to authentically represent what is learned through research and the artistic impulse to create a work of high aesthetic quality. This tension is perhaps most profound in projects incorporating arts-based methods of dissemination since the artistic work is given the task of translating existing findings into another medium.

## Conclusion

The ethics of doing ABHR has received little attention until recently (Boydell et al. 2012b). This chapter has provided an overview of some central ethical dilemmas that have arisen in everyday practice in both the creation and dissemination of research using various literary, performance, and visual art genres. It also includes a number of potential solutions to the challenges inherent in this work.

As we have noted in earlier work, a focus on the ethical challenges encountered in ABHR will move the field forward in terms of the creation of an evidence-based ethics as 'empirically driven studies, rather than principle-driven approaches alone, assist in enhancing our awareness of the key issues as they are experienced by the full range of salient participants' (Boydell et al. 2012b, p. 14). This will inform the development of new research ethics

policy and will also play a role in evolving research and creative practice (McDonald and Cox 2009).

Our own efforts in this area centre on generating creative responses to ethical challenges identified in health research, grounded in the perspectives and practices of researchers, artists, patients, and other research participants. We believe that such knowledge, appropriately translated into policy recommendations, will be of value in the governance of research ethics. It also has the potential to provide specific guidance to REBs in their review of ABHR proposals and to be helpful to researchers and artists embarking upon new collaborative work.

## References

Belliveau, G. (2007). Dramatizing the data: an ethnodramatic exploration of a playbuilding process. *Arts and Learning Research Journal*, **23**, 31–51.

Blackstone, M. Given, L., Levy, J., et al. [Social Sciences and Humanities Research Ethics Special Working Committee (SSHWC): a Working Committee of the Interagency Advisory Panel on Research Ethics (PRE)] (2008). *Research Involving Creative Practices: A Chapter for Inclusion in the TCPS*. Ottawa: Interagency Advisory Panel and Secretariat on Research Ethics.

Bosompra, K. (2007). The potential of drama and songs as channels for AIDS education in Africa: a report on focus group findings from Ghana. *International Quarterly of Community Health Education*, **28**, 127–151.

Boydell, K.M. (2011a). Making sense of collective events: the co-creation of a research-based dance. *Forum Qualitative Sozialforschung/Forum: Qualitative Social Research*, **12**(1), art. 5. Available at: <http://nbn-resolving.de/urn:nbn:de:0114-fqs110155> (accessed 18 October 2013).

Boydell, K.M. (2011b). Using performative art to communicate research: dancing experiences of psychosis. *Canadian Theatre Review*, **146**, 12–17.

Boydell, K.M. (2013). Using visual arts to enhance mental health literacy in schools. In: K. Tilleczek (ed.), *Youth, Education and Marginality*, pp. 229–240. Kitchener, ON: Wilfrid University Press.

Boydell, K.M., Gladstone, B.M., Volpe, T, Allemang, B., and Stasiulis, E. (2012a). The production and dissemination of knowledge: a scoping review of arts-based health research, *Forum Qualitative Sozialforschung/Forum: Qualitative Social Research*, **13**(1), art. 32. Available at: <http://nbn-resolving.de/urn:nbn:de:0114-fqs1201327> (accessed 18 October 2013).

Boydell, K.M., Volpe, T., Cox, S., et al. (2012b). Ethical challenges in arts-based health research. *International Journal of the Creative Arts in Interprofessional Practice*, Spring Suppl. Issue 11. Available at: <http://www.ijcaip.com/archives/IJCAIP-11-paper1.html> (accessed 18 October 2013).

Boydell, K.M., Jackson, S., and Strauss, J.S. (2012c). Help seeking experiences of youth with first episode psychosis: a research-based dance production. In: K.M. Boydell and H.B. Ferguson (eds), *Hearing Voices: Qualitative Inquiry in Early Psychosis*, pp. 25–44. Kitchener, ON: Wilfrid Laurier University Press.

Bourriaud, N. (2002). *Relational Aesthetics*. Paris: Presses du Reel.

Butler-Kisber, L. (2002). Artful portrayals in qualitative inquiry: the road to found poetry and beyond. *Alberta Journal of Educational Research*, **48**, 229–239.

Catalani, C. and Minkler, M. (2010). Photovoice: a review of the literature in health and public health. *Health and Education Behaviour*, **37**, 424–451.

Clark, A., Prosser, J., and Wiles, R. (2010). Ethical issues in image-based research. *Arts & Health: An International Journal for Research, Policy and Practice*, **2**, 81–93.

Colantonio, A., Kontos, P.C., Gilbert, J., Rossiter, K., Gray, J., and Keightly, M. (2008). After the crash: research-based theater for knowledge transfer. *Journal of Continuing Education in the Health Professions*, **28**, 180–185.

Cox, S., Townsend, A., Preto, N., Woodgate, R.L., and Kolopack, P. (2009). Ethical challenges and evolving practices in research on ethics in health research. *Health Law Review*, **17**, 2–3.

Cox, S.M., Lafrenière, D., Brett-Maclean, P. et al. (2010). Tipping the iceberg? The state of arts and health in Canada. *Arts & Health: An International Journal of Research, Policy and Practice*, **2**, 109–124.

Fleming, J., Mahoney, J., and Carlson, E. (2009). An ethnographic approach to interpreting a mental illness photovoice exhibit. *Archives of Psychiatric Nursing*, **23**, 16–24.

Fraser, D. and al Sayah, F. (2011). Arts-based methods in health research: a systematic review of the literature. *Arts & Health: An International Journal of Research, Policy and Practice*, **3**, 110–145.

Frith, H. and Harcourt, D. (2007). Using photographs to capture women's experiences of chemotherapy: reflecting on the method. *Qualitative Health Research*, **17**, 1340–1350.

Guillemin, M. and Drew, S. (2010). Questions of process in participant-generated visual methodologies. *Visual Studies*, **25**, 175–188.

Guillemin, M. and Gillam, L. (2004). Ethics, reflexivity and ethically important moments in research. *Qualitative Inquiry*, **10**, 261–280.

Herman, P.M. and Larkey, L.K. (2006). Effects of an arts-based curriculum on clinical trials attitudes and breast cancer prevention knowledge. *Health Education and Behavior*, **35**, 664–676.

Keen, S. and Todres, L. (2007). Strategies for disseminating qualitative research findings: three exemplars. *Forum Qualitative Sozialforschung/Forum: Qualitative Social Research*, **8**(3), art. 17. Available at: <http://www.qualitative-research.net/fqs/> (accessed 18 October 2013).

Knowles, J.G. and Cole, A.L. (eds) (2008). *Handbook of the Arts in Qualitative Research: Perspectives, Methodologies, Exemplars, and Issues*. Thousand Oaks, CA: Sage.

Kontos, P. and Naglie, G. (2006). Expressions of personhood in Alzheimer's disease: an evaluation of research-based theatre as a pedagogical tool. *Qualitative Health Research*, **17**, 799–811.

Lafrenière, D. and Cox, S.M. (2012). Comparing two methods of knowledge dissemination: the Café Scientifique and the artistic performance. *Sociology Mind*, **2**, 191–199.

Lafrenière, D. and Cox, S.M. (2013). 'If you can call it a poem': toward a framework for the assessment of arts-based works. *Qualitative Research*, **13**, 318–336.

Lafrenière, D., Hurlimann, T., Menuz, V., and Godard, B. (2012). Health research: ethics and the use of arts-based methods in knowledge translation processes. *International Journal of the Creative Arts in Interdisciplinary Practice*, Spring Suppl. Issue 11. Available at: <http://www.ijcaip.com/archives/IJCAIP-11-paper3.html>

Lafrenière, D., Cox, S.M., Belliveau, G., and Lea, G. (2013). Arts-based knowledge dissemination methods in health research: performing and displaying the human subject. *Journal of Applied Arts and Health*, **3**, 243–257.

Lapum, J., Church, K., Yau, T., David, A.M., and Ruttonsha, P. (2012a). Arts-informed research dissemination: patient's perioperative experiences of open heart surgery. *Heart Lung*, **41**(5), e4–e14.

Lapum, J., Ruttonsha, P., Church, K., Yau, T., and David, A.M. (2012b). Employing the arts as an analytic tool and dissemination method: Interpreting experiences through the aesthetic. *Qualitative Inquiry*, **18**, 100–115.

Levin, T., Scott, B.M., Borders, B. et al. (2007). Aphasia talks: photography as a means of communication, self-expression, and empowerment in persons with aphasia. *Topics in Stroke Rehabilitation*, **14**, 72–84.

McDonald, M. and Cox, S.M. (2009). Moving towards evidence-based human participant protection. *Academic Ethics*, **7**, 1–16.

Mienczakowski, J. (2003). The theater of ethnography: the reconstruction of ethnography into theater with emancipatory potential. In: Y.S. Lincoln and N.K. Denzin (eds), *Turning Points in Qualitative Research: Tying Knots in a Handkerchief*, pp. 415–432. Walnut Creek, CA: AltaMira Press.

Mitchell, G.J., Jonas-Simpson, C., and Ivonoffski, V. (2006). Research-based theatre: the making of I'm Still Here! *Nursing Science Quarterly*, **19**, 198–206.

Nisker, J., Martin, D.K., Bluhm, R., and Daar, A.S. (2006). Theatre as a public engagement tool for health-policy development. *Health Policy*, **78**, 258–271.

Parsons, J. and Boydell, K.M. (2012). Arts-based research and knowledge translation: some key concerns for health care professionals. *Journal of Interprofessional Care*, **26**, 170–172.

Parsons, J.A. and Lavery, J. (2012). Brokered dialogue: a new research method for controversial health and social issues. *BMC Medical Research Methodology*, **12**, 92, doi:10.1186/1471-2288-12-92

Pauwels, L. (2010). Visual sociology reframed: an analytical synthesis and discussion of visual methods in social and cultural research. *Sociological Methods Research*, **38**, 545–581.

Piko, B.F. and Bak, J. (2006). Children's perceptions of health and illness: Images and lay concepts in preadolescence. *Health Education Research*, **21**, 643–653.

Ponic, P. and Jategaokar, N. (2012). Balancing safety and action: ethical protocols for photovoice research with women who have experienced violence. *Arts & Health: An International Journal for Research, Policy and Practice*, **4**, 189–202.

Roberts, G., Somers, J., Dawe, J., et al. (2007). On the edge: a drama-based mental health education programme on early psychosis for schools. *Early Intervention in Psychiatry*, **1**, 168–176.

Sinding, C., Gray, R., Grassau, P., Damianakis, F., and Hampson, A. (2005). Audience responses to a research-based drama about life after breast cancer. *Psycho-Oncology*, **15**, 694–700.

Sonke, J. Rollins, J., Brandman, R. et al. (2009). The state of the arts in healthcare in the United States. *Arts & Health: An International Journal of Research, Policy and Practice*, **1**, 107–135.

Streng, J., Rhodes, M., Scott D., et al. (2004). Realidad Latina: Latino adolescents, their school, and a university use photovoice to examine and address the influence of immigration. *Journal of Interprofessional Care*, **18**, 403–415.

Thompson, N.C., Hunter, E.E., Murray, L., et al. (2008). The experience of living with chronic mental illness: a photovoice study, *Perspectives in Psychiatric Care*, **44**, 14–24.

Vaughn, L.M., Rojas-Guyler, L., and Howell, B. (2008). Picturing health: a photovoice pilot of Latina girls' perceptions of health. *Family and Community Health: The Journal of Health Promotion and Maintenance*, **31**, 305–316.

Walsh, A. and Ledgard, A. (2013). Re-viewing an arts-in-health process: For the Best. *Research in Drama Education: The Journal of Applied Theatre and Performance*, **18**, 216–229.

Wang, C.C. and Pies, C.A. (2004). Family, maternal, and child health through photovoice. *Maternal and Child Health Journal*, **8**, 95–102.

White, V. and Belliveau, G. (2010). Whose story is it anyway? Exploring ethical dilemmas in performed research. *Performing Ethos International Research Journal*, **1**, 85–95.

Wreford, G. (2010). The state of arts and health in Australia. *Arts & Health: An International Journal of Research, Policy and Practice*, **2**, 8–22.

# PART 2

# National and international developments in practice

12  **Seeking a common language: the challenge of embedding participatory arts in a major public health programme** *95*
Marsaili Cameron, Richard Ings, and Nikki Crane

13  **Arts for health in community settings: promising practices for using the arts to enhance wellness, access to healthcare, and health literacy** *103*
Jill Sonke and Jenny Baxley Lee

14  **Arts in healthcare settings in the United States** *113*
Jill Sonke, Judy Rollins, and John Graham-Pole

15  **Arts in healthcare in Uganda: an historical, political, and practical case study** *123*
Kizito Maria Kasule, Kizito Fred Kakinda, and Jill Sonke

16  **Siyazama in South Africa: Zulu beadwork, HIV/AIDS, and the consequences of culture** *129*
Kate Wells

17  **Arts and health in Australia** *135*
Gareth Wreford

18  **Addressing the health needs of indigenous Australians through creative engagement: a case study** *145*
Jing Sun and Nicholas Buys

19  **Arts and health initiatives in India** *151*
Varun Ramnarayan Venkit, Anand Sharad Godse, and Amruta Anand Godse

20  **A role for the creative arts in addressing public health challenges in China** *163*
Jing Sun and Nicholas Buys

21  **Culture and public health activities in Sweden and Norway** *171*
Töres Theorell, Margunn Skjei Knudtsen, Eva Bojner Horwitz, and Britt-Maj Wikström

22  **Talking about a revolution: arts, health, and wellbeing on Avenida Brasil** *179*
Paul Heritage and Silvia Ramos

23  **Case study: 'I once was lost but now am found'—music and embodied arts in two American prisons** *187*
André de Quadros

24  **Case study: lost—or found?—in translation. The globalization of Venezuela's El Sistema** *193*
Andrea Creech, Patricia A. González-Moreno, Lisa Lorenzino, and Grace Waitman

# Seeking a common language: the challenge of embedding participatory arts in a major public health programme

Marsaili Cameron, Richard Ings, and Nikki Crane

## Introduction

Who and what is art for? The question is hardly new, but it is never less than challenging. There is a growing body of evidence that creativity and the arts can make a significant difference to people's health and wellbeing—and also to how they feel about, and interact with, their neighbours. Clift (2012, p. 123) makes clear the significant role to be played by randomized controlled trials and systematic reviews in the evaluation of practical interventions designed to improve health. But he also highlights:

'[ . . . ] the many research questions that these cannot answer; questions such as: how does an intervention work; is it acceptable to potential participants; is it an appropriate intervention given participant needs; and are service users and other stakeholders satisfied with the intervention?'

This chapter describes an attempt to address some of these research questions in relation to the part played by the participatory arts in an innovative partnership programme for improving the health and wellbeing of some of the poorest communities in London.

In 2007, the UK Big Lottery Fund announced that it was giving just under £9.5 million to finance a new 4-year health and mental wellbeing programme called Well London. The successful application had come from the Well London Alliance, a group of agencies from different sectors across the capital that aimed to challenge the stigma of mental health issues and promote positive wellbeing, encourage healthier eating choices, and enable communities to provide opportunities for local people to become more active. A cornerstone of the Well London approach was to build and strengthen the foundations of good health and wellbeing in communities by significantly increasing community participation in activities that enhance health and wellbeing and by building individual and community confidence and sense of control.

Phase 1 of the Well London programme (2007–11) comprised 14 projects and extended over 20 of London's most disadvantaged areas. The boundaries of the projects often cut across the natural neighbourhoods of streets and estates (the term used in England to describe high-density housing developments). Projects were based around five themes: culture and tradition, healthy eating, mental health and wellbeing, open spaces, and physical activity. All projects had a remit to support community engagement and capacity building. The theme of culture and tradition was delivered through Be Creative Be Well, developed by Arts Council England, and one of the most ambitious grassroots arts and health programmes ever delivered in the United Kingdom. This initiative nurtured around 100 different small participatory arts projects across 20 of London's most disadvantaged areas. However, creativity in the Well London programme was not confined to Be Creative Be Well—creative approaches were embedded throughout.

Phase 2 of Well London started in 2012 and is due to finish in 2015. Some things remained the same as in Phase 1. For example, the community development approach underpinning the programme was retained as a key feature; as was the development of, and reliance on, volunteers within the local communities. But some substantial changes were made to how the programme was planned and how work was commissioned. It was agreed, for instance, that projects should work within what were seen as natural neighbourhoods; in many cases these took the form of housing estates. Another significant change was to the model of commissioning projects. Previously, the London-wide agencies who were partners in Well London had been actively involved in commissioning and supporting initiatives. They now stood back in favour of a system of local commissioning, where different agencies took the lead in different areas and shaped the activities to meet what they saw as local priorities. Local communities were introduced to participatory budgeting (a concept and approach described on the PB Network website: <http://www.pbnetwork.org.uk>), with the aim of directly involving local people in making decisions on the spending and priorities for a defined budget.

There has been both formal and informal learning associated with the programme. In 2010 Arts Council England commissioned an independent team, consisting of the present authors, to carry out an evaluation of Be Creative Be Well (Ings et al. 2012; Cameron et al. 2013). The aims of this evaluation were to:

◆ explore the range of benefits potentially associated with artists working in close collaboration with local communities

◆ share new learning about factors that help—and hinder—successful collaboration of this kind

◆ contribute to the growing dialogue between arts and health professionals

◆ offer recommendations on how to ensure that the commissioning process is most likely to give rise to work that will result in a sustainable legacy.

With its findings made available both to funders and practitioners, the evaluation was intended to complement other evaluative work, including the overall evaluation of Phase 1 of Well London by the University of East London and academic partners (available at <http://www.welllondon.org.uk/>). At the same time, informal, emergent learning has been shared across the Well London community in relation both to individual projects and to the overall delivery of the programme.

This chapter draws on both formal and informal sources to summarize several cycles of learning from this wide-ranging and innovative programme. First, we look briefly at what we found to be links between the process and outcomes of participatory arts work and creating the conditions for wellbeing.

## Joining in existing conversations

Our evaluation of Be Creative Be Well had as a starting point the belief that there is a potential link between evidence-based benefits for people from participating in arts activity and actions that have been shown to promote health and mental wellbeing. We set out to test this assumption through a close analysis of what

happened, in all its local detail, in a dozen projects run during the third year of Be Creative Be Well. We visited projects as they were taking place and, using semi-structured questionnaires, talked to artists, local people, and staff from other agencies in the community about what had been happening and what it felt like to be engaged in artistic activity (Fig. 12.1).

For theoretical underpinning to our inquiry, we turned to two frameworks that had emerged from intensive study of, on the one hand, wellbeing and, on the other, participatory arts. The first framework was the evidence-based 'Five Ways to Wellbeing' developed by the New Economics Foundation (NEF). Commissioned by the government, NEF reviewed the work of over 400 scientists working on different aspects of health and wellbeing. Based on this research, NEF produced a concept of everyday wellbeing, comprising two main elements: feeling good and functioning well (New Economics Foundation 2008, pp. 1–2).

> 'Feelings of happiness, contentment, enjoyment, curiosity and engagement are characteristic of someone who has a positive experience of their life. Equally important for wellbeing is our functioning in the world: experiencing positive relationships, having some control over one's life'.

These two main elements give rise to 'five simple actions which can improve wellbeing in everyday life': connect, be active, take notice, keep learning, give. The model based on these five actions indicates how each action engenders its own positive feedback and thus reinforces wellbeing. As an evaluation team, we noted that these five actions correspond closely to behaviours that can emerge in well-designed participatory arts projects.

The second, complementary framework came from the arts world and enabled us to make some key links between the discourses of health and the arts. The framework (509 Arts 2010) documented the process and potential benefits of participatory arts work through a study of several leading companies working in this way.

To these two frameworks we added another that might best be described as a 'wraparound' approach to the evaluation, presenting

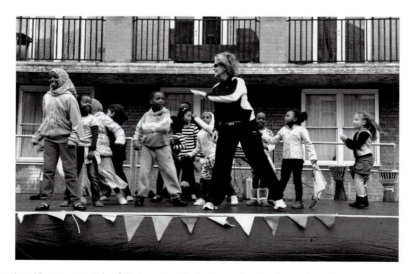

**Fig. 12.1** The New Global Image project, 'Connect: My Side of the Story', in Woolwich, used performing and creative arts to engage with the energies and interests of local people.

a vehicle for shared learning. Pawson and Tilley's (1997) model of 'realistic evaluation' offers the opportunity to show in precise terms how learning can lead to improved performance.

During Phase 2 of Well London, we held semi-structured interviews with a range of people who had been deeply involved in creative engagement aspects of the programme. We also invited them to comment on the findings of the evaluation. From this iterative process, we identified learning points and drew conclusions that acknowledge the real-life opportunities and threats for programmes such as this.

## What was learned that can inform future arts interventions?

Be Creative Be Well was a wide-ranging innovative programme that, at its most effective, was shaped by local conditions and local people. Throughout the programme, we found that participants in the arts projects cared very much about the quality of the experience they had. 'Quality' was defined in very different ways. The concept of professionalism was widely seen as a desirable and significant basis for a serious transaction between artist and project participants. Commitment by artists to high standards in how they worked with participants was seen to be mirrored in high expectations of artistic achievement on the part of participants. Other participants referred favourably to:

◆ the ability of individual artists to combine artistic/performance skills with passion to communicate their craft

◆ what might be called high production values in both workshops and performance; for example, good lighting, pleasing surroundings, high-quality instruments or materials

◆ the ability of project leaders, some of whom were not artists, to 'share their leadership' and thus instil a new confidence in participants (for example, in response to one project leader's disclaimer , 'I'm not an artist!', a participant responded at once, 'You're an artist with people')

Whatever their precise definition of quality, participants seemed to concur in what a good experience offered to them: care, attention, acknowledgement, and respect.

Interim findings of the evaluation were discussed at a series of artists' workshops staged during the programme. It emerged that several artists were conscious of the danger of losing sight of quality when working in community settings. The worst-case scenario was seen as approaching social contexts with a sense that virtually anything would do as long as people were 'contained' or 'entertained'. It was agreed too that an arts approach that is purely instrumental also militates against quality—for example where the artist is fixed on achieving 'x' aim and looks on art simply as a means of getting there. So, what seemed to count as 'quality' for artists working in a community setting? There was wide agreement that when artists put the art first and care about the standards of the emerging work, the result is much better—they inspire, move, and challenge people and help them to aspire to something.

Interestingly, quality of artistic practice is acknowledged to be an important issue during Phase 2 of Well London. In the course of the Be Creative Be Well initiative, Arts Council England offered support, guidance, and encouragement to all the artists involved. In Phase 2, this organization continues to support some artists and groups participating in Well London. It also encourages greater engagement with similar communities through strategic funding programmes, notably Creative People and Places, for which Be Creative Be Well effectively served as a pilot. But, since different agencies take the lead in different Well London areas, questions arise as to how local artists can in future be provided with appropriate support and encouraged to develop their skills further, and how local communities can be given access to wider cultural opportunities. One answer is seen to lie in forming partnerships with major arts organizations keen to explore what being a 'centre of excellence' could really mean in practice.

The experiences, challenges, and achievements of the programme reveal a great deal about how to make an arts intervention successful and sustainable. The following learning points are presented here in summary form. The initial quotations come from artists who led different projects visited by us. The reflections are taken from interviews with long-standing stakeholders in Well London who were asked during Phase 2 of the programme to comment on how well the recommendations had stood up to the test of time.

### Defining the community

'Communities are organic and define themselves; programmes [ . . . ] should reflect this.'

---

**Recommended**

*Commissioners/funders/sponsors*: Aim to select a self-defining community
*Artists*: Where possible, build on existing community resources

**Not recommended**

*Commissioners/funders/sponsors*: Set up projects across split sites

---

Reflections from Well London veterans:

◆ You need to really think about this complicated issue. For a start, bear in mind that there is likely to be a tension between reality and evaluation. Split sites are very difficult for everyone except researchers and funders.

◆ When you're working with the most disadvantaged communities, remember that there may be very little existing sense of community. People come and go all the time—sometimes from and to half way round the world. Life is fragmented, often fractured across racial and generational lines and between newcomers and established residents.

◆ The feeling that people are most likely to share is, 'I want to be in a community that I feel part of, and safe in'.

### Selecting the artist

'I'm realizing that working within the community presents a whole set of different issues from working in a school, which is my usual setting.'

**Recommended**

*Commissioners/funders/sponsors*: Ensure that artist teams have skills in community development as well as their specific practice

**Not recommended**

*Artists*: Set up an opposition between quality of artistic product and deep engagement with the community—the best projects seem to combine the two

Reflections from Well London veterans:

◆ Artists can only work well in this context if they have taken care to examine their own assumptions and acknowledge who they are.

◆ Local people may not know what they want at first. That doesn't mean that expectations shouldn't be high on all sides. Artist and community need to reflect together on, 'What can we do now that will continue to make a difference later?'

## Preparing the ground

'To plonk an artist in the middle of an estate and expect things to happen straightaway is unrealistic.'

**Recommended**

*Commissioners/funders/sponsors*: Ensure that artist teams are briefed as fully as possible on how decisions are made locally, or outside of the community, and who holds the power
*Commissioners/funders/sponsors/artists*: Make practical acknowledgement of the fact that it takes time to develop relationships and trust, and to establish what kind of activities local people would like to see and support
*Artists*: Pay careful attention to finding a venue that local people will be happy to attend

**Not recommended**

*Commissioners/funders/sponsors/artists*: Assume statistical demographic information will provide a clear picture of the communities involved
*Commissioners/funders/sponsors/artists*: Raise unrealistic expectations of the project among local people

Reflections from Well London veterans:

◆ Induction really does set the tone for what is to follow—work at getting it right.

◆ Be guided constantly by the question 'What is the point of providing services or activities that people neither need nor want?' Unless you include local people in design and delivery (and allow time to do so), few people will join in.

◆ Invite people in a way that makes them feel truly included.

◆ If you've offered something to the community, see it through!

## Demystifying the artistic process

'What I think is off-putting to everyone is actually talking about 'the arts''

**Recommended**

*Artists*: Begin by exploring participants' thoughts and feelings about their community and environment and focus on building on these
*Artists*: Reflect on the questions 'What difference do I hope to make?' and 'Why do I think what I'm planning to do will make that difference?'

**Not recommended**

*Artists*: Set out an agenda of 'we are going to make art'

Reflections from Well London veterans:

◆ Don't underestimate the importance of the 'sideways glance' when getting to know a community. Artists will find that ideas, thoughts, feelings, shapes, and forms will emerge throughout the process.

◆ It's OK for things to seem to be a muddle at the beginning; you don't have to understand everything all at once.

◆ Bring in other artists when you can. The community will benefit, and so will you. One of the joys of all this is creative collaboration (Fig. 12.2).

## Working with local structures

'Tenant and resident associations are supposed to be open to all and committed to representing all members' interests; but the truth of it here is that it's a club for members only.'

**Recommended**

*Commissioners/funders/sponsors/artists*: Make every effort to enlist the active support of local organizations—the 'familiar face on the estate' is often an invaluable aid to marketing the project
*Commissioners/funders/sponsors/artists*: Think through the role that project partners are expected to play and use that analysis to identify the most appropriate partners
*Artists*: Form mutually respectful and productive relationships with representatives of the local authority and other major agencies

**Not recommended**

*Artists*: Try to set up activities without the support of local organizations, programme sponsors or project partners

Reflections from Well London veterans:

◆ Artists and local coordinators need flexibility to act quickly and seize opportunities.

◆ Early effort must be put into ensuring clarity about governance—who's responsible for what, how, when? Then there need to be regular comings together locally where everyone, residents included, can reflect on issues and events. Artists can make such events stimulating and fun.

## Collaborative programming

'The YMCA has supported our dance programme—we created a couple of dance drama productions'.

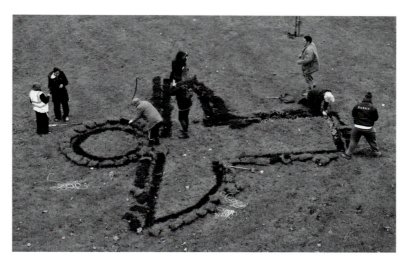

**Fig. 12.2** Tiger Monkey's '100 Angels' project, in Edmonton, London, attracted a wide variety of partners—from strategic to grass roots. Reproduced by kind permission of Bethany Clarke. Copyright © 2015 Bethany Clarke Photography.

**Recommended**

*Commissioners/funders/sponsors/artists*: Make every effort to create good conditions for collaboration and joint working
*Commissioners/funders/sponsors/artists*: Aim to develop opportunities for active and equal partnership
*Artists*: Be clear about your own contribution to the collaborative work—including the nature of the energy you bring—and be explicit about your aspirations for joint working

**Not recommended**

*Commissioners/funders/sponsors/artists*: Underestimate the challenges of bringing together very different discourses and approaches

Reflections from Well London veterans:

◆ Where projects are working together towards a common purpose, funders should treat a communications hub as essential infrastructure.

◆ If you're going to work together well, you need good spaces—physical and virtual—where you can get together and build relationships.

◆ Bear in mind that it can be hard for professionals to relinquish power—but a supportive role is just as important as a steering role.

## Building levels of engagement

'Posters and flyers don't work, but what else can I do?'

**Recommended**

*Artists*: In recruiting to the project, find good reasons for people to step out of their comfort zone on a cold night
*Artists*: Prioritize face-to-face encounters with local people and use 'ambassadors' when you can

**Not recommended**

*Artists*: Give in to the temptation of relying on conventional promotional approaches like flyers, posters, and newsletters—easily ignored and of little intrinsic interest, they are rarely effective for community arts projects

Reflections from Well London veterans:

◆ You may seem to get nothing but complaints when you start talking with people—but they will decrease in volume as people get to know you, and you'll often find that making small changes can make a big difference.

◆ Always aim for a coherent story, where possible linking up different activities going on locally. Remember to speak human!

◆ Glossy flyers will join the pizza leaflets on the way out of the door. Newsletters can be OK if they're of the 'What's on?' type, are produced by local people, and delivered in a personal way. Posters can be useful prompts.

## Using evaluation

'[ . . . ] having to go through the evaluation forms with people when they are getting bored and you just want to start the workshop. . .'

**Recommended**

*Commissioners/funders/sponsors*: Structure the programme in such a way that projects are allowed to set their own tempo and find their own sense of direction and purpose
*Artists*: Take opportunities to turn evaluation into a creative learning activity that has the potential to enhance your practice as well as the specific project

**Not recommended**

*Commissioners/funders/sponsors/artists*: Over-consult local people so that gaining feedback gets in the way of developing the work

Reflections from Well London veterans:

◆ Most programmes need several iterations to get it right. Evaluation has to be about real learning, even if that learning is difficult and perhaps embarrassing.

◆ Many people are scared about saying what's gone wrong in case the funder thinks, 'Well, they didn't know what they were doing.' Try to resist this fear; sometimes you need to change things completely.

◆ It's inevitable that you will want to differentiate new activities from earlier ones—but build constructively on their legacy.

## Leaving a legacy

'I would love this to be an art studio, with a couple of artists in residence.'

---

**Recommended**

*Commissioners/funders/sponsors*: Give priority to working with artists to identify how projects can be embedded systematically
*Artists*: Throughout the project, build on opportunities to pass on skills—including fundraising and advocacy skills

**Not recommended**

*Commissioners/funders/sponsors/artists*: Leave thinking about legacy until the last few months of the project

---

Reflections from Well London veterans:

◆ Be open about the fact that your programme will not last forever—and explore early on what is needed for the community to sustain the activity in a resource-starved environment.

◆ Support the group in welcoming new people and in developing reflective skills.

◆ Identify barriers to engagement and work with the community to plan sustainable solutions (e.g. DIY crèches to address issues of childcare).

## Conclusions

At one level, arts and health professionals do not need to seek too hard to find a common language through which to discuss, and plan to promote, the health and wellbeing of local communities. Studies associated with wellbeing and with the participatory arts offer findings and frameworks that are flexible and multidimensional, capable of being adapted to a variety of situations.

The inquiry that is the focus of this chapter presents an example of putting these frameworks to use. In doing so, we identified some key learning points for artists—and, crucially, for those who train, fund, and support artists—concerning the creation of meaningful art for and with the public, from initial commission to sustainable legacy.

An important indicative finding from our inquiry is that the quality of creative work matters. Improvements in health and wellbeing and greater engagement in the arts are closely intertwined: the better the creative engagement, the more likely it is to lead to healthy outcomes. A further significant finding is that the creative arts offer an effective means of encouraging and equipping local people to develop leadership skills and to take up new roles and responsibilities in their communities.

A real question remains, however, as to whether, in practice, the circle of discussion has been widened in a significant way. As one of the veterans of the programme put it:

'The arts offer a holistic, joined-up, fun approach to health promotion. Will people responsible for allocating funds understand that the arts are important to the delivery of public health programmes? Or will they carry on thinking that artists create a good sideshow while the health professionals do the serious stuff?'

Commissioners of services deserve a clear, coherent, and consistent narrative about the potential contribution of community arts to health and wellbeing. Knell and Taylor (2011, pp. 27–28) set out the underlying challenge:

'[ . . . ] to develop coherent (and challenging) accounts of the role art does, can and could play in helping us imagine and create more fulfilling lives in a better society'

A collaborative effort is needed to meet this challenge effectively, with trust and meaningful communication nurtured across the arts, health, and community development domains. Progress of this kind will enable the participatory arts to play their full part rather than remain a sideshow.

## References

509 Arts (2010). Elements of process and product. In *Adult Participatory Arts: Thinking it Through*, p. 20. London: Arts Council England.

Cameron, M., Crane, N., Ings, R., and Taylor, K. (2013). Promoting well-being through creativity: how arts and public health can learn from each other. *Perspectives in Public Health*, **133**, 52–59.

Clift, S. (2012). Creative arts as a public health resource: moving from practice-based research to evidence-based practice. *Perspectives in Public Health*, **132**, 120–127.

Ings, R., Crane, N., and Cameron, M. (2012). *Be Creative Be Well: Arts, Wellbeing and Local Communities*. London: Arts Council England. Available at: <http://www.artscouncil.org.uk/advice-and-guidance/browse-advice-and-guidance/be-creative-be-well-arts-wellbeing-and-local-communities-evaluation> (accessed 6 October 2013).

Knell, J. and Taylor, M. (2011). *Arts Funding, Austerity and the Big Society: Remaking the Case for the Arts*. London: Royal Society of Arts. Available at: <http://www.artscouncil.org.uk/media/uploads/pdf/RSA-Pamphlets-Arts_Funding_Austerity_BigSociety.pdf> (accessed 17 March 2015).

New Economics Foundation (2008). *Five Ways to Wellbeing: the Evidence*. London: nef. Available at: <http://www.neweconomics.org/publications/entry/five-ways-to-wellbeing-the-evidence> (accessed 6 October 2013).

Pawson, R. and Tilley, N. (1997). *Realistic Evaluation*. London: Sage.

# CHAPTER 13

# Arts for health in community settings: promising practices for using the arts to enhance wellness, access to healthcare, and health literacy

Jill Sonke and Jenny Baxley Lee

## Introduction

'The greatest social impacts of participation in the arts . . . arise from their ability to help people think critically about and question their experiences and those of others . . . It is in the act of creativity that empowerment lies, and through sharing creativity that understanding and social inclusiveness are promoted.'

Matarasso (1997, p. 79)

In this chapter we will consider models for arts and health programmes in community settings in different areas of the world, highlighting promising practices for using the arts to enhance wellness, access to healthcare, and health literacy. Through a lens of interdisciplinary theoretical frameworks we will explore the benefits and challenges of the arts and health in community settings in urban, rural, and developing communities around the world.

What is a community? As societies change in relation to widespread urbanization and globalization, the concept of community is also changing. Communities are frequently defined geographically, such as by neighbourhood, town, or region, but can also be defined by affiliations in relational terms, such as by shared histories, identities, and interests, regardless of geography or proximity (Luke and Xu 2011).

An understanding of the concept of community can provide arts and health professionals with an important basis for thinking about community populations, issues, and interventions. In a 2004 glossary of terms, the Word Health Organization (WHO) defines community as:

'a group of people, often living in a defined geographical area, who may share a common culture, values and norms, and are arranged in a social structure according to relationships which the community has developed over a period of time. Members of a community gain their personal and social identity by sharing common beliefs, values and norms, which have been developed by the community in the past and may be modified in the future. They exhibit some awareness of their identity as a group, and share common needs and a commitment to meeting them.'

Laverack (2011, pp. 113–120)

There is a growing emphasis on addressing the needs of members of rural communities. In the United States, urban bias in health planning and assessment is more widely recognized as an impediment to the development of effective health policies, and investment in rural health research and appropriate interventions for rural populations is on the rise (White House Rural Council 2013). Significant health disparities between urban and rural communities in many countries indicate a crucial need for interventions that can have an impact on health behaviours and reduce the incidence of preventable illnesses that are the most common causes of death in rural areas (Hartley 2004).

## Community-based arts and health practice

Use of the arts as a means to educate the public, foster social engagement and social change, and influence the behaviours of targeted populations has a long history. Arts-based health promotion has its historical roots in traditional cultures where story-telling, drama, and song are primary means for facilitating healing and enforcing the belief systems of a given culture. Anthropologist Ellen Dissanayake (2000) recognizes art and ritual activities as universal human actions that promote health for both individuals and communities. She asserts that the arts have had selective value in human evolution and that they promote cooperation, harmony, and unity among group members and enable our species to cope with difficult events such as illness. Art and art-making have also been shown to promote competence and self-efficacy (Evans 2008).

Due to their broad appeal and flexible application in a variety of contexts, the arts are well placed to affect social engagement, and to engage and empower residents by developing a stronger sense of place, decreasing social stress, increasing individual confidence, and facilitating understanding of relevant issues (McQueen-Thomson and Ziguras 2002; Ife and Tesoriero 2006). Social engagement has long been shown to support health (Cohen 2004; Cohen and Janicki-Deverts 2009; McHenry 2011), and participation in the arts and cultural activities has been demonstrated to improved wellbeing and even to extend life (Bygren et al. 1996, 2001).

Culture plays a vital role in alleviating social stress, which is a significant determinant of health. During a European Communities summit in 2005 the arts were considered as a means for addressing social inclusion. 'Effective access to and participation in cultural activities for all is an essential dimension of promoting an inclusive society' (European Commission 2005, p. 1). During an official US public assembly on 'Arts and Liveability', the city of Philadelphia served as an urban model for the value of cultural assets within marginalized or underserved pockets of the city: 'Philadelphia's social stress index for the early 2000s was strongly correlated with the cultural asset index, even controlling for per capita income. That is, even in low-income neighbourhoods, a high concentration of cultural assets was associated with a dramatic decline in social stress indicators' (Pierson 2010, pp. 13–15). The evidence presented in this convening presents a clear connection between the presence of culture and improved health outcomes due to reduced social stress.

# Wellness: health promotion and disease prevention

'An ounce of prevention is worth a pound of cure.'
Benjamin Franklin

According to the National Wellness Institute in the United States, wellness is an active process through which people become aware of, and make choices toward, a more successful existence (Hettler 1976). Health systems worldwide are emphasizing the need for health programmes that promote health and prevent disease. The concept of prevention is guiding health policy-makers and service deliverers to develop health programmes that engage and empower people outside healthcare settings and at various stages of their lives in a more integrated manner (Hanna et al. 2011; Laverack 2011). The arts are ideally suited for promoting this integrated approach. Numerous studies demonstrate that arts participation can affect health behaviour and promote wellness in individuals across the life course (Stuckey and Nobel 2010; Hanna et al. 2011; Camic and Chatterjee 2013).

The World Health Organization (1946) defines health as a 'state of complete physical, mental and social wellbeing, not merely the absence of disease or infirmity', reflecting a holistic view of both society and health. In this vein, health promotion is a core component of providing a holistic system of care for individuals living in communities. With healthcare costs rising in western countries in particular due to an ever-increasing population, shortages of healthcare providers, and economic instability, it is more essential than ever that cost-effective solutions for health promotion are identified.

Health trends indicate that the decrease in acute illness and significant increase in chronic, often preventable, disease is a primary driver behind rising healthcare costs, placing a heavier burden on both individuals and communities (World Health Organization 2005; Department of Health and Human Services 2009). An essential role within public health agencies, then, is to promote wellness through community health policy, disease prevention initiatives, workplace health promotion programmes, and access to care early in the illness process.

In light of this understanding, what is the role of promising practices in the arts and health for promoting wellness within communities? New research is demonstrating more clearly than ever that incorporation of the arts into health promotion programmes offers the potential to enhance health behaviours and outcomes (Carson et al. 2007; Stuckey and Nobel 2010; Clift 2012; Camic and Chatterjee 2013). As the literature demonstrates, engaging the arts for health promotion and wellbeing is no longer an *if* but a *when, where*, and *how*.

## Promising practices in wellness

### The Dance for PD programme

One of the community programmes in the arts in health that has had the most impact over the past decade is the Dance for PD programme in Brooklyn, New York. The programme developed organically in 2001 when the founder and executive director of the Brooklyn Parkinson Group (BPG), a support group for people with Parkinson's disease (PD), approached the Mark Morris Dance Group, an internationally acclaimed modern dance company, about bringing dance to members of the BPG. The resulting Dance for PD programme has grown into a widely replicated international model, with programmes in more than 100 communities in nine countries (Fig. 13.1).

The programme is based on the tenet that 'professionally-trained dancers are movement experts whose knowledge is useful to persons with PD' (Mark Morris Dance Group and Brooklyn Parkinson Group 2010). Professional dancers from the Mark Morris Dance Group offer weekly classes to people with PD in New York that integrate elements of modern and theatre dance, ballet, folk dance, tap, improvisation, and choreographic repertory in a safe and supportive professional dance environment. Programme leaders facilitate an aesthetic experience within the class that is challenging and socially engaging and that can provide physical and psychosocial benefits for the symptoms of PD.

As dance programmes for people with PD have grown in numbers over the past decade, a body of literature has begun to develop documenting some of the benefits of dance for this population. A pilot study of the Brooklyn Dance for PD programme found improved gait and resting tremor as well as positive contributions to participants' quality of life (Westheimer et al. 2011). In a review of the literature on dance and PD, Earhart (2009) notes that dance meets most, if not all, of the established required components for exercise for people with PD, and summarizes the literature to suggest that dance may be an effective strategy for improving balance, gait function, and quality of life.

More recent studies have found improvements in motor function, including in rigidity, hand movement, balance, stability, and facial expression (Heiberger et al. 2011; Houston and McGill 2013). Houston and McGill (2013) found strong adherence to the

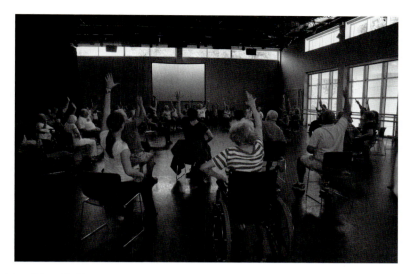

**Fig. 13.1**  Dance for PD teacher training, Gainesville, FL.
Reproduced by kind permission of David Leventhal, Director, Dance for PD, Mark Morris Dance Group, Brooklyn New York. Copyright © 2015 David Leventhal.

weekly programme and concluded that dance, due to its creative, social, and cultural nature, can be an effective motivator for engagement in physical activity, particularly for people who do not enjoy repetitive exercise regimes:

> 'The fundamentals of dancing and dance training—things like balance, movement sequencing, rhythm, spatial and aesthetic awareness, and dynamic coordination—seem to address many of the things people with Parkinson's want to work on to maintain a sense of confidence and grace in their movements. Although participants from all over the world tell us they find elements of the class therapeutic, the primary goal of our programme is for people to enjoy dance for dancing's sake in a group setting—and to explore the range of physical, artistic and creative possibilities that are still very much open to them.'
> David Leventhal, Dance for PD founding teacher, Brooklyn, NY

### TimeSlips, Wisconsin, United States

TimeSlips was established in 1996 to address quality of life among older adults with dementia. The programme engages improvisational storytelling within group activities in a method designed to reduce pressure on memory and maximize preserved abilities such as creativity. TimeSlips uses creative story-telling to help residents in nursing or care facilities communicate with each other, their care providers, and their family members. The success of the programme has led to training and certification programmes, and broad media attention.

A study of the TimeSlips programme reveals that individuals living in facilities that provided TimeSlips programmes were more engaged and alert than those individuals living in control facilities. In facilities that provided TimeSlips, more frequent staff–resident interactions, social interactions, and social engagement occurred. Staff who participated in the programme demonstrated more positive views of residents with dementia and valued residents more highly than did the staff in the control group staff (Fritsch et al. 2009). Additional studies demonstrate positive outcomes such as increased and improved socialization among peers and with care staff as well as enhanced quality of life.

In addition to providing evidence to substantiate the value and impact of creative expression, TimeSlips distinguishes itself as a method for engaging older adults through story in several notable ways. The programme offers a replicable, hence far-reaching, model that brings creative storytelling to bear among members of a generation who need an outlet to express themselves and be heard. It harnesses the power of technology, including an interactive web-based interface for story sharing and an online digital library, to bring stories to a wider audience and to train practitioners, while engaging and honouring the target audience.

### The Hip Op-eration Hip Hop Crew, Waiheke Island, New Zealand

The Hip Op-eration Hip Hop Crew of New Zealand is the 'oldest' hip-hop dance company in the world, though it was only established in 2012. At the time of writing, the Crew consisted of 36 members, ranging in age from 66 to 96 years. In August 2013, the Crew performed at the World Hip-Hop Championship Finals in Las Vegas, Nevada, delivering to a global audience the message that creativity is for people of all ages. While the original goal of the programme was to reduce the stigma of ageing, an additional focus on connecting seniors with younger people has emerged. The programme has attracted significant media attention, and has been featured on the front page of the *Wall Street Journal*, on the BBC, and is the focus of a feature film released in 2014 (see <http://www.hipop-eration.com/>).

While the programme only directly serves a small local population, its impact in communicating important messages that affect individual and societal health is significant. The media is drawn to the idea (and the visuals) of elderly adults doing hip-hop dance, and is spreading it messages rapidly to global audiences. The Hip Op-eration exemplifies the power of the arts to rapidly and broadly communicate health information. Through its wide exposure, the programme encourages participation in dance and active, creative ageing by older adults worldwide.

## Access to healthcare

While healthcare is simply unavailable to people in some areas of the world, in areas where it is available services are often underutilized. This lack of utilization relates to access issues such as cost of care and transportation, as well as social and cultural barriers. These barriers make it difficult to improve health and lead to significant disparities, particularly in rural areas. According to the WHO, nearly 90% of people living in countries with very high levels of vulnerability are not covered formally by any scheme or system. The challenge, then, to make healthcare, specifically essential procedures and medicine, accessible to all citizens is common to most countries (World Health Organization 2012).

Access to healthcare can be a difficult subject to articulate because it is such a nuanced concern, dependent upon a myriad of factors such as geographic region, economics, cultural beliefs and norms, and health behaviour patterns. Primary among obstacles to healthcare, yet perhaps more difficult to address, are the social and cultural disparities among groups of individuals living together in community. Every region has varying pockets of community members who are marginalized due to socio-economic status, disability, race, ethnicity, or sexual and/or gender identity.

Arts programmes that reduce social isolation among these underserved populations reduce barriers to healthcare by connecting people to systems, services, and community members. In fact, the arts are uniquely positioned to create a neutral hub across which seemingly disparate groups of people can come together to create solutions to accessing health and human services.

### Promising practices in access to healthcare

#### The Rowan, Antrim, Northern Ireland

The first of its kind in the region, the Rowan is a sexual assault referral centre located at the Antrim Area Hospital in Antrim, Northern Ireland (Northern Health and Social Care Trust 2013). The centre is open 24 hours a day, 365 days a year, and strives to provide a welcoming and non-discriminatory one-stop location for people who have experienced sexual assault. The centre uses the arts to create a welcoming environment and also to accomplish its mission of providing comprehensive care to promote recovery and wellbeing.

From the beginning of the design process for the centre's physical space and programming, a professional artist from ArtsCare, the national arts and health organization serving Northern Ireland, was engaged as a member of the design and planning team. The artist in residence, Helen Bradbury, facilitated arts workshops with the centre's service users, and developed a permanent exhibit of their work for the waiting and reception areas, as well as consultations areas. The exhibits serve to welcome visitors, create a more humane environment, and communicate to victims of sexual assault that they are not alone in their experience.

At the Rowan, as it does throughout Northern Ireland, ArtsCare realizes its mission to transform health and social care through creative activity. Upon entering the building, victims of sexual assault are greeted by a warm, colourful, and comforting display of art created by local people who have survived sexual assault. These works transform the space into a healing environment from entry to the building and throughout each room, including an installation of a local glass artist's work depicting the rising of the phoenix from the ashes. In this instance, the artist exemplifies the essence of survivorship, engaging the creative process and bringing artistic excellence to bear with a level of grace and humanity that transforms the environment (Figs 13.2 and 13.3).

In this programme, the arts provide service users with an opportunity for expression, and also create a bridge to health services. The Rowan's approach reminds us that the environment of care itself can be a barrier to healthcare if it is perceived as cold, unfamiliar, institutional, or threatening. In this case, the Rowan, as a referral centre, is the first point of contact for victims and is an essential link in the course of care for this population. The works of art at the Rowan give voice to survivors of sexual assault and provide a sense of safety, hope and connection for an individual entering the healthcare system, paving a more inviting way forward.

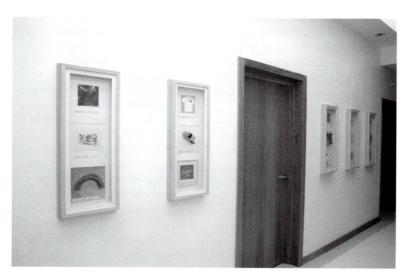

**Fig. 13.2** Art installations featuring the artwork of service users at the Rowan Sexual Assault Referral Centre, Northern Health and Social Care Trust, Antrim. Reproduced by kind permission of Karen Douglas. Copyright © 2015 Karen Douglas.

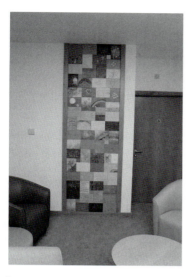

**Fig. 13.3** Art installation at the Rowan Sexual Assault Referral Centre, Northern Health and Social Care Trust, Antrim.
Reproduced by kind permission of Karen Douglas. Copyright © 2015 Karen Douglas.

### Tanpopo-no-ye, Nara City, Japan

Since 1973 Tanpopo-no-ye has provided global leadership in using the arts for 'caring', broadly defined, and for helping to develop a more caring society in Japan. Tanpopo's mission is centred on social inclusion and the concept of socializing art and 'artifying' society (Tanpopo-no-ye, not dated). The organization maintains art studio facilities in numerous locations that provide community members, including people with disabilities, with opportunities for connection and creative engagement. The organization cultivates community involvement in the lives of people with disabilities. Approximately 100 people with disabilities engage in art-making in the studios on a daily basis, and are supported by over 150 local volunteers who contribute through a variety of means, including cooking and art-making.

Tanpopo's programmes exemplify the concept of bringing people who are differently abled, ill, and in need of connection and services to the centre of communities, as opposed to the marginalization that commonly occurs. Tanpopo's Caring for Caregivers programme recognizes the needs of people who care for others, including professional and family caregivers. The programme started with a needs assessment that identified needs for acceptance of disability among family members and access to supportive doctors and other care services (Kable 2003). The programme developed a series of theatrical and literary performance works to present the needs of caregivers to the public, and also engages caregivers in arts workshops that provide connection and support. The programmes of Tanpopo-no-ye establish a network that links care providers with care users and community members to create a culture of inclusiveness, awareness, support, and access to needed services.

### Artes y Salud en Immokalee, Florida, United States

Artes y Salud en Immokalee is a partnership-based programme focused on improving access to healthcare and health literacy in a large rural community largely comprising migrant farm workers. Based on community composition and needs assessment, a group of community partners developed a set of arts programmes,

including weekly classes and seasonal festivals. The programme has documented its impact through research (unpublished), including a study of a weekly dance programme for adolescents that demonstrated improvements in body weight, physical activity, conduct, and pro-social behaviours.

Qualitative components of the study identified unexpected outcomes in addition to anticipated ones, including a sense of community pride, empowerment, and partnership with health providers that emerged from participation in the programme. The researchers also learned that parents were more committed to bringing their children to the health clinic because they were motivated by their child's enjoyment of the dance programme and the positive changes in behaviours that they could observe at home, such as increased physical activity. This resulted in increased utilization of clinic services and stronger relationships between residents and care providers. The connection of the primary-care providers to the dance programme appeared to increase willingness to participate and adherence with general healthcare recommendations (i.e. changes in diet and exercise). Additionally, children and parents alike developed recognition of the connections between cultural norms and health behaviours, such as over-eating.

### The Barefoot Artists, Pennsylvania, United States and Gisenyi, Rwanda

The Barefoot Artists is an organization dedicated to transforming communities around the world through art. In the Gisenyi region of Rwanda, the Barefoot Artists assembled a consortium of not-for-profit organizations including the Rwanda Red Cross, the Rwandan Village Concept Project, Engineers without Borders, and the University of Florida Center for Arts in Medicine, to address wellbeing in villages with survivors of the genocide. Within the multifaceted project, access to healthcare was identified as one need. While local clinics were available to provide health services, residents within walking distance were not utilizing services, and rates of preventable illness were high, as were maternal and infant death rates. To address this access issue, a project was developed that brought local artists and village residents to the local clinics to paint murals. In this way, residents became familiar with the clinics, made relationships with the medical staff, and felt a sense of connection and place in the clinics where they had painted murals. On-going health surveys have documented reductions in malaria, intestinal parasites, and mother and infant death following the project.

## Health literacy

Health literacy, in its most basic form, is defined as the function of reading health information and adhering to treatment—genuine literacy regarding one's health is not fully explored, and it is a limited view of the concept of health literacy. Nutbeam's three tiers of health literacy allow for further exploration of the concept by expanding the idea of literacy beyond basic functionality to include an individual's capacity to be critically informed about their illness and treatment (Nutbeam 2008). Health literacy is not about the need for more health information, but providing health information in a manner that is accessible across cultural and linguistic barriers (Day 2009; Singleton and Krause 2009).

A study by the US-based Institute of Medicine finds that nearly half of all American adults have difficulty understanding and using traditional health information, such as printed materials.

This difficulty is universal, especially in areas with a high concentration of individuals who are not literate, and results in a higher rate of hospitalization and healthcare costs (Nielsen-Bohlman 2004). Culture and creative media, including images, theatre, song, and dance, can give meaning to health information (Parker and Kreps 2005) and can significantly improve understanding, retention, and utilization of information, which is essential for addressing individual and public health needs.

McDonald et al. (2006) cite the arts as among the most effective tools for health education. Numerous international health agencies, such as United Nations Educational, Scientific and Cultural Organization (UNESCO), the Joint United Nations Programme on HIV/AIDS (UNAIDS), and the United Way, have adopted arts-based strategies for disseminating health information and effecting changes in health-related behaviours in rural communities throughout the world (Durden and Nduhura 2007). In an article examining the potential and use of visual arts, music, textile arts, performing arts, and literature in health education practice, the authors note the extensive history of the arts in effecting social change and in communicating culturally relevant health information. They also define six ways in which the arts can work in the service of health education: (1) to get people involved; (2) to facilitate the understanding of a community; (3) to change awareness and relay health education messages; (4) to bring attention to a health issue; (5) to promote community building; and (6) to promote healing itself.

Health information delivered through the arts can result in better use of benefits, better health outcomes, and reduced costs (Joint Commission 2007; Day 2009). According to the *UN Chronicle*, indications for excellence in health information delivery that may be particularly enhanced through the arts include: using images to communicate health information, creating a neutral and friendly environment, and adapting the delivery and content of the education to the local culture (Murthy 2009). The use of arts-based methodologies for enhancing the delivery of health information makes sense at every level.

## Promising practices in health literacy

### The Names Project—AIDS Memorial Quilt, California, United States

One of the best-known examples of the arts as a means for health education and awareness is the Names Project (<http://www.aidsquilt.org>), an AIDS memorial quilt, which began in 1987 and is still growing and travelling the globe to raise awareness. The project has been extremely effective in it mission to foster healing, raise awareness, and inspire action in the struggle against HIV and AIDS.

Knaus and Austin (1999) conducted a study assessing the impact of the quilt on students' perceptions of people with AIDS, self-efficacy, and awareness of risky behaviours associated with transmission of HIV/AIDS. The study demonstrated the efficacy of the quilt project in addressing issues centrally related to behavioural change in the college population.

### Gomeroi Gaayanggal, Tamworth, New South Wales, Australia

Gomeroi Gaayanggal (<http://www.newcastle.edu.au/research-and-innovation/centre/crs/mothers-and-babies/gomeroi/about-us>)is a unique arts and health programme addressing concern about low-birth-weight and premature infants in rural indigenous Australia. The programme uses the arts as a means of engaging expectant mothers and their families in a warm, welcoming environment, which features an art studio (Rae et al. 2009, 2011; Rae 2010, 2013). At Gomeroi Gaayanggal, pregnant mothers gather for art activities in which they connect with health practitioners and fellow community members to discuss nutrition, diet, and exercise in the context of community art-making.

In the case of Gomeroi Gaayanggal, healthcare staff identified a need for health literacy and for expectant mothers to come together to connect with other women, including their sisters and Elders, about their experience of pregnancy. The intergenerational nature of the programme and its effectiveness in conveying health information in an informal, creative environment make the model particularly special and promising. A local love of art-making and the opportunity for social connection bring the women together, resulting in access to essential health information and services. The women also produce works of art that engender a sense of pride, accomplishment, and empowerment.

### The SPREAD theatre programme, Rwanda

Rwanda is the most densely populated country in Africa, and family planning is highly underutilized, particularly in rural areas. With 3% of its population being HIV-positive, HIV remains a significant health concern (USAID 2012). The Sustaining Partnerships to Enhance Rural Enterprise and Agribusiness Development (SPREAD) project is a partnership between American and Rwandan universities and non-governmental organizations, including the National University of Rwanda, USAID, and Texas A&M University.

In Rwanda, coffee has been the leading export and one of the major sources of rural income, and thus the coffee industry was identified as a way in to address the health and wellbeing of residents. The SPREAD programme is focussed on and operates within the structure of a national coffee cooperative, recognizing that a cooperative's community engagement structure provides a mechanism for rapidly disseminating health information.

Within the project, the National University of Rwanda Theatre Troupe runs a theatre initiative through which over 100 coffee and pyrethrum farmers have been trained in community theatre. Recognizing that behavioural change is essential for changing health status, the farmers perform skits for their community members based on relevant health issues, including family planning, maternal and child health, nutrition, hygiene, sanitation, and HIV/AIDS prevention (Bucyensenge 2010). The farmers themselves identify the most pressing health issues and work with the theatre trainers to develop and learn to perform culturally relevant skits that they can use to educate their own communities. This person-to-person approach is unique and rapidly disseminates health information in an engaging and non-threatening way that community members can understand and will want to talk to others about.

In its mid-point evaluation in 2012, the SPREAD project reported improvements in personal and household hygiene, understanding and acceptance of family planning, increased uptake of voluntary HIV counselling and testing, increased use of condoms and other local health services, and shifts in gender norms affecting use of household revenue, alcohol use, and reproductive health (USAID 2012).

## Arts in Healthcare for Rural Communities, Florida, United States

In 2008, the arts in medicine programmes at the University of Florida (UF) implemented a statewide initiative to develop arts and health programmes in rural communities identified by the State of Florida as areas of critical concern. Improving health literacy was a major aim of the project. Over 5 years, 11 rural communities established arts and health programmes in Florida in partnership with the arts in medicine programmes at UF. The established programmes are self-sustaining and provide a diverse group of models for addressing rural health issues through the arts. These programme models are documented in a set of online resources in the Arts in Healthcare for Rural Communities Toolkit on the centre's website (<http://legacy.arts.ufl.edu/cam/rurallinks.aspx>).

Within the project, the Weems Arts in Medicine programme, Franklin's Promise Coalition, and the UF Center for Arts in Medicine's Theatre for Health Literacy team joined together to address health literacy among adolescents. The county's incidence of pregnancy and sexually transmitted infections among 15–19-year-olds is twice that of the state, and issues such as intimate partner violence and gender identity create significant health and social challenges. The Theatre for Health Literacy team comprises theatre, health education, sociology, and nursing students and professionals and is in residence on an annual basis providing immersive arts-based education to every middle- and high-school student in the county. The leadership team conducts a needs assessment in preparation for annual residencies, which provides a clear maxim for designing the content of theatrical skits and preparing the most up-to-date health resources and information.

In the class sessions, students enjoy humorous theatre activities such as dialogue among characters facing health issues. The students can contribute health questions anonymously, and participate in dialogue, writing, acting, and directing a portion of theatre themselves. Preliminary study data suggest that students are highly interested in the subject and are retaining health information presented in previous years. At the end of each residency, the team gathers data to understand the impact of the work. In response to the evaluative question 'Has your mind changed about anything today?' a student responded, 'To be honest, you guys have come here every year for the last three years, and every time, you guys have really impacted me, so YES IT HAS!'

## Asociación Ak'Tenamit, Guatemala City, Guatemala

Because of barriers in accessing healthcare, such as poverty, lack of access to education, and taboos about sexuality, the prevention and control of sexually transmitted infections such as HIV and AIDS in indigenous communities in Guatemala have proved to be a huge challenge. In light of the need for health information, Asociación Ak'Tenamit (http://www.aktenamit.org/)has developed methods of sharing vital health information, including the use of theatre in the Q'eqchi language and in Spanish to reach local communities and present characters dealing with sexual issues (Valladares 2011).

In partnership with organizations like Ak'Tenamit, UNESCO is strengthening and systematizing knowledge and best practices in the use of creativity and artistic expression in HIV and AIDS education as well as developing youth-friendly tools and materials (UNESCO 2005). At the time of writing, UNESCO Toolkits on Theatre for HIV Prevention in South America, Africa, and Asia Toolkits are available online (UNESCO 2005).

## Conclusion

As demonstrated in the examples included in this chapter, the arts are being employed successfully throughout the world as a way to engage community populations in improving wellbeing, health literacy, and access to healthcare services. This approach is by no means new, but as wellbeing and prevention become higher priorities in many health systems, the arts are being recognized and engaged with more frequently and are also being demonstrated through research to be effective interventions:

> By introducing their energy into a community, artists can—given the right conditions—set off a chain reaction, releasing people's own creative energies and making their full potential visible. Another important word here is 'play'. Artists model creativity as play and by involving people in play help to create a sense of wellbeing.
>
> Ings et al. (2012, p. 18)

As the field of arts and health grows, more partnerships are being developing between arts and public health professionals worldwide. Promising practice models are beginning to yield notable outcomes, and are providing reproducible structures for engaging the arts as low-risk and low-cost tools for engaging populations and improving health. While much more work is needed to document outcomes and define these promising practices as best practices, the discipline is making great strides. Partnerships are particularly important in this interdisciplinary work. As partnerships grow and are demonstrated to have an impact, networks will inevitably develop and be instrumental in disseminating models of best practice.

# References

Bucyensenge, J.P. (2010). Rwandan farmers to use theatre in promotion of family planning. *In2EastAfrica* [online]. Available at: <http://in2eastafrica.net/rwandan-farmers-to-use-theatre-in-promotion-of-family-planning/> (accessed 14 September 2013).

Bygren, L.O., Konlann, B.B., and Johansson, S. (1996). Unequal in death: attendance at cultural events, reading books or periodicals, and making music or singing in a choir as determinants for survival. *British Medical Journal*, **313**, 1577–1580.

Bygren, L.O., Konlann, B.B., and Johansson, S. (2001). Sustaining habits of attending cultural events and maintenance of health: a longitudinal study. *Health Promotion International*, **16**, 229–234.

Camic, P.M. and Chatterjee, H.J. (2013). Museums and art galleries as partners for public health interventions. *Perspectives in Public Health*, **133**, 66–71.

Carson, A., Chappell, N., and Knight, C. (2007). Promoting health and Innovative health promotion practice through a community arts centre. *Health Promotions Practice*, **8**, 366–374.

Clift, S. (2012). Creative arts as a public health resource: moving from practice-based research to evidence-based practice. Perspectives in Public Health, 132, 120–127.

Cohen, S. (2004). Social relationships and health. *American Psychologist*, **59**, 676–684.

Cohen, S. and Janicki-Deverts, D. (2009). Can we improve our physical health by altering our social networks? *Perspectives on Psychological Science*, **4**, 375–378.

Day, V. (2009). Promoting health literacy through storytelling. *OJIN: The Online Journal of Issues in Nursing*, **14**(3), art. 6, doi: 10.3912/OJIN.Vol14No03Man06

Department of Health and Human Services (2009). *The Power of Prevention*. Atlanta, GA: National Center for Chronic Disease Prevention and Health Promotion Available at: <http://www.cdc.gov/chronicdisease/pdf/2009-power-of-prevention.pdf> (accessed 5 August 2013).

Dissanayake, E. (2000). *Art and Intimacy: How the Arts Began*. Seattle: University of Washington Press.

Durden, E. and Nduhura, D. (2007). Use of participatory forum theatre to explore HIV/AIDS in the workplace: a research article. *Communicare: Journal for Communication Sciences*, **29**, 56–70.

Earhart, G.M. (2009). Dance as therapy for individuals with Parkinson disease. *European Journal of Physical and Rehabilitation Medicine*, **45**, 231–238.

European Commission (2005). *The Role of Culture in Preventing and Reducing Poverty and Social Exclusion*. Available at: <http://ec.europa.eu/employment_social/social_inclusion/docs/studyculture_leaflet_en.pdf> (accessed 7 September 2013).

Evans, J.E. (2008). The science of creativity and health. In: J. Sonke-Henderson, R. Brandman, I. Serlin, and J. Graham-Pole (eds), *Whole Person Healthcare, Volume 3: The Arts and Health*, pp. 87–105. Westport, CT: Praeger.

Fritsch, T., Kwak, J., Grant, S., Lang, J., Montgomery, R.R., and Basting, A.D. (2009). Impact of TimeSlips, a creative expression intervention program, on nursing home residents with dementia and their caregivers. *The Gerontologist*, **49**, 117–127.

Hanna, G., Patterson, M., Rollins, J., and Sherman, A. (2011). The arts and human development. The arts and human development: learning across the lifespan: National Endowment for the Arts, March 14, 2011, Washington, DC. [pdf] Available at: <www.arts.gov/pub/theartsandhumandev.pdf> (accessed 7 September 2013).

Hartley, D. (2004). Public health and health care disparities. *American Journal of Public Health*, **94**, 1675–1678.

Hettler, B. (1976). *The Six Dimensions of Wellness*. Stevens Point, WI: National Wellness Institute. Available at: <http://www.national-wellness.org/?page=six_dimensions> (accessed 14 September 2013).

Houston, S. and McGill, A. (2013). A mixed-methods study into ballet for people living with Parkinson's. *Arts & Health: An International Journal for Research, Policy and Practice*, **5**, 103–119.

Ife, J.W. and Tesoriero, F. (2006). *Community Development: Community-Based Alternatives in an Age of Globalisation*. Frenchs Forest, NSW: Pearson Australia.

Ings, R., Crane, N., and Cameron, M. (2012). *Be Creative, Be Well: Arts, Wellbeing and Local Communities*. London: Arts Council England. Available at: <http://www.artscouncil.org.uk/media/uploads/pdf/bcbw_final.pdf> (accessed 10 August 2013).

The Joint Commission (2007). *What Did the Doctor Say?: Improving Health Literacy for Patient Safety*. Washington, DC: The Joint Commission. Available at: < http://www.jointcommission.org/what_did_the_doctor_say/> (accessed 7 August 2013).

Kable, L. (2003). *Caring for Caregivers*. Washington, DC: Society for the Arts in Healthcare.

Knaus, C.S. and Austin, E.W. (1999). The AIDS memorial quilt as preventative education: a developmental analysis of the quilt. *AIDS Education and Prevention*, **11**, 525–540.

Laverack, G. (2011). Improving health outcomes through community empowerment: a review of the literature. *Journal of Health, Population and Nutrition*, **24**, 113–120.

Luke, N. and Xu, H. (2011). Exploring the meaning of context for health: Community influences on child health in South India. *Demographic Research*, **24**, 345–374.

McDonald, M., Antunez, G., and Gottemoeller, M. (2006). Using the arts and literature in health education. *International Quarterly of Community Health Education*, **27**, 265–278.

McHenry, A.J. (2011). Rural empowerment through the arts: the role of the arts in civic and social participation in the Mid West region of Western Australia. *Journal of Rural Studies*, **27**, 245–253.

McQueen-Thomson, D. and Ziguras, C. (2002). *Promoting Mental Health and Wellbeing Through Community and Cultural Development: A Review of Literature Focusing on Community Arts Practice*. Melbourne: VicHealth (Victorian Health Promotion Foundation) and The Globalism Institute (RMIT University).

Mark Morris Dance Group and Brooklyn Parkinson Group (2010). *Dance for PD*. Available at: <http://danceforparkinsons.org/about-the-program> (accessed 10 August 2013).

Martinez-Martin, P., Gil-Nagel, A., Gracia, L. M., Gómez, J.B., Martínez-Sarriés, J., and Bermejo, F. (1994). Unified Parkinson's disease rating scale characteristics and structure. *Movement Disorders*, **9**, 76–83.

Matarasso, F. (1997). *Use or Ornament? The Social Impact of Participation in the Arts*. Stroud: Comedia Publishing Group. Available at: <http://www.feisean.org/downloads/use-or-ornament.pdf>.

Murthy, P. (2009). Health literacy and sustainable development. *UN Chronicle*, **XLVI**(1,2). Available at: <http://unchronicle.un.org/article/health-literacy-and-sustainable-development/> (accessed 10 August 2013).

Nielsen-Bohlman, L., Panzer, A.M., and Kindig, D.A. (eds) [Committee on Health Literacy, Board on Neuroscience and Behavioral Health, Institute of Medicine] (2004). *Health Literacy: a Prescription to End Confusion*. Washington, DC: National Academies Press.

Northern Health and Social Care Trust (2013). *Northern Ireland's First Sexual Assault Referral Centre*. [online] Available at: <http://www.northerntrust.hscni.net/about/1814.htm> (accessed 10 September 2013).

Nutbeam, D. (2008). The evolving concept of health literacy. *Social Science and Medicine*, **67**, 2072–2078.

Parker, R. and Kreps, G.L. (2005). Library outreach: overcoming health literacy challenges. *Journal of the Medical Library Association*, **93**(4 Suppl.), S81.

Pierson, J. (2010). *Arts and Livability: The Road to Better Metrics*, pp. 13–15. [A report from the June 7, 2010 NEA Research Forum.]

Washington, DC: National Endowment for the Arts. Available at: <http://arts.gov/sites/default/files/Arts-and-Livability-Whitepaper.pdf> (accessed 15 September 2013).

Rae, K. (2010). Wearing someone else's shoes. *Medical Humanities*, **36**, 40–42.

Rae, K., Weatherall, L., Smith, R., and Mackay, P. (2009). The birth of Gomeroi Gaaynggal. *Aboriginal and Islander Health Worker Journal*, **33**(6), 3–5.

Rae, K., Weatherall, L., Naden, M., Slater, P., and Smith, R. (2011). Gomeroi Gaaynggal—moving forward. *Aboriginal and Islasnder Health Worker Journal*, **35**(6), 28–29.

Singleton, K. and Krause, E. (2009). Understanding cultural and linguistic barriers to health literacy. *OJIN: The Online Journal of Issues in Nursing*, **14**(3), art. 4, doi: 10.3912/OJIN.Vol14No03Man04

Stuckey, H.L. and Nobel, J. (2010). The connection between art, healing, and public health: a review of current literature. *American Journal of Public Health*, **100**, 254–263.

Tanpopo-no-ye (not dated). *About Tanpopo-no-ye*. Available at: <http://tanpoponoye.org/english/> (accessed 6 September 2013).

USAID (United States Agency for International Development) (2012). *Country Progress Report: Rwanda*. Available at: <http://www.unaids.org/sites/default/files/en/dataanalysis/knowyourresponse/countryprogressreports/2012countries/ce_RW_Narrative_Report%5B1%5D.pdf> (accessed 13 September 2013).

UNESCO (United Nations Educational, Scientific and Cultural Organization) (2005). *HIV and AIDS. Culturally Appropriate Responses. Using Theatre and Performing Arts*. Available at: <http://www.unesco.org/new/en/hiv-and-aids/our-priorities-in-hiv/human-rights/culturally-appropriate-responses/promoting-arts-and-creativity/theatre-and-performing-arts/> (accessed 5 August 2013).

Valladares, D. (2011). *Guatemala: Theatre as HIV Prevention Tool in Native Communities* [Inter Press Service News Agency]. Available at: <http://www.ipsnews.net/2011/04/guatemala-theatre-as-hiv-prevention-tool-in-native-communities/> (accessed 5 August 2013).

Westheimer, O., McRae, C., Henchcliff, C., et al. (2011). Dance for Parkinson's disease: a pilot investigation of effects on motor impairments and quality of life [abstract]. Poster presented at the MDS (Movement Disorder Society) 15th International Congress of Parkinson's Disease and Movement Disorders, 5–9 June 2011, Toronto, Canada.

White House Rural Council (2013). *Policy Initiatives*. Available at <http://www.whitehouse.gov/administration/eop/rural-council/policy-initiatives> (accessed 13 December 2013).

World Health Organization (1946). Preamble to the Constitution of the World Health Organization as adopted by the International Health Conference, New York, 19–22 June, 1946; signed on 22 July 1946 by the representatives of 61 States (*Official Records of the World Health Organization*, no. 2, p. 100) and entered into force on 7 April 1948.

World Health Organization (2005). *Preventing Chronic Diseases. A Vital Investment. Part 2 The Urgent Need for Action*. Available at: <http://www.who.int/chp/chronic_disease_report/contents/part2.pdf> (accessed 5 September 2013).

World Health Organization (2012a). *Addressing Inequities in Healthcare Coverage*. [online]. Available at: <http://www.who.int/pmnch/media/news/2012/implementation_addressing_inequities.pdf?ua=1> (accessed 10 August 2013).

World Health Organization (2012b). *Achieving Universal Access to Quality Health Care* [online] Available at: <http://www.who.int/pmnch/media/news/2012/implementation_universal_access.pdf> (accessed 10 August 2013).

# CHAPTER 14

# Arts in healthcare settings in the United States

Jill Sonke, Judy Rollins, and John Graham-Pole

## The overall state of the field

Arts in healthcare, arts in medicine, art for healing, arts and health—all these terms are used in the United States for the multidisciplinary field of healing through art. Until recently, the most often used term has been 'arts in healthcare', but with expansion into community health promotion 'arts and health' has gained favour and we will use it here.

The Joint Commission (for national accreditation), in partnership with Americans for the Arts (<http://www.americansfort-hearts.org/>) and the former Society for the Arts in Healthcare/Global Alliance for Arts and Health (GAAH) (https://www.art-sandhealthalliance.org), has conducted surveys of the prevalence and characteristics of arts programming in US healthcare institutions. From 2004 to 2007, the number hosting arts programmes rose from 43 to 49% (State of the Field Committee 2009). Over half have permanent or rotating displays, 45% public performances, and about a third activities for inpatients, outpatients, and staff. By 2008, patient programmes were more prevalent than environmental enhancements. Despite economic challenges, the number of not-for-profit arts organizations has increased to over 100,000 (Kushner and Cohen 2012), with many arts and health organizations included.

## Research in the United States

Research is under way in every area of the US arts and health field. The topic has been the focus of several Cochrane reviews, for example music therapy for people with dementia (Vink et al. 2004) and dance/movement therapy for improving psychological and physical outcomes in cancer patients (Brandt et al. 2011). The pace of publication is growing quickly, with most studies focusing on hospital-based interventions and programmes because engaging community members in art activities is less widespread in America than in Europe and elsewhere. While community-based research is the largest gap in the literature, we anticipate that this will soon be corrected in response to the goals of Healthy People 2020, an initiative of the US Department of Health and Human Services (USDHHS) that provides science-based national objectives for improving the health of all Americans. Every 10 years, Healthy People establishes benchmarks and monitors progress over time in order to: (1) encourage collaborations across communities and sectors, (2) empower individuals toward making informed health decisions, and (3) measure the impact of prevention activities (USDHHS 2013). Further, qualitative research is being increasingly recognized as an important complement to biomedical research methodologies.

We are seeing recent shifts in research directions, reflecting population characteristics and a greater awareness of the arts in public health. Our ageing population has increased, spurring greater interest in arts engagement by older adults. Researchers are studying the effects of arts engagement on quality of life and wellbeing for individuals of all ages, and one-third of the current funding of the National Endowment for the Arts (NEA) supports such studies in US communities (NEA 2013). Our increasingly multicultural society has prompted culture-specific arts and health programming, with more rigorous designs and long-term studies determining the impact of these and other arts and health interventions.

As the number of publications increases, US researchers are revisiting earlier research conclusions. For two decades, guidance for selecting hospital art has favoured realistic works depicting comforting images of nature and compassionate faces (Ulrich and Gilpin 2003). Nanda et al. (2010) reviewed studies of the impact of visual imagery on the trauma-related symptoms of combat veterans and guidelines on evidence-based art for civilian hospitals, and concluded that some existing guidelines might be contraindicated. For instance, a combat veteran with post-traumatic stress might see hidden dangers in paths leading to idyllic but ill-defined destinations.

Although curators are cautioned to avoid art with uncertain meaning (Ulrich and Gilpin 2003), some hospitals exhibit ambiguous, abstract art, citing narrative evidence of its aptness for healthcare settings. Rollins (2011) proposes a theoretical perspective of 'curiosity' as a framework for investigating the impact on health of more abstract forms of art.

Other means for creating healing environments are being explored. Researchers at Georgetown University Medical Center, Washington, DC are studying children's perceptions of child-friendly vintage photographs. A psychiatrist at the Walter Reed National Military Medical Center (WRNMMC), Bethesda, MD, is collecting artefacts such as old or unusual musical instruments for display in a behavioural health clinic, to compare perceptions of patients, families, and staff before and after the installation of items designed to distract by arousing curiosity.

Music, along with the visual arts, is a frequent research topic, with numerous studies showing its benefit to patients, families, and staff. An effective intervention across all ages, music was found to increase non-nutritive sucking of premature infants (Standley 2000) and to transcend physical symptoms and facilitate emotional expression for people in hospice care at the end of life (Hilliard 2007). However, findings from a University of Florida (UF) study suggest that music in healthcare settings may not always be beneficial (Sonke et al. 2015). Nurses in the study reported that they sometimes found that music distracted them from their work.

Because of the competitive structure of the US healthcare system, institutions remain focused on improving patient and staff satisfaction. According to Press Ganey, a consulting company that partners healthcare organizations to improve the overall patient experience, patient satisfaction directly affects the organization's reputation, operating revenue, and profit margin (Ganey 2005). We anticipate that measures of patient and hospital staff satisfaction will become frequent research endpoints.

With our growing number of disasters—natural and wilful—artists have been quick to provide assistance after major events such as terrorist attacks, hurricanes, floods, and earthquakes. The arts reached a new level of public support following the events of 11 September 2001, but optimal research methodologies need to be determined.

Despite the rapid expansion of arts and health reported by the State of the Field Committee (2009), arts-based research (ABR) has not grown in parallel. It seems vital to focus more on qualitative research and reclaim its original meaning of 'empirical research'—that derived from practical experience, not theory. The primary mandate of ABR is to explore narrative-based, personal experience to complement the conventional biomedical model that emphasizes quantitative data collection, derived from specific interventions for groups of patients with specific diagnoses, mostly within healthcare institutions. We are encouraging researchers and artists to produce empirical evidence to complement quantitative and epidemiological measures of evidence-informed practice and policy. For example, artists in

residence are often asked to keep field notes or to provide a written report of their observations after completing an arts session with patients, families, or staff. This realignment of priorities is particularly relevant to the growing focus on community-based creative arts and public health. Future directions in arts and health should involve both looking back and looking forward, and explore mixed quantitative and qualitative methods, to achieve the goals of Healthy People 2020.

## New directions in practice

A major shift in the US arts and health landscape in the past decade is evident in attention to the scope of practice and professionalism in the discipline. As more programmes are established in healthcare settings, providers are setting higher standards for artists and art programmes with regard to patient safety and professionalism. The divide in the disparate cultures of the arts and health notable in the early years, when many artists were struggling to understand healthcare culture and policies, is no longer acceptable, and artists employed by healthcare facilities must adhere to the same protocols as other health professionals and fully comply with their cultural and practical standards.

Over the past three decades, the field has emerged from a grassroots movement to a professional discipline, similar to yet distinct from the arts therapies. On-going discussion among professionals regarding similarities and differences in arts therapies and arts and health practices has highlighted the need for better definition of arts and health as a discipline, as well as standards of practice and boundaries of practice (Raw 2012). It is incumbent on arts and health professionals to clearly define the discipline, an on-going but incomplete process at the time of this writing.

The US arts and health literature is also expanding rapidly as clinicians and researchers recognize more widely the health benefits of the arts. The Arts in Healthcare Research Database, maintained by the UF Center for Arts in Medicine (UFCAM), has more than doubled its entries over each of the past 5 years. The increase in programmes and in research publications has created considerable momentum (Fig. 14.1).

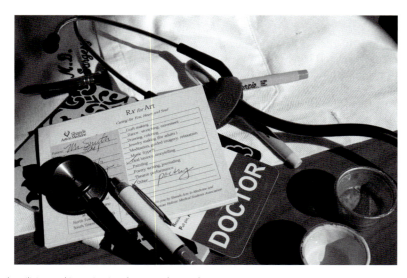

**Fig. 14.1** Clinicians are more actively utilizing and investigating the arts in hospital settings.

Current pay scales in the field are consistent with, or higher than, those of many allied health professions, suggesting a viable level of compensation for artists and administrators entering the field. In a 2010 GAAH survey, 220 arts and health professionals voiced a strong desire for higher pay scales and a need for graduate-level education and certification. The survey showed that while some artists and arts health administrators are paid as much as $120/hour, the median hourly pay rate was $31–40/hour (Parsonnet 2010).

While US arts and health has been primarily centred in healthcare settings since the 1980s, it is quickly expanding into community settings, in alignment with national priorities targeting public health, wellness, and prevention. Programmes like the Mark Morris Dance Group's Dance for PD are being replicated at a stunning pace, due to their popularity among participants and their compelling outcomes (Hackney and Earhart 2010; De Drue et al. 2012; Duncan and Earhart 2012). This programme, which started in Brooklyn, New York, in 2001, has been replicated in over 100 communities worldwide. Dance for PD has run teacher-training programmes in over 30 US states, and is developing a certification process for instructors. Arts and ageing, arts in the military, and arts in correctional institutions are also quickly gaining in prevalence.

## Arts across the life span

Newer technologies, such as functional magnetic resonance imaging (fMRI), are providing neurobiological information about engaging in art. For example, using fMRI, Limb and Braun (2008) discovered that when jazz musicians improvise, their brains turn off areas linked to self-censoring and inhibition and turn on those that let self-expression flow. Although knowledge is expanding rapidly, gaps about arts-based pathways and processes of human development remain. Unfortunately, although we acknowledge childhood as the foundation for lifelong learning and health, with arts enhancing development of the specific skills and behaviours of the 'whole child', widespread funding cuts are disrupting arts education in our schools (Bryant 2011). Research on benefits of art making in other important areas, such as helping children cope with normal stressors and those associated with illness, injury, disability, and healthcare experiences, are even less well developed (Hanna et al. 2011).

US health and education policy leaders are increasingly recognizing the need for strategies and interventions to address 'the whole person' (Hanna et al. 2011), and are adopting an integrated approach to policy development that reaches Americans at every stage of life, across generations, and in multiple learning contexts. The notion of lifelong learning is driving development of arts programming beyond childhood, perhaps the greatest application being in our fast-growing older population. Cohen's landmark study of the impact of cultural programmes on the physical, mental, and social health of older adults showed that those assigned to an intervention group (choral) reported higher physical health ratings, and fewer medications, doctor visits, falls, and other health problems than controls (Cohen et al. 2006).

The studies of Cohen and others have inspired arts and ageing programmes in all parts of the country, with resources to support them. Founded in 2001, the National Center for Creative Aging (NCCA) is dedicated to fostering understanding of the vital

**Box 14.1** Interagency Task Force on the Arts and Human Development membership roster

National Endowment for the Arts
Corporation for National and Community Service
US Department of Education
US Department of Health and Human Services
- ◆ National Institutes of Health
  - Office of Behavioural & Social Sciences Research
  - National Center for Complementary & Alternative Medicine
  - National Institute on Aging
  - National Institute of Child Health & Human Development
  - National Institutes of Health Library
  - National Institute of Mental Health
- ◆ Substance Abuse and Mental Health Services Administration

US Department of Veterans Affairs
National Endowment for the Humanities
Institute of Medicine (consulting member)
Institute of Museum and Library Services
National Science Foundation
Walter Reed National Military Medical Center

relationship between creative expression and healthy ageing, and developing programmes building on this understanding. In 2013, GAAH released *Bringing the Arts to Life: A Guide to the Arts and Long-term Care* (Rollins 2013a).

The National Endowment for the Arts (NEA)—an independent agency supporting artists and arts organizations—convened a Federal Interagency Task Force in the Arts and Human Development in 2011 to promote more research on the potential of the arts to foster health through creative expression across the life span. Members represent multiple units across the federal government (Box 14.1), and meet quarterly to share ideas and information about research gaps and opportunities. Activities to date include public webinars on compelling research and practice, a literature review of research on the arts and human development, and, in September 2011 in Washington, DC, the first ever National Academy of Sciences convening to review the current state of research on the arts, health, and wellbeing in older Americans.

## Arts in palliative care

Care of our ageing population is quickly expanding research and practice in arts for palliative care (Bertman 1999). The medical historian Guenter Risse (1999) tells of ostracized gay men dying of (as yet unidentified) AIDS in San Francisco General Hospital. These brothers' and lovers' music and painting, evoking laughter and tears, formed a poignant backdrop to their mutual caring until mutual death.

Loss takes many forms through our life spans: parts of oneself, significant others, material objects, and developmental deficits. Art in palliative care settings can focus its lens on existential meaning-making through self-expression, to ease the suffering of body, mind, and spirit (Graham-Pole and Lander 2009). Although both caregivers and receivers may well have recourse to optimal scientific knowledge, it is to their innermost thoughts and feelings that they look to sustain them in life-and-death situations. Humans crave inspiration and awe, and the qualitative narratives of palliative care resonate with and across cultures, serving as metaphors for everyone's loss of health, abilities, and, in due season, life itself.

The arts and art making lend themselves readily to the nuance and complexity implied in Stanworth's (2004) definition of palliative care: 'An approach that improves the quality of life of patients, and their families/significant others, facing the problems associated with life-threatening illness, through the prevention and relief of suffering by means of early identification, assessment, and treatment of pain and other problems: physical, psychosocial, and spiritual' (Stanworth 2004, p xvi). The values summarized by many hospices, most notably the Canadian Hospice Palliative Care Association (2013), suggest many possibilities for the arts to activate the interplay between the intrinsic value of life and of each autonomous individual, the natural process of death, the opportunities for self-actualization, and the need to address patients', families', and caregivers' suffering, expectations, needs, hopes, and fears (Stanworth 2004, p. 7).

Qualitative methodologies are peculiarly well suited to arts research and education in palliative care, and are becoming more and more accepted as complementing quantitative research with the dying and bereaved (Strang 2000; Morse et al. 2001). They represent a renaissance of the ancient marriage of science and art: it is no accident we use art to describe both the creation of works of beauty and the offering of skilled patient care, especially to the dying (Graham-Pole 2001, p. 165; 2005, p. 21). There is practical value in western healthcare's application of these methodologies to palliative care: they can have major impact on professional development, government funding, and public acceptance of both palliative care and of arts and health.

The concept of 'evidence-based medicine' has emanated from the increasing specialization of medical scientists (Rousseau 2006), who have come to regard quantitative evidence, especially the randomized clinical trial, as a gold standard. But in trying to eliminate confounds and observer bias, evidence-based medicine discounts a wealth of psychosocial, arts-based, and spiritual experience (White 2000; Stanworth 2004). Qualitative research ensures that participants in ABR bring the vital component of socially and culturally determined biases and positions to their meaning-making (Parker 2005).

## Arts and health in rural communities

Significant health disparities between urban and rural communities indicate a crucial need for interventions that can have an impact on health behaviours and reduce the incidence of preventable illnesses in rural areas (Jones 2009; Jones et al. 2009). While arts and health programmes have become prevalent in both urban and suburban settings in the United States (State of the Field Committee 2009), and their models have been widely documented, models for rural community programmes are still unavailable in the literature. However, some excellent programme models have been developed over the last 5 years, and their potential to benefit rural health is becoming increasingly evident.

Growing understanding of rural health disparities, social determinants of health (SDH), and the role of culture in affecting health behaviours is changing the way health programmes are designed for rural populations (World Health Organization 2008; National Prevention Strategy 2011; US Department of Health and Human Services 2012; Thomas et al. 2014). This broadening perspective, with its emphasis on rural culture in enforcing negative health behaviours (Hartley 2004; Thomas et al. 2014), presents an opportunity for the arts to become a tool for encouraging positive health behaviours. The arts reveal aspects of community life (Eisner 1991), affect changes in behaviour among individuals and communities (Burleigh and Beutler 1996), and promote competence and self-efficacy (Evans 2008).

An NEA survey (National Endowment for the Arts 2010) examining arts engagement in urban and rural communities confirmed clustering of arts organizations in urban areas, but revealed surprising consistency between urban and rural participation in personal creativity and 'informal' arts attendance. While formal activities, centred in museums and performing arts centres, are less available to rural residents, the latter participated more actively in activities such as singing in a choir. Clearly, rural settings are as viable as urban ones for arts and health programming.

Throughout the world, and for many decades, community health organizations have engaged street theatre, public murals, music, and arts-based social marketing to improve health and health literacy in rural areas (Lauby et al. 2010; Pelto and Singh 2010; Francis 2011; Muth 2011). Best practices demonstrate the importance of reflecting local culture and using interdisciplinary programmes based on local resources and needs assessment to guide the development of arts and health initiatives in rural communities. Three states—Oregon, South Dakota, and Florida—are currently making significant investment in such rural programmes.

In Oregon, Samaritan Health Services has developed the ArtsCare programme to serve populations in three counties. The programme supports 20 artists at 11 clinical sites in rural communities, and includes art-making, arts in the environment, and outcomes research and evaluation. The programme's survey studies have shown benefits to patient satisfaction, physical and emotional recovery, and the environment of care (Samaritan Health Services 2014).

Sanford Health, the University of South Dakota, and the South Dakota Arts Council are working together on an initiative to develop arts and health programmes throughout this predominantly rural state. Sanford Health initiated the Sanford Arts programme at their main hospital in Sioux Falls, and in 2008 expanded to include programmes at partner sites in Vermillion and Fargo, North Dakota (Sanford Health 2014).

In Florida, the University of Florida's Arts in Medicine Programs developed Arts in Healthcare for Rural Communities, with support from the State of Florida Division of Cultural Affairs, the Kresge Foundation, and the Florida Office of Rural Health. From 2008–12 the programme developed arts and health programmes in 11 rural communities, developing: (1) a unique model for developing arts and health programmes that can be replicated by other rural communities; (2) annual training programmes; (3) a national Arts in Healthcare for Rural Communities Network; and (4) print and online toolkits (UFCAM 2013).

This programme was shown to be a non-threatening means for healthcare systems (often viewed with mistrust in rural communities) to create more trusting relationships with residents (Moon 2012), increasing the use of healthcare services, and reducing costs of care associated with avoidance. These programmes can also enhance health literacy, health behaviours, and lifestyle choices, directly promoting health and wellbeing.

## Military-based programmes

In 2013, GAAH surveyed Veterans Administration Medical Centers (VAMCs), with 100 of the 140 medical centres responding. Nearly 80% reported providing arts activities for veterans and/or families and caregivers, either directly or in partnership with another organization. Currently, no data exist about arts programming prevalence for active service members and their families receiving care in military treatment facilities (MTFs).

In October 2011, the first National Summit: Arts in Healing for Warriors was held in Bethesda, MD at WRNMMC—the largest military medical centre in the United States and first destination in the continental United States caring for the wounded, ill, and injured from global conflicts—and the National Intrepid Center of Excellence (NICoE)—a unique Department of Defense institute for service members and their families dealing with traumatic brain injury and psychological health conditions. This marked the first time that different branches of the military had collaborated with civilian agencies to discuss how the arts can meet key health issues, from pre-deployment to homecoming.

Following the summit's success, in January 2012 Americans for the Arts and WRNMMC, in partnership with federal, military, not-for-profit, and private sector agencies, developed a 3-year National Initiative for Arts and Health in the Military, with the following aims:

1. to advance the policy, practice, and quality use of arts and creativity as tools for health in the military;

2. to raise visibility, understanding, and support of arts and health in the military; and

3. to make the arts as tools for health available to all active duty military, staff, family members, and veterans.

In November 2012, the Initiative held the Arts and Health in the Military National Roundtable in Washington, DC. Roundtable participants included 21 concerned and dedicated military, government, private sector, and not-for-profit leaders. The group recommended a 'blueprint for action' to ensure the availability of arts interventions for military personnel and their families, and to integrate the arts as part of the 'standard of care' in military hospitals as well as community settings across the country.

The Initiative held the National Summit: Arts, Health and Wellbeing Across the Military Continuum at WRNMMC in April 2013, considering the benefits of the arts across the entire military continuum: pre-deployment/active duty; re-entry/reintegration; veterans/VA and community systems; late life; families/caregivers; and members of the healthcare team. Military, health, and arts professionals were asked for ideas about how to make the arts part of military health, healing, and healthcare. Their recommendations, along with those of roundtable participants, are reflected in the publication, *Arts, Health and Wellbeing across the Military Continuum: White Paper and Framing a National Plan for Action* (Rollins 2013b).

One strong recommendation concerns the need for training artists beyond what is needed to work in civilian settings. The military, health, and arts fields represent distinct cultures, each with its own body of knowledge, terminology, philosophies, rules, and regulations. Artists need knowledge about military life, combat, and the impact of these issues on service members and their families.

In keeping with the focus of military leaders on readiness and resilience across the continuum of service, the Initiative proposes that arts programming be available to service members, veterans, and family members throughout their life span (Rollins 2013b). At some duty stations, creative arts therapists provide consulting services to active duty service members pre-deployment and concurrent with deployment. Operation Oak Tree, a programme of the Music Institute of Chicago's Institute for Therapy Through the Arts, offers creative arts therapies services for military families throughout their cycle of deployment.

For injured service members, re-entry occurs at a military treatment facility. Arts initiatives are integrated through rehabilitation or behavioural health services, the American Red Cross, occupational therapy, and elsewhere. Many of these initiatives include families. For example, artist-in-residence programmes provide arts experiences for service members, families, and staff at the bedside on WRNMMC's wards for wounded service members.

Community arts programmes are helping to ease the reintegration of returning service members into civilian life. In papermaking workshops throughout the United States, participants in the Combat Paper Project use their combat uniforms to create cathartic works of art. Workshop participants cut up their uniforms, beat them into pulp, and form them into sheets of paper. Using the apparently transformative process of papermaking, participants reclaim their uniforms as art, and express their experiences of military service. According to project co-founder Drew Cameron (2007), 'The story of the fiber, the blood, sweat and tears, the months of hardship and brutal violence are held within those old uniforms. . .. Reshaping that association of subordination, of warfare and service, into something collective and beautiful is our inspiration.' Other service members and their families benefit from the powerful healing, bonding, and socialization offered by a traditional music and dance project, Dancing Well: The Soldier Project.

Many VAMCs have robust arts programmes to meet the needs of veterans. The US Department of Veterans Affairs holds an annual arts competition and festival. An increasing number of facilities also employs music therapists. The National Center for Creative Aging is working with the VAMC in Washington, DC, to restructure and enhance its existing creative arts programme. At others, combat veterans from conflicts in Iraq and Afghanistan participate in From War to Home: Through the Veteran's Lens, a photovoice project sponsored by VA Health Service Research and Development.

Nearly a third of the 22 million veterans in the United States today are from the Vietnam era (US Census Bureau 2012). While troops returning from Iraq and Afghanistan are met today with a heartfelt 'welcome home and thank you', many Vietnam service members were in their time greeted with hostility and indifference. Increasingly, community arts organizations are reaching out to these and other veterans. Keene, New York's Creative Healing Connections programme, presents arts and healing retreats for active-duty and veteran women serving in any branch of service at any time. The Shakespeare Center of Los Angeles' Veterans in Art initiative hires veterans of all ages and abilities to receive on-the-job training and apprentice work in all aspects of a Shakespeare production (e.g. actors, technical directors, sound engineers, wardrobe assistants, prop managers).

Today, one in four dying Americans is a veteran (National Hospice and Palliative Care Organization 2013). To address the unique challenges that veterans may present at end of life, the National Hospice and Palliative Care Organization partnered with the US Department of Veterans Affairs in 2010 to create a programme called We Honor Veterans. This holds great promise as a valuable resource for artists serving dying veterans.

## Arts in health education and credentialing

As arts and health grows as a discipline and programmes become more widespread, attention to professionalism becomes vital. Currently in the United States, arts and health programmes are considered to be support services, and there is inconsistency in the name of the field, leading to confusion and a slowing down of development. In 2011, the GAAH board of directors spurred development of the Arts in Healthcare Certification Commission (AHCC), and in 2012 this five-member group of professionals in both arts and health and the arts therapies, including programme directors, educators, and artists, was established. The group has begun work on national certification for artists practising in healthcare settings, piloting a national examination in 2014, and anticipating certification to be in place in 2016. The certification is intended for professional artists seeking work in healthcare settings, and is designed to test knowledge and skills related to patient safety, ethics, and other practice-related topics.

This process reflects movement toward establishing a defined healthcare discipline, with the intention that the field becomes identified as an allied health profession, aligning it with approximately 80 other professions involved in the delivery of health-related services, such as occupational therapists, arts therapists, and child life specialists (American Dental Education Association 2013). The terminal degree for arts and health practitioners is currently an MA, but as scholarship develops a PhD will become the terminal degree for academic professionals.

Development of certification has spurred the standardization of ethics and practice. In 2009, GAAH charged a committee of board members and field leaders with developing a set of ethics for guiding practice in the field, which is being used to guide the AHCC in the same undertaking. While there are no published standards of practice, they are emerging with some consistency in academic and training programmes, such as those offered by the UFCAM, the University of Oregon, and the Creative Center at University Settlement, reflecting best practices identified for over a decade by organizations including the NEA (National Endowment for the Arts 2008). The need for education has also been widely recognized (Moss and O'Neil 2009), and there is a quickly emerging landscape of educational options.

Numerous accredited educational institutions are developing academic programmes to meet the increasing demand for education and training among current and new practitioners (Box 14.2). Currently, there is one degree programme offered at an accredited university, the University of Florida's Master of Arts in Arts in Medicine, and there are several certificate programmes, one master's degree concentration, and many individual courses and training programmes. In reviewing global best practices, Moss and O'Neil (2009) identified the UFCAM as the sole best practice

---

**Box 14.2** Current programmes of study at accredited US universities

University of Oregon

- Master of arts (MA) in arts administration with a concentration in arts in healthcare management: 72-quarter-hour residential programme

University of Florida (Center for Arts in Medicine)

- Certificate in arts in healthcare: 12-credit undergraduate residential or low-residence programme
- Certificate in dance in healthcare: 14-credit undergraduate residential programme
- Graduate certificate in arts in medicine: 12-credit online programme
- Graduate certificate in arts in public health: 12-credit online programme
- Master of arts (MA) in arts in medicine: 35-credit online programme

The New School for Public Engagement

- Creative arts and health certificate: nine courses + 150 fieldwork hours, undergraduate

Leslie University (Institute for Arts and Health)

- Advanced professional certificate in arts and health: 15 credits, post-baccalaureate or post-masters

Five Branches University, California Graduate School of Traditional Chinese Medicine

- Certificate of expressive arts in mind–body medicine: 9 units/135 hours of study

---

programme in the United States for training artists to work in health. This study identified significant gaps in training for artists outside of the arts therapies, and recommended development of master's-level courses of study that include research as a catalyst for further professionalism of the field.

Individual courses not associated with certificate or degree programmes are offered at University of New Mexico, Georgetown University, San Francisco State University, University of Minnesota, and Baylor University, among others. Excellent training programmes are offered by the Creative Center at University Settlement, the University at Buffalo, and the National Center for Creative Aging.

## Art and public health

In 1912, the field of public health was defined as 'the science and art of preventing disease, prolonging life, and promoting health through the organized efforts and informed choices of society, organizations, public and private, communities and individuals' (Winslow 1920). Eighty years later, the definition had become even more comprehensive, holistic, and community-oriented: 'Optimal health requires an integration of physical, mental, spiritual, and environmental wellbeing. . . . a means to living a successful and satisfying life' (Pelletier 1992). Yet conventional medicine, especially perhaps in the US health system, maintains to this day its narrow focus on highly sophisticated and costly diagnosis and treatment of individual diseases and illnesses within healthcare (better termed illness-cure) institutions.

So it is hardly surprising that the US arts and health movement has until recently been largely confined to healthcare institutions. GAAH's membership and programming are largely confined to healthcare facilities, and receive most of their funding from institutional operating budgets. The State of the Field Committee's 2009 report demonstrated that some form of arts programming exists in almost 50% of all US healthcare institutions, and is 60% funded by operating budgets. US hospitals freely admit to using their valuable art collections as marketing strategies (Hathorn and Nanda 2008), with their art market being valued in 2012 at between $300 million and $1.3 billion.

This is in direct contrast with the situation in other countries, for example Australia, Canada, and the United Kingdom, where profit is less of a driving force (Mills and Brown 2004). In those countries arts and health has a less institution-based focus, and has reached out much more to vulnerable and marginalized groups within society at large, including the young and older people at risk, those with addictions and other psychosocial problems, and people in hospice and palliative care settings. The US literature also contains minimal recognition of art as a SDH. Matarasso's (1997) UK study on the public health impact of participating in the arts is, to our knowledge, the first comprehensive research on this subject. This study furnished substantial evidence that participating in arts-based activities has significant benefits for both societal and individual health and wellbeing. A subsequent report published by the Royal Society for Public Health (RSPH 2013) provided further evidence of the impact and significance of arts and health research and policy.

The association of art with community, celebration, festivals, and healthy human pleasure had initially been highlighted in the World Health Organization (WHO) Commission on the Social Determinants of Health, the 1986 Ottawa Charter for Health Promotion defining health as 'a positive concept emphasizing social and personal resources, as well as physical capacities. . .'. (WHO 1986). Yet the WHO Commission continues to stress the deficit language of disease, ill-health, and social inequities in its list of fundamental conditions and resources for determinants of health (WHO 2012); notably, it fails to specifically identify art and art making by name as a SDH.

In *Use or Ornament?* François Matarasso (1997) claims a central position for the impact of arts on public health: 'Rather than the cherry on the policy cake, to which they are so often compared, they should be seen as the yeast without which it fails to rise to expectations' (Matarasso 1997, p. 10). Art making provides the stickiness binding a community, creating 'interdependency, tolerance and respect. The making of these values is a cultural process' (Mills 2003, p. 9). Participatory art making is the cultural 'means by which citizens acquire the skills, language and connectedness to engage in these processes' (Mills 2003, p. 9). The integration of communal art-making activities into healthcare settings should be at the heart of SDH public policy, not something to be addressed *after* achieving the many other SDHs sited by the WHO.

In launching Healthy People 2020 (USDHHS 2013), the US Department of Health and Human Services has placed its primary emphasis on community-based initiatives. Its four stated goals are to: (1) attain high-quality, longer lives free of preventable disease,

disability, injury, and premature death; (2) achieve health equity, eliminate disparities, and improve the health of all groups; (3) create social and physical environments that promote good health for all; (4) promote quality of life, healthy development, and healthy behaviours across all life stages. In doing so, Healthy People 2020 is acknowledging the ancient history in public health of using art to prevent illness, or—better—promote wellness. The Hippocratic oath, dating from the fifth century BC, and still affirmed by newly graduating American physicians, states in part: 'I will preserve the purity of my life and my arts . . . If I keep this oath faithfully, may I enjoy my life and practice my art, respected by all humanity . . .' (Edelstein 1943, p. 56). Despite the pervasive influence of Cartesian and Newtonian thinking on modern healthcare, how could anyone who is either a giver or receiver of healthcare consider medicine any less an art than a science?

Art for public health has an even more ancient history among the world's indigenous peoples, who represent the majority of our global population. 'Feasting and gifting rituals . . . singing, dancing, drumming, weaving, basket making, and carving were simultaneously . . . creative expression, religious practice, ritual . . . and markers of governance structures and territorial heritage . . . maps of individual and community identity and lineage' (Muirhead and de Leeuw 2012). This legacy underscores the primal significance and value of art as it infuses the global work of health promotion, education, research, and activism. Art has, from time immemorial, furnished the 'stickiness' that binds a community together, creates mutual care, and promotes individual and societal productivity. Participatory art is the 'cultural means by which citizens acquire the skills, language and connectedness to engage in these processes' (Mills 2003). In today's world of paucity of food, shelter, employment, and education, we should not resign ourselves to awaiting a magical diagnosis and cure of such pandemic ailments, but take every opportunity to proclaim the crucial value of art, side-by-side with every other SDH that the WHO upholds.

Although not overtly stated, the goals of Healthy People 2020 clearly underscore this vital importance of art to the US public health system. Repeated research has shown the value of arts to: (1) ably complement conventional medical treatment of chronic physical and psychological health conditions; (2) improve physical environments and reduce workplace stress and burnout; (3) enhance relationships in diverse work settings, with higher employee retention; (4) reduce reliance on pharmaceutical medications; (5) measurably improve workplace performance, cooperation, and mutual support, notably in healthcare settings; and (6) accelerate recovery from many illnesses, with consequently reduced strain on the healthcare system.

This large body of research has been primarily quantitative in scope and methodology, but many cross-cutting expressions of arts-based human creativity, as applied to public health, readily lend themselves to qualitative as well as quantitative research (Knowles and Cole 2008). This applies to every multifaceted arts and health activity that seeks to achieve societal as much as individual healing, together with popular and professional education and activism (Fig. 14.2).

The overwhelming evidence from global arts-based activities and experiences indicates that human beings are hard-wired to make art (Dissanayake 1992), and perhaps this explains the extraordinary paradox that no national, regional, or local government, whatever its degree of social and economic development,

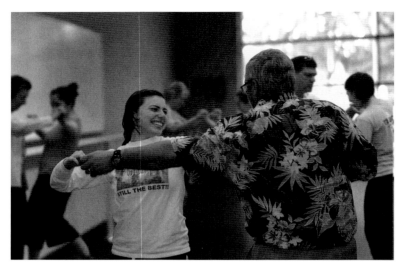

**Fig. 14.2** An intergenerational dance programme in Florida is the subject of current research.
Reproduced by kind permission of Jill Sonke. Copyright © 2015 Jill Sonke.

has declared and celebrated art as a cardinal determinant of public health, or taken comprehensive and far-reaching action to reflect this cumulative and compelling evidence.

This leads us to several specific recommendations for incorporating art into public health, and promoting global wellness in the American healthcare system. First, we should activate a universal movement to *name* art as a SDH, endorsed by health professionals, educators, researchers, policy-makers, and social justice practitioners. Secondly, we should develop and implement multicultural professional and popular education, together with qualitative and quantitative research, to deepen and broaden public understanding of arts and health as a positive SDH, not confined to healthcare and educational settings but embracing our whole society. Finally, we should integrate each and all of the above-named leaders to design, coordinate, promote, and adequately fund local, regional, national, and global arts and health programmes.

# References

American Dental Education Association (2013). Allied health professions overview. Available at: <http://explorehealthcareers.org/en/field/1/allied_health_professions> (accessed 10 August 2013).

Bertman, S.L. (1999). *Grief and the Healing Arts.* Amityville, NY: Baywood.

Brandt, J., Goodill, S., and Dileo, C. (2011). Dance/movement therapy for improving psychological and physical outcomes in cancer patients. *Cochrane Database of Systematic Reviews,* Issue 10, CD007103, doi: 10.1002/14651858.CD007103.pub2

Bryant, J. (2011). *Starving America's Public Schools: How Budget Cuts and Policy Mandates are Hurting our Nation's Students.* Washington, DC: National Education Association.

Burleigh, L. and Beutler, L. (1996). A critical analysis of two creative arts therapies. *The Arts in Psychotherapy,* **23**, 375–381.

Cameron, D. (2007). About Combat Paper. Available at: <http://www.combatpaper.org/about.html> (accessed 6 December 2013).

Canadian Hospice Palliative Care Association (2013). *A Model to Guide Hospice and Palliative Care.* Available at: <http://www.chpca.net/media/319547/norms-of-practice-eng-web.pdf> (accessed 17 January 2014).

Cohen, G., Perlstein, S., Chapline, J., Kelly, J., Girth, K., and Simmens, S. (2006). The impact of professionally conducted cultural programs on the physical health, mental health, and social functioning of older adults. *The Gerontologist,* **46**, 726–734.

De Dreu, M.J., Van der Wilk, A.S.D., Poppe, E., Kwakkel, G., and Van Wegen, E.E.H. (2012). Rehabilitation, exercise therapy and music in patients with Parkinson's disease: a meta-analysis of the effects of music-based movement therapy on walking ability, balance and quality of life. *Parkinsonism and Related Disorders,* **18**, S114–S119.

Dissanayake, E. (1992). *Homo Aestheticus: Where Art Comes From and Why.* Seattle, WA: University of Washington Press.

Duncan, R.P. and Earhart, G.M. (2012). Randomized controlled trial of community-based dancing to modify disease progression in Parkinson disease. *Neurorehabilitation and Neural Repair,* **26**, 132–143.

Edelstein, L. (1943). *The Hippocratic Oath: Text, Translation and Interpretation.* Baltimore, MD: The Johns Hopkins Press.

Eisner, E. (1991). *The Enlightened Eye: Qualitative Inquiry and the Enhancement of Educational Practices.* New York: Macmillan.

Evans, J.E. (2008). The science of creativity and health. In: J. Sonke-Henderson, R. Brandman, I. Serlin, and J. Graham-Pole (eds), *Whole Person Healthcare: Volume 3: The Arts and Health,* pp. 87–105. Westport, CT: Praeger.

Graham-Pole, J. (2001). The marriage of art and science in health care. *Yale Journal of Biology and Medicine,* **74**, 21–27.

Graham-Pole, J. (2005). The 'S' in SOAP: exploring the connection. *Journal of Poetry Therapy,* **18**, 165–170.

Graham-Pole, J. and Lander, D. (2009). Metaphors of loss: an appreciative inquiry. *Arts & Health: An International Journal for Research, Policy and Practice,* **1**, 74–88.

Francis, D.A. (2011). Using forum theatre to engage youth in sexuality, relationship and HIV education. In: D. Francis (ed.), *Acting on HIV: Using Drama to Create Possibilities for Change,* pp. 15–28. Rotterdam: Sense Publishers.

Hackney, M.E. and Earhart, G.M. (2010). Effects of dance on gait and balance in Parkinson's disease: a comparison of partnered and non-partnered dance movement. *Neurorehabilitation and Neural Repair,* **24**, 384–392.

Hanna, G., Patterson, M., Rollins, J., and Sherman, A. (2011). *The Arts and Human Development.* Washington, DC: National Endowment for the Arts.

Hartley, D. (2004). Public health and health care disparities. *American Journal of Public Health,* **94**, 1675–1678.

Hathorn, K. and Nanda, U. (2008). *A Guide to Evidence-based Art.* Concord, CA: The Center for Health Design.

Hilliard, R. (2007). The effects of Orff-based music therapy and social work groups on childhood grief symptoms and behaviors. *Journal of Music Therapy,* **44**, 123–138.

Jones, C., Parker, T., Aheam, M., Mishra, A., and Variyan, J. (2009). Health status and health care access of farm and rural populations. *Economic Information Bulletin No. (EIB-57).* Washington, DC: US Department of Agriculture.

Jones, C., Parker, T., and Ahearn, M. (2009). Taking the pulse of rural health care. *Amber Waves,* **7**, 10–15.

Knowles, J.G. and Cole, A.L. (2008). *Handbook of the Arts in Qualitative Research.* Thousand Oaks, CA: Sage.

Kushner, R. and Cohen, R. (2012). *National Arts Index.* Washington, DC: Americans for the Arts.

Lauby, J.L., LaPollo, A.B., Herbst, J.H., et al. (2010). Preventing AIDS through live movement and sound: efficacy of a theater-based HIV prevention intervention delivered to high-risk male adolescents in juvenile justice settings. *AIDS Education and Prevention,* **22**, 402–416.

Limb, D. and Braun, A. (2008). Neural substrates of spontaneous musical performance: an fMRI study of jazz improvisation. *PLoS ONE,* **3**(2), e1679, doi: 10.1371/journal.pone.0001679.

Matarasso, F. (1997). *Use or Ornament? The Social Impact of Participation in the Arts.* Stroud: Comedia [online]. Available at: <http://www.feisean.org/downloads/use-or-ornament.pdf> (accessed 15 August 2013).

Mills, D. (2003). Cultural planning—policy task, not tool. *Artwork Magazine,* **55**, 7–11.

Mills, D. and Brown, P. (2004). *Art and Wellbeing: A Guide to the Connections Between Community Cultural Development and Health, Ecologically Sustainable Development, Public Housing and Place, Rural Revitalisation, Community Strengthening, Active Citizenship, Social Inclusion and Cultural Diversity.* Sydney, NSW: Australia Council for the Arts.

Moon, L. (2012). Arts in healthcare for rural hospitals and communities. Graduate Thesis, Drexel University, Philadelphia, PA.

Morse, J.M., Swanson, J.M., and Kuzel, A.J. (eds) (2001). *The Nature of Qualitative Evidence.* Thousand Oaks, CA: Sage.

Moss, H. and O'Neill, D. (2009). What training do artists need to work in healthcare settings? *Medical Humanities,* **35**, 101–105.

Muirhood, A. and de Leeuw, S. (2012). *Art and Wellness: The Importance of Art for Aboriginal Peoples' Health and Healing.* Prince George, BC: National Collaborating Centre for Aboriginal Health (NCCAH). Available at: <http://www.nccah-ccnsa.ca/publications/lists/publications/attachments/26/art_wellness_en_web.pdf> (accessed 9 August 2013).

Muth, W. (2011). Murals as text: a social-cultural perspective on family literacy events in US prisons. *Ethnography and Education,* **6**, 245–263.

Nanda, U., Gaydos, H., Hathorn, K., and Watkins, N. (2010). Art and posttraumatic stress: a review of the empirical literature on the therapeutic implications of artwork for war veterans with posttraumatic stress disorder. *Environment and Behavior,* **42**, 376–390.

National Endowment for the Arts (2008). *Arts in Healthcare: Best Practices.* Available at: <http://nevadaculture.org/nac/dmdocuments/ArtsinHealthcare_handouts.pdf> (accessed 1 September 2013).

National Endowment for the Arts (2010). *Come as You Are: Informal Arts Participation in Urban and Rural Communities.* Available at: <http://www.creativecity.ca/database/files/library/nea_100.pdf> (accessed 1 September 2013).

National Endowment for the Arts (2013). *ArtWorks: Research.* Available at: <http://apps.nea.gov/grantsearch/searchresults.aspx> (accessed 5 September 2013).

National Hospice and Palliative Care Organization (2013). *We Honor Veterans: Achievements 2012.* Alexandria, VA: National Hospice and Palliative Care Organization.

National Prevention Council (2011). *National Prevention Strategy*. Washington, DC: US Department of Health and Human Services, Office of the Surgeon General.

Parker, M. (2005). False dichotomies: EBM, clinical freedom, and the art of medicine. *Journal of Medical Ethics, Medical Humanities*, **31**, 23–30.

Parsonnet, K. (2010). Pay scales for artists and coordinators working in the arts and health field. Global Alliance for the Arts and Health. Available at: <http://www.thesah.org/doc/SalaryScalesForArtistsInHealthcare_reduced.pdf> (accessed 3 August 2013).

Pelletier, K.R. (1992). Mind-body health: research, clinical, and policy applications. *American Journal of Health Promotion*, **6**, 345–358.

Pelto, P.J. and Singh, R. (2010). Community street theatre as a tool for interventions on alcohol use and other behaviors related to HIV risks. *AIDS and Behaviour*, **14**, 147–157.

Press Ganey (2005). The importance of patient satisfaction. Available at: <http://medpractice.pressganey.com/the-importance-of-patient-satisfaction-pages-176.php> (accessed 1 September 2013).

Raw, A., Lewis, S., Russell, A., and Macnaughton, J. (2012). A hole in the heart: confronting the drive for evidence-based impact research in arts and health. *Arts & Health: An International Journal for Research, Policy and Practice*, **4**, 97–108.

Risse, G.B. (1999). *Mending Bodies, Saving Souls*. Oxford: Oxford University Press.

Rollins, J. (2011). Arousing curiosity: when hospital art transcends. *Health Environments Research and Design Journal*, **4**, 72–98.

Rollins, J. (2013a). *Bringing the Arts to Life: A Guide to the Arts and Long-term Care*. Washington, DC: Global Alliance for Arts and Health. Available at: <http://thesah.org/doc/Bringing_the_Arts_to_Life_ebook.pdf>

Rollins, J. (2013b). *Arts, Health and Wellbeing Across the Military Continuum: White Paper and Framing a National Plan for Action*. Washington, DC: Americans for the Arts.

Rousseau, D.M. (2006). Is there such a thing as 'evidence-based medicine'? *Academy of Management Review*, **31**, 256–269.

RSPH (2013). *Arts, Health and Wellbeing Beyond the Millennium*. London: Royal Society for Public Health. Available from <https://www.rsph.org.uk/en/policy-and-projects/areas-of-work/arts-and-health.cfm>

Samaritan Health Services (2014). Arts in health program integrates art and healing. Available from <http://www.samhealth.org/communitysupport/pages/artscareprogram.aspx> (accessed 6 February 2014).

Sanford Health (2014). Sanford Arts. Available from: <http://www.sanfordhealth.org/services/sanfordarts> (accessed 6 February 2014).

Sonke, J., Pesata, V., Arce, L., Carytsas, F.P., Zemina, K., and Jokisch, C. (2015). The effects of arts-in-medicine programming on the medical-surgical work environment. *Arts & Health: An International Journal for Research, Policy and Practice*, **7**, 27–41.

Standley, J.M. (2000). The effect of contingent music to increase non-nutritive sucking of premature infants. *Pediatric Nursing*, **26**, 493–495, 498–499.

Stanworth, R. (2004). *Recognizing Spiritual Needs in People Who Are Dying*. Oxford: Oxford University Press.

State of the Field Committee (2009). *State of the Field Report: Arts in Healthcare 2009*. Washington, DC: Society for the Arts in Healthcare.

Strang, P. (2000). Qualitative research methods in palliative medicine and palliative oncology—an introduction. *Acta Oncologica*, **39**, 911–917.

Thomas, T.L., DiClemente, R., and Snell, S. (2014). Overcoming the triad of rural health disparities: how local culture, lack of economic opportunity, and geographic location instigate health disparities. *Health Education Journal*, **73**, 285–294.

Ulrich, R.S. and Gilpin, L. (2003). Healing arts: nutrition for the soul. In: S.B. Frampton, L. Gilpin, and P.A. Charmel (eds), *Putting Patients First: Designing and Practicing Patient-centered Care*, pp. 117–146. San Francisco: John Wiley and Sons.

University of Florida Center for Arts in Medicine (2013). Arts in healthcare for rural communities toolkit. Available at <http://www.arts.ufl.edu/cam/ruralLinks.aspx> (accessed 9 September 2013).

US Census Bureau (2012). Veterans by selected period of service and state. *Statistical Abstract of the United States: 2012*, table 520. Available at: <http://www.census.gov/compendia/statab/2012/tables/12s0520.pdf> (accessed 17 August 2013).

US Department of Health and Human Services (2010). Disparities—Healthy People 2020. Available at: <http://www.healthypeople.gov/2020/about/disparitiesabout.aspx> (accessed 29 August 2013).

US Department of Health and Human Services (2013). Healthy People 2020. Available at: <http://healthypeople.gov/2020/default.aspx> (accessed 4 September 2013).

Vink, A., Bruinsma, M., and Scholtlen, R. (2004). Music therapy for people with dementia. *Cochrane Database of Systematic Reviews*, Issue 4. art. no. CD003477, doi: 10.1002/14651858.CD003477.pub2.

White, G. (2000). Soul inclusion: researching spirituality and adult learning. In: A. Jackson and D. Jones (eds), *Researching Inclusion: Proceedings of the 30th Annual SCUTREA Conference, University of Nottingham, 3–5 July 2000*. Nottingham: School of Continuing Education, University of Nottingham. Available at: <http://www.leeds.ac.uk/educol/documents/00001469.htm> (accessed 1 February 2014)

Winslow, C.A. (1920). The untitled fields of public health. *Science*, **51**, 23–33.

World Health Organization (1986). *Ottawa Charter for Health Promotion*. Copenhagen: WHO. Available at: <http://www.phac-aspc.gc.ca/ph-sp/docs/charter-chartre/pdf/charter.pdf> (accessed 15 August 2013).

World Health Organization (2008). *Closing the Gap in a Generation: Health Equity Through Action on the Social Determinants of Health*. Geneva: WHO.

World Health Organization (WHO) (2012). *Summary Report: World Conference on Social Determinants of Health, Rio de Janeiro, Brazil, October, 2011*. Geneva: WHO. Available at: <http://www.who.int/sdh-conference/resources/conference_summary_report.pdf> (accessed 7 July 2013).

# CHAPTER 15

# Arts in healthcare in Uganda: an historical, political, and practical case study

Kizito Maria Kasule, Kizito Fred Kakinda, and Jill Sonke

## Introduction to arts in healthcare in Uganda

Although there is relatively little published, or even written, regarding the use of the arts for healing in Uganda, oral history, long-standing cultural practices, and works of art themselves confirm that the arts have been used in health practices since at least the pre-colonial era. Indeed, the arts have been integral to healing practices throughout Africa for centuries. A look into the traditional healing practices of cultures throughout the African continent reveals a broad array of rituals that use the arts as a means for transcendence, diagnostic discovery, affirmation, treatment, and for communication across human and spiritual realms (Janzen 2000; Sonke 2011). While history itself does not legitimize arts-based rituals as promoting health, it does present the ubiquitous connection of the arts to healing practices, and individual anthropological studies document the structures, meaning, and utility of many such rituals (Ghent 1994; Freidson 1996). In Uganda, the arts have a long history of being central to healing practices that fall under the realm of traditional healing. Uganda also has a unique history among nations in using the arts in biomedical settings. While the majority of formal arts and health programmes had their origins in the 1980s and 1990s, programmes in Uganda began in the 1960s.

This chapter will provide a brief overview to illustrate the roles that the arts have held in traditional healing practices in the pre-colonial and colonial periods in Uganda, and will also highlight some notable arts programmes that are operating within or in partnership with biomedical health services and in communities. Programmes focusing on HIV/AIDS awareness and prevention will be addressed as an area of specialization in arts and health in Uganda.

## The arts and healing in pre-colonial Uganda

Pre-colonial arts and health practices were holistic in nature, often performance based, and involved both physical and spiritual structures. While we will speak here in the past tense in reference to this time period, it is important to note that many of these practices are still used today in Uganda.

For pre-colonial Ugandans, one's personality was not independent of the world of the living or the dead. For a person to be complete in life and health, he or she had to be connected not only to those who were living but also to the ancestors in the world of the dead (Mbiti 1990). Art was commonly used as a manifestation of the invisible forces related to health and protection, and as a representation of the Creator, who would be invoked for healing. Art forms such as painting and sculpture, music, dance, and drama were blended and used simultaneously depending on the nature of an illness. Some practices were seasonal and others spontaneous in response to the needs of an individual or a whole community.

Widespread misunderstanding regarding African healing arts stems from a predominantly western perspective in anthropological studies. The implication in many publications is that Africans believed in magical and superstitious powers that did not really exist. For many Africans, the art of healing has never been associated with magic or superstition as termed by western scholars and missionaries. For example, the Baganda people of Uganda believe that whatever happens in the universe is made possible by the supreme God through his assistants, the saints. Because God is invisible, there was need to create objects through which his powers could be manifested and invoked for healing. Similarly, in the case of disease caused by ancestors or spirits, which were invisible, it was believed that these invisible powers could become visible and be interacted with through the arts.

Body painting was commonly involved in healing practices in pre-colonial times. Bodies were painted in various colours and patterns to symbolize the spiritual powers needed for healing. Paintings made on bodies, as well as on rock walls, surfaces of houses, or on the ground were used to counter the powers of evil that caused illness or misfortune. Clay, sand, soil and plant dyes were used to produce colours specific to particular symptoms or situations. Among the Baganda of Uganda, children suffering from smallpox were painted a white colour made from a mixture of white clay and ashes. The Bagisu of eastern Uganda used white clay, ash, and red earth to paint the bodies of boys being circumcised to ease pain during circumcision and to quicken the healing of the wound (Roscoe 2005). Performance, such as music, dance, and drama, was often incorporated into these rituals.

The Omugelegejo ceremony is one of the most ancient and important healing ceremonies of the Baganda people in Uganda (Ssempangi 2013). The ritual involves performance of actions that symbolize the breaking of taboos and capture healing power in a symbolic artwork called a jembe. The ritual involves both diagnostic and curative elements, and results in the creation of a sacred object, a horn that is decorated with red, white, and black beads symbolizing blood, brotherhood and protection. After the Omugelengejo ceremony has been performed and the execution of the art object completed, the art object is kept in a fine backcloth and then covered in two baskets or hung on a wall of the family or clan shrine.

## The colonial period (1894–1962)

A decade prior to the establishment of Uganda as a British Protectorate in 1894, Christian missionaries came to Uganda for the purpose of converting Africans to Christianity. One of the first pursuits of the missionaries was to rid tribes of their gods and ancestral spirits. Objects of art and arts-based healing practices were misunderstood by the missionaries, who did everything possible to destroy art objects and healing practices, which they associated with African traditional religions and viewed as pagan. While most objects of healing art were destroyed by missionaries, some were hidden away by natives (Kizito 2003). For community members, these objects were deeply rooted in cultural and religious meaning related to healing.

Newly converted Africans themselves often assisted in the destruction of African arts related to healing. Significant artefacts were lost in this process. For instance, in 1885 Princess Nalumaansi of the Buganda Kingdom, keeper of the royal umbilical cord art treasures of the children of the Kabakas' of Buganda, set fire to the royal umbilical cords under the influence of the missionaries.

As a consequence of such acts, revered art works used in healing were either burned or shipped to European museums. This destruction continued unabated through the colonial period. Fortunately, a few Africans remained faithful in private to the use of art in healing. These individuals lived as 'Christians by day and Africans by night', and were able to assist with reconstructing the history of the use of arts in healing in the pre-colonial East African society.

As we have shown, the arts have been widely engaged in healing practices in Ugandan culture. Music, dance, and drama were used to invoke ancestors and spirits to come to aid the afflicted and to ease psychological distress. Despite the commonality of arts-based healing practices, when Uganda was colonized little was done to incorporate the arts into newly developing biomedical clinics run by missionaries and the new government. Changes in society were apparent, as those who engaged openly in traditional healing practices were deemed backward or un-Christian.

The Second World War contributed to hardship in the country, including increased poverty, physical and psychological illness, and disability. In response to the growing need for health services for individuals affected by war and for a healthy workforce to fulfil colonial economic objectives, the British government established hospitals and clinics between 1945 and the 1950s. Mulago Hospital was built in Kampala as a main referral hospital to undertake treatment, research, and training. In government hospitals, British biomedical approaches were employed. While improvements in health resulted, many Ugandans felt that biomedical treatment was incomplete, as it did not address issues dealing with culture and traditional religion, which could only be addressed through the use of traditional arts. During this time many Ugandans utilized biomedical care while engaging in traditional practices in private (Ssempagi 2013).

In 1938, Makerere University in Kampala established the Margaret Trowell School of Art. By the 1950s, it was noted that, while the arts were not encouraged in patient care, medical staff at Mulago Hospital were influenced by Margaret Trowell to engage in the arts as a hobby that supported their own wellbeing. In 1958, Professor Cecil Todd from the Margaret Trowell School of Art introduced the concept of using the arts for therapeutic purposes with the ill. He proposed the concept to medical officials at Butabika Hospital, a large psychiatric hospital on the outskirts of Kampala. Todd's request was controversial and did not yield results until 1967 when the arts were formally introduced into biomedical care for the first time.

## The arts and health in post-colonial Uganda to the present

In 1969, the first exhibition of art by patients from Butabika Hospital was presented to the public. This exhibition was sponsored by the Uganda National Association for Mental Health, the Makerere University School of Art, and the Makerere University Department of Psychiatry. In his written comments in the catalogue, Professor Todd praised the works of art and emphasized the importance of art as an means of communication for this population, citing the arts as 'a bridge thrown across a gulf to give us access to a world which invites our exploration' (Asbjorg and Mardsen, 1969).

By 1969, the use of art at Butabika Hospital had become a recognized therapy for treating patients. There were two appointed 'art therapists' on the staff and there was a clearly established process of using art in patient care. The exhibition of 1969 also spurred recognition by the Uganda National Association of Mental Health that arts can be an effective component of treatment.

The progress made in this arena in the 1960s was largely halted by the ascendance to power of Idi Amin in 1971. At this point, many expatriates who were involved in the use of art at Butabika and Mulago hospitals left the country. As local manufacturing abated, art supplies became very expensive, and use of the arts in healthcare waned. Sadly, Amin's cruel reign from 1971–79 was a time when the Ugandan people could have benefited greatly from the arts in healthcare settings.

After the fall of Amin and during Obote's second government, public health projects involving the arts were commissioned by UNICEF, the Uganda Ministry of Health, and other agencies. These projects focused on the use of the arts in disease awareness, prevention, and health literacy. The graphic arts were in greater demand than ever as numerous health campaigns involving posters were launched, and many Ugandan studio artists gained employment. The effectiveness of theatre, music, and dance in addressing public health concerns spurred their integration into government health campaigns, including performances commissioned by the Ministry of Health.

Today in Uganda, the ratio of biomedical practitioners to the population is approximately 1:20,000 compared with traditional healers at 1:200 (Aboo 2011). Studies report that about 80% of Ugandans rely on traditional medicine due to a lack of access to and/or acceptance of biomedical treatment, and the arts remain central to traditional healing practices. Despite the setbacks of the late twentieth century in the integration of the arts into medical care, over the past two decades formal programming in healthcare settings and in communities has again been on the rise. After the National Resistance Army came into power in 1986 and formed the National Resistance Movement government, which is currently still in power, it embarked on the rehabilitation of national hospitals, including Butabika Hospital. At Butabika Hospital, new art studios and programming have been re-established under the Department of Occupational Therapy.

Several arts programmes operate at Mulago Hospital, including arts activities provided to patients in the main hospital by artists from the Uganda Art Consortium and the Margaret Trowell School of Industrial and Fine Arts, and a full-scale art programme in the Infectious Disease Institute (IDI) clinic. The IDI programme has transformed the clinic's waiting area into a working art studio, and features a full-time professional artist who assists patients in art-making and exhibiting the works produced. A study of the IDI programme found that patients visiting the clinic before the art programme was implemented were twice as likely to fear catching an infection as those who came after the intervention (Neema 2012). The study also found that the creative arts intervention helped to build self-esteem, improved communication, positively affected stigma surrounding HIV/AIDS, and dramatically improved the ambiance in the clinic environment.

Many outstanding programmes are operating in communities throughout Uganda, using the arts to address significant health issues as well as underlying or causal factors, including poverty, access to clean water, and war trauma. The Ntuuha Drama Performers, a group developed in 1994 by students of Makerere University's Department of Music, Dance, and Drama, specializes in using theatre to address HIV, reproductive health, and other public health concerns. The group works primarily in the Kabarole and Bundibugyo districts in western Uganda, and has created satellite programmes in five other regions. The group works in collaboration with the Ministry of Health and uses both traditional and puppet theatre, which can help to engage participants by reducing the stigma associated with human actors (Kilian 2002).

A project in the remote and highly underdeveloped Karamoja region, entitled Karamoja in the Eyes of her Children, used the arts to engage children in dialogue concerning the needs and future of their region. The project's needs assessment phase garnered 2411 paintings and drawings by children which were analysed to determine how young people see their region. The project identified alcoholism, domestic violence, corruption, and poverty as key issues, and helped to focus an arts-based education campaign, utilizing participatory theatre and the visual arts, to address these and resulting health issues.

Freedom in Creation (FIC) uses the arts to empower war-affected and at-risk communities, with a focus on access to clean water. The programme engages community members in the arts for therapeutic purposes and to teach skills and principles related to water hygiene. Through weekly 3-hour art classes led by FIC volunteers, including teachers, pastors, artists, and community elders, FIC raises funds to provide participating communities with water and educational infrastructures. FIC also hosts art exchanges between children and adults in the international community to encourage a sense of commonality as opposed to difference, peace building, and connection.

These are just a few of many notable examples of outstanding and impactful arts and health programmes in Uganda. While the issues that these programmes address span a range of health concerns, HIV/AIDS remains a primary concern in Uganda and truly cutting-edge work is emerging from both grassroots and formal organizations as well as from individual artists.

## Arts and health programmes for addressing HIV/AIDS

As of 2013, 1.4 million people were living with HIV in Uganda (UNAIDS 2013). HIV has been a major health concern in Uganda since the mid 1980s. The highest rate of infection among adults in Uganda was documented in 1992 at 18.5%. Due to a strong government response to the epidemic, the rate dropped to 5% in 2000. In 2005, prevalence increased to 6.4%, and in 2011 to 6.7% (Uganda AIDS Commission 2012). While the rate of transmission is generally stabilized, it is still quite high and remains a major national health concern.

In addition to the strong government campaign led by President Museveni to address the AIDS epidemic, the decline in transmission of HIV in Uganda can be linked to a unique level of community-based education and awareness activity—much that specifically engaged the arts, and most commonly music. In a study of music and HIV in Uganda, Gregory Barz (2006) documents how music has been used in addressing HIV as both education and medicine. Barz describes how, since the start of the epidemic, Ugandans have 'sung' their response to HIV. Using music, dance, and drama, Ugandans have raised awareness and spread information about the disease, and have consoled one another in these times of great suffering and loss.

Music, dance, and dramatic performances focused on HIV education have emerged from many health programmes and within communities. Outstanding examples among the multitude of such programmes include the Bwakeddampulira AIDS Patients Educational Team in Masindi, the People with AIDS Development Association (PADA) in Iganga, the Uganda Art Consortium, BUDEA in Buwolomera Village, Gordon Healing Arts in Kampala, The AIDS Support Organization (TASO) Drama Group at Mulago Hospital in Kampala (see <https://tasomulagodrama.wordpress.com/taso-mulago-drama-group/>), the Friends of Ruwenzori and the Kitojo Integrated Development Association in the Kabarole District, the Voluntary Service trust Team in the Luwero district, and the Good Shepherd Support Action Centre in Kampala.

The programmes presented by these groups use music and performance to engage audiences and deliver strong messages through their content. A song performed by PADA begins, 'Someone wants to kill you . . .' and goes on to address HIV through the metaphor of the luggage brought by a visitor that is too heavy to lift. After establishing the memorable metaphor, the song goes on to speak directly about HIV symptoms and prevention (Barz 2006, p. 19).

Many of these programmes are run by and include artists living with HIV themselves. The TASO Drama Group at Mulago Hospital comprises mostly individuals who are HIV positive. The members volunteer their time and present HIV/AIDS education through performances in schools and communities throughout the region. The group focuses on positive living, using the arts to convey messages that encourage lifestyles that prevent the spread of HIV and convey encouragement to those infected with the disease.

Artists from the Uganda Art Consortium volunteer their time to provide therapeutic arts activities to HIV/AIDS patients, children orphaned by AIDS, street children, hospital patients, and psychiatric patients in the Kampala area. The programme provides direct services to these populations and sells works of art to support the artists themselves and the programming.

Individual artists are also making an impact in the fight against HIV in Uganda. Lilian Nabulime uses sculpture, in the context of a social practice, for HIV awareness and prevention (Nabulime and McEwan 2011) (Fig. 15.1). Nabulime demonstrates that sculpture can be instrumental in educating people about HIV, particularly 'in communities with high rates of illiteracy and in which discussion of sexuality remains largely taboo' (Nabulime and McEwan 2011, p. 276). Her impactful work using sculpture to educate people in rural Ugandan communities is based in her understanding that 'In order to be effective, HIV/AIDS awareness initiatives need to reflect the lived experiences of people living with HIV/AIDS and communicate coherent messages that are precise, easy to remember, and able to transcend educational, linguistic and cultural differences' (Nabulime and McEwan 2011, p. 279). Nabulime's radical use of soap sculptures representing human genitals and HIV infection effectively engages people and spurs lively dialogue regarding the causes and prevention of HIV.

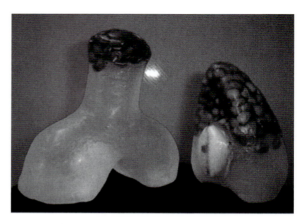

**Fig. 15.1** Soap sculptures created by Lilian Nabulime.
Reproduced by kind permission of Dr Lilian Mary Nabulime. Copyright © 2015 Lilian Mary Nabulime.

## Conclusion

The programmes noted here, as well as many others, are beginning to formally demonstrate their impacts through more formalized research and evaluation. The leadership of the Ministry of Health and Makerere University have done much to spur growth of the field in Uganda. While Uganda faces similar challenges to every nation in building arts and health programmes, it also provides many excellent models for programmes worldwide.

## References

Aboo, C. (2011). Profiles and outcomes of traditional healing practices for severe mental illnesses in two districts of Eastern Uganda. *Global Health Action*, **4**, 7117–7131.

Asbjorg H. and Mardsen, U.T. (1969). *Art as Therapy, an Exhibition of Psychotic Art, Butabika Hospital, Kampala*. Exhibition Catalogue.

Barz, G.F. and Wooten, J.T. (2006). *Singing for Life: HIV/AIDS and Music in Uganda*. New York: Routledge.

Friedson, S.M. (1996). *Dancing Prophets: Musical Experience in Tumbuka Healing*. Chicago: University of Chicago Press.

Ghent, G. (1994). *African Alchemy: Art for Healing in African Societies*. Moraga: Saint Mary's College of California.

Janzen, J.M. (2000). Theories of music in African Ngoma healing. In: P. Gouk (ed.), *Musical Healing in Cultural Contexts*, pp. 46–66. Aldershot: Ashgate.

Kilian, A. (2002). *HIV/AIDS Control in Kabarole District*. Eschborn: Deutsche Gesellschaft für Technische Zusammenarbeit. Available at: <http://www.afronets.org/files/gtz-aids-brochure-uganda.pdf> (accessed 20 September 2013).

Kizito, M. (2003). The Renaissance of Contemporary Art at Makerere University Art School. PhD thesis, Makerere University, Kampala.

Mbiti, J.S. (1990). *African Religions and Philosophy*. Portsmouth, NH: Heinemann.

Nabulime, L. and McEwan, C. (2011). Art as social practice: transforming lives using sculpture in HIV/AIDS awareness and prevention in Uganda. *Cultural Geographies*, **18**, 275–296.

Neema, S., Atuyambe, L.M., Otolok-Tanga, B., et al. (2012). Using a clinic based creativity initiative to reduce HIV related stigma at the Infectious Diseases Institute, Mulago National Referral Hospital, Uganda. *African Health Sciences*, **12**, 231–239.

Roscoe, J. (2005). *The Baganda: An Account of Their Native Customs and Beliefs*. Whitefish, MT: Kessinger Publishing.

Sonke, J. (2011). Music and the arts in health: a perspective from the United States. *Music and Arts in Action*, **3**, 5–14.

Ssempangi, K. (2013). Personal interview regarding PhD thesis on Omugelengejo, 3 July 2013.

Uganda AIDS Commission (2012). *Global Aids Response Progress Report, Country Progress Report: Uganda*. Available at: <http://www.unaids.org/sites/default/files/en/dataanalysis/knowyourresponse/countryprogressreports/2012countries/ce_UG_Narrative_Report%5B1%5D.pdf> (accessed 9 September 2013).

UNAIDS (2013). *Uganda Country Overview*. Available at: <http://www.unaids.org/en/regionscountries/countries/uganda/> (accessed 9 September 2013).

# CHAPTER 16

# Siyazama in South Africa: Zulu beadwork, HIV/AIDS, and the consequences of culture

Kate Wells

## Introduction to Siyazama in South Africa

The Siyazama Project has been a most insightful rural crafts and HIV/AIDS intervention, in that through the merging of creative art, health, and anthropological disciplines some very complex, modern, disconcerting, supernatural, but very human, stories have been revealed. These stories, in three-dimensional beaded form, including dolls and tableaus, have clearly demonstrated complex translations of other realities, and in so many cases of a paranormal nature (Fig. 16.1). This, I believe, has occurred as a result of the central focus of the project, which has been to impart information about HIV/AIDS to a small group of female makers of beaded cloth dolls and jewellery who reside in deep rural villages in KwaZulu-Natal, South Africa.

This chapter includes a brief history of the project, and the expert beadworkers, as well as details of the current international interventions in which the project finds itself today. I will describe how the rural beadworkers bravely and collectively began to deal with an impending, and mysterious, epidemic using their expert bead-working abilities as their weapon of choice.

When Celani Nojeza, a beadworker in the project, handed me a beaded cloth tableau in 2003, which spoke at length of the all-powerful *umpundulu* bird, I was intrigued. The tableau depicted two small children sitting at one end, and addressing them both was a *sangoma* or traditional healer. Here was a tableau about a huge, dangerous bird. But there was no bird to be seen! I asked Celani where the bird was, and she told me you cannot see it—it is an invisible bird.

The story told a sad tale of how the children had been playing, and on returning home for dinner they found both their parents missing. Where were their parents? The *sangoma* related that the powerful *umpundulu* bird had kicked them and they were both dead. She described the bird as being enormous with huge feet. Slapping her butt, and indicating the place where the bird kicks most often, she also told me that if the victim is a child it is most likely that the child will turn green.

This was by no means the last I was to hear about *umpundulu*. Rather it was just the start of many supernatural stories about this powerful, mythical, and much feared bird, stories of which continued to emerge through the Zulu rural women of the *Siyazama* project.

Throughout the world art has long been used as a tool for cultural, political, social, and economic change. Add to this 'health', and in my case as with the Siyazama Project, add AIDS, a catastrophic disease fuelled by and embedded in everyday normal human behaviour. In short, in Siyazama we use art as a means to inform, communicate, and cascade awareness of AIDS, with all of its cultural, political, social, and economic ramifications, challenges, and disruptions.

There is much evidence to show that South Africa, the most developed and industrialized country in Africa, is facing a huge hurdle with AIDS alone. According to the UNAIDS report for 2012 (UNAIDS 2012) sub-Saharan Africa remains most severely affected, with nearly 1 in every 20 adults (4.9%) living with HIV, and accounting for 69% of the people living with HIV worldwide. Gender inequality drives the epidemic in southern Africa, and HIV continues to profoundly affect women and girls across all regions. Because of the lower socio-economic, political, and cultural status of women, augmented by the power imbalances between men and women, many women and girls have little capacity to negotiate sex, insist on the use of condoms, or otherwise take steps to protect themselves from HIV (Wells 2009; UNAIDS 2012).

The sheer scale of need is evident, as only 40% of all those needing anti-retroviral therapy are receiving it. A decade and a half ago, when the Siyazama Project had just been inaugurated, nobody was on treatment. In South Africa, HIV/AIDS is a public health crisis of major proportions. It is still very rare to hear that somebody has died of AIDS. Indeed, bodies of people with AIDS are mostly handled with unease, and are generally associated with pollution (Henderson 2012).

South Africa, in 2015, finds itself within a milieu of contradictions. On one hand we have the voice of the late Nelson Mandela claiming that 'each one of us is intimately attached to the soil of this beautiful country'. Yet all of this beauty coexists within a complexity of economic, social, and cosmological inequalities that have an impact at numerous levels.

Aggravating this palpable inequality are typically misunderstood ideas around the looming threat of malicious and invisible supernatural forces. The democratic government has embraced all the trappings of a liberal modern state which attempts to look after its citizens—from the standpoints of both security and prosperity. Yet notions of the 'secret ministrations of evil people seeking

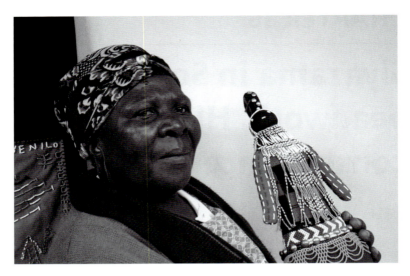

**Fig. 16.1** Tholiwe (Gogo) Sitole with her beaded cloth doll.
Reproduced by kind permission of Kate Wells. Copyright © 2015 Kate Wells.

harm for others or illicit profit for themselves by means of powers loosely designated as witchcraft' are endemic (Ashforth 2001, p. i). These invisible forces, and beings, often termed familiars, tend to wreak havoc amongst rural populations in particular, but are also well known for their mischievousness by the younger, modern population.

## Early beginnings

It was in 1996 that I began my first creative involvement with a small group of rural traditional craftswomen, and it was 2 years later in 1998, with funding through the British Council, that we employed the red ribbon logo as the metaphoric vehicle for engaging in AIDS educational workshops. At this early stage the group of craftswomen comprised four mothers and their daughters, collectively amounting to 13 females in total. Two of the daughters have since passed away. When the creative bead design workshops were first set up numerous other rural women joined us. It was the arrival of this new disease that sparked increased energy within the beadworkers of KwaZulu-Natal, and also provided the Siyazama Project with its brand identity.

The scenario within which the rural craftswomen of Siyazama live is one in which their government has been of little help because it has perpetuated the mystery of AIDS with confusing and inconsistent signals about HIV and its links to AIDS (Leclerc-Madlala 2005). In the words of Nelson Mandela in 2011 'We have failed to take HIV/AIDS seriously. That failure is a betrayal of our struggle for social justice and hope for our society.' Partly because of the culturally accepted polygamous insistence of men, in KwaZulu-Natal, AIDS has been termed 'the disease of men with money and women without'. South African President Jacob Zuma is a good example of this. He has five wives—not to mention his casual girlfriends.

My initial craft developmental work was driven by a great curiosity about rural craft and rural craftspeople in KwaZulu-Natal, the province in which I live and which has been my research domain for over 20 years.

## The Siyazama Project: a living innovation project

It was very early on in the Siyazama Project, following an initial evaluation study addressing issues about better understanding of HIV/AIDS, that it became clear that the rural women beadworkers were vulnerable due to cultural beliefs, and this was also keeping them mostly silent on matters of intimacy and sex. Further topics which emerged included the role of traditional healers *izangoma* (traditional doctors or diviners), the loss of the close-knit bond between twins if one is HIV positive, views on wide-scale virginity testing, polygamy, rape, AIDS orphans, *ubuthakathi* (witchcraft), and a variety of cultural behavioural prescriptions of avoidances and taboos termed *hlonipha*. Most historical and anthropological accounts of the Zulu emphasize the importance of the system of *hlonipha* in daily rural life (Krige 1936; Bryant 1949) and it is Raum (1973) who described *hlonipha* as a social function within Zulu-regulated behaviour that directly results in one's inability to discuss matters of intimacy. This practice of *hlonipha* as a moral code of behaviour still applies today. The most dangerous aspect of this is that, if married, one is largely unable to negotiate for condom use if one suspects infidelity or AIDS, and therefore to be married as a Zulu woman means that one is in a high-risk situation (Wells 2009).

It is also well documented that the crisis of rape in South Africa is out of control. Without a doubt, the large-scale levels of poverty entrench certain practices such as selling sex for a bundle of wood, a loaf of bread, or even for mobile phone airtime.

Amongst the most significant ethnographic studies undertaken in South Africa are those by researchers Leclerc-Madlala and Wojcicki (as cited in Nattrass 2004, p. 146). Their research describes the unacceptably high level of sexual violence against women. Claiming this situation to be 'endemic' and one in which rape is sometimes considered 'a normal recreational activity', these researchers clearly make the point that any intervention which aims to promote behavioural change must look into the sexual culture of the community or the society under study.

I quickly discovered that the communication mode in which the rural craftswomen were skilled—beadwork—had long been used by women in KwaZulu-Natal as a mode of communication to circumvent the Zulu cultural taboo on discussion of matters of emotional and sexual intimacy, *hlonipha*. It was Frank Jolles (1991) and Mthethwa (1988) (as cited in Wells 2006), both renowned beadwork researchers, who attempted to decode and interpret beadwork messages, and explained that a singularly literate style could never be sanctioned in beadwork. Mthethwa's theory, based on his findings, is that the historical function of beadwork was meant to transmit love messages secretly. As love messages are considered a very private matter in Zulu tradition, or *hlonipha*, it would not be advisable to send love messages which 'lack secrecy', i.e. making use of modern writing forms.

This system of restraints is felt by many Zulu to be an essential identifying marker of Zulu culture and its preservation viewed as vital to the maintenance of ethnicity. Much has been recorded on the notion concerning the complex so-called 'language' of beadwork (Twala 1954; Levinson 1965; Brottem and Lang 1973; Schoeman 1975; Grossert 1978; Mthethwa 1988; Jolles 1994; Preston-Whyte 1994; Magwaza 1999; Van Wyk 2003). Seemingly, most of this literature appears as the result of a paper written in 1906 by a missionary in Zululand named Reverend Franz Mayr. In his notes he recorded his observations and interviews about bead colours (Fig. 16.2). Of special interest was his reference (Mayr 1906, p. 162) to the fact that 'the natives have given each colour of beads a special name and meaning: and they have invented a kind of language of colour, whereby they can convey their thoughts from one to the other without speaking'. A beadwork producer in Siyazama states:

> 'This doll making has a specific purpose to us, as the Zulus. The dolls we make symbolize our culture, the way we dress and the way our grandparents used to dress. It's like we are continuing our dress code so that our grandchildren will see how we used to dress. We choose the colours according to age. The young ladies and the older women do not wear the same colours and we always do it that way.'

In the Valley of a Thousand Hills beaded cloth doll making exists in a slightly different capacity and form from the tradition of the Msinga beaded cloth doll makers. This three-dimensional craft form is the beaded cloth sculptures or tableaus made by the rural craftswomen who reside in this valley. These soft cloth beaded tableaus were directly fostered by Jo Thorpe, Director of the African Art Centre in Durban. She encouraged the beadworkers to continue with this most unique art form from the very first time Sizakhele Mnchunu-Nojiyeza brought a tableau in to sell in the early 1980s. Indeed many of these sculptures were made to produce a 'shock' response rather than to entertain, according to Preston-Whyte (1991, p. 67), and have became well known for their social commentary. This art form created a fresh insight into the world of the 'other' and provided tourists with a new opportunity to encounter a mysterious and unknown world.

Nonetheless, whilst economic growth and personal developmental are evident for the Siyazama producers, it is on closer inspection that one sees there is still much that needs to be understood. This includes the role that jealousy plays amid the workers of Siyazama Project and the powers of the supernatural forces. Bonagani, Lobolile's oldest daughter and an accomplished young beadworker, had joined us in London in 2003 at a Siyazama Project exhibition. For several years after this trip, she was ill. Once she had recovered, she amazed all of us by obtaining her driving licence, buying a small truck and beginning a very successful cupcake business. One can only imagine how much jealousy this gave rise to in her remote homeland village. Indeed, it's virtually impossible to keep secretive about successes in crowded villages.

This jealousy is completely understandable, considering the varying levels of financial insecurity in communities which are suffering much with poverty-stricken lifestyles and uncontrolled disease. Food is scarce and finding work can be difficult, if not impossible, for many. When one is showing signs of success it is perfectly possible that jealousy from others, neighbours, workmates, will emerge. Ashforth (2001) believes that the epidemic of AIDS has festered into becoming an epidemic of witchcraft. When there is wide-scale suspicion and secrecy in a community as AIDS continues to threaten all, problems of 'illness and death can easily transform matters of public health into questions of public power', and therefore identification and punishment of the people thought responsible might result in a type of witch hunt. The range of punishments may include beatings, illness, and even death. Indeed, in such an environment it is perfectly reasonable to accept that HIV/AIDS is nothing more than witchcraft.

It is at this desperate, confusing, stage that myths can provide an alternative mode of knowing. Like most non-western societies the Zulu perceive illness in a different manner to the narrow western biomedical idea of illness. According to Berglund (1976) the Zulu also do not view the finality of death as the end of life. Rather, immediately after death the spirits of the ancestor's *amadlozi* take an active and curious interest in the lives of the living. The ancestor's *amadlozi* are believed to be paying attention to everything concerning the day-to-day activities and thoughts of the living. Accordingly they also expect a continual degree of interaction and acknowledgement from the living. This conviction implies a softening of the division between life and death, which subsequently makes death an event of lesser effect than is the case in western societies.

The *sangoma* in Zulu culture is also known as a type of doctor or diviner. Often female, they have the power to connect and link with the ancestors, interpret spirit messages, and make these

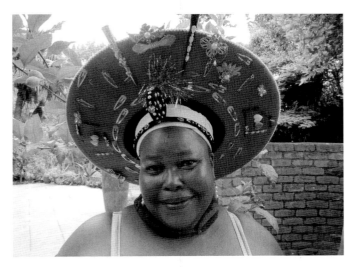

**Fig. 16.2** Lobolile Ximba proudly wearing her traditional wedding hat liberally decorated with glitzy adornments.

known to the living. They also have the ability to understand both the spirit world and the supernatural beyond the conception of ordinary people. Krige (1936, p. 297) explains that 'the doctor is, however, more than a link between the spirits and their decedents; he is the protector of society. He can smell out the evil people who have acquired power to work evil on their neighbours.'

One of our very best beadworkers in the Siyazama Project, and the only daughter of Tholiwe Sitole, was Kishwhepi. Her quality and workmanship was unsurpassed by all in the project. In the third series of design development workshops with the Swedish 'Editions in Craft' team of Renee Padt and Ikko Yokoyama, and design workshops with the Swedish all-female designer group FRONT, she was asked to submit a story which was meaningful to her, and this story would be beaded onto her story vase. She offered the following story:

> 'The one bad thing my husband did was to take another wife. He stays at my house some days, other days he is with his other wife. Some days are not good, and I am not satisfied, but other days I just don't care and just let things be. I am not accepting it, but I didn't have a choice.'

Three short months after completing the beading of her story vase she died very suddenly. Due to the unexpected nature of her death, some disclosed to me that they suspected poisoning, possibly by the new wife, or at least from somebody who was jealous of her. The debate on her death went on for a while. It was confirmed within a short time that *umpundulu* had indeed played a role.

## Conclusion

Through their beadwork practice in Siyazama the rural craftswomen have been enabled to demystify and unravel the cosmology of their own culture as rural women. They have also had to alter their position and focus, whist learning to adapt and to question significant components of their culture. This change occurred with little interference but became a vital necessity once the topic of sexual practice was raised in the AIDS workshops. Several told of how they were able to make their beadwork artefacts 'talk' through whatever means they deemed fit for the purpose. Through this methodology they claimed that they did not have to 'talk' themselves. But, importantly, this process allowed them to uphold their affinity to their esteemed culture and to deal

with AIDS, which was, and still is, classified as completely and dangerously taboo.

Nonetheless, a prevailing trend was that the Siyazama women, and most especially those from the middle to older generation, felt more confident to teach and help others rather than being enabled to help themselves in the face of AIDS. One of our leading beadworkers made a poignant statement about 'helping others to open their eyes', and 'cascading her newfound knowledge on AIDS' has clearly brought her confidence and empowerment. She says it has made her think differently, and more deeply.

If, as the literature recounts, the traditional beadwork has hidden codes, meaning, and symbolism, then this is partly what has assisted these vulnerable women to become aware of a virus which is slowly killing thousands in their communities.

Addressing cultural complexities and defining notions of supernatural occurrences through the arts, as the Siyazama women have done and continue to do, could not have been more surprising to me, or to others. I will always appreciate these first-hand insights into the range of cultural intricacies and challenges the women have to navigate through, and know well that all ambitions to empower rural women in KwaZulu-Natal must understand that there are precarious cultural beliefs and practices which can be obstacles in their lives and lifestyles.

My work in Siyazama has revealed the chasms and gaps that exist for meeting the health needs of poor communities in South Africa, and more emphatically in KwaZulu-Natal. Today in South Africa some of the most pressing needs are healthcare expectation, healthcare reception, healthcare understanding, and methods of healthcare information dispersal. It is my belief that visual communication methods, such as those in the Siyazama Project, can play a vital role in communities struggling to have these needs met. Methods of visual communication can represent culturally sensitive and traditionally resonant forms of engaging with people and are potentially capable of effectively transmitting powerful and important health messages. The challenge is to fully realize the extent to which this valuable characteristic of traditional craft making can be exploited as a tool for getting across health messages.

The Siyazama Project is indeed adding to this understanding by revealing new records of belief systems, some of which are clearly dangerous but still as relevant and prevalent as they were decades ago.

# References

Ashforth, A. (2001) AIDS, witchcraft, and the problem of power in post-apartheid South Africa. Occasional Papers of the School of Social Science 10 (unpublished). Available at: <https://www.sss.ias.edu/files/papers/paperten.pdf>

Berglund, A. (1976). *Zulu Thought-Patterns and Symbolism*. Bloomington and Indianapolis: Indiana University Press.

Brottem, B. and Lang, A. (1973). Zulu beadwork. *African Arts*, **6**(3), 8–13, 64, 83–84.

Bryant, A.T. (1949). *The Zulu People*. Pietermaritzburg: Shuter and Shooter.

Grossert, J.W. (1978). *Zulu Crafts*. Pietermaritzburg: Shuter and Shooter.

Henderson, N. (2012). *A Kinship of Bones: AIDS, Intimacy and Care in Rural KwaZulu-Natal*. Amsterdam: Amsterdam University Press.

Jolles, F. (1994). Contemporary Zulu dolls from KwaLatha: the work of Mrs. Hluphekile Zuma and her friends. *African Arts*, **27**(2), 54–69.

Krige, E. (1936). *The Social Systems of the Zulu's*. London: Longmans Green.

Leclerc-Madlala, S. (2005). *Reflections on Women's Leadership in the Context of the Second Phase HIV/AIDS*. Agenda 2005: Durban.

Levinson, R. and Levinson, M. (1965). Symbolic significance of traditional Zulu beadwork. *Black Art*, **3**, 29–35.

Magwaza, T. (1999). Function and meaning of Zulu female dress: a descriptive study of visual communication. Unpublished PhD thesis, University of KwaZulu-Natal, Durban.

Mayr, F. (1906). Language of colours amongst the Zulus expressed by their beadwork ornament; and some general notes on their personal adornments and clothing. In: E. Warren (ed.), pp. 159–165. *Annals of the Natal Government Museum*. London: Adlard and Son.

Mthethwa, B. (1988). Decoding Zulu beadwork. In: E.R. Sienaert and A.N. Bell (eds), *Catching Winged Words, Oral Traditions and Education*. Durban: University of KwaZulu-Natal.

Nattrass, N. (2004) *The Moral Economy of AIDS in South Africa*. Cambridge: Cambridge University Press.

Preston-Whyte, E. (1991) Zulu bead sculptors. *African Arts*, **24**(1), 64–76, 104.

Preston-Whyte, E. (1994). *Speaking with Beads/Zulu Arts from South Africa*. Johannesburg: Thames and Hudson.

Raum, O. (1973). *The Social Functions of Avoidances and Taboos among the Zulu*. Berlin: Walter De Gruyter.

Schoeman, H. (1975). *The Zulu*. Cape Town: Purnell and Sons.

Twala, R. (1954). Beads. Fascinating secrets of Zulu letters. Stories behind patterns and colours of the language of beads. Editorial. *Sunday Times*, 14 February 1954.

UNAIDS (2012). *2012 UNAIDS Report on the Global AIDS Epidemic*. Available at: < http://www.unaids.org/en/resources/documents/2012/20121120_UNAIDS_Global_Report_2012 >

Van Wyk, G. (2003). Illuminated signs: style and meaning in the beadwork of the Xhosa-and Zulu-speaking peoples. *African Arts*, **36**(3), 12–33, 93–94.

Wells, K. (2006). Manipulating metaphors: an analysis of beadwork craft as a contemporary medium for communicating on AIDS and culture in KwaZulu-Natal. Unpublished PhD thesis, University of KwaZulu-Natal, Durban.

Wells, K. (2009). Dolls with jobs: a compelling response by traditional KwaZulu-Natal craftswomen in an era of HIV/AIDS. In: D. Budryte, L. Vaughn, and N. Riegg (eds), *Feminist Conversations: Women, Trauma, and Empowerment in Post-Transitional Societies*, pp. 101–109. Lanham: University Press of America.

# CHAPTER 17

# Arts and health in Australia

## Gareth Wreford

## Introduction to arts and health in Australia

Australia's National Arts and Health Framework (NAHF), released in 2013, is endorsed by all Australian arts ministers and health ministers (ICH 2013b). The historical influences that led to this moment inform the shape of the NAHF and its arts-driven agenda to engage with the health sector. Connections between diverse areas of arts and health practice have emerged since the 1970s along with Australia's strong community arts movement and the increasing role of government patronage with the establishment of the Australia Council as a statutory authority in 1975 (Throsby 2001). While a historical absence of published material about arts and health and an effective central reference point for what does exist is acknowledged, the practice strengthened through the 1980s and 1990s aided by the establishment of four independent state health promotion agencies. From the 1990s the sector took its first steps to develop national perspectives and approaches as an identifiable community of interest. The last decade has been one of growth and consolidation in the sector through evaluation, conferences, peak bodies and awards, university research centres, and government policy development.

The central issue the NAHF seeks to address is the desire of the arts and health movement to increase recognition and support for creativity by health agencies (Mills 2013). This desire is influenced by a genuine belief in the multiple points of connection between creativity and health alongside limited arts funding, making it necessary for artists to seek new resources. Artists also report that arts and health programmes only exist so long as there are arts funding sources to support them (Mills and Brown 2004), making the development of policy a priority for the sector. The very limited evidence of arts and health funding patterns across governments arguably makes it difficult to take a definite position on whether arts or health agencies could be doing more, and testing 'government commitment and levels of support' is one of the questions the NAHF has set out to address (Mills 2011, p. 5).

The NAHF is the expression of a community of interest that defines itself as 'Creating arts and health experiences to improve community and individual health and wellbeing' (Putland 2010, quoted in ICH 2013b, p. 6). This statement of intent also makes arts and health relevant to the majority of Australians who perceive the benefits of the arts (Australia Council 2010).

Although any attempt at defining a community of interest involves some degree of reduction, Putland's recent background work for the NAHF is a useful starting point. Putland has identified the following five categories of arts and health practice (Putland 2012, p. 2):

- arts in healthcare design
- arts programmes (performance, exhibitions) in healthcare services
- art therapy (visual, dance, music, drama)
- arts and humanities in health professional education, and
- community based (participatory) arts

### Arts in healthcare design

While environmental design of hospital and health environments has a long history (Price 2010), in Australia the government-funded practice of incorporating art into major public buildings, including hospitals, is more recent, with Tasmania establishing the Art for Public Buildings Scheme (now the Artsite Scheme) in 1979 (Frankham 2005; Arts Tasmania 2013). Australian practice has also been significantly influenced by Peter Senior's work in the United Kingdom (Marsden 1993; Francis 2007) and Roger Ulrich's US study into the effects of interior design on wellness (Ulrich 1991).

In addition to the breadth of art and design in healthcare practice profiled by Sally Marsden in *Healthy Arts* (Marsden 1993), Marily Cintra is a leading Australian arts worker who coordinates public art and cultural planning for healthcare facilities (Australia Council 2007b). Cintra's post-occupancy evaluations demonstrate high levels of support for public art programmes (HARC 2013). The last 15 years has seen an unprecedented level of investment in health infrastructure supporting arts in health design (IADH 2013). Recent Australian examples of best practice like the Royal Melbourne Children's Hospital and Queensland Children's Hospital have designers and curators working from the earliest stages of a project and include major pieces of commissioned contemporary artwork (Cormack 2012).

### Arts programmes in healthcare services

Taking the approach of the creative industries and innovation to the arts and healthcare services Pagan et al. (2008) surveyed the widespread use of creative activities in healthcare settings. Within these creative activities professional artists are mostly included in healthcare services by way of art collections and artist in residence programmes (Fig. 17.1).

International trends recognizing the role of art in patient recovery led to the establishment of Sydney's Westmead Hospital

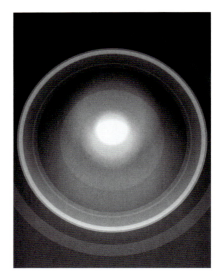

**Fig. 17.1** BrightHearts App (iOS), heart-rate controlled relaxation training application (still image from interactive application).
Reproduced by kind permission of Sensorium Health Pty Ltd. Copyright © 2015 Sensorium Health Pty Ltd.

collection in 1978. The subsequent neglect and rediscovery of Westmead's collection demonstrates how easily art can be sidelined by health-focused administrators without a strong arts partner (Barclay and James 2009). A recent and highly successful partnership model established in 2009 in the regional New South Wales (NSW) town of Orange is an arts and health programme that includes works from the regional gallery being exhibited at the town's general hospital and Broomfield Psychiatric Hospital. More of the gallery's collection is now displayed and seen by an additional 300,000 people per year (Orange Health Service 2013).

Another recognized model of arts in healthcare is artist in residence programmes (Price 2010). Since the mid 1980s artists have successfully gained grants and employment in healthcare settings. The first was at Larundal Psychiatric Hospital in Melbourne in 1984 (Sutton 2005) closely followed by other examples. The Prince Charles Hospital, Brisbane, established in 1989 (Marsden 1993) is significant as a residency based on health support rather than arts funding (Price 2008) with instrumental support from the state arts and disability organization Access Arts Queensland. Residencies continued to gather pace over the next decade to the point that Queensland Artsworkers Alliance published a guide on arts residencies for healthcare (Price 1998). Recent significant centres of activity that have influenced the development of the NAHF include Arts in Health at Flinders Medical Centre in Adelaide founded in 1996 (Putland 2009) and the music therapy programme at the Royal Melbourne Hospital founded in 1997 (RMH 2013).

## Art therapy

The aim of art therapy is primarily diagnostics and treatment, with little regard for aesthetics (Lloyd et al. 2007) and it receives minimal attention in the NAHF. Therapy is supported through the health sector and receives no national arts funding (Australia Council 2007a). Interestingly where professional artists are involved in therapeutic settings, for example at Melbourne's Splash Studios which offer an arts programme as part of a

recovery-orientated mental health service, the employment of artists is credited with the success of the programme (O'Brien 2003). Other therapy-centred organizations like the Dax Centre, Melbourne, and the Creative Expression Centre for Arts Therapy (CECAT), Perth, have evolved over time to build a strong community profile and make a major contribution to arts and health practice.

The Dax Centre houses the world's third largest collection of art produced by psychiatric patients after the Prinzhorn Collection in Heidelberg, Germany, and the Musee de l'Art Brut in Lausanne, Switzerland (Dax Centre 2013). While psychiatrist Eric Cunningham Dax is recognized as a pioneer in art therapy he had little interest in aesthetics, seeing 'painting as an expression of the particular sort of illness' (Cunningham Dax, cited in Radio National 1997). This position eventually shifted, reflecting broader societal changes and arts influences.

Cunningham Dax began collecting works soon after arriving in Melbourne from England in 1951 to head Victoria's Mental Hygiene Authority with responsibility for all asylums and services. By the 1980s, with most of the old institutions closing their doors as people with mental illness were de-institutionalized, Cunningham Dax found a home for the various works, and this became known as the Cunningham Dax Collection (Radio National 2007). The shift to an arts focus strengthened in 2010 with the development of a curatorial guide to the ethical issues associated with exhibiting works by people with mental illness (Jones et al. 2010). Since 2011 the renamed Dax Centre has been a curated collection and an accredited museum with a strong education focus 'promoting art and creativity for the promotion of good mental health and wellbeing' (Dax Centre 2012, p. 5).

Cunningham Dax also influenced the establishment of CECAT in Western Australia in 1968 (CECAT 2008). CECAT provides a stepped programme that includes 'individual and group art psychotherapy, open art studios and art classes, [and] a TAFE [Technical and Further Education] certificate in art and design' (Government of Western Australia 2013). CECAT also partners the Western Australian arts and disability organisation DADAA WA to provide community support and professional development to artists (CECAT 2008).

## Arts and humanities

The medical illustrations of Thomas Bock in Hobart, dating from 1824, mark the 'earliest western interactions between the Arts and Medicine' in Australia (Price 2010, p. 11). With the advances in photography from WW1 and film technology the field of medical illustration expanded to incorporate these new media. The Australian Institute of Medical and Biological Illustrators, founded in 1976, exists as a networking and professional development body for this specialized occupation (AIMBI 2013). New technology and the capacity to re-imagine the human body led to a 1996 conference, exhibition and forum 'Art, Medicine and the Body' at the Perth Institute of Contemporary Art with a series of related articles forming a special issue of *Artlink* magazine (Artlink 1997). The possibilities of biomedical illustration and education have continued to expand with three-dimensional computer animation technology as used by the Melbourne-based Walter and Eliza Hall Institute (WEHI) to produce award-winning animations of 'ideas about science that are impossible to observe and difficult to visualise' (WEHI 2013) (Fig. 17.2).

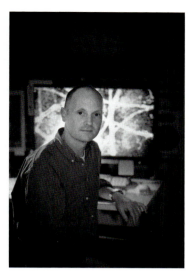

**Fig. 17.2** Biomedical Animator Drew Berry at the Walter and Eliza Hall Institute.

The personal experience of medical professionals and their many anecdotal stories of creativity and its influence on careers and the health of patients remains a largely untold part of the arts and health movement. Visible signs of activity include an Australian doctor's orchestra established in 1993 (ADO 2013), a doctors art festival held annually since 2009 (McKenzie 2009), the short-lived *Arts and Medicine* magazine launched in 2004 (Arts and Medicine Magazine 2004), and two special arts issues of the *Australian Medical Observer* magazine in 2009 (AMO 2009) and 2010 (AMO 2010). In addition the role of art in creating better doctors and as a part of healthcare is receiving recognition in university courses (Edwards 2006; University of Sydney 2013) with visual arts also being used to improve observation and empathy (Thomson 2009).

## Community based arts/arts and health

Community based arts and arts and health have historical influences in trade union movement concerns about class, i.e. who creates and attempts to establish a vernacular Australian culture (Cassidy 1983; Australia Council 1985). These concerns were partially formalized in the period following the election of Gough Whitlam's federal Labor government in December 1972 and the establishment of the Australia Council for the Arts with a Community Arts Committee (CAC). The earliest grants of the CAC supported a research study to assess the feasibility of establishing an Arts Access organization based on the US model of Hospital Audiences Incorporated (Australia Council 1974; Arts Access Victoria 2013). Throughout the 1970s and 1980s the Australia Council and various state arts funding authorities continued to fund a range of community-based arts activities (Hawkins 1993).

From the late 1980s energy shifted in some states to arts activity funded under the banner of health promotion. Influenced by the 1986 Ottawa Charter for Health Promotion (WHO 1986) state government health promotion organizations were established between 1987 and 1995 in Victoria, South Australia, Western Australia, and the Australian Capital Territory (Healthpact 2006). Each agency included a focus on arts sponsorship and the

promotion of health messages. By the late 1990s all four agencies moved from using arts to promote health messages towards supporting projects based on the value of arts participation for marginalized groups. As the language of participation and wellbeing became part of health some community arts practice also shifted to become more discipline-based as it sought to establish itself within health.

## First national steps

Although gradual and uneven the convergence of arts and health through the 1990s saw the first developments towards national perspectives and approaches. These developments show the ongoing role of the Australia Council as a supporter of organizations and activities in the broad community arts field and the international flow of ideas among arts workers. Peter Senior, Director Arts for Health, Manchester, UK, visited Melbourne in 1989 for a series of lectures and meetings hosted by Arts Access Victoria (DADAA 1992). In 1992 the newly formed DADAA National Network (now Arts Access Australia) held its first national conference in Brisbane on arts, health, and disability. The conference delegates carried a recommendation to 'develop a national strategy to integrate arts into the health sector' (DADAA 1992).

In 1993 Arts Access Victoria, published Sally Marsden's *Healthy Arts: A Guide to the Role of the Arts in Healthcare*. In 1994 Queensland held the first national Arts in Health conference (Woodhams and Bishop 1995) in the same month as the release of Creative Nation, Australia's first national cultural policy. Additional resources and models of practice designed for advocacy include Arts on Fire, a national model project for integrating people with a mental illness into the community through arts activity (Radbourne et al. 1995) and Creating Social Capital, the first Australian longitudinal evaluation of social impacts (Williams 1995) that influenced Matarasso's seminal UK study *Use or Ornament?* (Merli 2002). Then the election in 1996 of a conservative coalition federal government saw an effective 6% cut to the budget of the Australia Council (Parliament of Australia 1996), reducing its capacity to support new national arts and health-related strategies.

In these challenging times two Queensland arts workers established the Australian Network for Arts and Health (ANAH) in 1997. The ANAH closed in 2004, citing a shift from arts in healthcare settings to a broader focus on wellbeing that duplicated resources with the national community arts portal ccd. net (Clifford and Kaspari 2003), although ccd.net subsequently closed in 2006 (ccd.net 2013). In attempting to use instrumental arguments to support a diverse range of practice the ANAH fell between the arts sector and the health sector without sufficient support from either to be sustainable, and offers a counterpoint to the later UK experience with the National Network for Art and Health that lasted for 6 years from 2000 to 2006 (Dose 2006).

## Evaluation

Discussion about instrumental evaluation of arts and health for gaining support from health agencies reveals the influence of community arts in the arts and health movement (Pettigrew 2009) and a power relationship that favours health (Mills 2004).

The initial lack of interest from arts agencies in evaluating health impacts is related to resistance from artists who are concerned about instrumental evaluation (Mills 2004; Kelaher et al. 2008). This resistance can also be more subtly expressed as a preference for the less overtly instrumental language of wellbeing (Mills and Brown 2004; Putland 2007).

The danger that artists see is the potential for instrumental impacts to become the basis for funding, while not recognizing the broader role that art plays as a pillar of a healthy society (Hawkes 2001; Thiele and Marsden 2003). This tension between art for art's sake and art for social policy purposes is not easily resolvable because working in arts and health means negotiating different knowledge systems (Mills and Brown 2004) and funding from 'health promotion, is by definition, based on instrumental principles' (Putland 2008, p. 270).

In 2004 the Cultural Ministers Council (CMC), a government forum for state, territory, and federal arts ministers, published *Social Impacts of Participation in the Arts and Cultural Activities* (CMC 2004). The rationale for the report includes interest in social impacts as a potential justification for arts funding, though despite much anecdotal evidence it found 'little data to support the hypotheses' (CMC 2004, p. 10). Data here are being assessed from a health perspective in which evidence often means quantitative data generated through randomized controlled trials and qualitative research is dismissed as anecdotal.

Parallel to the CMC work one of its member agencies, the Australia Council, published *Art and Wellbeing*, the first national examination of the systemic connections between community arts and a diverse range of sectors including health and social inclusion conceptually linked through wellbeing (Mills and Brown 2004). *Art and Wellbeing* signalled a shift in the community arts sector based on a more sophisticated understanding of research and evaluation that moved beyond binary quantitative or qualitative understandings. The sector also started to strengthen its case through additional publications including a selection of the best international and Australian research in *Proving the Practice* (Lewis and Doyle 2008).

Other notable evaluation studies include Craemer's (2009) economic appraisal demonstrating the cost-effectiveness of arts activities, particularly for mild to moderate depression. Also, as part of the development of the NAHF, the Australian Health and Hospitals Association reviewed the best international and Australian evidence for arts and healthcare from clinical to community settings, finding significant support for arts and health practice (Fenner et al. 2012). As a result of this activity the arts and health movement is more assertive about the fitness for purpose of evaluation, noting the significant differences between large-scale epidemiological studies, clinical, and therapeutic settings and small-scale community projects, while arguing that each contributes to 'the development of a robust evidence base' (Putland 2012, p. 3). Putland also argues, quoting Clift, that the consistency of anecdotal and qualitative findings should be recognized as 'serious personal testimony' (Putland 2012, p. 9).

## National consolidation

The discussion about evaluation is closely related to a necessary and successful period of national consolidation in the arts and health field that emerged alongside the initial work of the ambitious and under-resourced ANAH. Writing in 2003, VicHealth, the health promotion agency for Victoria, stated that there is a 'community of interest' though 'no recognisable arts and health sector, nor the resources that generally sit with a sector, such as peak bodies for research or to lobby for interests, professional development or peer networking' (VicHealth 2003, p. 42). Ironically, for the arts and health sector, some of the generous state and territory-based funding for health promotion, like VicHealth, may have initially limited the development of national approaches. That the NAHF has its origins in the community arts sector is driven by that sector's established track record of success in developing partnerships outside of the arts (Throsby 2010). Within this context the early to mid 2000s saw some significant attempts to provide a framework for the breadth of practice beyond community arts through conferences, peak bodies, awards, university research centres, and government policy. After multiple starts and some failures many of these efforts remain relevant and support the development of the NAHF.

### Conferences

Inspired by UK conferences, held since 1999, Marily Cintra developed and produced the 2003 Synergy: Arts, Health and Design World Symposium. Without the necessary resources no papers were published, limiting the impact of this seminal event. It is remembered as the conference that brought Dr Rosalia Staricoff, the director of research at Chelsea and Westminster Hospital Arts, to Australia along with many other international speakers (Morgan 2003).

While community arts-related conferences were held regularly (CDN 2013) the next dedicated national arts and health events all took place in 2008. In one 5-week period the Arts Access Australia network and two university arts and health research centres, at the University of Newcastle and the UNESCO Observatory Multi-disciplinary Research in the Arts at the University of Melbourne, each held their inaugural arts and health conferences. Australia's second international arts and health conference The Art of Good Health and Wellbeing followed in November 2009. This conference is now an annual event and brings key UK and US leaders in arts, health, and creative ageing to Australia (ACAH 2013).

### Peak bodies and awards

The NAHF is supported by a great many arts partners and health partners, with its policy agenda, advocacy, and partnership development being driven by the Institute for Creative Health (ICH 2013a,b,c), previously known as the Arts and Health Foundation. Established in 2006, the Arts and Health Foundation soon split, with the Foundation continuing and a new organization, Arts and Health Australia, forming. The Arts and Health Foundation then rebranded as the Institute for Creative Health (ICH) in 2013. The change with the ICH was to concentrate on building the evidence base for arts and health (Mills 2013). The ICH also sponsors national arts and health awards and does so with the support of Creative Partnerships Australia, the government organization established to increase private sector support for the arts (Creative Partnerships Australia 2013). In 2012 Arts and Health Australia in turn rebranded to the Australian Centre for Arts and Health (ACAH). Since 2009 the ACAH has produced the annual Art of Good Health and Wellbeing conference and its rebranding is intended to develop a stronger focus on networking and advocacy. The ACAH annual conference is also

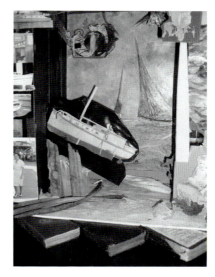

**Fig. 17.3** Liz's memory of her father.
Reproduced by kind permission of Neal Price. Copyright © 2015 Neal Price.

the platform used to promote its national arts and health awards (ACAH 2013).

There are more recent additions to the Australian arts and health landscape, including the Australian Institute for Patient and Family Centred Care (AIPFCC) that aims to transform people's experience of healthcare through partnerships and cultural change including high-quality integrated art, architecture, and design (AIPFCC 2013). The AIPFCC has collaborated with a national theatre company HealthPlay to present works and discussion forums about health issues (HealthPlay 2013). Another organization, the Arts Health Institute (AHI), brings creativity to care settings for the elderly and, reflecting Australia's ageing population, has grown rapidly since 2011. The AHI held its first conference in Sydney in September 2013 (AHI 2013). Similarly the Brisbane-based Creative Ageing Centre, founded by Neal Price in 2011, supports creativity and self-expression among older people in care (CAC 2013) (Fig. 17.3).

## University centres

Australia has an increasing number of university centres interested in cross-disciplinary practice, research, dissemination of evidence, journals, and networking. While it is difficult to determine their resonance within arts and health practice these collaborative approaches do illustrate attempts to link disparate areas of practice as well as the nature of a university system driven by competition for students, fees, and research dollars. Some have had a tenuous existence, like the ArtsHealth Centre for Research and Practice at the University of Newcastle that opened in 2006 and subsequently closed, with the university currently maintaining an interest in arts and health through its Collaborative Environments for Creative Arts Research group (CeCAR 2013).

Ongoing centres of interest include the UNESCO Observatory Multi-disciplinary Research in the Arts at the University of Melbourne, established in November 2006. The UNESCO Observatory publishes a refereed e-journal and produced a community health and arts conference in 2008 (UNESCO Observatory 2013). In addition the Young and Well Cooperative

Research Centre is a significant partnership-driven research centre investigating the creation of online digital media, mental health, and young people (YAWCRC 2013). Other noteworthy centres are the Art, Science and the Body Research Cluster at the Royal Melbourne Institute of Technology (RMIT), with an interest in topics that include the design of sound for health and wellbeing (RMIT 2013), and the Art and Design of Health and Wellbeing Cluster (ADHWC) at the University of South Australia, with a broad brief to positively influence the health and wellbeing of individuals and communities (2013).

## Government policy

The development of the NAHF is informed by work at the Australia Council and pioneering efforts in South Australia. The emergence of creative ageing as a field of interest in arts and health policy in NSW may also prove influential for the future of the NAHF.

### The Australia Council

After a restructure in 2004 the Australia Council held a lengthy consultation process to determine future directions for community arts and cultural development. The final consultation report included a recommendation that 'health and wellbeing' be one of three 'National Leadership Initiatives' (Dunn 2006, p. 16). In addition the Australia Council developed an internal paper *Strategy Options in Arts and Health* (Australia Council 2007a) that influenced the development of its community partnerships section (Australia Council 2009a) and cultural engagement framework (Australia Council 2009b). In keeping with the national leadership focus of the 2006 Dunn report the Australia Council provided resources to the then Arts and Health Foundation to canvas the development of a NAHF. The Australia Council is also part of the official working group that drafted the NAHF.

### Arts SA/SA health partnership commitment

This state arts and health agency partnership commitment was the first arts and health interagency policy agreement in Australia (Arts SA 2008). The commitment reflects the influence of the UK prospectus for arts and health developed a year earlier (ACE 2007) and the strength of arts and health practice in South Australia, including the Flinders Medical Centre (Fig. 17.4).

### National cultural policy

The election of the federal Labor government in 2007 brought plans for a new Australian cultural policy and, in 2013, shortly before losing an election, Labor released Creative Australia. The Creative Australia policy included a commitment to:

'Develop an Arts and Health Framework with state and territory governments to recognise the health benefits of arts and culture and to provide an agenda for activity.'

Australian Government (2013)

### The National Arts and Health Framework

The NAHF began its formal life with endorsement by arts ministers under a federal Labor government that consistently spoke of the need for the arts to make itself relevant to other portfolios (Westwood 2012). With the election of a conservative coalition government in 2013 the NAHF was untroubled by the incoming coalition arts

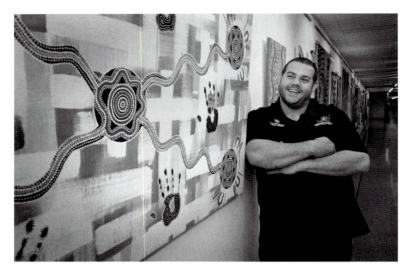

**Fig. 17.4** 'Community Consultation' painting by Allan Sumner.
Reproduced by kind permission of Flinders Medical Centre. Copyright © 2015 Flinders Medical Centre.

minister highlighting intrinsic values (Brandis 2013) and had coalition support in subsequently gaining endorsement by health ministers. The NAHF describes current practice, outlines future directions for government consideration, and identifies health promotion, healthcare, and community wellbeing as outcomes of arts and health (ICH 2013b). By including and synthesizing intrinsic and instrumental areas of arts and health practice the NAHF may be that rare example of a policy that enjoys bipartisan support. This support also marks a new degree of recognition for and independence of arts and health from its community art origins.

While the NAHF is significant, the coalition government has also committed to a commission of audit process to review expenditure with a view to making cuts across government (Greber and Anderson 2013), similar to the previous 1996 process (Griffiths 2013) that included cuts to the arts budget. While the future is difficult to predict with certainty a focus on intrinsic values of the arts within budget constraints may see increasing promotion of the 'relevance' of heritage art forms (Australia Council 2011) looking to deepen engagement with the community. Rather than being a conservative or elitist trend this shift is likely to be recast as popular—a democratization of culture using the techniques of cultural democracy (Matarasso 2013). This approach could favour an arts and health sector that is now broader than its community art origins, with demonstrated support from the coalition government. In terms of overall levels of cultural funding since 2000 the coalition is the equal of Labor (Eltham 2013), with coalition funding historically skewed towards single areas of interest (Craik 2007). Potential support available within health portfolios will also be tested as the NAHF switches focus to the development of action plans within each jurisdiction (ICH 2013c).

### NSW creative ageing

The reality of an ageing population has seen an increasing level of government interest in ageing issues. The 2012 NSW Ageing Strategy recognizes creative ageing (FACS 2013), as does a subsequent Arts NSW discussion paper on the development of a state cultural policy (Arts NSW 2013). Creative ageing in NSW is understood as the 'intersection between Arts and Health programs, strategies and policies which support people as they get older' (NSW Government 2013). In 2013 the NSW Department of Family and Community Services (FACS) sponsored a creative ageing forum that brought together FACS, the NSW Ministry of Health, and Arts NSW with national and international experts to inform future policy development aligned with the NSW Ageing Strategy.

## Conclusion

The growth and consolidation of the arts and health movement over the last 20 years is represented by the NAHF. Current strengths in the arts and health movement that will drive its future include:

- the increased profile of the sector through conferences and practice
- a more robust evidence base combined with broad public support for the benefits of arts participation
- greater comfort with evaluation and a willingness to negotiate instrumental arguments for support from health partners
- better networks, partnerships, and multidisciplinary collaborations across the arts sector and the health sector
- the emergence of creative ageing as a field of practice
- an organized and effective peak advocacy organization in the Institute for Creative Health
- successful bipartisan engagement and policy support across government arts and health portfolios

With these strengths and the momentum that created the NAHF, arts and health may flourish even as the focus on state arts and health action plans occurs in the context of efficiencies and savings across all levels of government. Continued advocacy backed by evidence that utilizes the diverse network of partners established by the ICH will be essential to fully realize the vision of securing recognition and resources for arts and health. Within the current political and economic environment the NAHF is well positioned as a new platform to support the Australian arts and health sector.

# References

ACAH (Australian Centre for Arts Health) (2013). Australian Centre for Arts and Health—the not for profit peak body for the arts and health sector in Australia. Available at: <http://www.artsand-health.org.au/latest-news/australian-centre-for-arts-and-health---the-new-nfp-peak-body-for-the-arts-and-health-sector-in-aust.html> (accessed 12 October 2013).

ACE (Arts Council of England) (2007). *A Prospectus for Arts and Health*. Available at: <http://www.artscouncil.org.uk/publication_archive/a-prospectus-for-arts-and-health/> (accessed 12 October 2013).

ADHWC (Art and Design of Health and Wellbeing Cluster) (2013). University of South Australia Art and Design of Health and Wellbeing Cluster. Available at: <http://www.unisa.edu.au/research/industry-partners/strategic-research-partnerships/research-and-innovation-clusters/art-and-design-of-health-and-wellbeing-cluster/> (accessed 12 October 2013).

ADO (Australian Doctors Orchestra) (2013). The Australian Doctors Orchestra. Available at: <http://www.ado.net.au/ado/public/history.aspx> (accessed 12 October 2013).

AHI (Arts Health Institute) (2013). Arts Health Institute. Available at: <http://www.artshealthinstitute.org.au/> (accessed 12 October 2013).

AIMBI (Australian Institute of Medical and Biological Illustration) (2013). AIMBI. Available at: <http://www.aimbi.org.au/> (accessed 12 October 2013).

AIPFCC (Australian Institute for Patient and Family Centred Care) (2013). Homepage. Available at: <http://www.aipfcc.org.au> (accessed 16 December 2013).

AMO (Australian Medical Observer). (2009). *Annual Arts Issue*. St Leonards, Sydney.

AMO (Australian Medical Observer). (2010). *Annual Arts Issue*. St Leonards, Sydney.

Artlink (1997). Special issue on art and medicine. *Artlink: Australian Contemporary Art Quarterly*, **17**. Available at: <http://www.artlink.com.au/issue.cfm?id=1720> (accessed 12 October 2013).

Arts Access Victoria (2013). Our history. Available at: <http://artsaccess.com.au/about/about-aav/who-we-are/> (accessed 12 October 2013).

Arts and Medicine Magazine (2004). Launch issue. *Arts and Medicine Magazine*. Sydney: imedia asia pacific.

Arts NSW (2013). *Discussion Paper: Framing the Future: Developing an Arts and Cultural Policy for NSW*. Available at: <http://www.arts.nsw.gov.au/wp-content/uploads/2013/04/revised-web-version-final-25-oct-2013.pdf> (accessed 16 December 2013).

Arts SA (2008). *Arts and Health: Partnership Commitment Between the Department of Health and Arts SA*. Adelaide: Arts SA.

Arts Tasmania (2013). *The Tasmanian Government Art Site Scheme—History*. Available at: <http://www.arts.tas.gov.au/about_us/history/the_tasmanian_government_art_site_scheme> (accessed 22 April 2015).

Australia Council (1974). *A Community Arts Compost 23–25 August 1974 Macquarie University*. Sydney: Australia Council.

Australia Council (1985). *Working Art: A Survey of Art in the Australian Labour Movement in the 1980's*. Art Gallery of NSW.

Australia Council (2007a). *Strategy Options in Arts and Health*. Sydney: Australia Council.

Australia Council (2007b). *Artist Honoured for Creative Contribution to Community Health*. Available at: <http://australiacouncil.gov.au/news/media-centre/media-releases/artist-honoured-for-creative-contribution-to-community-health-2/> (accessed 22 April 2015).

Australia Council (2009a). *Community Partnerships*. Available at: <http://2014.australiacouncil.gov.au/grants-2012/fundingguide/cp> (accessed 22 April 2015).

Australia Council (2009b). *Cultural Engagement Framework*. Available at: <http://www.australiacouncil.gov.au/about/cultural-engagement-framework/> (accessed 22 April 2015).

Australia Council (2010). *More Than Bums on Seats: Australian Participation in the Arts*. Available at: <http://www.australiacouncil.gov.au/workspace/uploads/files/research/full_report_more_than_bums_on_-54325919b74d6.pdf> (accessed 22 April 2015).

Australia Council (2011). *Understanding Community Relevance: A Discussion Paper*. Available at: <http://www.australiacouncil.gov.au/workspace/uploads/files/research/understanding_community_releva-5432545d57e08.pdf> (accessed 22 April 2015).

Australian Government (2013). National Cultural Policy—Creative Australia. *8.1.3 Regional Development and Social Dividends Through Community-Based Arts and Cultural Programs: What Happens Next*. Available at: <http://creativeaustralia.arts.gov.au/archived/module/ creative-australia-pathways/theme-connecting-to- national-life-for-a-social-and-economic- dividend/pathway-regional-development-and-social-dividends-through-community-based-arts-and-cultural-programs/regional-development-and-social-dividends-through-community-based-arts-and- cultural-programs-what-happens-next-2/> (accessed 12 October 2013).

Barclay, S. and James, P. (2009). Not the main game: art collections in hospital spaces: the Westmead experience. *Australasian Journal of ArtsHealth*, **1**, 78–89.

Brandis, G. (2013). The Coalition's vision for the arts. Speech 20 August 2013. Available at: <http://au.artshub.com/au/news-article/opinions/arts/the-coalitions-vision-for-the-arts-196364> (accessed 12 October 2013).

CAC (Creative Ageing Centre) (2013). Homepage. Available at: <http://creativeageingcentre.com.au/> (accessed 12 October 2013).

Cassidy, S. (1983). *Art and Working Life in Australia: A Report Prepared for the Australia Council*. Sydney: Australia Council.

ccd.net (Community Cultural Development on the Net) (2013). Arts health and wellbeing. Available at: <http://www.ccd.net/about/health.html> (accessed 12 October 2013).

CDN (Cultural Development Network) (2013). Past events—conferences. Available at: <http://www.culturaldevelopment.net.au/category/past-events/conf/> (accessed 12 October 2013).

CeCAR (Collaborative Environments for Creative Arts Research) (2013). Homepage. Available at: <http://www.newcastle.edu.au/research-and-innovation/centre/education-arts/cecar/about-us> (accessed 12 February 2014).

CECAT (Creative Expression Centre for Arts Therapy) (2008). *Art Spoken: 1968–2008 40 Years of Art Therapy in Mental Health in WA*. Perth, WA: Department of Health.

Clifford, S. and Kaspari, J. (2003). Australian Arts and Health 1997–2003: a six year perspective. *Artwork*, **57**, 10–13. Available at: <http://www.ccd.net/pdf/art57_6years_arts_health.pdf> (accessed 12 October 2013).

CMC (Cultural Ministers Council) (2004). *Social Impacts of Participation in the Arts and Cultural Activities: Stage Two Report—Evidence, Issues and Recommendations*. Canberra: Cultural Ministers Council. Available at: <http://culturaldata.arts.gov.au/publications/statistics_working_group/cultural_participation> (accessed 12 October 2013).

Cormack, E. (2012). Contemporary art in healing environments. *ArchitectureAU*. Available at: <http://architectureau.com/articles/contemporary-art-in-healing-environments/#img=0> (accessed 12 October 2013).

Craemer, R. (2009) The arts and health: from economic theory to cost effectiveness. *UNESCO Observatory e-journal*, **1**(4). Available at: <http://education.unimelb.edu.au/__data/assets/pdf_file/0003/1105815/craemer.pdf> (accessed 12 October 2013).

Craik, J. (2007). *Re-Visioning Arts and Cultural Policy: Current Impasses and Future Directions*. ANU e-press. Available at: <http://press.anu.edu.au?p=61151> (accessed 10 April 2014).

Creative Partnerships Australia (2013). About us. Available at: https://www.creativepartnershipsaustralia.org.au/about-us/ (accessed 12 October 2013).

DADAA National Network (1992). National Artability Conference: Crossing the Boundaries 15–17 October 1992. Conference report. Unpublished.

Dax Centre (2012). *Annual Report 2012*. Available at: <http://www.daxcentre.org/wp-content/uploads/2012/02/thedaxcentre_annual-report_lr.pdf> (accessed 12 October 2013).

Dax Centre (2013). History. Available at: <http://www.daxcentre.org/about-us/history/> (accessed 12 October 2013).

Dose, L. (2006). National Network for the Arts in Health: lessons learned from six years of work. *Journal of the Royal Society for the Promotion of Health*, **126**, 110–112.

Dunn, A. (2006). *Community Partnerships Scoping Study Report*. Surry Hills, NSW: Australia Council. Available at: <http://2014.australiacouncil.gov.au/__data/assets/pdf_file/0007/33973/Directions_and_opportunities_discussion_paper.pdf> (accessed 22 April 2015).

Edwards, H. (2006). Adding another string to their bow is music to doctors' ears. *Sydney Morning Herald*, 11 June. Available at: <http://www.smh.com.au/news/national/adding-another-string-to-their-bow-is-music-to-doctors-ears/2006/06/10/1149815358785.html> (accessed 12 October 2013).

Eltham, B. (2013). Arts funding: which party gives more? *ArtsHub*. Available at: <http://www.artshub.com.au/news-article/features/all-arts/arts-funding-which-party-gives-more-195988> (accessed 10 April 2014).

FACS (NSW Department of Family and Community Services) (2013). *NSW Ageing Strategy*. Available at: <http://www.adhc.nsw.gov.au/about_us/strategies/nsw_ageing_strategy> .(accessed 16 December 2013)

Fenner, P., Rumbold, B., Rumbold, J., and Robinson, P. (2012). Is there compelling evidence for using the arts in health care? *Deeble Institute Evidence Brief No 4*. Available at: <http://ahha.asn.au/publication/evidence-briefs/there-compelling-evidence-using-arts-health-care> (accessed 12 October 2013).

Francis, S. (2007). *Churchill Fellowship Report on Arts in Health*. Available at: <http://www.artsaccessaustralia.org/resources/research-and-reports/350-churchill-fellowship-report-on-arts-in-health> (accessed 12 October 2013).

Frankham, N. (2005). *Claiming Ground; Twenty-Five Years of Tasmania's Art for Public Buildings Scheme*. Hobart: Quintus. Available at: <http://ecite.utas.edu.au/57623> (accessed 12 October 2013).

Government of Western Australia (2013). Art therapy for mental health recovery. About Creative Expression Centre for Art Therapy (CECAT). Available at: <http://www.health.wa.gov.au/arttherapy/cecat/index.cfm> (accessed 12 October 2013).

Greber, J. and Anderson, F. (2013). Abbott told to cut soon and deep. *Australian Financial Review*, 10 September. Available at: <http://www.afr.com/p/national/abbott_told_to_cut_soon_and_deep_s1k7q3y1o07ldvpnyzix3h> (accessed 12 October 2013).

Griffiths, E. (2013). Nothing out of bounds to Commission of Audit, Tony Abbott says. Australian Broadcasting Commission, 5 September. Available at: <http://www.abc.net.au/news/2013-09-05/tony-abbott-happy-for-open-book-audit-of-spending/4937416> (accessed 12 October 2013).

HARC (Health Arts Research Centre) (2013). Available at: <http://www.harc.org.au/harc/index.html> (accessed 22 April 2015).

Hawkes, J. (2001). *The Fourth Pillar of Sustainability: Culture's Essential Role in Public Planning*. Melbourne: Common Ground Publishing.

Hawkins, G. (1993). *From Nimbin to Mardi Gras: Constructing Community Arts*. Sydney: Allen & Unwin.

Healthpact (2006). *Healthy Canberra: Community Stories Celebrating 10 Years of Health Promotion*. Australian Capital Territory: Healthpact.

HealthPlay (2013). The company. Available at: <http://www.healthplay.com.au/the-company/> (accessed 16 December 2013).

IADH (International Academy of Design and Health) (2013). *Welcome to the International Academy of Design and Health*. Available at: <http://www.designandhealth.com/> (accessed 12 October 2013).

ICH (Institute for Creative Health) (2013a). *The National Arts and Health Framework*. Available at: <http://instituteforcreativehealth.org.au/national-rural-health-conference-endorses-national-arts-and-health-framework/> (accessed 12 October 2013).

ICH (Institute for Creative Health) (2013b). *Framework*. Available at: <http://instituteforcreativehealth.org.au/doing/advocacy/> (accessed 22 April 2015).

ICH (Institute for Creative Health) (2013c). *Framework Unifies Sector in Cause for Better Health*. Available at: <http://instituteforcreative-health.org.au/framework-unifies-sector-in-cause-for-better-health/> (accessed 16 December 2013).

Jones, K., Koh, E., Veis, N., White, A. (2010). *Framing Marginalised Art*. Available at: <http://www.daxcentre.org/wp-content/uploads/2012/02/framingmarginalisedart.pdf> (accessed 12 October 2013).

Kelaher, M., Curry, S., Berman, N., et al. (2008). Structured story telling in community arts and health program evaluations. In: A. Lewis and D. Doyle (eds), *Proving the Practice: Evidencing the Effects of Community Arts Programs on Mental Health*, pp. 148–164. Freemantle, WA: DADAA Inc.

Lewis, A. and Doyle, D. (eds) (2008). *Proving the Practice: Evidencing the Effects of Community Arts Programs on Mental Health*. Freemantle, WA: DADAA Inc.

Lloyd C, Wong S,R., and Petchkovsky, L. (2007). Art and recovery in mental health: a qualitative investigation. *British Journal of Occupational Therapy*, **70**, 207–214.

McKenzie, S. (2009). Doctors' artistic talents on show at inaugural Doc Art Festival. *Medical Observer*. Available at: <http://www.medicalobserver.com.au/news/doctors-artistic-talents-on-show-at-inaugural-doc-art-festival> (accessed 12 October 2013).

Marsden, S. (1993). *Healthy Arts: A Guide to the Role of Arts in Health Care*. Melbourne: Arts Access.

Matarasso, F. (2013). All in this together: the depoliticisation of community art in Britain, 1970–2011. In: E. van Erven (ed.), *Community, Art, Power: Essays from ICAF 2011*. Rotterdam: ICAF. Available at: <https://parliamentofdreams.files.wordpress.com/2013/08/2013-all-in-this-together-matarasso.pdf>

Merli, P. (2002). Evaluating the social impact of participation in arts activities. A critical review of François Matarasso's *Use or Ornament? International Journal of Cultural Policy*, **8**, 107–118.

Mills, D. (2004). Review of Evaluating Community Arts and Wellbeing—an evaluation guide for community arts practitioners. *Artwork*, **59**, 43–44.

Mills, D. (2011). Joining the policy dots: strengthening the contribution of the arts to individual and community health and wellbeing. Submission. *National Cultural Policy Discussion Paper*. Available at: <http://creativeaustralia.arts.gov.au/assets/arts-health-foundation.pdf> (accessed 12 October 2013).

Mills, D. (2013). Address to the 12th National Rural Health Conference, Adelaide, Monday April 8. Available at: <http://instituteforcreativehealth.org.au/wp-content/uploads/2013/05/address-to-12th-national-rural-health-conference-published-version-on-letterhead-amended.pdf> (accessed 12 October 2013).

Mills, D. and Brown, P. (2004). *Art and Wellbeing*. Sydney: Australia Council.

Morgan, J. (2003). Healing art and the medicine in music. *Sydney Morning Herald*, 8 February. Available at: <http://www.smh.com.au/articles/2003/02/07/1044579930534.html> (accessed 12 October 2013).

NSW Government (2013). Invitation Creative Ageing Forum—15 November 2013. Unpublished.

O'Brien, A. (2003). *The Secret Life of Splash: Putting Words to a Visual Experience*. Melbourne: Neami.

Orange Health Service (2013). Arts + health. Available at: <http://www.orangeartsandhealth.org.au/about.html> (accessed 12 October 2013).

Pagan, J., Higgs, P., and Cunningham, S. (2008). *Getting Creative in Healthcare. The Contribution of Creative Activities to Australian Healthcare.* ARC Centre of Excellence for Creative Industries and Innovation. Available at: <http://eprints.qut.edu.au/archive/00014757/> (accessed 12 October 2013).

Parliament of Australia (1996). Parliamentary library, budget review 1996–97. Detailed portfolio reviews, communications and the arts, August 1996. Canberra.

Pettigrew, C. (2009). Current Evaluation Practice in the Field of Community Cultural Development: A Report to Community Cultural Development NSW. Sydney: University of Technology Sydney. Unpublished.

Price, N. (1998). *Artist Residencies for Health Care: A Guide for Health Care Institutions Developing and Implementing Artist Residency Programs.* Brisbane: Queensland Artsworkers Alliance.

Price, N. (2008). Without the labels: narratives of a diagnosed culture. In: A. Lewis and D. Doyle (eds) (2008). *Proving the Practice: Evidencing the Effects of Community Arts Programs on Mental Health*, pp. 46–59. Freemantle, WA: DADAA Inc.

Price, N. (2010). First Aid Kit for Cultural Health and Wellbeing. A Journey with Art and Survivors of Health Institutions. Australia Council–Community Cultural Development Arts Fellowship 2007. Unpublished.

Putland, C. (2007). Art and community-based health promotion: lessons from the field. In: H. Keleher, B. Murphy, and C. MacDougall (eds), *Understanding Health Promotion*, pp. 299–312. Melbourne: Oxford University Press.

Putland, C. (2008). Lost in translation: the question of evidence linking community-based arts and health promotion. *Journal of Health Psychology*, **13**, 266–276.

Putland, C. (2009). *Arts in Health at FMC: Towards a Model of Practice.* Wayville: Christine Putland.

Putland, C. (2012). *Arts and Health—A Guide to the Evidence. Background Document Prepared for the Arts and Health Foundation Australia.* Available at: <http://instituteforcreativehealth.org.au/wp-content/uploads/2013/07/evidenceguidefinal.pdf> (accessed 12 October 2013).

Radbourne, J., Leong, C., Price, N., and Gerrand, D. (1995). Arts on Fire: integrating people with mental illness into the community through community based arts activity. A report for the Federal Department of Health and Human Services. Brisbane: Access Arts. Unpublished.

Radio National (2007). *Art in the Asylum: Orphans of the Art World? Part 1 of 2 (The Cunningham Dax Collection)*, Saturday 13 October. Available at: <http://www.abc.net.au/radionational/programs/allinthemind/art-in-the-asylum-orphans-of-the-art-world-part-1/3230500> (accessed 12 October 2013).

RMH (Royal Melbourne Hospital) (2013). Music therapy at the Royal Melbourne Hospital. Available at: <http://www.rmh.mh.org.au/music-therapy/w1/i1001366/> (accessed 12 October 2013).

RMIT (Royal Melbourne Institute of Technology) (2013). *Designing Sound for Health and Wellbeing.* Available at: <http://www.rmit.edu.au/research/research-institutes-centres-and-groups/research-centres/centre-for-art-society-and-transformation/publications/designing-sound-for-health-and-wellbeing/> (accessed 22 April 2015).

Sutton, K. (2005). A study of the Mater Children's Hospital tile project. Unpublished masters thesis, Australian Catholic University, Fitzroy, Victoria. Available at: <http://dlibrary.acu.edu.au/digitaltheses/public/adt-acuvp105.11092006/02whole.pdf> (accessed 12 October 2013).

Thiele, R. and Marsden, S. (2003). *Engaging Art: The Artful Dodger's Studio.* Richmond, Melbourne: Jesuit Social Services.

Thomson J. (2009). Art for medicine's sake. Can visual art be used to boost the observational skills of medical students? *Medical Observer*. Available at: <http://www.medicalobserver.com.au/news/art-for-medicines-sake> (accessed 12 October 2013).

Throsby, D. (2001). Public funding of the arts in Australia—1900 to 2000. *1301.0—Year Book Australia, 2001*. Canberra: Australian Bureau of Statistics. Available at: <http://www.abs.gov.au/ausstats/abs@.nsf/previousproducts/1301.0feature%20article302001?opendocument&tabname=summary&prodno=1301.0&issue=2001&num=&view=> (accessed 12 October 2013).

Throsby, D. (2010). *Do You Really Expect to get Paid? An Economic Study of Professional Artists in Australia.* Available at: <http://www.australiacouncil.gov.au/workspace/uploads/files/research/do_you_really_expect_to_get_pa-54325a3748d81.pdf> (accessed 22 April 2015).

Ulrich, R. (1991). Effects of interior design on wellness: theory and recent scientific research. *Journal of Health Care Interior Design*, **3**, 97–109.

UNESCO Observatory (2013). *Melbourne UNESCO Observatory of Arts Education.* Available at: <http://education.unimelb.edu.au/about_us/specialist_areas/arts_education/melbourne_unesco_observatory_of_arts_education> (accessed 22 April 2015).

University of Sydney (2013). Arts in health. Available at: <http://sydney.edu.au/courses/uos/BETH5207/arts-in-health> (accessed 12 October 2013).

VicHealth (2003). *Creative Connections: Promoting Mental Health and Wellbeing Through Community Arts Participation.* Carlton, Vic: Victorian Health Promotion Foundation.

WEHI (Walter and Eliza Hall Institute) (2013). *WEHI.TV.* Available at: <http://www.wehi.edu.au/wehi-tv/wehitv> (accessed 22 April 2015).

Westwood, M. (2012). Council's new chief wants to lead from behind in support of cultural life. *The Australian*, 25 September, 17.

WHO (World Health Organization) (1986). *The Ottawa Charter For Health Promotion.* Available at: <http://www.who.int/healthpromotion/conferences/previous/ottawa/en/index.html> (accessed 12 October 2013).

Williams, D. (1995). *Creating Social Capital: A Study of Long-term Benefits From Community Based Arts Funding.* Adelaide: Community Arts Network of South Australia.

Woodhams, L. and Bishop, M. (eds) (1995). *The Arts In Health: Exploring The Role of Arts in Health: Conference Papers.* Toowoomba, Qld: Darling Downs Regional Health Authority.

YAWCRC (Young and Well Cooperative Research Centre) (2013). *About.* Available at: <http://www.youngandwellcrc.org.au/about/> (accessed 22 April 2015).

# CHAPTER 18

# Addressing the health needs of indigenous Australians through creative engagement: a case study

Jing Sun and Nicholas Buys

## The mental illness and chronic disease prevention needs of Aboriginal and Torres Strait Islander people

Aboriginal and Torres Strait Islander people suffer from a higher prevalence of mental illness and chronic disease than non-indigenous Australians (Australian Bureau of Statistics 2008). They also typically die younger and are more likely to experience disability and a reduced quality of life because of ill-health (Australian Bureau of Statistics 2008). Their disadvantaged health status is demonstrated by the high prevalence of social and emotional difficulties, and obesity and overweight (Priest et al. 2012; Schultz 2012).

The annual direct medical cost of treatment for Aboriginal and Torres Strait Islander people due to mental illness and chronic disease is AU$112.4 million or 10% of the total admitted patient expenditure (AIHW 2010). Traditional treatment approaches have had limited success, primarily because they fail to take into account cultural issues such as identity, kinship and family influences, and connection to community (AIHW 2008). Furthermore, poor health literacy, coupled with low help-seeking behaviour and reluctance to access primary healthcare services offered by the Aboriginal Community Controlled Health Services (CCHSs) contributes to the ongoing high prevalence of mental illness and chronic disease (Australian Bureau of Statistics 2008). The mechanisms involved in shaping the development and treatment of mental health problems and chronic illness have not been comprehensively addressed in previous research in this population (Australian Bureau of Statistics 2008).

Increasing international evidence indicates that wellbeing and health are related to resilience (Ong et al. 2006). Resilience involves both individual-level factors, such as self-esteem, self-efficacy, readiness to learn, and positive social identity, and socio-cultural factors, including family, community, and environmental supports. Resilience factors provide a 'buffer' for exposure to disease risks and are linked to a positive quality of life and wellbeing (Bartley et al. 2010). These benefits are not simply the result of the absence of mental and/or physical illness but are also due to positive mental health and community social capital and social support (Masten 1994). The concepts of resilience and capability are centrally concerned with positive adaptation, protective factors, and 'assets' that moderate the effects of risk factors (Bartley et al. 2010), including in relation to chronic illnesses.

Participation in arts-based activities have been shown to build resilience (Sun et al. 2013). Choral singing, as one such activity, is an expressive and creative experience that involves body–mind coordination, muscle movement, and breathing skills. It is one of the most valuable and significant human arts activities and plays a critical role in improving peoples' physical and mental health and promoting social functioning and spiritual meaning (Clift et al. 2008; Clift and Morrison 2011). Choral singing can be one resource for developing family coherence, social capital, and social support. It is a cost-effective approach to health promotion in communities (Sun and Buys 2013a,b,c).

It has been argued that resilience theory may underpin the mechanisms through which choral singing activities help the individual in coping with mental illness and chronic disease (Sun and Buys 2013a,b,c). This includes the development of individual-level coping resources and characteristics such as self-esteem, self-efficacy, the ability to 'bounce back' quickly, positive mood and feelings, aspiration, purpose in life, physical health, and a sense of spiritual meaning in life. Singing also enhances the 'social context', interacting with individual-level factors to provide coping resources. Social–contextual factors include support from family members, friends, and community, as well as developing social capital such as trust and a sense of safety in the community, and increased health-service utilization (Sun and Stewart 2007). However, there are no comprehensive studies on the role of choral singing in building resilience to cope with health problems in Aboriginal and Torres Strait Islander populations.

## A community singing programme in the Aboriginal and Torres Strait Islander population

A case study of a community singing programme was conducted by a Griffith University research team (Sun and Buys 2013a,b,c), in conjunction with the Queensland Aboriginal and Islander Health Council (QAIHC) and a number of CCHSs in Queensland, Australia. The project team established five community singing groups, including two urban, one regional, and two rural groups, which involved 235 participants. The programme combined annual health assessments with a weekly singing rehearsal in each community. The CCHSs conducted and coordinated the intervention programmes, including rehearsals and regular joint singing performances in the five communities. The 2-hour singing sessions were held weekly for 18 months and consisted of physical warm-up exercises, breathing and tension-releasing techniques, social interaction, and singing. Participants were encouraged to practise at home between rehearsals and were involved in the selection of songs with the musicians. A more detailed description of the methods and intervention protocol used in the case study may be found in Sun and Buys (2013b,c).

Evaluations of participants' health occurred during the intervention, with health assessments conducted at the beginning of the programme (baseline) and 18 months after the completion of the programme. Control-group participants were also assessed at the follow-up assessment session. Continuous recruitment for baseline assessments and follow-up assessments was undertaken between October 2009 and December 2012. Assessment of mental and physical health was carried out using standard measures in each community. Mental health and psychological distress were measured by the Indigenous Risk Impact Screen (IRIS), which has been validated in the Aboriginal and Torres Strait Islander population (Schlesinger et al. 2007). The brief resilience scale was used to assess an individual's ability to bounce back and recover from stress (Smith et al. 2008). Social connectedness was measured by a scale involving 10 questions related to sense of connectedness

to society, friends, and environment (Lee et al. 2001). Social support (McCubbin et al. 1987) was measured using eight questions relating to perception of the quality and number of friendship networks, and feelings of trust in the local community. Risk factors for chronic disease, including hypertension, depression, and overweight and obesity were based on the results of participants' recent health checks by the CCHSs, as well as anthropometric measures such as height, weight, waist and hip circumference, and blood pressure.

## Results of the evaluation

The results of the evaluation found that community singing provided significant benefits to resilience, mental health, health behaviour, access to health services, and social connection and social trust. Table 18.1 indicates that fewer participants had psychological distress and fewer engaged in smoking behaviour at the end of the 8-month intervention. There were also significantly increased levels of resilience, increased sense of social connectedness and social support, and an increased number of visits to Aboriginal health services and other types of health services.

### Community singing provided benefits to individual-level resilience characteristics

Singing appeared to benefit individuals' resilience through cognitive benefits and decreased life stress, increased confidence and self-esteem, and positive changes in attitude and mood. For example, one participant stated:

> 'Well, that's part of the therapy of it. I mind it less and less as I go and the possibilities of some of these songs, getting away from the TV a bit, it's good, it's great. If we get a good choir—when we get a good choir going some of the songs we sing have been phenomenal. Be a good sound. It'll rock this place once we got going I can tell you.'

A comparison was also made between the number of stressful life events reported pre- and post-intervention in both the singing and control group participants. While pre-intervention there was no significant difference in the number of stressful life events,

**Table 18.1** Benefits of the singing programme to Aboriginal and Torres Strait Islander people

|  | Intervention group | | |
|---|---|---|---|
|  | Pre-intervention (n = 117) | Post-intervention (n = 108) | P |
| Psychological distress |  |  | 0.02 |
| Normal n(%) | 53 (45.2%) | 67 (61.7%) |  |
| Abnormal n(%) | 64 (54.8%) | 41 (38.3%) |  |
| Resilience M(SD) | 5.28 (1.79) | 6.38 (2.02) | <0.005 |
| Sense of connectedness M(SD) | 33.00 (12.07) | 34.65 (9.58) | 0.05 |
| Social support M(SD) | 3.70 (1.68) | 3.81 (1.46) | 0.05 |
| Smoking |  |  |  |
| No n(%) | 81 (69.4) | 87 (80.4) | 0.05 |
| Yes n(%) | 36 (30.6) | 21 (18.6) |  |
| Number of times visiting Aboriginal Health Services M(SD) | 4.82 (11.11) | 8.92 (22.66) | 0.02 |
| Number of times visiting any health service M(SD) | 6.47 (20.09) | 9.06 (19.85) | 0.002 |

there was a significant reduction in these events for the singing group post-intervention. Reduction of stress through the singing programme was a significant achievement, as stress adversely affects the health of Aboriginal and Torres Strait Islander people, and has traditionally been a difficult area to successfully treat. Many participants in the singing group explained that that enjoyment of singing is connected with cognitive and emotional health benefits, and reported feeling 'high' or 'happy':

'The harmony, the voice and the vibration that people carry is lifted and is flowing. That's just so healing and positive. The positiveness in that and the potential of that energy that is being put into that song, goes into the universe you know. It just goes out of the, you know . . .'

Singing was also viewed as a means to reduce stress. Comparisons between the singing and control groups using quantitative data, as well as interview data from group leaders and CCHS health workers, revealed that participants benefited from the programme, particularly in terms of promoting their sense of self-esteem, self-confidence, learning, purpose in life, and their capacity to deal with stress. The singing programme also assisted participants in their recovery from stressful and adverse events, and enabled them to cope with challenging life situations (Fig. 18.1). Our results therefore suggest that group-based singing has become an important resource that can be used as a means to reduce stress and promote individual-level resilience in Aboriginal and Torres Strait Islander people.

## Singing promotes social interaction and social capital within the community

The social benefits of singing reported by participants include increased friendships, empowerment, greater appreciation for diversity, and connection to the broader community and the participants' own history. Through singing, participants made active choices to establish friendships and social relationships with others within their singing group, as well as with family and community members, including CCHS staff and local musicians. They gained positive life experiences, which shaped these positive relationships, through weekly rehearsals, joint rehearsals, workshops, performances, and events, together with community singing groups. This is indicated by the many ways in which participants sought new friendships and established friendships with others in their own communities, as well as in external communities:

'It helped me make a lot more friends and people who I'd known already, know them even better and to get along a lot more easier and happy with them, because it makes you feel better when you're singing.'

Singing groups are therefore a powerful means through which Aboriginal and Torres Strait Islander people can become active agents in making social changes in relation to their positive sense of identity and community life, which in turn leads to them seeking and receiving family and community-level support. In addition to the level of social support, group singing also benefits social capital (Putnam 1993), with our study showing that social capital can be generated by such groups in Aboriginal and Torres Strait Islander communities. This result highlighted that the singing programme is an important avenue for providing more opportunities to establish trust among Aboriginal and Torres Strait Islander people, and an important means to develop friendships for those who struggle socially. Friendship and building community trust was a prominent theme:

'It is very beneficial. That's the biggest reason why I wanted this to happen, because of all the disharmony in the community, the different tribal groups. At least we can talk to each other about anything. I think that's a start. That's what everybody else in this community needs to see. Every one of us can be friends and be really close and really, really be there for each other. This is what we need for this . . . It's like part of the process of healing for the community.'

## Improved health behaviours

Over the intervention period, participants demonstrated a significant increase in participation in physical activities and other activities with health benefits, such as extra exercise by

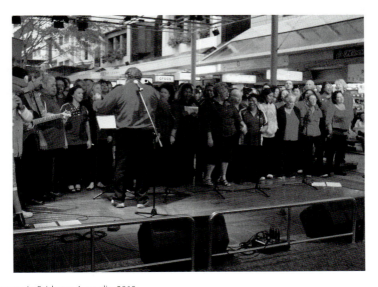

**Fig. 18.1** Mental health week performance in Brisbane, Australia, 2010.
Reproduced by kind permission of Jing Sun. Copyright © 2015 Jing Sun.

walking, swimming, jogging, and sports, as well as arts-related activities such as sewing, crafts, painting, dancing, and additional performances. As a result participants demonstrated significantly improved health behaviour. For example, 12% of participants in the intervention group stopped smoking compared with none in the control group (Fig. 18.1). They also demonstrated a significant increase in participation in exercise activities on an individual basis and community exercise, whereas there was a significant decrease in the proportion of participants in the control group who engaged in these activities. The participants in the intervention group felt more socially connected than those in the control group, and this may have made a significant contribution to their improvement in health behaviour and increased their participation in other exercise and arts experiences.

### Community singing to prevent chronic disease by promoting resilience

There was a significant association between the benefits of community singing and the reduction in poor health behaviours in the singing groups, and this association was attained through the promotion of resilience factors (e.g. self-efficacy, self-esteem, and self-confidence, and increased social support and social connectedness). From a socio-ecological perspective, it is evident that the possession of resilience makes it easier to acquire other social and personal resources, competencies, and social connectedness, as well as to actively make health choices such as stopping smoking and increasing exercise (Sun and Buys 2013a). This supports the idea that community singing can be an important resource for building and promoting resilience by building self-esteem and self-efficacy, enabling people to cope with stressful life events, and improving social and emotional wellbeing. Singing programmes are an enjoyable health-promotion activity, empowering Aboriginal and Torres Strait Islander people to take action at both the individual and the community level to improve their health. This has significantly facilitated their accessing of Aboriginal CCHS primary health services for the purposes of preventing chronic disease and promoting health. These factors have led to a reduction of symptoms of chronic disease and of risk factors. For example, one participant stated:

> I actually lost about 33 kg since October . . . So I feel better in myself because it's amazing how many people put you down because of your weight. So my metabolism's working better now. Yes, and that's happened with my depression. As I said, going out and singing I'm doing what I like doing.

### Increasing the use of primary health services

From a socio-ecological perspective, health services are also an important social support for people with health problems. The availability and quality of such services, and the ability or willingness of individuals to access them, are important determinants of health and health inequalities in all societies. This is particularly true in Aboriginal and Torres Strait Islander communities, where people feel 'shame' in accessing the non-indigenous health services because they see them as a part of an alienating and dominant culture. The Aboriginal

and Torres Strait Islander community singing programme has changed participants' perceptions of the CCHS, and they now see this service as culturally appropriate and feel comfortable accessing it, feeling they are treated as equals by CCHS staff. Access to CCHSs significantly increased at the post-intervention assessment in this study (Fig. 18.1), while the use of hospital services decreased. Thus, the participants in the singing group appeared to be making better use of the medical services that they had traditionally refused to access.

### Reducing the sense of social inequality

Most participants felt that the singing programme accepted everyone regardless of their different backgrounds, including those who were homeless, illiterate, unemployed, or had no singing experience. This experience broke down the barriers and obstacles to communication and interaction between the members in each community and significantly promoted participants' sense of community connectedness (Fig. 18.1), friendship, sense of community support (Fig. 18.1), and social trust and has helped promote social inclusion in the communities. For example:

> 'For people it stops loneliness. I know a lot of elderly ladies there and they're on their own and coming and meeting with all of us. Acceptance. There is one fellow there, he's got a learning disability and we all accept him. He can't read. He's a joy to have around and we all love him. Accepting each other for who we are and embracing our differences. It's non-judgmental and it's really good. We embrace everybody. They make you feel at home. So, yes, it has beneficial effects for everybody.'

Both male and female members of the singing group thought that unstructured activities in general, and singing in particular, were appealing as these activities not only addressed the mental health and chronic disease prevention needs of both individuals and the community, but also reflected and enhanced the cultural identity and kinship characteristics of the Aboriginal and Torres Strait communities (Fig. 18.2).

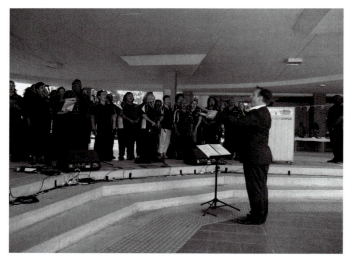

**Fig. 18.2** Social inclusion week performance conducted by Jonathan Welch in Brisbane, Australia, 2011.
Reproduced by kind permission of Jing Sun. Copyright © 2015 Jing Sun.

## Conclusion

Findings from our case study indicate that the community singing programme played an important role in promoting resilience in the following ways:

◆ improved psychological, mental, physical, health behaviour, family and social support,

◆ increased access to Aboriginal CCHSs at the primary-health-care-service level, and

◆ reduced access to acute hospital-based tertiary health care.

The significant association between the benefits of community singing and the prevention of chronic disease and depression by reducing the development of risk factors related to chronic disease was possibly related to improved resilience, which acts as a pathway between community singing and the prevention of chronic disease outcomes.

The findings of the case study provide further evidence that individual-level resilience factors such self-esteem and self-confidence, and contextual-level factors such as friends and community support are important factors influencing health outcomes (Sun et al. 2012). The community singing programme had an impact on these factors, and this has in turn significantly reduced risk factors (e.g. smoking) for the chronic diseases present in the Aboriginal and Torres Strait Islander people. The mechanism underpinning this effect may relate to the fact that community singing not only addresses factors at the individual level but also social factors such as family, kinship, and community health and social-support services, and facilitates access to other primary preventive health services within a culturally appropriate context.

## References

AIHW (2008). *Australia's Health 2008.* The eleventh biennial health report of the Australian Institute of Health and Welfare. Canberra: AIHW. Available from: <http://www.aihw.gov.au/WorkArea/DownloadAsset.aspx?id=6442453674> (accessed 26 February 2014).

AIHW (2010). *Expenditure on health for Aboriginal and Torres Strait Islander people 2006–07: an analysis by remoteness and disease.* Canberra: AIHW. Available from: <http://www.aihw.gov.au/publication-detail/?id=6442468394> (accessed 26 February 2014).

Australian Bureau of Statistics (2008). *4704.0–The Health and Welfare of Aboriginal and Torres Strait Islander Peoples, 2008.* Canberra: Australian Bureau of Statistics. Available from: <http://www.abs.gov.au/ausstats/abs@.nsf/allprimarymainfeatures/ae9ff832a4f230ebca25773000183239?opendocument>

Bartley, M., Schoon, I., Mitchell, R., and Blane, D. (2010). Resilience as an asset for healthy development. In: A. Morgan, M. Davies, and E. Ziglio (eds), *Healthy Assets in a Global Context: Theory, Methods, Action,* pp. 101–116. New York: Springer.

Clift, S. and Morrison, I. (2011). Group singing fosters mental health and wellbeing: findings from the East Kent 'singing for health' network project. *Mental Health and Social Inclusion,* **15**, 88–97.

Clift, S., Hancox, G., Staricoff, R., and Whitmore, C. (2008). *A Systematic Mapping and Review of Research on Singing and Health Non-Clinical Studies.* Canterbury: Canterbury Christ Church University College.

Lee, R.M., Draper, M., and Lee, S. (2001). Social connectedness, dysfunctional interpersonal behaviors, and psychological distress: testing a mediator model. *Journal of Counseling Psychology,* **48**, 310–318.

McCubbin, H.I., Paterson, J., and Glynn, T. (1987). Social support index. In: H.I. McCubbin, A.I. Thompson, and M.A. McCubbin (eds), *Family Assessment: Resiliency, Coping and Adaptation: Inventories of Research and Practice,* p. 389. Madison, WI: University of Wisconsin Publishers.

Masten, A.S. (1994). Resilience in individual development: successful adaptation despite risk and adversity. In: M.C. Wang and E.W. Gordon (eds), *Educational Resilience in Inner-city America: Challenges and prospects,* pp. 141–149. Hillsdale, NJ: Lawrence Erlbaum.

Ong, A.D., Bergeman, C.S., Bisconti, T.L., and Wallace, K.A. (2006). Psychological resilience, positive emotions, and successful adaptation to stress in later life. *Journal of Personality and Social Psychology,* **91**, 730–749.

Priest, N., Baxter, J., and Hayes, L. (2012). Social and emotional outcomes of Australian children from Indigenous and culturally and linguistically diverse backgrounds. *Australian and New Zealand Journal of Public Health,* **36**, 183–190.

Putnam, R. (1993). *Making Democracy Work: Civic Traditions in Modern Italy.* Princeton, NJ: Princeton University Press.

Schlesinger, C.M., Ober, C., McCarthy, M.M., Watson, J.D., and Seinen, A. (2007). The development and validation of the Indigenous Risk Impact Screen (IRIS): A 13-item screening instrument for alcohol and drug and mental health risk. *Drug and Alcohol Review,* **26**, 109–117.

Schultz, R. (2012). Prevalences of overweight and obesity among children in remote Aboriginal communities in central Australia. *Rural and Remote Health,* **12**, 1872.

Smith, B.W., Dalen, J., Wiggins, K., Tooley, E., Christopher, P., and Bernard, J. (2008). The Brief Resilience Scale: assessing the ability to bounce back. *International Journal of Behavioral Medicine,* **15**, 194–200.

Sun, J. and Buys, N. (2013a). Effectiveness of a participative community singing program to improve health behaviors and increase physical activity in Australian Aboriginal and Torres Strait Islander people. *International Journal of Disability and Human Development,* **12**, 297–304.

Sun, J. and Buys, N. (2013b). Improving Aboriginal and Torres Strait Islander Australians' wellbeing using participatory community singing approach. *International Journal of Disability and Human Development,* **12**, 305–316.

Sun, J. and Buys, N. (2013c). Participatory community singing program to enhance quality of life and social and emotional wellbeing in Aboriginal and Torres Strait Islander Australians with chronic diseases. *International Journal of Disability and Human Development,* **12**, 317–323.

Sun, J. and Stewart, D. (2007). Development of population based resiliency measures in the primary school setting in Australia using exploratory and confirmatory factor analysis. *Health Education,* **107**, 575–599.

Sun, J., Buys, N., Tatow, D., and Johnson, L. (2012). Ongoing health inequality in Aboriginal and Torres Strait Islander Population in Australia: stressful event, resilience, and mental health and emotional wellbeing difficulties. *International Journal of Psychology and Behavioral Sciences,* **2**, 38–45.

Sun, J., Zhang, N., Buys, N., Zhou, Z.Y., Shen, S.Y., and Bao, J.Y. (2013). The role of Tai Chi, cultural dancing, playing a musical instrument and singing in promoting physical and mental health in Chinese older adults: a mind–body meditative approach. *International Journal of Mental Health Promotion,* **15**, 227–239.

# CHAPTER 19

# Arts and health initiatives in India

Varun Ramnarayan Venkit, Anand Sharad Godse, and Amruta Anand Godse

## Introduction to art and health in India

We begin with an overview of the traditions of Indian art forms including music, dance, theatre, fine arts, and yoga. The traditional literature and various schools that practise these art forms have rich cultural intricacies that focus on aspects of physical and mental health. We then proceed to give an overview of the present health status of India in order to understand the role of arts-based interventions. We then evaluate these art forms separately to document practice, research, and organizational initiatives. There is increasing attention from users and clients in urban settings towards such initiatives. We end by documenting research and training opportunities as well as setting the stage for the future of arts and health in India.

The chapter is a compilation and interpretation of data collected by the authors through various methods. Literature was reviewed using traditional and modern texts, and research journals in the area of arts and health, stress, music therapy, dance therapy, fine arts, and yoga. We conducted in-depth interviews with experts and eminent practitioners based in Pune, Mumbai, Delhi, and Bangalore, some of the main metropolitan cities of India. The work of published therapists and practitioners has been mentioned throughout the text with references, and the work of upcoming or unpublished practitioners is listed in Table 19.1. Telephone interviews and an online questionnaire were used to investigate the following topics:

◆ philosophy and nature of the art form

◆ background of the artist/practitioner

◆ application of the art form

◆ therapeutic potential of the art form

◆ research undertaken—published and unpublished

Data were collected and interpreted to understand the current practices in arts and health in India. All the respondents interviewed for this chapter have had formal training in at least one Indian classical or western art form. This, in conjunction with their academic background (psychology or psychiatry) and, at times, familiarity with principles of other western art forms or bodies of knowledge, has helped them explore the therapeutic potentials of their medium.

## Overview of art in India

In India the word *kala* is used to mean art, and it is believed in Hindu mythology that Lord Krishna possessed 64 *kalas*. The 64 art forms are mentioned in various texts such as *Sukranitisara*, *Kamasutra*, and *Kadambari* to name a few. These include a wide range of art forms like singing (*Geetam*), musical instruments (*Vaadyam*), dancing (*Nartanam*), theatricals (*Naatya*), painting (*Alekhya*), and so on (Monroe 2000).

According to the *Rgveda* (an ancient Indian text) all truth, goodness, and beauty emanates from the Lord. Art is eternal, unending. The expressed consciousness of the beauty of God is called Art. According to the *Brahmasutra* (another ancient Indian text), art is expressing the concept of God with form (*saakaar*) or without form (*niraakaar*), direct or indirect. Humans express themselves through art, and the creative energy of God, which they receive in a limited form, is art (Veereshwar and Sharma 2001). The Vedic literature including all four *Vedas, Rgveda, Samveda, Yajurveda*, and *Atharvaveda*, are where the roots of all knowledge and also art are found (Radhkrishnan 1989). India is a country of great geographical and cultural diversity with intricately developed performance art that can be broadly classified as music and dance, of which *Abhinaya* (the art of expression, role-play also known as drama) was also an intricate part. The *Sangeet Ratnakar* (a traditional text on Indian music) says that music comprises three elements—singing, musical instruments, and dancing (Sharma 2006)—showing the inseparable nature of these art forms.

Religions such as Buddhism, Jainism, Islam, and Sufism have distinct art traditions and different perspectives on the idea of God. When it came to India between the eighth and eleventh centuries even monotheistic Islam interacted creatively with Hinduism to produce versions of Sufism in which many saints and endless songs mediated between the human and the divine (Chakravarthi 2010). In order to give a more detailed picture, this chapter will focus mainly on arts practices influenced by the Hindu tradition. Tribal art in India is well established. Tribal folklore, tales, songs, craft, wood carvings, music, and dance strongly represents tribal life. The various aspects of life (economic, social, conjugal, and sacred), thoughts, and nature are represented in tribal art. In other words, folklore is the mirror of tribal culture (Vidyarthi and Rai 1976). Traditional folk or tribal art, namely music, dance, and drama, has played an important role in harmonizing and providing a vent for social outbursts relating to caste, creed, religion, and language issues (Haldar 2012).

All Indian ceremonies, marriages, festivals, and religious and community centres are associated with some sort of artistic expression such as dances and songs (Haldar 2012). The *Palkhi*

**Table 19.1** List of therapists and practitioners interviewed for this chapter with training in the field of art therapy

| No. | Name | Qualification | Area of work | Contribution |
|---|---|---|---|---|
| 1. | Mrs Vidya Chikte | Arts-based therapist, school counsellor | Children suffering from autism, learning difficulties, ASD, PDD, speech, visual, and hearing impairment | Development of communication skills, healthy emotional awareness, greater understanding of their physical and social environment, positive changes in four domains (self-expression, cognitive, motor, and composite) |
| 2. | Mr Arthur Fernandez | Arts-based therapist, psychologist | Special needs groups—children with special needs | Commendable movement in the self-expression, cognitive, motor, and composite domains of participants |
| 3. | Mrs Natasha D'Cruz | PhD, psychologist, art therapist | ADHD, ODD, mood disorders, anxiety disorders, addictions, learning issues as well as growth and personal, and professional development | Cognitive, affective, behavioural, biological as well as social benefits such as restoring or encouraging cognitive growth and ability, helping or healing the ability to express emotions, modifying deviant or encouraging social behaviour and helping social skills, increasing confidence, helping with coordination, increasing neurotransmitter activity through aerobic activity, and increasing overall fitness |
| 4. | Ms Aarti Sinha | Counselling psychologist, music therapist | Schizophrenia, mood disorders, and mental retardation | Increased cognitive, behavioural and motor functioning/development, emotional and social development (expression), improvement of communication skills, impulse control, appropriate response generation, and an increase in self-esteem and confidence |
| 5. | Mrs Suchitra Date | MA medical psychiatry, Bharatnatyam dancer, dance therapist | Patients with Parkinson's, children of HIV patients, senior citizens, children with autism, children with polio | Reduced dependence on appendages, reduced risk of accidents, increase in expression, confidence and interaction |
| 6. | Mrs Anubha Doshi | Clinical psychologist, art-based therapist | Children with special needs—ADHD, autism, Down syndrome | Reduced stress levels as reported by participants, development of speech |
| 7. | Dr Nikita Mittal | Dance movement therapist | Children with special needs | Reduced stress levels as reported by participants, development of speech |
| 8. | Ms Devika Shekar | Dance movement therapist | Children with special needs | Reduced stress levels as reported by participants, development of speech |
| 9. | Mrs Sushma Deshpande | Drama therapist, activist | Rural women, sex workers and the LGBT community in and around Pune | Increased participation of women in rural development, higher confidence levels and awareness |
| 10. | Mr Pankaj Meethbhakre | Clinical psychologist, drama therapist | General population | Increased unconditional positive regard, empathy, congruence, acceptance, and emotional awareness |
| 11. | Ms Tia Pleiman | Art therapist | School children, pre-schoolers, and adolescents | Left and right brain stimulation, expression of emotive content and communication of ideas, feelings, dreams, and aspirations through art |
| 12. | Mrs Susan Khare | Visual art therapist | Children, parents, women's groups, and remedial teachers | Facilitated expression, tool for special educators, stress reduction |

ASD, autism spectrum disorder; PDD, pervasive developmental disorders; PD, Parkinson's disease; ADHD, attention deficit hyperactivity disorder; ODD, oppositional defiant disorder; LGBT, lesbian, gay, bisexual, and transgender.

pilgrimage and *Ganpati* festival of *Maharashtra*, the *Durga Puja* of West Bengal, and the *Kumbha Mela* of Allahabad are all examples of some of the many large-scale Indian festivals in which group drumming processions, group devotional singing, and community dances are a major part (Sharma 2007).

### Indian perspective on health

*Sushruta Samhita*, a traditional Indian text in the field of Ayurveda describes health as *Svastha*, which means 'to be established' (*stha*) 'in oneself' (*sva*). Someone whose physiological functions (*dosha*) and metabolism (*agni*) are in the state of equilibrium with a cheerful mind, clarity of intellect, and contented senses is said 'to be established in oneself' (Morandi and Fave 2013).

Health was believed to be conditioned by balance of three primary fluids or *doshas* (literally 'defects') in the body: wind (*vata*), gall (*pitta*), and mucus (*kapha*). There were five separate 'breaths' or 'winds' which controlled the main bodily functions. When these vital factors were operating harmoniously, the body was inhabited by the vital soul (*jiva*), as distinct from the innermost soul (*atman*), and enjoyed health (Leslie 1976).

### Overview of current health issues in India today

According to the World Health Organization (WHO), the per capita expenditure on health in 2011 increased by US$40, showing an increased awareness about health issues and disease prevention among the population (World Health Organization 2012). The WHO estimated that cardiovascular disease, chronic respiratory disease, and other chronic diseases caused 28, 7, and 8%, respectively, of deaths in people of all ages in India in 2005 (World Health Organization 2012). With rapid economic development and increasing westernization of lifestyle in the past few decades the prevalence of 'lifestyle diseases' such as hypertension, diabetes, mellitus, cardiovascular disease, and obesity has reached alarming proportions among Indians (Pappachan 2011). Stress is now known to cause or exacerbate a great deal of illness. The US Centers for Disease Control and Prevention estimated that stress accounted or 75% of all doctor's visits and 90% of all primary healthcare visits (Salleh 2008). Lifestyle interventions have shown definite benefit in the management and prevention of lifestyle diseases in large-scale studies (Pappachan 2011). Arts-based techniques can be classified as non-pharmacological or lifestyle interventions.

According to the Global Health Observatory, there are only 0.33 mental health outpatient facilities per 100,000 people in India, demonstrating a great disparity in the attention towards and facilities for mental healthcare (World Health Organization 2012). Mental health in India focuses more on the biomedical nature of disorders, despite research-based evidence for emphasis on their biopsychosocial nature (Joshi 2005). The current understanding, having a curative basis, neglects the role of social determinants, which are vital components of wellbeing, in the causes and outcomes of mental illness and distress. A holistic understanding of mental health would require promotion of the curative and preventive aspects of healthcare. Hence, there is a policy-level need for emphasis on culturally relevant support systems using traditional or modern arts-based practices as healing tools.

Given this background of art and health in India, the next section will highlight the five main areas of research and their connection to health and wellbeing.

## Music and health

Classical music is divided into Indian classical and *Carnatic* (Menon 1995). The vocal tradition has many *Gharanas* (schools of thought) and instrumental music is equally diverse, including stringed instruments (e.g. the *sitar, sarod*, and *sarangi*), percussion instruments (e.g. the *tabla, mridangam*, and *pakhwaj*), and wind instruments (e.g. the flute). Apart from these traditional Indian instruments, as a recent development for the purpose of therapy India has adopted many western instruments such as the drum kit, the guitar, the violin, and the piano. There exists a strong culture of devotional group singing in India, which depending on its heritage includes regional practices, namely *Abhangas, Bhajans, Bhatiyalis, Kirtan, Quawwali*, and *Shabad* (Kumar 2003). Community singing, for example *Kirtans, Bhajans*, and *Hari Kathas*, has great potential to bring people together irrespective of their caste, creed, or colour (Haldar 2012).

Traditionally, the Indian healing systems of *Nadayoga* (yoga of sound) and *Ragachikitsa* (healing through music) prescribed listening to certain *ragas* (roughly translated as musical scales) to cure ailments like anxiety, anorexia, arthritis, and insomnia (Sundar 2007). Specific ragas are known to have therapeutic value, for example *Rag Bageshriis* that is claimed to help insomnia (Menen 2005). In current practice, therapy integrates both traditional and modern ways of healing, focusing on active participation and experience. Concepts in Indian classical music have been formulated in order to promote and propagate health and wellbeing in practitioners, and to some extent the audience. References to the effects of certain ragas on physiological conditions have been found in ancient Indian texts (Menen 2005). In Indian classical music there is an ideal time of the day to perform a certain *raga* (Joshi 1977). For instance, *Desi-Todi* is one of the ragas appropriate for the late morning and the raga *Yaman* is for the late evening. Use of ragas at the appropriate times with their melodic patterns, colourful ascents and descents, and harmonious relationships creates a meditational state of mind (Prajnananda 1979). One study indicated that such use of music reduces state and trait anxiety and depression and also induces a relaxed physical state (Gupta and Gupta 2005).

Indian classical music has two basic elements, *Raga* and *Taal. Raga* is the basis of melody. The other elements of *Raga* are *Naad*, which is sound, *Swar*, which is made up of whole and half notes, and *Shruti* which are microtones. The aim of *Raga* is to elicit *rasa* which is the emotional and psychological response of the performer and listener. *Rasa* is also referred to as the 'aesthetic delight'.

*Taal*, the second element, is the basis of rhythm. There are various groupings of rhythmic beats. *Taal* is the very basis or pulse of music. Similar to *Raga* and *Rasa, Taal* is also associated with moods, for example: *Chatusram* (beat cycle of 4), devotional and happy times; *Tisram* (beat cycle of three), festivity; *Khandam* (beat cycle of five), anger and frustration, *Misram* (beat cycle of seven), romantic and joyous; and *Sangeernam* (beat cycle of nine), confusion (Kumar 2003).

The use of music as therapy has been prevalent in Indian culture and is now widely used in physiological illnesses, psychological disorders, adjustment problems, and for development in marginalized populations. However, the principle behind the application of the art form in therapy is different when dealing with different populations. In most cases music therapy is used as an alternative or complementary to existing medical treatment. In India, for example, therapists have claimed success in using music for pain management during colonoscopy (Harikumar et al. 2006). Another study describes positive effects of soft instrumental music while dealing with anxiety and depression (Gupta and Gupta 2005). A practice-based report studied the potential of group drumming as therapy for young female commercial sex workers in Mumbai, India and found that the use of group drumming and music provides participants with an opportunity to elicit genuine responses and embark on a therapeutic process (Venkit et al. 2013). Research studies on traditional Indian healing methods and modern music therapy have found music therapy to be a non-medical modifier of the treatment of illness and disease in clinical settings (Sundar 2007).

## Practical initiatives in music and health

Researchers have found that listening to certain kinds of tunes, notes, and rhythms can lead to physiological changes in the body of the listener in the form of elevated neurotransmitters and altered hormonal levels (Krumhansl 1997; Gupta and Gupta 2005; Menon and Levitin 2005). Such therapy sessions involve listening to recordings or live pieces of specific ragas, generally (but not necessarily) rendered by the therapist. These changes in the body are said to help treat diseases. One of the interviewees for this chapter, *pandit* Shashank Katti, a sitar player, music therapist, and founder of the Sur Sanjeevan Centre for Music Therapy, has dedicated a great deal of his time to conducting lecture demonstration programmes, workshops, treatment sessions, and training courses at Sur Sanjeevan. The trust works in collaboration with Ayurvedic doctors and prescribes sessions of listening to particular ragas in addition to the natural medication, depending on the ailment. He has observed positive changes in the areas of arthritis, acidity, migraine headaches, diabetes, liver disease, asthma, hypertension, stress, schizophrenia, and dementia. He believes this process is therapeutic because ragas were traditionally formulated with its health benefits in mind.

Dr Shekhar Kulkarni, an oncology physician and musician, is undertaking research to determine which tunes and harmonies can help control nausea during chemotherapy. Since music helps the secretion of dopamine, which in turn builds the immune system response, he has started to prescribe listening sessions for his cancer patients along with chemotherapy sessions and has begun to research the effect of music on longer survival of cancer patients. Most of the therapists using music therapy do so in conjunction with other allopathic medication.

Music therapy has found wide application in the treatment of autism. Institutions such as Action for Autism, Autism Care, Assam Autism Centre, and the Sampoorna Music Therapy Centre (SMTC) have found improvement in communication in autistic children after introducing music therapy. Ganesh Anantharaman of SMTC found that practising music encouraged children to make eye contact and interact with the therapist, and to build sustained attention. Researchers believe that this is possible because listening to music engages the affective/emotional part of the brain rather than the cognitive/rational part. Autistic children find music/musical gestures and musical movements a better channel of communication than language-based interactions.

The World Centre for Creative Learning Foundation (WCCLF), founded by drum circle facilitator Zubin Balsara, offers a basic guide for using music for working with autistic children and certification courses in Arts Becomes Therapy (ABT). This has led to the emergence of many therapists in India who are working with special needs groups.

Taal Inc., an organization started by Varun Venkit, a clinical psychologist, master practitioner in neurolinguistic programming, and drum circle facilitator, uses rhythm to work with various populations. It is dedicated towards positively influencing health and wellbeing using rhythm, music, and the arts, and has done so by providing regular drum circles for special needs populations, open communities, and by also documenting these processes to be able to further the acceptance and credibility of the use of arts in promoting a better sense of health and wellbeing. The populations with which Taal Inc. has worked include children with learning disabilities, alcohol and drug addicts, and minor and adult commercial sex workers; corporate training is also offered.

Music therapy has been used for marginalized or economically disadvantaged populations including children living in slums (with or without their parents), children caught committing petty crimes, and children in remand homes and other institutions. Dharavi Rocks is one such musical initiative which was started by Acorn Foundation in Mumbai for the children of Asia's largest slum, Dharavi. This band of children performs music from junk instruments, spreads a message about their heritage, and acts as a good social example of exercising the right choice and raising their standard of living. Organizations like Music Basti (Delhi), Sing a Smile (Mumbai), and Audience of One (Mumbai) believe in the importance of art in the overall development of a child, and work in conjunction with municipal schools or with institutions which house such at-risk children. Their aim is to foster creativity in children through activities such as discussion about lyrics and song writing. They believe that through music training one can encourage qualities such as taking initiative, conversation, expression, and confidence. Their sessions typically include music practitioners conducting activities such as singing and song-writing with the children. Most organizations have reported that they do not have any published results since they do not have the resources necessary to conduct research.

## Dance and health

Dance in India is divided into two broad classes: classical and folk. The most popular Indian traditional or classical dances are *Bharatnatyam, Kathak, Kathakali, Odissi, Kuchipudi, Mohiniyattam*, and *Manipuri* (Narayan 2005). According to *Abhinay Darpan* (an ancient text written by Acharya Nandikeshwar), traditional basic dance elements revolve around 'Abhinay' (the 'bodily expression' in any Indian dance form, also known to be the soul of the performance). It is further categorized in four types: *Angika*, the physical aspect, especially gestures and postures; *Vachikabhinaya*, the use of language in or for the dance performance; *Aharyabhinaya*, the external expression, mood, and background as conveyed by costume, make-up, accessories, and sets; and *Satvikabhinaya*, the psychological expression as shown in the eyes in particular, and as a whole by the entire being of the performer. This type of *abhinaya* revolves around nine *Rasas*;

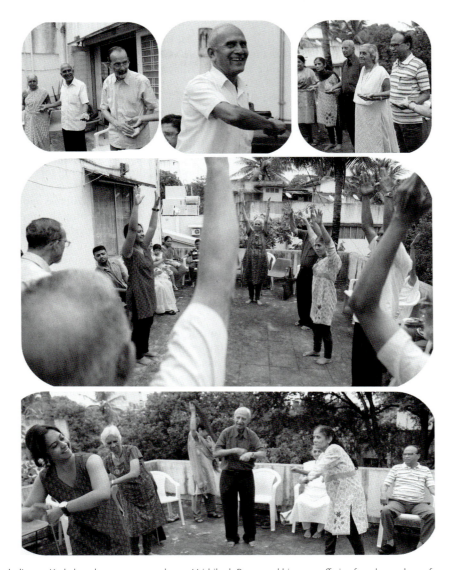

**Fig. 19.1** Dance for Parkinson's disease. Kathak and contemporary dancer Hrishikesh Pawar and his team offering free dance classes for people with Parkinson's disease in collaboration with an orthopaedic and rehabilitation hospital in Pune, India.
Reproduced by kind permission of Hrishikesh Pawar. Copyright © 2015 Hrishikesh Pawar.

namely love (*Shringar*), humour (*Hasya*), pathos (*Karuna*), anger (*Rudra*), heroism (*Vir*), terror (*Bhayanaka*), disgust (*Veebhatsa*), wonder (*Adbhuta*), and peace (*Shantam*, which was added later) (Kumar 2003). These elements form aspects of visual beauty and aesthetics traditionally offered as worship to Lord Shiva or Natraja (Sinha 2006) (Fig. 19.1).

The underlying essence of Indian dance is *Bhakti* (devotion), and its practice was considered a high form of meditation that transcends entertainment and facilitates sublime joy (Narayan 2005). In his *Natya Shastra* (a detailed handbook of Indian drama), Bharata, the founder of the Indian theatrical arts, highlighted the importance of expression of emotions and moods such as love, anger, terror, comedy, pity, and joy serving as a natural vent (Divyabha 2011).

The Indian folk dance tradition is vast. Tribal dances among the Bhils from western India, the Oraons from Jharkhand, and the Santhals from eastern India, and many others, are divided into three broad categories: war and hunting dances, sacred dances (circle dances typically around an idol), and social dances (linked with seasonal festivals, marriages, funerals, etc.) (Haldar 2012). The purpose of these dances, apart from entertainment, has been to bring people together.

## Practical initiatives in dance and health

Dance today serves as a strong medium for work on behavioural issues: newer definitions include dance as a unique physical discipline in which emotional, psychological, spiritual, intellectual, and creative energies can be unified and harmonized (Kashyap 2005). Kashyap has worked at rehabilitation treatment centres, half-way houses, hospitals, special schools (for the mentally challenged and hearing and visually impaired), and addiction treatment centres, and with therapists training to use dance as a metaphor. Dance prompts people to have a dialogue with their bodies. Dance therapy aims to address suppressed memories in the body that hamper progress and to increase wellbeing, self-awareness, and mental health (Kashyap 2005).

Hrishikesh Pawar is a professional Kathak and contemporary dancer. He has set up a centre for contemporary dance and works on promoting contemporary dance and physical theatre as a new way of communicating through the human body. He also represents the Pune chapter of the US-based Dance for PD (Parkinson's disease) project where he offers free dance classes for people with Parkinson's disease in partnership with an orthopaedic and rehabilitation hospital in Pune (Pawar 2010). The programme has also been an important catalyst in creating active, engaged Parkinson's communities where there were none. Pawar says that 'In the act of dancing together, people learn, talk, and inspire each other to explore their creative and physical potential through group singing, yoga, and fitness classes that complement their dance training.' The therapeutic goals of this project are dynamic control of balance, reduction of tremors, improving cardiovascular endurance, practice of functional movements, providing attention cues, increasing confidence, and fostering community involvement.

Not much research work or interventions are being undertaken in the field of dance/movement therapy with regards to different populations since most of the research is funded by the therapists themselves. Formal and popular dance training institutions like the Terence Lewis dance academy and Shiamak Davar's dance studio and lesser known dance companies like Arts in Motion and Dance All are now giving dance training and encouraging the values of giving back to society and working for underprivileged groups.

## Drama and health

*Abhinaya* or drama has traditionally existed as a part of Indian classical dance but has come into its own over the years. Drama therapy is a form of creative arts therapy that works on spontaneity and creativity, and uses techniques of theatre exercises to explore the human mind: story-telling, image making, 'personograms' (making an image using one's body), and role-play, to name a few. Drama therapy has been applied in hospitals, old people's homes, special schools, prisons, and where there is a need to help people cope with new realities (Uppal 2006).

Culturally, folk dramas have been providing a healthy environment for rural and urban masses, as seen in the *Nautankis* of Bihar and *Jatras* of Bengal. Drama, being a product of the masses and having undergone an unconscious process of evolution through the creative genius of the people, represents different trends in society in their true colours (Haldar 2012).

With respect to special needs populations, drama has immense potential to break through stereotypes about participants' abilities. This experience is both educational and therapeutic. Drama therapy has shown positive changes in dealing with real-life problems (socio-drama), serving as a vent for aggression, violence, and frustration (psycho-drama) by providing social and moral training, seeking expression that is unique to each and every individual, and, especially for children's groups, discovering own hidden impulses through concepts of play (Uppal 2006).

### Practical initiatives in drama and health

Anand Chabukswar, a drama therapist and one of respondents for this chapter, has conducted theatre exercises, role-play, and story-telling with special needs populations and has reported his results. He describes his experiences of theatre in search of healing in India (Chabukswar 2009).

Valliappan, an artist-activist who has been diagnosed with paranoid schizophrenia, is a success story validating the therapeutic power of art. She has started an institution called 'The Red Door' that mentors and offers peer support for patients with schizophrenia and other psychological disorders using story-telling, fine arts (painting), and martial arts. The aim is to reach out to young people at grass-roots level and provide them a network of care and support, thereby reducing their chances of reaching a severe psychotic state. Thus, drama is a platform that continues to raise awareness of severe mental illness and reduce stigma and discrimination along with addressing the importance of everyday mental health. Her aim is to reduce dependence on medication. This further strengthens the use of drama, since street theatre exercises, proscenium, and pantomime exercises improve listening, problem solving, physical coordination, and physical fitness. This medium acts as a tool for catharsis, communication, awareness, and empathy (Uppal 2006).

Organizations like Velvi, which offers training programmes in theatre, arts, music, and dance for people with autism spectrum disorders, and Budhan Theatre, an organization comprising marginalized de-notified tribes that use theatre for community development, are evidence of theatre being helpful in the development of skills for coping more effectively with life's real problems (Uppal 2006). According to Dr Parsuram Ramamoorthi, founder of Velvi, drama therapy is the process of systematizing the cathartic and therapeutic effects of drama on a specific group of people with the intention of healing. It helps people cope with their mental and physical conditions (Ramamoorthi and Nelson 2011). They have worked at rehabilitation homes with prisoners, children with autism spectrum disorders, and tsunami survivors.

Natyashala Charity Trust, a Mumbai-based organization that aims to provide physical, intellectual, social, emotional, and spiritual support to children with special needs and special educators, has existed for over two decades and has managed to set up a strong financial support structure (governmental, private, and foreign) for sustenance of their arts-based programmes.

## Yoga and health

The word yoga is derived from the Sanskrit word *yuj*, meaning to yoke or unite. It is one of the six orthodox systems of Indian philosophy (Iyengar 1966). This art form originated in ancient India and has many different schools of thought, though all of them strive to achieve one goal—to attain a state of permanent peace. Recent traditions and practices of yoga can be traced back to the *Sutras* (aphorisms or axioms) of Patanjali, *Upanishads*, *Vedas* (ancient Indian texts), and the *Bhadwad Gita*, which evolved into different paths, namely, *Hath Yoga* (path of physical discipline), *Bhakti Yoga* (realization through devotion to God), *Karma Yoga* (realization through work and duty), *Jnana Yoga* (realization through knowledge), and *Raja Yoga* (path of conquering mind) (Iyengar 1966). The *Sutras* were the earliest, and still the most profound and enlightening study, of the human psyche (Fig. 19.2).

In India the relation that obtains between religion and medicine is importantly different from that of the dominant tradition of the Anglo-European world where science and religion tend to be treated separately. Among the world traditions, classical yoga is a useful starting point for inquiry into the relationship of medical and religious health because it connects the cultivation of physical and psychological health with spiritual wellbeing and it exemplifies the idea of religious liberation as healing (Fields 2002).

Patanjali's writing became the basis for a school of yoga referred to as *Ashtanga Yoga* (eight-limbed yoga). This eight-limbed concept is a core characteristic of practically every *Raja Yoga* variation taught today: the eight limbs are *Yama* (abstentions), *Niyama* (observances), *Asana* (postures for meditation), *Pranayama* (control of breath), *Pratyahara* (control of senses), *Dharana* (concentration), *Dhyana* (meditation), and *Samadhi* (liberation) (Iyengar 1966).

Traditional Indian healing systems like yoga and Ayurveda have been welcomed globally and have been given scientific endorsements for their therapeutic value (Sundar 2007).

One of the oldest schools of yoga that has spread all over the world was started by B. K. S. Iyengar, disciple of the late Krishnamacharya (Krishnamacharya Yoga Mandiram, Chennai)

who emphasized the aesthetic and therapeutic elements of yoga. His institute, the Ramamani Iyengar Memorial Yoga Institute in Pune, conducts regular yoga classes for the general public, medically ill patients, and trainee teachers. The institute also publishes books and conducts research. B. K. S. Iyengar Guruji (2001) says:

> Yoga is a fine art and seeks to express the artist's abilities to the fullest possible extent. While most artists need an instrument, such as a paintbrush or a violin, to express their art, the only instruments a yogi needs are his body and his mind.

Hence, yoga as an art is a life-long process that is rewarded with personally (physical, mental, emotional, and spiritual) fulfilling experiences, and is aesthetic as a result of one's practice being refined to its optimum potential.

## Practical initiatives in yoga and health

Renowned institutions like Kaivalyadham (yogic hospital and healthcare centre), Lonavala, Swami Vivekananda Yoga Anusandhana Sansthana, Bengaluru, Bihar School of Yoga, Munger and Yogavidyadham, Nashik offer, apart from regular

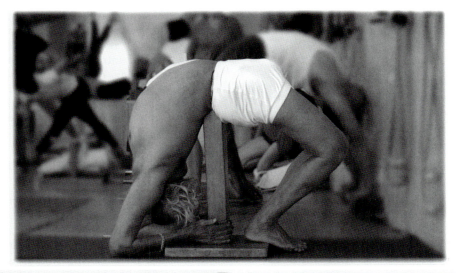

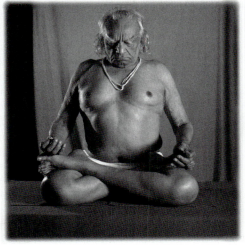 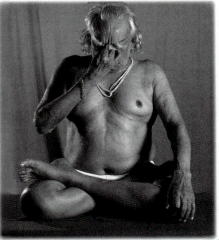

**Fig. 19.2** Yoga, derived from '*yuj*', meaning 'to yoke' or 'unite'. The late Sri Yogacharya B. K. S. Iyengar demonstrating (from top to bottom) the 'upward bow' and two breathing techniques in the 'lotus position'.

yoga classes, teacher training programmes and courses in yoga therapy that address physical and psychological disorders such as musculoskeletal, nervous, metabolic, respiratory, cardiovascular, and immunity issues.

Various studies of the effects of yoga have already been documented by many researchers and it has been found that yoga has physical benefits (Thombre, et al. 1992; Raub 2002; Khattab et al. 2007; Woodyard 2011). In yoga, a specific set of *Asanas* are practised and researched to cure not only physical illnesses but also mental conditions like mood and anxiety disorders (Da Silva et al. 2009), depression (Woolrey et al. 2004), insomnia (Khalsa 2004), and post-traumatic stress disorder (Mehta 2011).

The V. V. M. Research Centre (the Art of Living's alcohol and drug de-addiction unit inspired by the spiritual figure Sri Sri Ravi Shankar) has started many yoga and *Pranayama* programmes in prisons and juvenile homes across the country in Tihar, Jharkhand, Andhra Pradesh, Indore, and Udaipur to reach goals of total abstinence and enrich their quality of life (VVM Research Centre 2003).

Godbole, a senior yoga therapist and one of interviewees for this chapter, said that yogic concepts such as understanding the body's vital points (*Marma),* energy channels, and breathing techniques are used in martial art forms like *Krushniyavidya* (the ancient martial art form used by Lord Krishna). This practice helps in understanding and overcoming one's fears by building self-confidence. Its benefits are similar to those of other Indian martial art forms like *Kalaripayattu* (the ancient martial art form of Kerala). A study indicated that the respiratory functions of *kalaripayyatu* practitioners were better than a control group (Chandran et al. 2004). The Indian School of Martial Arts has been recognized by the Government of India and the Indian Sports Council as an ideal training centre for *kalaripayyatu* and *kalarichikilsa*, which is a parallel science to Ayurveda for healing (Indian School of Martial Arts 2005).

There are some commonalities between yoga and dance—alertness of the mind and full involvement in one's own postures—that creative movement therapist Tripura Kashyap uses in her practice while working on issues such as awareness and wisdom of the body showing the interconnectedness of art.

## Fine arts and health

The great Nobel laureate Rabindranath Tagore says 'Literature, music and the arts are all necessary for the development of and flowering of a student to form an integrated, total personality' (Uppal 2006). Art therapy is a powerful tool that helps one to get in touch with feelings through the creative process. Sometimes art is an easier form of expression for patients than verbalizing their pain. Creative expression improves self-esteem, self-awareness, and personal growth, and also provide a sense of mastery (Jahagirdar 2012).

Art education brings a better balance between cognitive and emotional development (Khadri 2011) and is also one of the most accessible expressive art forms. Hence the use of fine arts, painting, drawing, sketching, and colouring seems to be widespread in Indian schools (rural and urban), day care homes, and institutions for special populations, but empirically speaking, only a select few institutions and therapists have contributed to its academic development.

## Practical initiatives in fine arts and health

The Pomegranate Workshop is a venture that was set up to develop and deliver learning methods that focus on experiential learning and self-expression in children and adults. On their roster they have practising professionals in the areas of visual art (contemporary artists), language arts (published writers), performing arts (theatre actor-directors), maths, science, and design to construct a variety of modules (The Pomegranate Workshop 2013). The Assam Autism Foundation day care centre and the Muktangan de-addiction rehabilitation centre also have a range of arts-based interventions to address the needs of their respective populations. Sujata Dharap, one of the respondents for this chapter, is an artist and muralist who started the Amber Creative Club in 1981 with the main aim of wellbeing through art (painting, pottery, sculpture). Expression and catharsis through art is the main focus area apart from increasing self-confidence, communication, social skills, and concentration. Susan Khare, visual art therapist and another respondent for this chapter, is a member of the foundation course in expressive and creative arts therapies offered by the Studio for Movement Arts and Therapies, Bengaluru. She has trained many therapists working in the field today and believes that there is not enough value placed on visual art in the educational system. The United Nations Children's Fund (UNICEF) along with the Metamorphosis Group in Chattisgarh have introduced many arts interventions such as painting, sketching, music, drama, and photography to work with children who have suffered violence and orphaned children in *Ashramshaalas* (rural residential schools), child-friendly spaces that offer a protective environment for the child to grow up (UNICEF India 2010).

## Research and training in arts and health

On a governmental level, institutions such as the Lalit Kala Academi (National Academy of Fine Arts), the National Council for Education Research Trust (NCERT), and the Indian Council for Mental Health do recognize and endorse the importance of propagating the arts with an emphasis on their application in the area of health and wellbeing. Non-governmental organizations (NGOs) such as The Music Therapy Trust of India, New-Delhi (TMTT) and the Mumbai Education Trust (MET) offer a post-graduate diploma and certificate courses in music therapy. MEWSIC, the Brett Lee Foundation, has helped with financial support of TMTT courses with a vision of making music freely available to every child in the country. Nada (the Centre for Music Therapy), Chennai, apart from research work and organizing music therapy conferences, offers a distance learning course in music therapy. The World Centre for Creative Learning Foundation, Pune, being the most structured and comprehensive arts therapy organization in India, offers a course called 'Arts Become Therapy' which is aimed at providing professional social workers, counsellors, caregivers, and psychologists with a healing model that they can apply in a therapeutic setting. WCCLF has successfully trained more than 100 arts-based therapists who are working in at the grass-roots level in various NGOs across the country (World Centre for Creative Learning Foundation 2001).

Apart from organizational initiatives, experienced arts practitioners and therapists are training young artists to spread awareness of the importance of research and practice for arts in health in India.

## The future of arts and health in India

Based on the current scenario it is evident that the health culture in India is pluralistic in nature since people have access to various medical systems. These systems are used, either simultaneously or sequentially, for a single ailment or for different ailments. In the building of modern India, it was visualized that the traditional, indigenous practices along with their practitioners would gradually give way to modern medicine as modern education and healthcare facilities spread through the country. The latter did happen, but the indigenous systems did not disappear. Instead, a medical pluralism based on a hierarchy of medical systems has emerged (Abraham 2005). An overview of the role of expressive arts in society today shows the innate potential of these art forms if they are given due credit. For this more work needs to be done to highlight the benefits of arts and health.

Even though documentation of therapy work is on the rise there is a need for structured archival and practice- and evidence-based reports to ensure progressive development of this field.

Students in India today have greater access to art therapy conferences and practitioners and therapists are steadily gaining acceptance from psychologists and counsellors as complementary caregivers for certain special needs populations, showing an increase in the acceptance of the power of arts as therapy.

However, there is a need for stronger institutionalization by means of accredited certification courses in universities to increase the number of art therapists able to work with the large number of people who will benefit from these interventions and to facilitate the experience of the therapeutic potential of the arts in a country where it is inherent.

## Conclusion

Art forms have been and continue to be an integral part of rural and folk cultures in India. However, with many cross-cultural influences, young people in rural and urban settings need to be shown the health and social benefits of the existing ways of life. There is a growing increase in the awareness of the therapeutic potential of the arts among the upper middle class, which needs to be nurtured into a systematic, structured, and academic effort to spread the arts as far and wide as possible.

## Acknowledgements

This chapter on 'Arts and health initiatives in India' would not have been possible without the tireless efforts of our team: Miss Kohinoor Darda, Miss Mrinmayi Kulkarni, Mr Swatcchanda Kher, Miss Rajeshwari Baxi, Mr Kaustubh Tambhale, Miss Nupur Moudgill, and all at Taal Inc. We would like to extend warm thanks to our expert therapists, practitioners, and all the responding institutions, particularly the Ramamani Iyengar Institute of Yoga, for all the information they imparted.

## References

Abraham, L. (2005). Indian systems of medicine (ISM) and public healthcare in India. In: L.V. Gangolli, R. Duggal, and A. Shukla,(eds), *Review of Healthcare in India*, pp. 187–224. Mumbai: CEHAT.

Chabukswar, A. (2009). Making, breaking and making again: theatre in search of healing in India. In: S. Jennings (ed.), *Dramatherapy and Social Theatre: Necessary Dialogues*, pp. 117–128. New York: Routledge Publications, Taylor and Francis.

Chakravarthi, R. (2010). The soul of India. In: R. Chakravarthi (ed.), *Exploring the Life, Myth and Art of India*, pp. 6–9. New York: Rosen Publishing Group.

Chandran, C.K., Nair, R.H., and Shashidhar, S. (2004). Respiratory functions in Kalaripayattu practitioners. *Indian Journal of Physiology and Pharmacology*, **48**, 235–240.

Da Silva, T.L., Ravindran, L.N., and Ravindran, A.V. (2009). Yoga in the treatment of mood and anxiety disorders: a review. *Asian Journal of Psychiatry*, **2**, 6–16.

Divyabha (2011). History of Indian drama. *Journal of Department of Applied Sciences and Humanities*, **9**, 27–30.

Fields, G. (2002). *Religious Therapeutics; Body and Health in Yoga, Ayurveda and Tantra*. Delhi: Motilal Banarasidass.

Gupta, U. and Gupta, B.S. (2005). Psychophysiological responsivity to Indian classical music. *Psychology of Music*, **33**, 363–372.

Haldar, A.K. (2012). *Evaluation Study of Tribal/Folk Arts and Culture in West Bengal, Orissa, Jharkhand, Chhatisgrah and Bihar*. Available at: <http://planningcommission.gov.in/reports/sereport/ser/ser_folk2211.pdf> (accessed 20 February 2014).

Harikumar, R., Raj, M., Paul, A., et al. (2006). Listening to music decreases need for sedative medication during colonoscopy: a randomized, controlled trial. *Indian Journal of Gastroenterology*, **25**, 3–5.

Indian School of Martial Arts (2005). Kalari/ Kalaripayattu. Available at: <http://www.kalari.in/kalaripayattu.htm> (accessed 15 August 2013).

Iyengar, B. (1966). *Light on Yoga*. New Delhi: Harper Collins.

Iyengar, B. (2001). *Yoga: The Path to Holistic Health*. London: Dorling Kindersley.

Jahagirdar, R. (2012). Art therapy. Available at: <http://psychiatrist-frompune.blogspot.in/2012/08/art-therapy.html> (accessed 25 September 2013).

Joshi, G.N. (1977). *Understanding Indian Classical Music*. Mumbai: Taraporevala.

Joshi, A. (2005). Mental health in India: review of current trends and directions for future. In: L. Gangolli, R. Duggal, and A. Shukla (eds), *Review of Health Care in India*, pp. 127–136. Mumbai: CEHAT.

Kashyap, T. (2005). *My Body My Wisdom*. New Delhi: Penguin Books.

Khadri, S.V. (2011). Satyam Shivam Sundaram—philosophy of Indian art. Available at: <http://commentary.kalaparva.com/2011/05/satyam-shivam-sundaram-philosophy-of.html> (1 September 2013).

Khalsa, S.B.S. (2004). Treatment of chronic insomnia with yoga: a preliminary study with sleep wake diaries. *Applied Psychophysiology and Biofeedback*, **29**, 269–278.

Khattab, K., Kattab, A.A., Ortak, J., Richardt, G., and Bonnemeier, H. (2007). Iyengar yoga increases cardiac parasympathetic nervous modulation among healthy yoga practitioners. *Indian Journal of Physiology and Pharmacology*, **4**, 511–517.

Krumhansl, C.L. (1997). An exploratory study of musical emotions and psychophysiology. *Canadian Journal of Experimental Psychology/Revue Canadienne de Psychologie Expérimentale*, **51**, 336–353.

Kumar, R. (2003). *Essays on Indian Music*. New Delhi: Discovery Publishing House.

Leslie, C. (1976). *Asian Medical Systems*. Los Angeles: University of California Press.

Mehta, R. (2011). *Yoga Rahasya*. Pune: RIMYI.

Menen, R. (2005). *The Miracle of Music Therapy*. New Delhi: Pustak Mahal.

Menon, R. (1995). *The Penguin Dictionary of Indian Classical Music*. Australia: Penguin Group.

Menon, V. and Levitin, D.J. (2005). The rewards of music listening: response and physiological connectivity of the mesolimbic system. *NeuroImage*, **28**, 175–184.

Monroe, P. (2000). *Encyclopaedia of History of Education*. New Delhi: Cosmo Publications.

Morandi, A. and Fave, A.D. (2013). The emergence of health in complex adaptive systems: a common ground for Ayurveda and western science. In: A. Morandi and A.N. Narayanan Nambi (eds), *An Integrated View of Health and Wellbeing: Bridging Indian and Western Knowledge*, pp. 163–188. Dordrecht: Springer Science and Business.

Narayan, S. (2005). *The Sterling Book of Indian Classical Dances*. New Delhi: New Dawn Press.

Pappachan, M.J. (2011). Increasing prevalence of lifestyle diseases: high time for action. *Indian Journal of Medical Research*, **134**, 143–145.

Pawar, H. (2010). Hrishikesh Centre of Contemporary Dance. Available at: <http://www.hrishikeshpawar.com/project.php?page=project> (accessed 23 September 2013).

Prajnananda, S. (1979). *Music: Its Form, Function and Value*. New Delhi: Munshiram Manohalal Publishers.

Radhkrishnan, S. (1989). *Indian Philosophy, Vol. 1*. New York: Oxford India Paperbacks.

Ramamoorthi, P. and Nelson, A. (2011). Drama education for individuals on the autism spectrum. In: S. Schonmann (ed.), *Key Concepts in Theatre/Drama Education*, pp. 177–181. Rotterdam: Sense Publishers.

Raub, J.A. (2002). Psychophysiologic effects of Hatha Yoga on musculoskeletal and cardiopulmonary function: a literature review. *Journal of Alternative and Complementary Medicine*, **8**, 797–812.

Salleh, R.M. (2008). Life event, stress and illness. *Malaysian Journal of Medical Sciences*, **15**, 9–18.

Sharma, M. (2006). *Tradition of Hindustani Music*. New Delhi: Deep Printers.

Sharma, M. (2007). *Musical Heritage of India*. New Delhi: A. P. H. Publishing Corporation.

Sinha, A. (2006). *Let's Know Dances of India*. New Delhi: Star Publications.

Sundar, S. (2007). Traditional healing systems and modern music therapy in India. *Music Therapy Today*, **8**, 397–407.

The Pomegranate Workshop (2013). The Pomegranate Workshop. Available at: <http://www.tpw.in/> (accessed 20 July 2013).

Thombre, D.P., Balakumar, B., Nambinarayanan, T.K., Thakur, S., Krishnamurthy, N., and Chandrabose, A. (1992). Effect of yoga training on reaction time, respiratory endurance and muscle strength. *Indian Journal of Physiology and Pharmacology*, **36**, 229–233.

UNICEF India (2010). Photo essay: art based therapy—nurturing expression, healing minds. Available at: <http://www.unicef.org/india/reallives_7866.htm> (accessed 24 August 2013).

Uppal, S. (ed.) (2006). *National Focus Group on Arts, Music, Dance and Theatre*. New Delhi: National Council of Educational Research and Training.

Veereshwar, P. and Sharma, N. (2001). *Aesthetics*. Meerut: Krishna Prakashan.

Venkit, V.R., Godse, A.A., and Godse, A.S. (2013). Exploring the potentials of group drumming as a group therapy for young female commercial sex workers in Mumbai, India. *Arts & Health: n International Journal for Research, Policy and Practice*, **5**, 132–141.

Vidyarthi, L.P. and Rai, B.K. (1976). Folklore, art and craft of the tribals. The Tribal Culture of India, pp. 308–342. New Delhi: Concept Publishing Company.

VVM Rehabilitation Centre (2003). V. V. M. Rehabilitation Centre. Available at: <http://www.vvmrc.com/> (accessed 25 September 2013).

Woodyard, C. (2011). Exploring the therapeutic effects of yoga and its ability to increase quality of life. *International Journal of Yoga*, **4**, 49–54.

Woolrey, A., Myers, H., Sternlieb, B., and Zeltzer, L. (2004). A yoga intervention for young adults with elevated symptoms of depression. *Alternative Therapies in Health and Medicine*, **10**, 60–63.

World Centre for Creative Learning Foundation (2001). Home page. Available at: <http://wcclf.org/> (accessed 1 June 2013).

World Health Organization (2012). India. Available at: <http://www.who.int/countries/ind/en/> (accessed 20 February 2014).

# CHAPTER 20

# A role for the creative arts in addressing public health challenges in China

Jing Sun and Nicholas Buys

## Introduction to the creative arts and public health in China

Chronic diseases, including hypertension, cardiovascular diseases, cancer, diabetes, chronic obstructive pulmonary disease (COPD), and growing rates of dementia, have become significant public health problems in China. While cardiovascular disease remains the leading cause of death, the incidence of diabetes and hypertension has also increased, affecting more than 20 million Chinese people (Tang et al. 2013). Chronic diseases disproportionately affect people of low socio-economic status, with the 2008 Chinese National Health Services Survey demonstrating that the prevalence of chronic diseases was 23% among rural low-income populations compared with a population average of 17% (World Bank 2011). This is due to the fact that people of low socio-economic status affected by chronic disease are either not seeking care or are seeking inexpensive but inappropriate care, primarily due to limited finances (Tang et al. 2013).

At the same time increasing numbers of the population are suffering from chronic diseases (Lee 2004). Chronic diseases are associated with psychosocial difficulties such as depression and chronic stress, social problems such as social isolation or disconnection, and physiological abnormalities such as abnormal levels of metabolic factors, blood glucose, and cholesterol, and high blood pressure. All of these factors contribute to negative health outcomes, creating a significant public health challenge, a burden on health services, and a concomitant increase in medical expenditure in China (Chen et al. 2008; Tang et al. 2013). Culturally appropriate intervention programmes to address these problems are therefore an urgent priority for the country.

It has been proposed that positive adaptation, protective factors, social support, and health services, if used as assets, can moderate the impact of health risk factors, and that resilience is a major factor in this process (Sun and Buys 2013a). Resilience is defined as an 'interactive process of individual characteristics and the social context through which an individual can successfully adapt to stressful circumstances despite risk and adversity' (Masten 1994, p. 3). This perspective implies that wellbeing and health are significantly affected by an individual's social context and are a function of the quality of the relationships between an individual's resilience characteristics, such as self-esteem, self-confidence, self-efficacy, coping abilities, their family, and available social supports (Sun and Buys 2013a). In this context, arts-based activities have been found to build resilience in individuals, and therefore have the potential to affect health and wellbeing (Sun and Buys 2013a; Sun et al. 2013). They can alleviate the burden of chronic disease by engaging people in physical activities and social interaction (Sun et al. 2013), and can therefore be used as important public health resources, responding to the population's needs and contributing to a reduction in stress and depression (Clift 2012; Sun and Buys 2013a,b,c).

Over the past decade, public health professionals have begun to look at how the arts might be used in a variety of ways to promote mental health, increase social interaction and social connectedness, develop resources for social support, reduce symptoms, and change risky health behaviours (Clift and Morrison 2011; Clift et al. 2013; Sun and Buys 2013b). Given the ubiquity of creative expression, with its relative ease of engagement, minimal dependence on equipment and economic status, and convenience, it is vital to investigate the ability of creative arts to promote sustainable health outcomes (Cohen et al. 2007; Clift 2012; Sun et al. 2013).

In this chapter we report on the findings of one such investigation in China. It outlines the forces influencing the need for an arts-based approach to health management, the importance of cultural participation to the population, common cultural activities, and their benefits, and then describes a study that investigated the link between creative arts and health. We argue that arts-based activities, as a form of creative endeavour, have the potential to inform such intervention programmes by building resilience in individuals, enabling them to better manage and cope with their chronic conditions. This is the first research in China to investigate this important area.

## Forces influencing the need for engagement with the creative arts

With urbanization, industrialization, and a growing population, new social and environmental factors have emerged in China which have an impact on health and social wellbeing. In this changing context, consideration of the role of participation in the creative arts to promote health and wellbeing is warranted. More effective ways to create and share meaning between individuals, promote health, and prevent chronic illness are vital if China is to make the successful transition to a modern state. These forces and the role of creative activities are explored in this section.

### Urbanization and industrialization

China's rapid urbanization and industrialization are characterized by the large-scale migration of people from the countryside to the rapidly expanding urban areas. The percentage of China's population living in urban areas reached 51.27% in 2011, surpassing the rural population for the first time (Li et al. 2012). Rapid urbanization has changed living conditions: people are living in high-density housing and there are poor sanitary conditions, air and noise pollution from construction and transportation, and soil and water pollution caused by inadequate waste disposal. People's lifestyles have also changed, with an increasing reliance on cars and computers, resulting in reduced physical activity (Friel et al. 2011; Li et al. 2012). High-calorie fast food is more accessible and is therefore being increasingly consumed. Furthermore, the faster-paced urban lifestyle creates high levels of mental stress, which can adversely affect physiological, psychological, and behavioural processes (Li et al. 2006). These factors, combined with unhealthy behaviours such as smoking and high alcohol consumption, contribute to the increased prevalence of cardiovascular diseases, hypertension, weight problems, and obesity (World Bank 2011). Engagement in creative arts activities is one means by which Chinese people can adapt and adjust themselves to these environmental, social, and lifestyle changes, helping them to cope with stress and anxiety.

### The ageing population and demands on healthcare

China has a fast-growing ageing population, with approximately 147 million people aged between 55 and 64 years (10.9% of the total population) and 122 million older adults aged 65 years and over (9.1% of the total population). In 2013 the median age was 35.9 years (male 35.2, female 36.6)—in 1964 the median age was 20.2, 15 years less. By 2015, there will be over 200 million elderly people in China, increasing to 300 million in 2027 and 400 million in 2050 (China National Bureau of Statistics 2012). By the end of 2050, one-fifth to one-third of China's population will be aged 65 or over and the proportion of people aged 80 in the population will increase to 9% (it was 1% in 2005) (Mai and Chen 2013). Due to its strict population policies, China's fertility rate is very low. The introduction of the 'one-child policy' in 1976 means that the first 'one-child' generation is approaching old age, leading to an increasing number of older adults who are living alone.

The rapid increase in older people, particularly those aged 80 years or more, has resulted in changes in family household structure (Mai et al. 2013), posing a number of challenges. The primary challenge is 'fixing' a social and health system that is ill-prepared to cater for the needs of an ageing population. The number of older people with chronic diseases has increased exponentially, with those who are poor and living in rural areas having the least access to quality healthcare, exacerbating mortality rates and decreasing longevity (World Bank 2011). There is

an urgent need in China to solve the problems related to ageing through public health initiatives and sustainable economic and social development. Recent studies suggest a connection between people's mental and physical health and opportunities to express themselves creatively and participate in the cultural traditions of their communities of origin (Cohen et al. 2006, 2007). This finding necessitates research to address the role that the creative arts can play in the health and wellbeing of Chinese communities.

## Cultural participation in the general Chinese population

Arts and cultural activities play a significant role in the lives of Chinese adults, their children, and society in general. Arts activities, from crafts and projects in the home, to opera singing and Chinese folk dancing, are deeply valued by the population. These activities are pursued in a wide variety of ways, and reflect the cultural identity of the nation. The vitality of Chinese artistic and cultural life is a critical indicator of the quality of life (QoL) of its people. Arts activities involve the individual act of creating, acting, or observing and receiving and the communal act of sharing with others, evoking a range of psychological, social, spiritual, and physical responses (Cohen et al. 2006, 2007; Clift 2012). The opportunity to engage with others intensifies the experience and provides a valuable means to express feelings, participate in a social activity, manage anxiety and depression, and develop a sense of social connectedness and trust (Sun et al. 2013). Whether this involves reliving moments by singing a favourite song, acting, dancing, or reflecting on visits to art exhibitions or travel, such creative processes help people to explore the experience more deeply and benefit from different perspectives. Frequency of participation is a key indicator of the importance people place on the arts activities they pursue.

With the rapid ageing of the population in China, the transmission of artistic and cultural identity and knowledge is critical. Arts programmes are therefore a culturally appropriate method of encouraging Chinese people to be more physically active, socially participative, and psychologically and emotionally healthier and more resilient (Sun et al. 2013). Such programmes have the potential to play a vital role in encouraging Chinese people to participate in health services, to increase their exercise levels, and to promote social inclusion and social and emotional wellbeing (Sun and Buys 2013a). Anecdotal evidence indicates that participation in cultural groups is attracting interest and gaining momentum in China, largely through unstructured efforts in the local community. While most of these groups are organized by community volunteers, in recent years governments in economically developed areas have begun to support such activities as a means to enrich the lives of older adults.

## Traditional cultural activities

There are a number of traditional activities that express the cultural capital of China, and have the potential to improve the wellbeing of participants.

### Tai Chi

Tai Chi is an ancient Chinese art/exercise. It involves slow and controlled movements, deep and relaxed breathing, and correct

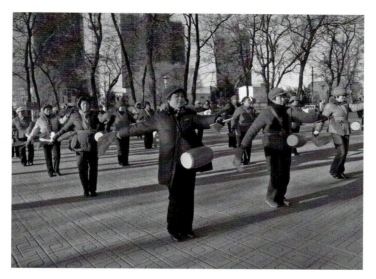

**Fig. 20.1** Chinese folk dancing in Beijing, China.
Reproduced by kind permission of Jing Sun. Copyright © 2015 Jing Sun.

posture, all enacted within a state of awareness and concentration. In the three studies that have specifically studied Tai Chi in patients with coronary heart disease this exercise had both physiological and psychological effects, lowering blood pressure (Channer et al. 1996), increasing exercise capacity (Zheng 2004), improving B-type natriuretic peptide levels, and increasing disease-specific QoL (Zheng 2004).

## Chinese folk dance

Chinese folk dance is a fundamental element in ethnic tradition, religion, customs, and cultural and historical narratives. China has 56 ethnic groups, and each has its own set of folk dances. Each type of folk dance has accompanying costumes, and the skilful use of props such as fans, handkerchiefs, long silks, tambourines, coloured sticks, coloured umbrellas, and coloured lanterns

strengthens the quality of the artistic performance. In addition, the combination of songs and dances promotes full expression of daily life and culture (Figs 20.1 and 20.2).

## Playing Chinese musical instruments

Ancient China was characterized by a wealth of musical instruments and classical compositions. The erhu, guzheng, guqin, xun, and pipa, are typical traditional Chinese musical instruments. Playing a musical instrument is an enjoyable activity and a form of self-expression. It not only requires individuals to exert physical effort, but also gives them the chance to develop skills and creativity (Bittman et al. 2005). Playing a musical instrument has physical benefits because it increases the aerobic capacity of the body and exercises fine motor skills. It also has psychological benefits, reducing stress levels through the

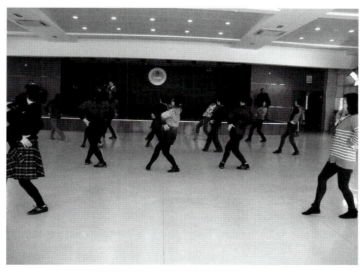

**Fig. 20.2** Traditional folk dancing indoors.
Reproduced by kind permission of Jing Sun. Copyright © 2015 Jing Sun.

action of the neuroendocrine system, which is related to emotional wellbeing (Bittman et al. 2005).

### Chinese opera singing and choral singing

For nearly a century, Yue opera, Shanghai opera, and Cantonese opera singing have been favoured by Chinese people. They blend well with vocal music, poems, folk songs, and Chinese musical instruments. These operas are innovative and self-enriching. The effects of group singing have been investigated in population groups such as people with enduring mental health issues (Clift and Morrison 2011), people with COPD (Clift et al. 2013), and Aboriginal and Torres Strait Islander people in Australia (Sun and Buys 2013a,b,c).

## Arts and health in China: a research study

The majority of studies using Tai Chi, dance, musical instruments, and singing with various age groups have been conducted in western countries. No quasi-experimental methods or randomized controlled trials using these arts activities to examine the prevention of chronic disease have been conducted in China. Indeed most reports about the impact of arts-based programmes in China have been anecdotal. The following account describes an intervention conducted in China that used arts-based activities to improve psychological and mental health, the sense of community connectedness, and overall health status in older people. The intervention was evaluated through a randomized controlled trial conducted collaboratively between Griffith University, Australia and the Changshu Center for Disease Control and Prevention. Changshu City was chosen because it is a heavily urbanized area with a significant population of older adults on low incomes.

Following a survey of peoples' arts preferences, four primary arts activities were chosen for the intervention: (1) meditation-based Tai Chi, (2) dancing, (3) playing a musical instrument, and (4) singing. These activities included different styles of Tai Chi, Yue opera, Shanghai opera, Cantonese opera singing, Chinese dancing, and playing a musical instrument—all are considered culturally important vocal, musical, and performing art forms in China, and all require body–mind coordination, memory, movement planning ability, and a sense of mind, body, and hand control. In these forms of expression, arts modalities and creative processes are used during intentional interventions to foster health and prevent or ameliorate chronic disease.

Seven hundred and fifteen adults aged 45 and over were selected to participate in the study. The study targeted people who had not previously experienced any engagement with the creative arts. All participants recruited into the study had chronic diseases or related risk factors. Most had achieved an educational level of 10 years or less, and had an income level less than 10,000 Chinese Yuan per year. Two groups were compared in this study: an intervention group who participated in one of the four primary creative arts activities ($n = 436$) and a control group ($n = 279$) who only participated in 'passive activities' involving history, literature, and/or computing. Attendance at these activities was for approximately 2 to 3 hours per week on average over a 12-month period. Most participants attended the activities on a regular basis for 12 months, meaning that attendance became habitual and part of their lifestyle. The length of

**Table 20.1** Participation in creative arts activities

|  | No. of participants | Mean time (hours per week) |
|---|---|---|
| Tai Chi | 53 | 3.53 |
| Musical instruments | 98 | 3.03 |
| Chinese folk dance | 99 | 3.78 |
| Singing | 186 | 2.00 |
| History, literature, and computing (control group) | 279 | 2.00 |

the classes was the same for both the intervention and control groups. The activities in which participants engaged are shown in Table 20.1.

Data were collected to measure the health benefits associated with the four creative engagement activities, as well as their impact on resilience. Two survey instruments were developed and validated through the study. The Health Benefits Questionnaire has 46 Likert-scale questions loading on six factors: (1) executive function, (2) social skills, (3) psychological health (Clift et al. 2007), (4) spiritual health (Clift et al. 2007), (5) physical health, and (6) self-esteem. The Resilience Survey has 37 questions and consists of six factors related to individual-level resilience (Friborg et al. 2003, 2005): (1) self-efficacy, (2) communication and social skills, (3) goals and aspirations, (4) self-esteem, (5) family support, and (6) friend support. Data were also collected on biomedical measures to comprehensively evaluate the benefits for peoples' health of engagement with the creative arts. These measures included triglycerides, blood glucose, total cholesterol, high-density lipoprotein cholesterol, and low-density lipoprotein cholesterol, as well as anthropometric measures including body mass index, systolic and diastolic blood pressure, and waist and hip circumferences.

## Health benefits of creative arts in the Chinese population

It is evident from the findings from this project that participation in these activities has a profound impact on physical, psychological, and social functioning. The benefits range from improved psychological and physical health and social and spiritual outcomes, to the building of resilience through increases in self-esteem and the ability to recover from stress. The degree of benefit depends on the art form. Among the range of arts engagement activities in the programme, Tai Chi and all types of opera singing and choral singing groups had a greater benefit on psychological functioning than other types of arts activities. Participants in Tai Chi, all dancing groups (including Latin dance, Chinese folk dance, and ballet), and all opera singing and choral singing groups also experienced benefits to their health-related QoL in all the areas measured. The music and instrument-playing group experienced significant benefits only in their psychological health. Resilience levels significantly improved in adults who participated in the intervention. These improvements are presented in Table 20.2 and described in more detail in the text.

**Table 20.2** Changes in health and wellbeing measures after participation in a creative arts-based activity: mean differences between post and pre intervention

| Health benefits | Tai Chi (n = 53) | Dancing (n = 99) | Musical instruments (n = 98) | Singing (n = 186) | Control (n = 279) |
|---|---|---|---|---|---|
| Executive function | +7.22* | +3.13* | +2.69 | +0.94 | +2.26 |
| Social skills | +3.21** | +1.50* | +2.35* | +1.69* | +0.21 |
| Psychological | +0.64 | +0.72 | +1.68* | +0.89* | −2.03*** |
| Spiritual | +2.23* | +1.10 | +2.73** | +1.20* | −0.66 |
| Physical | +2.45*** | +1.97*** | +2.40*** | +1.96*** | −0.16 |
| Self-esteem | +1.78* | +0.91* | +1.67* | +0.86 | −1.38** |
| Total health benefits | +17.53** | +9.30* | +13.50* | +7.53* | −1.77 |

Statistical significance: $*P < 0.05$; $**P < 0.01$; $***P < 0.001$.

A plus sign (+) indicates increased performance at 12 months' post-intervention and a minus sign (−) indicates a decreased score at 12 months' post-intervention.

## Psychosocial functioning

Participation in Tai Chi and dancing appeared to improve psychological functioning in a range of areas including working memory, inhibition of control and negative emotions, planning and organization, flexibility, and increased social and community participation. Participants had improved capacity to remember routine activities and take medications, organize their time, and attend appointments with friends, doctors, and for chosen activities. They also demonstrated more desire to engage in social activities such as meeting with friends and extra activities such as volunteering in the community. It may be that stimulation from these activities engages and promotes neuronal plasticity in brain areas such as the prefrontal lobes. Executive functioning is believed to be modulated by this brain region (Welsh and Pennington 1988).

## Physical health

All of the creative arts activities improved physical health in areas that included energy levels, physical capacity, blood pressure, weight, and breathing. These activities are meditative by nature and have an element of aerobic exercise, resulting in feelings of improved general health and wellbeing.

## Psychological and spiritual health

Consistent with previous findings in this area (Bittman et al. 2005; Koelsch et al. 2010) psychological and spiritual health is improved through arts-based activities, particularly those involving playing a musical instrument and singing. Playing a musical instrument and singing also improve mood, increasing positive emotions such as happiness as well as decreasing negative emotions (such as anger, sadness, and anxiety ratings) in the music-making and singing group. Social skills and a sense of meaning in life were improved with Tai Chi, dancing, and playing a musical instrument, and there was a significant impact on self-esteem. Relationships among family members and friendships were also improved, a stronger sense of a purpose of life developed, higher feelings of self-worth were held, and an increased sense of competence to solve problems and difficulties was noted. The aerobic nature of the activities such as Tai Chi, dancing, playing a musical instrument, and singing may improve mind–body coordination, accounting for the impact of these activities on these health areas.

## Physiological and biomedical markers

Dance and Tai Chi can have a significant impact on health, lowering the incidence of metabolic syndrome, decreasing systolic and diastolic blood pressure, body mass index, and waist circumference. In addition, dancing reduces triglyceride (mmol/L) levels related to lipid profiles. Participants in the dancing and Tai Chi groups had much lower rates of overweight and obesity than other groups, including those involved with a musical instrument and singing. This suggests that the vigorous exercise associated with dancing and the moderate exercise associated with Tai Chi are effective in reducing overweight and obesity, and lowering high blood pressure (see Table 20.3).

Cultural dancing and Tai Chi may be more likely to appeal to older people, who are at high risk of being overweight or obese, suffering from depression, and/or experiencing a decline in brain function. Dancing had the strongest effect on reducing metabolic syndrome, a finding which may guide future public health interventions to address the prevention and management of chronic disease. Tai Chi was seen to be effective in reducing negative feelings and promoting executive function of the brain, while playing a musical instrument assists in promoting mental health in people suffering from stress, depression, and anxiety.

## Promoting resilience

Engagement in creative arts, particularly Tai Chi and singing, improves self-efficacy, social skills, goals, and aspirations, and self-esteem at an individual level, as well as family and community support (see Table 20.4). Twelve months after the intervention, participants felt more positive in these areas, with positive feelings and confidence about completing and conducting tasks, planning for the future, and increasing confidence in their own abilities. In addition, participation in arts activities improved relationships and connections with family members and friends. Such participation provides older Chinese adults with an opportunity to strengthen friendship networks and community support through group activities. Dancing and playing a musical instrument also improved peoples' aspirations and life goals, leading to more positive feelings of self-worth. The building of resilience in this way is important as it assists older adults to better cope with chronic disease in a situation where it is perceived that managing such conditions is challenging.

**Table 20.3** Changes in metabolic factors and lipid profiles: means (standard deviations)

| Meditative versus Control | Tai Chi (n = 53) | | | Dancing (n = 99) | | | Control (n = 279) | | |
|---|---|---|---|---|---|---|---|---|---|
| | Pre test | Post test | Difference | Pre test | Post test | Difference | Pre test | Post test | Difference |
| 1. HDL | 1.56 | 1.50 | −0.06 | 1.55 | 1.63 | +0.08 | 1.59 | 1.55 | − 0.04 |
| | (0.48) | (0.30) | | (0.46) | (0.35) | | (0.58) | (0.41) | |
| 2.Triglyceride (mmol/L) | 1.86 | 2.08 | +0.22 | 2.21 | 1.85 | −0.36* | 1.51 | 1.54 | + 0.03 |
| | (1.18) | (1.31) | | (1.46) | (0.77) | | (1.57) | (0.53) | |
| 3.LDL | 2.60 | 2.59 | −0.01 | 2.98 | 2.80 | −0.18 | 2.81 | 2.74 | − 0.07 |
| | (0.85) | (0.76) | | (0.77) | (0.80) | | (1.04) | (0.72) | |
| 4. SBP | 132.10 | 119.88 | −12.22*** | 130.26 | 120.47 | −9.79*** | 133.77 | 132.75 | − 1.02 |
| | (16.51) | (15.19) | | (15.29) | (14.50) | | (16.15) | (14.35) | |
| 5. DBP | 84.47 | 76.65 | −7.82*** | 85.91 | 77.49 | −8.42*** | 81.60 | 79.56 | − 2.04 |
| | (8.94) | (8.41) | | (9.29) | (8.17) | | (7.56) | (8.07) | |
| 6. Waist circumference | 83.01 | 80.35 | −2.66* | 82.34 | 74.59 | −7.75*** | 82.47 | 82.00 | − 0.47 |
| | (10.93) | (5.38) | | (12.75) | (6.76) | | (8.50) | (9.00) | |
| 7. BMI | 25.45 | 23.85 | −1.60*** | 24.94 | 22.25 | −2.69*** | 23.79 | 23.85 | + 0.06 |
| | (3.86) | (2.23) | | (4.35) | (3.06) | | (3.05) | (3.11) | |

Statistical significance: *$p$ < 0.05; **$p$ < 0.01; ***$p$ < 0.001. Positive sign (+) indicates increased performance at 12 months post intervention, and negative sign (−) indicates decreased score at 12 month post intervention

## Implications of creative arts engagement in China

This research project demonstrated that arts-based interventions can promote resilience and reduce risk factors related to chronic disease in older Chinese adults. This is particularly so for those factors related to metabolic abnormalities. Interventions that are enjoyable, have a meditative element, and require moderate to vigorous exercise, appear to have wide application in health promotion and primary healthcare. They are relatively low-cost and can be conducted in many settings, such as parks or community centres. Most participants in the case study had less than 10 years of education, yet there was 99% compliance with the programme, indicating that they found it enjoyable and sustainable. This suggests that arts-based interventions are suitable for people with a range of educational levels and socio-economic backgrounds, including those adapting to the newer urban lifestyle as well as older populations with a high prevalence of chronic disease who require social support and increased exercise levels. Further, they can be used to promote mental health and prevent the deterioration of mental health.

**Table 20.4** Changes in measures of resilience after participation in a creative arts-based activity: mean differences between post and pre intervention

| Resilience | Tai Chi (n = 53) | Dancing (n = 99) | Musical instruments (n = 98) | Singing (n = 186) | Control (n = 279) |
|---|---|---|---|---|---|
| Family relationship | +2.64** | +0.96 | +1.54 | +2.27*** | −0.13 |
| Self-efficacy | +3.06*** | +1.22 | +1.23 | +2.55** | −0.10 |
| Social skills | +3.14** | +1.47 | +0.58 | +2.11** | −0.20 |
| Friend support | +2.83** | +0.85 | +1.22 | +1.99*** | −0.01 |
| Planning and goal aspiration | +2.50*** | +1.59*** | +1.53*** | +2.17*** | +0.26 |
| Self-esteem | +4.38** | +3.75*** | +3.54* | +4.10*** | +0.07 |
| Total resilience | +18.57*** | +9.85*** | +9.64* | +15.04*** | +1.05 |

Statistical significance: *$P$ < 0.05; **$P$ < 0.01; ***$P$ < 0.001.

A plus sign (+) indicates increased performance at 12 months' post-intervention and a minus sign (−) indicates a decreased score at 12 months' post-intervention.

## Conclusion and recommendations

When attempting to change unhealthy lifestyles by encouraging people to engage in more physical activity and eat a healthy diet, a cultural shift often precedes institutional structures or policy-making. This project has brought about a cultural shift using arts and community development: there has been movement from a focus on encouraging community members to attend and watch the arts, to community members actively participating and taking 'control of their cultural direction and development'. Creative arts programmes are a sustainable approach to health promotion, with a high rate of compliance and ongoing participation. Such programmes, based as they are in the everyday community environment, promote a friendly and sociable culture that is accepting of all participants, regardless of their age, education, or socio-economic status. This is important, given that many existing short-term interventions in clinical settings have low compliance levels due to the potentially alienating, non-social nature of medical treatment environments. Given the study design used in this project, its results may be generalized to other areas or regions in China, but this needs to be tested in further research studies.

Creative arts activities promote individual resilience and are therefore powerful approaches for improving self-esteem and increasing the coping and disease management abilities of people suffering from chronic disease. They also strengthen family and social support, and increase peoples' awareness and usage of health services. For these reasons, the use of creative engagement in the prevention of chronic disease should be advocated, particularly as these resources are at the disposal of every community. However, greater health and government organizational support is required if they are to be more extensively and effectively deployed. Artists employed with government funding should be integrated into health promotion and public health fields as an important 'new' workforce in the area of prevention and management of chronic disease.

## References

Bittman, B. B., Berk, L., Shannon, M., et al. (2005). Recreational music-making modulates the human stress response: a preliminary individualized gene expression strategy. *Medical Science Monitor: International Medical Journal of Experimental and Clinical Research*, **11**(2), BR31–BR40.

Channer, K.S., Barrow, D., and Barrow, R. (1996). Changes in haemodynamic parameters following Tai Chi Chuan and aerobic exercise in patients recovering from acute myocardial infarction. *Postgraduate Medicine*, **72**, 349–351.

Chen, R., Hu, Z., Wei, L., Qin, X., McCracken, C., and Copeland, J.R. (2008). Severity of depression and risk for subsequent dementia: cohort studies in China and the UK. *British Journal of Psychiatry*, **193**, 373–377.

China National Bureau of Statistics (2012). *China Statistical Yearbook 2012*. Beijing: China Statistics Press.

Clift, S. (2012). Creative arts as a public health resource: moving from practice-based research to evidence-based practice. *Perspectives in Public Health*, **132**, 120–127.

Clift, S. and Morrison, I. (2011). Group singing fosters mental health and wellbeing: findings from the East Kent 'singing for health' network project. *Mental Health and Social Inclusion*, **15**, 88–97.

Clift, S., Hancox, G., Morrison, I., Hess, B., Kreutz, G., and Stewart, D. (2007). Choral singing and psychological wellbeing: findings from English choirs in a cross-national survey using the WHOQoL-BREF. In: A. Williamon and D. Coimbra (eds), *Proceedings of the International Symposium on Performance Science 2007*, pp. 201–207. Utrecht: Association Européenne des Conservatoires, Académies de Musique et Musikhochschulen (AEC).

Clift, S., Morrison, I., Skingley, A., et al. (2013). *An Evaluation of Community Singing for People with COPD*. Canterbury: Sidney De Haan Research Centre for Arts and Health, Canterbury Christ Church University.

Cohen, G.D., Perlstein, S., Chapline, J., Kelly, J., Firth, K.M., and Simmens, S. (2006). The impact of professionally conducted cultural programs on the physical health, mental health, and social functioning of older adults. *The Gerontologist*, **46**, 726–734.

Cohen, G.D., Perlstein, S., Chapline, J., Kelly, J., Firth, K.M., and Simmens, S. (2007). The impact of professionally conducted culturally programs on the physical health, mental health and social functioning of older people—2 year results. *Journal of Aging, Humanities and the Arts*, **1**, 5–22.

Friborg, O., Hjemdal, O., Rosenvinge, J.H., and Martinussen, M. (2003). A new rating scale for adult resilience: What are the central protective resources behind healthy adjustment? *International Journal of Methods in Psychiatric Research*, **12**, 65–76.

Friborg, O., Barlaug, D., Martinussen, M., Rosenvinge, J.H., and Hjemdal, O. (2005). Resilience in relation to personality and intelligence. *International Journal of Methods in Psychiatric Research*, **14**, 29–42.

Friel, S., Akerman, M., Hancock, T., et al. (2011). Addressing the social and environmental determinants of urban health equity: evidence for action and a research agenda. *Journal of Urban Health*, **88**, 860–874.

Koelsch, S., Offermanns, K., and Franzke, P. (2010). Music in the treatment of affective disorders: an exploratory investigation of a new method for music-therapeutic research. *Music Perception: An Interdisciplinary Journal*, **27**, 307–316.

Lee, L. (2004). The current state of public health in China. *Annual Review of Public Health*, **25**, 327–339.

Li, X., Stanton, B., Fang, X., and Lin, D. (2006). Social stigma and mental health among rural-to-urban migrants in China: a conceptual framework and future research needs. *World Health and Population*, **8**, 14–31.

Li, X., Wang, C., Zhang, G., Xiao, L., and Dixon, J. (2012). Urbanisation and human health in China: spatial features and a systemic perspective. *Environmental Science and Pollution Research International*, **19**, 1375–1384.

Mai, Y., Peng, X., and Chen, W. (2013). How fast is the population ageing in China? *Asian Population Studies*, **9**, 216–239.

Masten, A.S. (1994). Resilience in individual development: successful adaptation despite risk and adversity. In: M.C. Wang and E.W. Gordon (eds), *Educational Resilience in Inner-city America: Challenges and Prospects*, pp. 141–149. Hillsdale, NJ: Lawrence Erlbaum.

Sun, J. and Buys, N. (2013a). Improving Aboriginal and Torres Strait Islander Australians' wellbeing using a participatory community singing approach. *International Journal of Disability and Human Development*, **12**, 305–316.

Sun, J. and Buys, N. (2013b). Effectiveness of a participative community singing program to improve health behaviors and increase physical activity in Australian Aboriginal and Torres Strait Islander people. *International Journal of Disability and Human Development*, **12**, 297–304.

Sun, J. and Buys, N. (2013c). Participatory community singing program to enhance quality of life and social and emotional wellbeing in Aboriginal and Torres Strait Islander Australians with chronic diseases. *International Journal of Disability and Human Development*, **12**, 317–323.

Sun, J., Zhang, N., Buys, N., Zhou, Z.Y., Shen, S.Y., and Bao, J.Y. (2013). The role of Tai Chi, cultural dancing, playing a musical instrument and singing in promoting physical and mental health in Chinese older adults: a mind–body meditative approach. *International Journal of Mental Health Promotion*, **15**, 227–239.

Tang, S., Ehiri, J., and Long, Q. (2013). China's biggest, most neglected health challenge: non-communicable diseases. *Infectious Diseases of Poverty*, **2**, 7.

Welsh, M.C. and Pennington, B.F. (1988). Assessing frontal lobe functioning in children: view from developmental psychology. *Developmental Neuropsychology*, **4**, 199–230.

World Bank (2011). *Toward a Healthy and Harmonious Life in China: Stemming the Rising Tide of Non-communicable Diseases*. World Bank Report Number 62318-CN. East Asia and Pacific Region. Available at: <http://www.worldbank.org/content/dam/Worldbank/document/NCD_report_en.pdf>

Zheng, J.Q. (2004). The effect of Tai Chi on coronary heart disease rehabilitation in the elderly. *Chinese Journal of Rehabilitation Theory and Practice*, **10**, 429–430.

# CHAPTER 21

# Culture and public health activities in Sweden and Norway

Töres Theorell, Margunn Skjei Knudtsen,
Eva Bojner Horwitz, and Britt-Maj Wikström

## Introduction to culture and public health activities in Sweden and Norway

This chapter builds on a recent review of research on cultural activities for health promotion in Norway and Sweden (Cuypers et al. 2011). Our aim in this chapter, however, is to provide the reader with some illustrations of the wide range of ongoing activities in Sweden and Norway concerning culture and health.

The development of international research with regard to culture and health has had a profound influence in Norway and Sweden. For instance, the formation of choirs was mentioned in a public health context in the United Kingdom, the United States, Australia, Indonesia, Venezuela, Israel, Palestine, and Germany as an instrument for creating increased cohesiveness and improved health (e.g. Cohen 2009; Clift et al. 2010; De Quadros and Dortewitz 2011). A Nordic network for music, culture, and health, based in Helsinki, has been established with regular meetings on culture and health for researchers, health practitioners, and politicians taking place annually in rotation between Denmark, Norway, Sweden, Iceland, and Finland.

This chapter will show that there is extensive interest in research on cultural activities and health in both Norway and Sweden, ranging from musical activities, theatre and dance, to the visual arts and literature. The examples we describe are mainly regional (counties and municipalities) with very few of them organized on a national level. First of all we will describe the political status of cultural activities and health in the two countries. Although Sweden and Norway are similar countries and have similar historical experiences there are some important differences. Both countries have been dominated during the post-war era mainly by social democratic policy; however, during the most recent period Norway has had social democratic governments while Sweden has had a more conservative government. A short overview of politics will be followed by a description of Swedish and Norwegian activities focused on women and also in three life periods: the school years, working age, and old age.

## The Swedish and Norwegian contexts

### Sweden

In 2000 the Swedish Governmental Commission on Public Health (Year 2000 Public Health Commission; see SOU 2000) published its future plans for public health work in Sweden. The commission was initiated by a social democratic government. The final document has a chapter on the importance of cultural activities. The report had been preceded by several years of scientific summaries and political negotiations, with the political discussions taking place at three levels: state, county, and municipality. For the first time in this kind of official document, cultural activity was mentioned as an important vehicle for public health work. The publication of the document was followed by a series of political processes. Prompted by this publication many counties and municipalities seriously considered the use of cultural activities in public health work. At the same time there was lively international activity in the field, both in public health work and in research.

With a new Swedish government the national authorities continued to stress the potential of cultural activities in health promotion and the need for both research (humanistic as well as biological and psychological) and evaluations in this field (Year 2009 Cultural Politics Commission; see SOU 2009). Several regional evaluations have been launched as a result of this commission. In addition there has been coordination between the ministries for culture and for health and social security (including national health insurance). This has resulted, for example, in three regional evaluations of the effects of cultural participation for patients on sick leave and also as a potential means for decreasing sick leave. The southern region (Skåne) is coordinating research on cultural participation and rates of sick leave nationally and there are evaluations going on in Skåne as well as in the north (Västerbotten) and in the west (Halland). An example of such activities will be described later (in Cultural activities during three age periods/Working age) (Bygren et al. 2009). This interest from the government was prompted by the high rates of sick leave during the period 1997–2003. However, these initiatives have not so far resulted in any specific permanent financial support. The National Board of Public Health produced a position paper for research (National Board of Public Health 2005) but has since then not given priority to it.

The Swedish Parliament started the Society for Culture and Health in 2007. This has organized seminars and served as a political pressure group for a continuous dialogue between politicians, researchers, and producers of cultural activities. It is also disseminating knowledge in the field and stimulates financial support of cross-disciplinary research (see

<http://www.kulturradet.se/>).The parliamentary society also collaborations closely with the Centre for Research on Culture and Health at the University of Gothenburg, which has organized several national panel discussions (<http://www.ckh.gu.se/>) (see Bjursell and Westerhäll 2008).

## Norway

During the years 1997–99 the Norwegian Government started a number of projects in the area of culture and health in order to test the potential of cultural activities for health promotion and illness prevention. There were several reasons for this. In the early 1990s social researchers had encouraged private and public organizations to make systematic evaluations of the effects of cultural activities. There was an increasing prevalence of what was labelled 'diseases of society' (Hjorth 1994). Increasing sickness absence in Norway—as in Sweden—prompted the need to search for new strategies, while increasing wealth in Norway did not seem to result in improved health equity (Elstad 1985). In addition, national surveys showed that participation in cultural activities was less common among lower social classes (Kulturdepartementet 1992). The UNESCO project during the World Decade for Cultural Development (1988–98) also contributed to the increased attention to culture and health interventions from the points of view of public health and culture policy (UNESCO 1996).

The initiative in Norway reached a peak in the years 1997–99 when the government decided to assign 15 million Norwegian crowns during a 3-year period to development work in the field of cultural activity and health. Twenty municipalities and counties took part in this project. The governmental initiative was monitored by a national advisory committee for cultural activity and health with its central node at the Centre for Culture, Health, and Care in Levanger. When the national project came to an end the national agencies left responsibility to regional and local actors. After this, initiatives in the field were taken on at regional and local levels.

One example has been the initiative for cultural activity and health in Nord-Trøndelag county as well as in the municipalities of Porsgrunn, Bergen, Trondheim, and some boroughs in Oslo. During later years national agencies have facilitated regional and municipal work by means of different new laws and official instructions. This development was reinforced in response to the increasing numbers of elderly people as well as increasing socio-economic differences in cultural activity and health. One example is the Cultural Walking Stick and the cross-disciplinary centre for Culture, Health, and Care in Levanger—both of which would not have materialized without strong regional and local engagement and financial input. As part of the Cultural Walking Stick project, Levanger municipality has organized several development projects in which music, dance, and visual arts have been used for health promotion and disease prevention among the elderly. One of the driving forces in the establishment of music therapy in homes for patients with dementia has been Audun Myskja (2012), who has developed music therapy techniques as well as controlled scientific studies in dementia care. A clear trend during later years is that activities in the field of culture and health which were previously confined mainly to the psychiatric sector are nowadays a visible part of governmental initiatives in public health work in general. Today there are laws in Norway (on public health and

on culture) as well as official instructions that can be used as arguments for increased utilization of cultural activities in both health promotion and in care.

Epidemiological results from the HUNT study (Cuypers et al. 2012) have been used as arguments in regional strategies and plans. For instance, initiatives have taken into account that, according to HUNT, some municipalities have few cultural activities and poorer public health compared with other areas. This has been an argument for allocating more resources to those areas. The county initiatives have stimulated several developmental projects such as Culture for Life, Writing for Life, and Singing as Health Promoting Work.

Comparing Norway and Sweden, the Norwegian national agencies coordinating regional and municipal cultural activities with national ones have been maintained to a greater extent than in Sweden. The emphasis in cultural national policy in Norway has been less on the elite and more on public interests in cultural activities (Åse Kleveland 2012, unpublished) and also less on commercial sustainability than in Sweden. One example is the national Swedish Organization for Concerts (National Concerts) which was founded in 1968 but disbanded by the government in 2010. It had organized music performances across Sweden, particularly in the genres of chamber music, choir, and art music as well as jazz and folk/world music. Its Norwegian counterpart, Concerts Norway, has a similar history, although it has more wide-ranging tasks, among them to organize school concerts in the whole of Norway. It was established in 1967 to stimulate regional music communities and is still active.

## National statistics on cultural activities in Sweden and Norway

Statistics Sweden, the national agency for population statistics, has been producing valuable statistics on cultural activities in the Swedish adult population at 8-year intervals since the early 1970s (see Chapter 8). Unfortunately production of these kinds of statistics has decreased since 2006 and information on cultural participation is therefore less extensive during more recent years than previously.

A very large data base has been created in Nord Trøndelag in northern Norway with data on cultural activities in the population. This study is affiliated to Trondheim University and comprises data collected in 1984–86, 1995–97, and 2006–08 on 125,000 Norwegians representing the average citizen. Extensive data on health parameters and on cultural activities from this study will provide unique possibilities to establish relationships between cultural activity and health (Krokstad et al. 2012). The Swedish Twin Registry is being used for a study of the importance of genetics and cultural experiences during childhood/adolescence for the development of musicality as well as the development of other kinds of cultural competence. In this study, which is based upon 8000 twins aged between 27 and 54, the researchers will examine the importance of cultural experiences during childhood and adolescence for the development of emotional competence.

## Experiences from music therapy as a stimulus for the field in general

In Norway there is a strong tradition of supporting various forms of music therapy. Theoretical and practical development of such forms of therapy has taken place under the guidance of Even Ruud

(1997) in Oslo and has an been inspiration for all the Nordic countries. Rune Rolvsjord and Christian Gold have established a music therapy research group at Bergen University in Norway. Their teaching programme and their development of music therapy theory has also been of importance to all the Nordic countries. The researchers in this group have published qualitative as well as quantitative evaluations of the health effects of several kinds of music therapy. For instance, they have recently published a study of 144 patients (in Norway, Austria, and Australia) with non-organic mental disorders and low therapeutic motivation who were randomly allocated to 'treatment as usual' and music therapy, respectively. The results show that music therapy was clearly better for improving collaboration with psychiatric therapy than 'treatment as usual' (Gold et al. 2013). In Stockholm a school of music therapy has been established at the Royal College of Music.

At a regional university hospital in Trondheim (Vaag et al. 2012), all hospital staff were offered participation in a rock music choir project which ended in a public concert. This seemed to appeal particularly to certain groups (middle-aged women and those with a lower level of education). This is of interest since many cultural activities appeal only to those with higher education. Questionnaire data indicated beneficial effects on mental health among the participants. From a public health point of view it is important to find diversified cultural activities that appeal to large proportions of employees (see Chapter 8 for more details on this project).

The Royal College for Higher Music Education in Stockholm has also been active in the field of formal music therapist training and music therapy research for many years and has been of major importance for work on the use of musical activities in rehabilitation and psychotherapy (see Hammarlund 1993; Paulander 2011).

A Swedish centre has examined the influence of nature-based vocational rehabilitation in a specially designed rehabilitation garden (Pálsdóttir et al. 2013). Significant changes were measured regarding perceived occupational values in daily life, symptoms of severe stress, and return to work. Both the rate of return to work and symptoms of severe stress were significantly associated with a change in everyday occupation. In the interviews, participants explained that after the rehabilitation programme they had a slower pace of everyday life and that everyday occupations were more often related to nature and creativity. This could be interpreted as nature-based rehabilitation inducing changes via meaningful tasks in restorative environments, leading to a positive change in the perceived value of everyday occupations. These findings have prompted discussions in Sweden on the importance of experiences in nature for health promotion in general.

Norwegian researchers have also investigated the potential of nature–culture–health (NaCuHeal) activities in terms of their health promoting properties. Research from three evaluation studies focused on how art, music, nature, and culture have a beneficial impact on health and wellbeing (Bratt-Rawden and Tellnes 2011). The first evaluation study described the subjective experiences of people taking part in NaCuHeal activities at the National Centre for NaCuHeal in a Norwegian municipality. The second evaluation study highlighted the extent and way in which people use folk-medical practice, administered in a non-professional setting, in modern culture to maintain, improve, or change their health status. The third evaluation presented results from a study conducted by the Eastern Norway

Research Institute in collaboration with a rehabilitation centre between 2008 and 2009. The three evaluations were based upon 90 ethnographic interviews and open narratives from men and women with long-term illness. The main finding was that NaCuHeal experiences may help participants construct a meaning, identify coping mechanisms, and revitalize their resourcefulness. Hidden resources were awakened and participants felt good about themselves—the salutogenic factors in a person's life are strengthened. These studies indicate how art, music, and NaCuHeal activities may have a beneficial effect on health and wellbeing (Bratt-Rawden and Tellnes 2011).

Volunteering in a Norwegian municipality has been examined in relation to cultural and health determinants (Lorentzen et al. 2012). Members of voluntary associations are engaging in unpaid work, offering their time to assist with cultural activity groups and organizations. Multiple logistic regression was used in order to assess the statistically independent impact of the volunteering component, with the results pointing to links between volunteering, culture, and wellbeing.

## Cultural activities and women

An evaluation of the effects of cultural activities for women with burnout syndrome has recently been performed in Stockholm within the framework of the project 'Culture Palette in Healthcare Centres'—culture activities for women with burnout. This was a controlled study carried out in ambulatory healthcare. The aim of the programme was to decrease symptoms of exhaustion, improve self-rated health, and increase the sense of coherence by means of cultural activities. It was hoped that if there were scientifically unequivocal findings from the evaluation of this programme it would stimulate the establishment of new forms of cultural activity programmes in healthcare centres for women with burnout. In this project the expertise of different culture producers was utilized and musicians, dancers, actors, visual artists, and movie experts acted as culture 'introducers'. The joint effect of these 'culture health palettes' has been evaluated in four healthcare centres in greater Stockholm, partly by means of standardized questionnaires and partly by means of qualitative interviews. Participating women were aged between 25 and 65 and all had a diagnosis of burnout syndrome (or, according to Swedish terminology, exhaustion syndrome) with extreme fatigue, cognitive symptoms, and sleep disorders arising after long-lasting stress. Other symptoms include pain, irritability, and lack of concentration.

The activities took place at the healthcare centre once a week for 3 months. The following activities were included:

◆ Interactive theatre: an experienced actor introduced poetical texts and poems and then initiated and participated in discussions with the participants regarding the thoughts, emotions, and experiences evoked by the texts.

◆ Movies: after a movie performance a movie expert initiated discussions among the participants about the experiences and thoughts evoked by the movie.

◆ Vocal improvisation (under the guidance of a performance artist and pianist): after musical improvisation the participants painted a picture showing the emotions, thoughts, and pictures evoked during the improvisation.

◆ Exploring dance: participants improvised dance movements under the guidance of a dance therapist and teacher of rhythm. The dance movements were staged according to the situation in the room and with focus on bodily awareness. Afterwards the group participants discussed their experiences during dance.

◆ Mindfulness and contemplation: participants contemplated and practised mindfulness with an experienced instructor. After this thoughts, emotions, pictures and body sensations were discussed in the group.

◆ Cultural show: after a theatre performance including music, song, and dance with the theme of food and bodily awareness the participants discussed their thoughts regarding the body and the food with the actor.

Sessions in each of the six different programmes lasted for 90 minutes. Four different healthcare centres tested each programme on two consecutive occasions. After 2 weeks with one programme there was a new programme for the next 2 weeks, and so on. This means that each participant experienced each programme on two consecutive occasions. Accordingly each person was offered 12 occasions to participate during a 3-month period. Interviews and the distribution of standardized questionnaires took place before the start as well as 3 and 6 months later. There were no more cultural activities after 3 months. A control group (without cultural activities) was followed in a parallel way during the whole process. Randomization to experimental and control groups took place at each healthcare centre. The selection of healthcare centres took into account socio-economic characteristics and the unemployment rate in the area.

Standardized scales were used for the assessment of exhaustion, sense of coherence, self-rated health, and alexithymia. Self-figure drawings were used for qualitative analyses.

The results showed decreased exhaustion, improved self-rated health, and decreased alexithymia (accordingly an improved ability to differentiate feelings). An unexpected finding was that the healthcare staff also benefitted.

This project has aroused interest throughout Sweden. It is likely that it will spread to many areas in Sweden and perhaps also to the other Nordic countries. Developing and adapting cultural programmes so that they fit these kinds of patients could cross-fertilize healthcare and culture production. The cultural activities that were offered to these women could help them understand what makes them vital, confirmed, curious, healthy, and creative. Above all, the project illustrated that there could be synergistic effects within the whole caring system.

## Cultural activities during three age periods

Cultural activities are of potential importance for health promotion in childhood, during the occupationally active years, and in older age. There are activities in the field for all the three age groups, and several examples show how counties have been stimulated by international discussions to start cultural activities for health promotion. Governments have been supportive in several of these projects.

### School years

There have been several interesting trials of cultural interventions in school-age children. One of the most interesting projects is 'Vi slår på trummor, inte på varandra' [We beat drums, not one another] which took place during a whole school year in Skåne in southern Sweden. All children had one lesson every week during which they were taught to play drums. This project may have been stimulated by an American project reported by Bittman et al. (2004, 2005) who showed that patients in dementia care and the care staff both benefitted from drums with dancing. Reduced sick leave and staff turnover were observed.

In the 'We beat drums' project positive effects were shown on both language and mathematics scores as well the proportion of pupils reaching high school standard, particularly in the year preceding high school (a 28% increase for that group). In addition, reduced problems with petty vandalism (such as burning litter

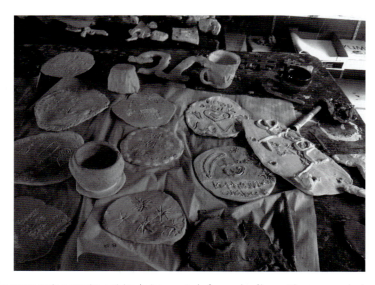

**Fig. 21.1** Ceramic objects produced by teenagers in a creative activity during a period of a couple of hours. The teenagers had no previous experience or knowledge of moulding clay.
Reproduced by kind permission of Töres Theorell. Copyright © 2015 Töres Theorell.

bags) were observed in the school. This project was supported both financially and administratively by the county (Göteborgs-Posten 2013) (Fig. 21.1).

Depression is increasing globally, and it is estimated that it will be one of the conditions causing the greatest burden of disease in 2030. Exercise is considered to be an active strategy for preventing and treating depression and anxiety in adults and school-aged children. Participation in physical activities can also improve self-esteem. An organized, non-competitive, leisure-time intervention is considered beneficial for increasing physical activity in the young. Dance is a well-established and popular form of physical activity, particularly for young women. In a social context, dance might serve as a protective factor in preventing mental illness and reducing the severity of psychosomatic symptoms. 'Dance for Young People' (Duberg et al. 2013) was a successful Swedish project intended to decrease the incidence of psychological symptoms. Through the school healthcare system, 171 girls between the ages of 13 and 18 with psychosomatic symptoms, tiredness, or depressive symptoms were recruited for this intervention, which took place in 75-minute sessions twice a week after school for 8 months. Randomization took place before the start. The control group had to wait while the intervention was ongoing in the intervention group and also during the follow-up. This means that participants in the control group only had normal curriculum. A significant beneficial effect on self-rated health was observed in the dance group compared to the control group not only 12 months after the start (i.e. 4 months after end of the intervention) but also 20 months after baseline. Dancing may accordingly be a preventive measure to decrease the incidence of psychological symptoms in young girls.

An interesting example of cultural activities designed for a community with clear implications for long-term health in young people is the activity in Namsos, a town north of Trondheim. Namsos experienced violent destruction in 1940 during the Second World War. Most of the buildings were destroyed and, most importantly, serious conflicts arose between families who had supported the Germans ('Quislings') and families who supported the opposition. These conflicts still have a tendency to poison the atmosphere in the town. A rock music centre, Rock City, the national resource centre for pop and rock in Norway, opened in Namsos in 2011, and the internationally known rock musician Åge Aleksandersen has been engaged in creating an improved social atmosphere and helping young people in Namsos work through these kinds of conflicts, for instance by means of participation in the production of a rock musical about family conflicts caused by war experiences.

## Working age

One example showing activities in this field for people of working age is the KROKUS project in Västernorrland County in northern Sweden. This project (or rather group of projects) was designed for people of working age. The idea was that cultural activities organized at or through the workplace may increase cohesiveness and also stimulate creativity. The county politicians saw the possibility of combining the interests of regional industries with those of regional culture producers, such as theatres, dance companies, orchestras, and jazz bands, in health promotion. Several pilot projects were started with financial support from government funds, one of which was evaluated by our research group (Theorell et al. 2007). In a pilot study of four large workplaces in the county, cultural activities occurred in the workplace once a week during working hours for a period of 3 months. Standardized questionnaires were used for the assessment of working conditions (self-reported psychological demands, decision latitude, and social support from workmates and superiors) and health (symptoms of depression and exhaustion as well as sleep disturbances) before the start and after 3 months. In addition, on these occasions blood samples were drawn for the assessment of endocrine and immune system parameters. On each occasion participants were asked to rate their emotional state on a visual analogue scale before and after the cultural activity. Separate scales were used for joy–sadness, relaxation–tension, and alertness–fatigue. There was no control group in this pilot study, so inferences about causality cannot be made. However, the results showed that participants who had more positive reactions than others to the events were also those who had the most favourable development of mental health and immune system parameters during the 3-month study period (Theorell et al. 2009).

The KROKUS project (Hartzell and Theorell 2007) was based upon the collective principle that cultural activities organized through workplaces—preferably during working hours and for as many employees as possible—create the optimal basis for improved cohesiveness and creativity. One of the conclusions was that there has to be a diversity of cultural activities since employees have different preferences. Another initiative supported by the Swedish Union of Local Government Officers, the Swedish National Council for Cultural Affairs, the Assurance Company Förenade Liv, and the local county council was based upon the idea that the possible health effects of cultural activities offered to individual employees in medical care should be evaluated (Bygren et al. 2009). This was designed as a randomized controlled trial. There were 51 employees in the municipality of Umeå (a university city in northern Sweden) randomly allocated to the intervention group and 50 to the control group. Both groups of participants had assessments performed prior to starting and 2 months later. In the intervention group the participants could choose which activity they wanted to participate in once a week for the 8 weeks of the study. Using standardized questionnaires (SF-36, Short Form Health Survey) the research demonstrated that participants in the cultural activities group had a more favourable development of physical health, social functioning, and vitality during the study period than participants in the control group. No differences in the development of physiological variables (immunoglobulin and cortisol) were observed. The intervention and follow-up period of 8 weeks is relatively short; longer interventions together with longer follow-up periods of at least a year would be of interest to ascertain whether longer involvement in a cultural activity is sustainable and, if it is, what impact it might have on health.

The project in Umeå was also part of a regional initiative in three counties to explore the feasibility of introducing 'physician recipes for culture' as part of the government's focus on the potential benefits of cultural activities in relation to preventing sick leave. The target group for the 'culture recipes' comprised patients on long-term sick leave. Initial small-scale qualitative follow-up evaluations showed that cultural activities had a vitalizing effect on these patients. Larger evaluations of activities for the prevention of sick leave by means of cultural activities are ongoing. Scientific proof of this would require large samples, comparable control groups, and long follow-up periods of more than a year. The latter is particularly important since effects on sick leave patterns are notoriously slow to show up. The usual follow-up period of a year or less is too short for such effects. The project in Skåne is planned to include 200 participants and will continue until December 2014. Effects of the cultural activities on the participants will be compared with referents who are not offered such activities (see <http://www.skane.se/sv/webbplatser/valkommen_till_vardgivarwebben/utveckling__projekt/sjukskrivningsprocess/rehabiliteringsgarantin/kultur-pa-recept-20/>).

There have also been initiatives in other parts of Sweden to revitalize workplaces by means of cultural activity. The county surrounding Gothenburg, Västra Götaland, has been active in this field. A good example is the Västra Skådebanan (approximately translated as 'theatre route in the western region'). This organization has existed since 1974 and is financed from both national and regional sources. Its goal is to stimulate cooperation between culture producers and employers. One of the reported findings from companies participating in 'Airis', an evaluation project, is that companies who have participated in the culture programmes have had a decrease in sick leave resulting in financial savings amounting from €30,000 to €130,000 during the project year, depending on the size of the company. Although these projects have not been designed as randomized controlled trials they seem to point at the health promoting potential of cultural activities. In the Airis project (Areblad 2010), the period of cultural activity was preceded by 2 months during which a 'culture producer' (mostly an artist but sometimes a composer or someone with another artistic occupation) had discussions with representatives of different groups of employees and management. During this period the cultural activities in the company were tailored to the particular needs and possibilities of the organization. This is a very important principle for successful introduction of cultural activities in the workplace.

### Older age

A Norwegian study of art communication in mental healthcare was conducted on a geropsychiatric ward at a university hospital. Health professionals used semi-structured art dialogues to communicate with patients via works of art. The findings of the study are based on verbatim quotations regarding the experiences of the health professionals in communicating with their patients. Two main categories were identified: the physical domain and the caring domain. Dialogues about figurative as well as non-figurative art forms were found to stimulate and evoke memories; for some patients, these dialogues were an essential step in promoting wellbeing as well as more-being. The dialogues were essential because they provided a key to the patients' inner worlds through associations with artworks. The main conclusion was that both figurative and non-figurative art can open doors to a dialogue with a patient (Ingeberg et al. 2012).

The approach of Ingeberg et al. (2012) was based on an earlier study in which health professionals had dialogues about visual art with patients (Wikström 2003). 'Talking about pictures' was a project for the care of people with dementia. A summary with instructions has been produced in a collaboration between the Fearnley Museum of Art in Oslo and the Museum of Modern Art in Stockholm, using the art collections in the two museums (Kaplan Collections 2013). A booklet was produced within the framework of this programme for use with framed reproductions of objects in the collections. It presents proposals for questions and topics for dialogues based upon the pieces of art. These can be used for support and inspiration when the caring staff discuss the pictures with the patients.

In the 1990s, Wikström et al. (1993) had carried out a randomized controlled trial intervention study concerning the effects of visual stimulation provided in the form of pictures. Pictures for the intervention group were selected based on individual taste and methods in scientific research in art psychology on aesthetic reactions to and perception of art. The paintings were selected because they represented different aesthetic preferences and emotions which may arise in an untrained spectator who is not familiar with academic artistic codes and interpretations of artworks. Two paintings were selected to suit the spectator's taste and the remaining six had an increasing degree of difficulty. The choice of pictures was based on the knowledge that patterns are assumed to be interesting when they contain information that cannot be absorbed immediately but is likely to be absorbed relatively quickly through perceptual and intellectual efforts. Complexity, ambiguity, and variability are associated with high uncertainty and it is important that the levels of information content and uncertainty in a painting are neither to high nor too low, i.e. they should be in balance with the onlooker's ability to perceive a painting.

The study found a significant improvement in the positive mood parameters, happiness, peacefulness, satisfaction, and calmness, and the negative parameters low-spirited, unhappiness, and sadness. Systolic blood pressure decreased and improvement was seen in subjects' medical health status with regard to reported dizziness, fatigue, pain, and the use of laxatives.

The Structure Funds of the European Union financed a health promotion project exploring the effects of visual arts in the work environment. This project was built upon widely recognized high-quality artworks, each of which represented a personal theme with high artistic integrity. The task was to present such a piece of art in a particular room during a specified time period in a number of workplaces. Among other things, indoor architecture, motifs, stimulation, and colour effects were studied and observations were made regarding effects on creativity and when the pieces of art were observed. One of the results from the observations was that pieces of art were often of importance during telephone conversations (Sandström and Wikström 2008).

## Conclusion

With support from commissions from national governments in Sweden and Norway, many regional and municipal projects have started in the field of arts and health in both countries. They comprise the elderly, people of working age, and children as well as all forms of art: visual arts, music, dance, theatre, and writing. Some scientific evaluations have been performed but most of the evaluations have been administrative. The field is rapidly gaining popularity and attention.

# References

Areblad, P. (2010). Creating a sustainable basis for cooperation between workplaces and the cultural sector: case TILLT in Västra Götaland. In: *Creative Economy and Culture in the Innovation Policy*, pp. 55–61. Helsinki: Ministry of Education, Finland.

Bittman, B.B., Snyder, C., Bruhn, K.T., et al. (2004). Recreational music-making: an integrative group intervention for reducing burn-out and improving mood states in first year associate degree nursing students: insights and economic impact. *International Journal of Nurse Education Scholarship*, 1, art. 12.

Bittman, B.B., Berk, L., Shannon, M., et al. (2005). Recreational music-making modulates the human stress response: a preliminary individualized gene expression strategy. *Medical Science Monitor*, 11, BR31–BR40.

Bjursell, G. and Westerhäll, L. (eds) (2008). *Kulturen och Hälsan*. Stockholm: Santérus Förlag.

Bratt-Rawden, K.B. and Tellnes, G. (2011). The benefits of nature and culture activities on health, environment and wellbeing: a presentation of three evaluation studies among persons with chronic illness and sickness absence in Norway. In: H. Nordby, R. Rønning, and G. Tellnes (eds), *Social Aspects of Illness, Disease and Sickness Absence*, pp. 199–222. Oslo: Oslo Academic Press.

Bygren, L.O., Weissglas, G., Wikström, B.M., et al. (2009). Cultural participation and health: a randomized controlled trial among medical care staff. *Psychosomatic Medicine*, 7, 469–473.

Clift, S., Hancox, G., Morrison, I., Hess, B., Kreutz, G., and Stewart, D. (2010). Choral singing and psychological wellbeing: quantitative and qualitative findings from English choirs in a cross-national survey. *Journal of Applied Arts and Health*, 1, 19–34.

Cohen, G. (2009). New theories and research findings on the positive influence of music and art on health with ageing. *Arts & Health: An International Journal for Research, Policy and Practice*, 1, 48–62.

Cuypers, K.F., Knudtsen, M.S., Sandgren, M., Krokstad, S., Wikström, B.M., and Theorell, T. (2011). Cultural activities and public health: research in Norway and Sweden. An overview. *Arts & Health: An International Journal for Research, Policy and Practice*, 3, 6–26.

Cuypers, K., Krokstad, S., Lingaas Holmen, T., Skjei Knudtsen, M., Bygren, L.O., and Holmen, J. (2012). Patterns of receptive and creative cultural activities and their association with perceived health, anxiety, depression and satisfaction with life among adults: the HUNT study, Norway. *Journal of Epidemiology and Community Health*, 66, 698–703.

De Quadros, A. and Dortewitz, P. (2011). Community, communication, social change: music in dispossessed Indian communities. *International Journal of Community Music*, 4, 59–70.

Duberg, A., Möller, M., and Taube, J. (2013). Dans kan ge unga skydd mot psykisk ohälsa. *Läkartidningen*, 110, 1539–1541.

Elstad, J.I. (1985). Helseulikheter mellom sosiale klasser. *Tidsskrift for Samfunnsforskning*, 26, 29–51.

Gold, C., Mössler, K., Grocke, D., et al. (2013). Individual music therapy for mental health care clients with low therapy motivation: multicentre randomised controlled trial. *Psychotherapy and Psychosomatics*, 82, 319–331.

Göteborgs-Posten (2013). Trummor gör skolan lugnare [Drums calm the school down]. *Göteborgs-Posten*, 29 September 2013.

Hjorth, P.F. (1994). Om samsykdommene. I: Helse for alle! Foredrag og artikler. *Utredningsrapport*, nr. U1-1994, pp. 75–85. Oslo: Statens Institutt for Folkehelse.

Krokstad, S., Langhammer, A., Hveem, K., et al. (2012) Cohort profile: the HUNT Study, Norway. *International Journal of Epidemiology*, 42, 968–977.

Hammarlund, I. (1993). Musikterapiutbildningen vid Musikhögskolan i Stockholm: Från enstaka kurs till musikterapiutbildning [From single courses to formal music therapist training]. In: *Musikterapi [Music Therapy]*. Stockholm: Svenska Förbundet för Musikterapi [Swedish Society for Music Therapy].

Hartzell, M. and Theorell, T. (2007) KROKUS http://lvn.se/upload/regional%20utveckling/kultur/krokus/rapport-krokus%20feb%2007.pdf),

Kaplan, F. (2000). *Art, Science and Art Therapy: Repainting the Picture*. London: Jessica Kingsley.

Kulturdepartementet [Norwegian Ministry of Culture] (1992). St. meld. nr. 61 (1991–1992). *Kultur i Tiden*, pp. 41–49. See: <http://www.folk2.no/>

Lorentzen, B., Wikström, B-M., and Jonanger, P. (2012). Volunteer participation in a Norwegian municipality; cultural and health determinants for participation. In: G. Tellnes (ed.), *Nature-Culture-Health 25-Years*. Oslo: Oslo University.

Pálsdóttir, A.M. Grahn, P., and Persson, D. (2014). Changes in experienced value of everyday occupations after nature-based vocational rehabilitation. *Scandinavian Journal of Occupational Therapy*, 21, 58–68.

Paulander, A.-S. (2011). Meningen med att gå i musikterapi? [Why does it make sense to go through music therapy?] Doctoral thesis, Musikhögskolan, Stockholm.

Myskja, A. (2012). Integrated music in nursing homes—an approach to dementia care. Doctoral thesis, Bergen University.

Ruud, E. (1997). Music and the quality of life. *Nordic Journal of Music Therapy*, 6, 86–97.

Sandström, S. and Wikström, BM. (2006) Konstinsatsen, en utvecklingsmodell: Konstinsatser i arbetsmiljö. [The art intervention, a model for development: Art interventions at work.] *Slutrapport Konstkrets (Final report)* Norrbottens läns landsting. Diarienummer 113-6395-02 inland, 304-19757-03 kust. <www.konstkretsen.net>.

SOU (2000). Hälsa på lika villkor [Health on equal conditions]. Stockholm: Commission of the Swedish Government.

SOU (2009). 16 Kulturutredningen [Commission on culture]. Stockholm: Commission of the Swedish Government.

Theorell, T., Hartzell, M., and Näslund, S. (2009). A note on designing evaluations of health effects of cultural activities at work. *Arts & Health: An International Journal for Research, Policy and Practice*, 1, 89–92.

Tones, K. and Green, J. (2004). *Health Promotion; Planning and Strategies*. London: Sage.

UNESCO (1996). Report from the International Conference on Culture and Health, Oslo, Sept 1995. Oslo: The Norwegian National Committee of the World Decade for Cultural Development.

Vaag, J., Saksvik, P.Ö., Theorell, T., Skillingstad, T., and Bjerkeset, O. (2012). Sound of wellbeing—choir singing as an intervention to improve wellbeing among employees in two Norwegian county hospitals. *Arts & Health: An International Journal for Research, Policy and Practice*, 5, 93–102.

Wikström, B.M. (2003). Health professionals' experience of paintings as a conversation instrument: a communication strategy at a nursing home in Sweden. *Applied Nursing Research*, 16, 184–188.

Wikström, B.-M., Theorell, T., and Sandström, S. (1993). Medical, health and emotional effects of art stimulation in old age. *Psychotherapy and Psychosomatics*, 60, 195–206.

# CHAPTER 22

# Talking about a revolution: arts, health, and wellbeing on Avenida Brasil

Paul Heritage and Silvia Ramos

## Introduction to arts, health, and wellbeing on Avenida Brasil

Avenida Brasil relentlessly resists Rio de Janeiro's spectacular beauty as its four-lane highway cuts northwards through 27 neighbourhoods of the city's poorest suburbs, each congested metre pushing further from the allure of the iconic beaches of Ipanema and Copacabana. From deep in the heart of Rio's docklands to the extreme outer limits of the city—from Benfica to Caju, from Deodoro to Santa Cruz, from Manguinhos to Irajá, from Guardalup to Coelho Neto—Avenida Brasil is one of Rio de Janeiro's essential arteries. It takes citizens from the heart of the city to its margins, not only to the formal neighbourhoods but to the dozens of unofficial communities—*favelas*—that line the highway's industrial landscape. Avenida Brasil was designed to connect the city with its peripheries, and remains a symbol of the flow as well as the enduring divisions of Rio de Janeiro today. As drivers hustle into chaotic lanes to leave the city centre, they catch a glimpse of Rio's former colonial splendour glistening in the hillside above the Avenida. This is the magnificent neo-Gothic palace that at the turn of the twentieth century was home to Oswaldo Cruz—the Brazilian epidemiologist and public health champion. The same reforming zeal that in 1906 inspired Rio's mayor Pereira Passos to open up the city with a road to connect the centre to the northern suburbs (a highway that eventually became Avenida Brasil), also brought Oswaldo Cruz into the public domain when he became director of public health with responsibility for reducing the frequent and fatal epidemics that devastated the city. The legacy of Passos and Cruz is imprinted in Rio's seemingly eternal quest to refigure and improve itself. This chapter will indicate how present-day cultural organizations emerging from Rio de Janeiro's peripheral territories propose a radical vision of art's role in transforming the health of the city and its citizens with the same passion to reconnect the city with itself.

On 12 September 2013 Rio de Janeiro's current mayor, Eduardo Paes, travelled up Avenida Brasil to inaugurate a new hostel for homeless adolescents who have issues with drug and alcohol dependence. The hostel is situated in the northern suburb of Bonsucesso and is part of the city council's programme known as Projeto Casa Viva/Living House Project. With a capacity for 20 young people aged between 12 and 17 years, the hostel provides health and education services as well as a framework of cultural, sporting, and leisure activities. The initiative by the Municipal Secretariat of Social Development is based on an intersectorial approach that involves medical, social welfare, education, and therapeutic interventions, and is dependent for its execution on a partnership with Viva Rio, one of Rio's leading non-governmental organizations (NGOs). Its collaborative, multi-agency approach is far removed from the authoritarian, invasive tendencies of Passos and Cruz's reforms with their compulsory vaccination and forced rehousing campaigns. In November 1904 Oswaldo Cruz's initiatives brought rioters onto the streets of Rio de Janeiro for the so-called Vaccine Revolt which resulted in over 30 deaths, hundreds of injured, and almost 1000 people taken prisoner (most of them exiled to Acre on the fledgling Brazilian republic's Amazonian border with Bolivia). Public health was a violent business at the beginning of the twentieth century. Over the following 100 years, civic authorities have learnt many lessons about the need for community dialogue in their implementation of measures to ensure 'good' public health, but it is worth noting that in June 2013 Rio's streets once again echoed with the sound of violent protests, in part invoked by a state in conflict with its citizens about how to create and shape a city that can provide health and wellbeing for all. The issues are as potent and zealously fought today as when Passos and Cruz opened up the city to a new century.

When mayor Paes met the young people in their hostel at 43 Cardoso de Moraes Street in Bonsucesso on 12 September 2013, he demonstrated just one way in which the state seeks to intervene in a current epidemiological crisis: the drama of chemical dependence and the accompanying devastation of lives lost to the violence of the gang and gun crime which accompanies illicit drug trafficking. Of course, the city has other responses that are more directly interventionist, especially in the fields of public security and criminal justice, but the publicized visit by the mayor seeks to show the city providing access to services that can reconnect a young person with their family, their community, their society. But what happens when the community itself is not integrated into that society? When the community is characterized as part of the problem that is 'causing' the crisis and seen as 'outside' any possible solution? For many residents of the improvised communities that line the Avenida Brasil as it stretches out from the port that brought their ancestors to the city, their designation as *favelados*—people who live in *favelas*—has characterized them in such a way that they have already been demonized as a threat to the wellbeing of the civic body. This chapter brings voices from arts and cultural organizations which have emerged as a vital force within these communities over the last two decades to offer a new hope of resilience in public health. Our aim in this chapter is to test how far and in what way the 'public health' paradigm resonates within the discourse that these groups use to frame their activities.

Over the last two decades Brazil has radically improved its public health profile. It has significantly reduced infant mortality rates, eradicated or brought about effective control of most infectious and parasitic diseases, and created a public policy to confront the AIDS/HIV epidemic that is considered by many to be one of the most advanced in the world. At the same time, this has been accompanied by the emergence of a problem that interconnects issues of public health, public security, and culture: the extremely high rate of death by violent causes, especially among young people. Every year over 50,000 people are murdered in Brazil, 40,000 die in traffic accidents, and 10,000 commit suicide. Since the 1990s, Brazil has consistently been placed among the top 10 countries with the highest rate of homicide per capita.

### There is an age, colour, and place for death in Brazilian cities

Brazilian murder victims are predominantly young people, in particular young black men who live in the *favelas* and peripheral communities of urban centres. While death by external (non-natural) causes represents 9.9% of deaths in the rest of the Brazilian population, 72.3% of the deaths of young people between 15 and 24 years are the result of external causes. Only 3% of deaths in the rest of population are the result of homicides, whereas they account for almost 40% of the deaths of young people aged between 15 and 24. With 54.8 homicides per 100,000, young people are 273 times more likely to be murdered in Brazil than in the UK or Japan (Waiselfisz 2013).

The total number of homicides in Brazil over the last decade exceeds the violent death rate of many countries at war. Between 2004 and 2007 the number of people killed in the world's 12 major conflicts was 169,574 (Global Burden of Armed Violence 2008), while over the last 4 years 206,005 people were murdered in Brazil. The racial bias of lethal violence is strongly evident, especially amongst victims aged between 15 and 24. Young white men represent 22.8% of the homicide victims and young black men 76.9% (Waiselfisz 2013).

There is no fair or equal distribution of homicides across Rio de Janeiro. At different ends of the Avenida Brasil it is clear that the homicide rates in the poorest neighbourhoods can often be 10 to 20 times the rates in the richest zones. There is an age, colour, and place for death in Brazilian cities, which helps to explain and understand how these deaths are socially perceived. The victims are young and black, living in poor neighbourhoods that are excluded from the centre of the metropolitan region. Some commentators classify the problem of intentional lethal violence in Brazil in terms of a 'public health problem' that is 'epidemic' and 'structural' (Mir 2004; Minayo 2005). Racial activists and other commentators (Soares 2006) characterize the homicides as a form of 'genocide' because of their strong impact on young black men. Others call attention to the 'epidemic of indifference' (Roque 2013), analysing the complacency of successive Brazilian governments and the everyday acceptance of the problem by general society when faced with the unremitting and seemingly inextricable nature of the tragedy.

### The *favelas*

According to the 2010 census undertaken by the Instituto Pereira Passos there are 763 *favelas* on the hillsides and borderlands of Rio de Janeiro, housing an approximate population of 1.4 million people, which represents 22% of the 6.3 million inhabitants of the city. Almost 800 communities have been established outside the official geography of the city, improvised and named by their own inhabitants. To visit Rio's *favelas* is to confront complex, heterogeneous realities. The particular characteristic of each community depends on the city zone in which it is located, the historic moment from which it emerged, the presence or absence of recent urbanization programmes, and the strength or weakness of community organizations. Despite the differences and distinctions that are obscured by the single word *favela*, they all have in common an exceptionally low level of public service delivery.

Rio's *favelas* have for over a century formed an influential a part of the city's mythology as well as its reality. For the first half of the twentieth century the hillside communities were often celebrated as a source of the poetry and musicality of the city, idealized for the dignity of a harmonious life. The unsustainability of such myths became increasingly apparent from the 1970s onwards as internal migration from the north-east of Brazil swelled the improvised communities as the country nose-dived into economic decline. The subsequent decades of abandonment allowed a vacuum that from the 1980s onwards has been occupied by organized crime in the form of rival drug gangs and corrupt police *milícias* (groups of armed police—current and former serving officers—who run violent crime operations). While the history of those who live in the *favelas* is marked out by a refusal to accept the ways in which they are characterized by the places they inhabit, the strength of the stigmatization is pervasive.

For almost four decades the heartbeat, pulse, respiration, physical articulation, and sanity of Rio de Janeiro has been measured by its collective capacity to heal the wounds of its own civil conflict. The scars and fissures on the body politic of the city are profoundly evident in social statistical data but also in the degraded imaginary of the city. In the face of the social exclusion and extreme poverty of so many of those who live there, it has become increasingly difficult to maintain the cultural myths that were for so long built into the supposed dialogue and transit between the *favela* and the official fabric of the city through popular music, performance, literature, and iconography. This chapter traces a different route in approaching the arts organizations that have emerged from within these communities in the last 20 years as agents of transformation with a diagnosis of hope.

## First person plural

In 2009 Rio de Janeiro created a new form of community policing that by 2013 had been implemented in 33 strategically significant *favelas*. The Pacification Police Units—known in Brazil as the Unidades de Polícia Pacificadora (UPPs)—have been officially credited with disarming the drug gangs within those 33 communities. As a consequence of this perceived disarmament, the state has established a permanent, local police presence in each of the 'pacified' communities. The relative success of this experience is measured by the state in the reduction of homicide rates (often to zero) and the near elimination of the daily shoot-outs between drug traffickers and police or between drug traffickers of rival gangs. Unfortunately, at the time of writing the social programmes are not keeping pace with the public security advances which may in time put the pacification process at risk.

Throughout these last decades of lethal tension that has fatally enmeshed Brazilian cities, a distinctive cultural phenomenon emerged which offered an alternative to the seemingly pre-destined narrative of violence that threatened the survival of young people in *favelas*. Rio de Janeiro began to be aware of arts organizations made up of young *favelados* that remained focused on cultural activity within these territories. Many of these groups arose as a specific response to the violence, the stigma of the young black man, and the exclusion and abandonment of their communities from the fabric of the city. In a context where youth culture and youth movements had previously been the exclusive terrain of university students who fought against the military dictatorship in Brazil (1964–85) it was the first time in which groups of young people from the *favelas* spoke in the first person. These were not philanthropic NGOs led by intellectuals to 'help' young people. There was no longer someone else at the microphone telling the media, civic society, and governments that young poor people from the *favelas* are the major victims of violence rather than the criminals. Young black *favelados* were now producing their own ideas, sounds, images, and visions of Brazil. These new organizations constructed a model for young people in which the shame of being black and living in a poor neighbourhood was substituted by a eulogy of Afro-Brazilian culture and a pride in belonging to a certain community. They express their vision through diverse aesthetic languages such as music, theatre, dance, circus, and cinema, producing the ideas and perspectives of young people from the *favelas* through an intensive use of the body and its emotions. The alternative images these young people are producing challenge the stereotypes of criminality and failure associated with their social class, race, and location. Some of them speak openly about their commitment to construct alternative lives outside of the paradigms of criminality with its strong material and symbolic attractions. Other groups refuse to situate their energies in what they see as a false and imposed dilemma of 'crime versus art', preferring instead to talk about the production of artistic excellence as the basis by which they break stereotypes and stigmas. By whatever means, and for whatever purpose, all these initiatives seek to 'act' not only in their own local communities but also in other contexts, seeking visibility as much for social and political impact as for the seduction of commercial success. All of them speak of art; all of them speak of citizenship.

Two decades since their emergence, the collective experiences of young people from peripheral communities constitute a field that continues to produce a new national agenda about and for Brazil. They appear daily in the media, are the intermediaries of government, lecture at universities, are employed as consultants to business, and advise social organizations. They represent probably the most vibrant and innovative part of modern Brazilian culture.

These fiercely independent groups, collectives, and actions share a combined cultural and artistic DNA in the material and symbolic production of a means to increase participatory citizenship and reduce inequality. They regard themselves and other young people from their own communities as potent and not dependent, needing only the means, methodologies, and technologies to turn ideas into projects and thus transform their territories.

Walkway 23 crosses Avenida Brasil as it reaches the far end of Rio's northern suburbs on an accentuated curve before the highway doubles back west along the outer limits of the city's frontiers. The concrete bridge with its green metal structures takes pedestrians back and forth across eight lanes of sometimes hurtling, often snarled-up, traffic. Here, in the communities of Parada de Lucas and Vigário Geral, Grupo Cultural AfroReggae run two of their five cultural centres based in *favelas* across Rio de Janeiro.

## Grupo Cultural AfroReggae

*Salve a arte que nos salva* [Long live the art that enables us to live]
from AfroReggae's mission statement.

AfroReggae leads over 70 arts projects in communities across Rio de Janeiro in partnership with municipal and state governments, produces its own national cable television programmes, broadcasts digital radio, advises businesses looking to develop social programmes from its office in the main financial district area of São Paulo, generates significant income from its own commercial artistic activity, and sells hard-edged sponsorship deals to national and multinational brands. Its annual turnover is in excess of £10 million. AfroReggae currently has nine professional bands that play a range of music from samba to reggae to *baião*, as well as a circus group whose members have graduated to the Cirque du Soleil and a range of professional dance and theatre groups. The main band—which also bears the name AfroReggae—has played the Carnegie Hall, opened the Rolling Stones concert on Copacabana Beach, given a series of critically acclaimed performances on the main stage of the Barbican Centre in London, and toured to India, China, France, and Germany.

The origins of the formation of AfroReggae will forever be associated with the execution by the police of 21 inhabitants of the *favela* of Vigário Geral on 29 August 1993. The site where the massacre took place is just a 15-minute walk from AfroReggae's cultural centre in Parada de Lucas, but it is a journey that is only possible because of what AfroReggae has achieved over two decades. Vigário Geral is a neighbouring *favela*, accessed by a 200-m passageway that separates the two communities. For almost 30 years, the two communities were caught in a lethal combat that resulted from their 'occupation' by two rival drug factions. The path between them became known as the Gaza Strip and was controlled at either end by heavily armed gang members. Although children from both communities attended the school that stands in the common ground between them, this no-man's-land was deserted as night fell when even a dog that appeared beneath the shot-out street lights would be fired on by both sides. Nothing moved for over 25 years until AfroReggae opened up cultural centres in both communities. The process by which the pathway itself was eventually opened involves many symbolic and real moments of failure and success, but by August 2013, residents could pass safely from Parada de Lucas to Vigário Geral because the art that AfroReggae invokes in their mission statement is the art that saves lives (Fig. 22.1).

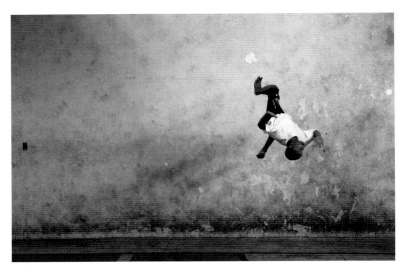

**Fig. 22.1** Participant in a project with young people in a juvenile detention centre led by AfroReggae and People's Palace Projects (Rio de Janeiro, 2010). Reproduced by kind permission of Ratão Diniz. Copyright © 2015 Ratão Diniz.

The preservation of life and the reduction of risk have been at the heart of AfroReggae's enterprise for the last 20 years. The success of AfroReggae in preventing young people from entering the drug factions and in providing alternative lives for gang members who want to leave is widely talked about in the Brazilian and international media. AfroReggae's teams are important mediators in the ongoing tensions between the communities and the different armed forces that variously dominate, occupy, and secure their territories. But behind the headline stories that are more commonly told (see Yudice 2003; Heritage 2009; Jovchelovitch 2012), there are everyday instances of how AfroReggae's work impacts on the behaviour and attitudes of those who participate in their programmes and projects. Here AfroReggae's joint artistic directors Roberto Pacheco (Beto) and Johayne Hildenfoso (Jô) explore together the multiple ways in which they are building bridges between the creative arts and the health and wellbeing of the young people with whom they work:

Beto: From the beginning we have worked with the bodies of young people, so there's no way of escaping questions of health and wellbeing. But in the *favela*, I've learned that the work I do is like the body itself: it has its own aesthetic, its own way of exercising which I have to define and adapt. The 'body' in the *favela* tends to be undernourished . . .

Jô: . . . not only eating what it shouldn't but sometimes having nothing to eat at all. We push those bodies to the limits with high-energy rehearsals knowing that at times they are extremely badly fed, often simply because they don't know good eating habits. So we adapt to address these habits and they adapt, and that's how all our work develops.

Beto: Do we bring change to their bodies? One small but important difference is that they've started to wear shoes. In the *favela* the youngest children spend a lot of time barefoot, and even into adolescence they'll favour flip-flops for everyday footwear. At any time here you can be stepping on rat and dog shit and a whole lot else besides. Any small cut will get infected. So for all our classes, workshops and performances we always get them to put something on their feet. Art education together with health education.

Jô: Health and aesthetics is what our work is about. I can remember right at the beginning when we first started, no-one arrived for the drumming or theatre workshops having freshened up with their teeth cleaned. When you're performing together in close proximity, talking directly at someone, embracing them—you've got to be smelling good at the start even if you are sweating as you do it. I've sent whole groups home to shower, scrub, and change. I can remember when I had to sit a group down to cut their nails together one by one. And it is always the public performances that change things the most. Always the same speech the day before: 'Tomorrow we've got people coming to see you perform here, you've got to look good ok? No flip-flops, best clean clothes, come looking beautiful'.

Beto: For some of them as they develop into more mature performers with the groups this will mean some radical lifestyle changes as they think about their bodies and what they will need to do to care for them.

Jô: It's about personal responsibility: 'I am an artist, I am part of a group; I have to look after myself because I am going to be on stage.'

Beto: We used to have more rules. For many years we had a 'no alcohol' rule at any time, even for those old enough to drink. Walk down these streets and you will see men and women—their brothers, fathers, sisters, mothers, cousins—sat at improvised bars in the streets with a beer or *cachaça* in their hand the whole day long. AfroReggae asks for a behaviour that runs counter to the culture of the *favela*. Even though the absolute ban on all alcohol drinking has been lifted we still push them to take personal responsibility. And there is still a zero tolerance policy of drugs inside or outside of the company.

Jô: Absolutely explicit. You can't use drugs and be part of AfroReggae. But we don't just throw people out because we find out they've been smoking a spliff with friends on a Saturday night.

Beto: We talk, make sure he knows it has to stop and we keep talking. AfroReggae has its own social welfare team, employing monitors to work with the young people in all of our cultural centres. Health and wellbeing issues are part of their daily interaction with the young people.

Jô: Talks on AIDS, SDT, pregnancy, drugs, etc. It's part of our routine activities alongside the workshops on theatre, dance, percussion, guitar, singing, circus, DJ, violin . . .

Beto: And we can see the changes. Adolescent pregnancies used to be the norm in Vigário Geral *and* in AfroReggae. But now a difference has opened up and you can see those young women who are not with AfroReggae have another sort of behaviour. They are at the mercy of the drug traffickers and anything that is likely to do them harm: they drink, smoke, and get pregnant. They are the same age as our young women but with a series of health problems in addition to becoming pregnant. The young women who are with AfroReggae are trying to look after themselves.

Jô: And that's why we are so demanding, because otherwise we would have lost so many of them.

Beto: But we've also changed. It used to be that when someone got pregnant they had to leave the group. Now we find ways for the groups themselves to support young women who become pregnant to stay part of AfroReggae, because getting pregnant for these young women is so caught up in their lives in the *favela*. If she gets pregnant, her life is transformed. Sometimes it seems that having a child is the limit of her horizon. If she has a partner, she'll stay with him until he leaves and then her mother and grandmother step in and so she gets fixed in her place.

Jô: But we've also got beautiful examples of young people from different AfroReggae groups who have kids together, live together, look after them really well, get them into school.

Beto: That's the transformation that we've worked hard to achieve.

Jô: A young woman who works for us in an administrative or artistic team, is likely to be the only person with a regular income in her family. So she's pregnant and her mother, her father, and the father of the child are all unemployed. AfroReggae is securing that family with one minimum salary and all the social, psychological support we can give to that young woman.

Beto: AfroReggae provokes them. It provokes us. We are not satisfied with simple transformations.

Jô: To sustain all these activities in the *favela* is in itself revolutionary. I don't know how to say it any differently. The mission of AfroReggae is not just to take young people away from an idle, unhealthy life in the *favela* that puts him or her at risk of involvement in the drug trade.

Beto: It is to not to stop them smoking, drinking, getting pregnant too young—although we hope that will be a consequence. It is for them to become better citizens, take a critical attitude: to be a revolutionary in society, in the city. We know that it is not enough to 'take them out' of where they are. The world that those young people meet outside their *favela* is full of lions and we are responsible for helping them to survive out there. We have to continue provoking them as they provoke us.

Jô: AfroReggae operates at its best when it convinces a young person that to come from a *favela*—to be black and beautiful—is a good thing and has its own energy. They learn that they have a force that comes through playing their drum or their violin that will in turn create a new image of other young people from the *favela* for the rest of the city. That's the revolution. Before there was either the bad guy from the *favela* who was a drug trafficker or the well-behaved, good-looking *favelado* who assimilated the looks and behaviour of the non-*favela* kid. AfroReggae produced a new character who didn't exist before. He wears the *favela* clothes and hair-style but plays drums or makes theatre. She is not afraid and tells the truth about the city.

Beto: AfroReggae produces a new player in the city who redefines and recuperates the potential force of the *favela* . . .

Jô: And this is reproduced in every moment of our work. You need that attitude in a drum rehearsal, to understand why a lecture on AIDS is important for you and how you're going to project that revolution through your dance performance. It's in every little piece of us.

Beto: The strength we have is that we pay attention.

Jô: Life stories. Histories. Trajectories. Telling our stories to each other. That's how we care for each other. AfroReggae is a way of looking after each other.

The essential characteristic of AfroReggae as identified by Pacheco and Hildefonso, is borrowed from the idea of community within the *favela* itself. In the absence of an effective state welfare system, the improvised communities that grew up in the aftermath of the abolition of slavery needed to create affective communities of care. This perspective remains at the very least a forceful part of the *favela*'s cultural mythology, if not a real part of the social infrastructures by which residents survive. Although AfroReggae is unique in its scale and ambition, its mission and achievements are reflected in a myriad of community-based organizations across Rio's peripheries that activate the care and attention that residents can give to each other through arts practices. The preservation of certain social spaces and the protection of those who live there are bound up in shared cultural traditions that bond individuals as residents of particular communities *before* they are citizens of the wider city. Such communities have historically been haunted by the impermanence of their lives through the irregularity of building constructions, lack of civic infrastructure, precarious healthcare and sanitation, and the weakness of the public security apparatus. In such contexts, the arts have taken on a role that belies their marginalization as entertainment and goes far beyond their commercialization as a product. A belief in the arts as a potential act of resistance to whatever threatens the health and wellbeing of individuals and their communities can be traced across the city in projects, programmes, and organizations as diverse and complex as Brazilian cultural identity itself.

The health indicators identified by Pacheco and Hildefonso stretch from the smallest, most intimate gestures to life-saving actions played out in contexts of extreme violence and risk. The promotion of wellbeing is imagined as part of the DNA of AfroReggae, delivered as much by its mission, methodology, and social organization as in the deliberate content of specific programmes to address particular health issues. While there are cognitive processes being stimulated by AfroReggae as it seeks to encourage young people to change habits and behaviours that are deemed unhealthy, their intervention might be more appropriately seen as a form of artistic vaccination. One hundred years after Oswaldo Cruz vaccinated Rio de Janeiro against yellow fever and bubonic plague, AfroReggae has developed its own unique form of protecting communities from the life-threatening conditions that decimate and degrade them. It understands, as the pioneers of public health knew at the beginning of the twentieth century, that defence and protection is more effective than the attempt to 'cure' and that improving the health of individuals is intrinsically linked to reforming the city itself.

## Crescer e Viver: to grow and to live

'The wellbeing of young people—every aspect of how their emotional and physical health is defined and preserved—has been at the centre of our mission since the beginning.' Junior Perim stakes out a bold vision for his circus company Crescer e Viver. Combining art and social transformation under the big top of its circus tent, the organization is located back at the other end of the Avenida Brasil in the centre of Rio de Janeiro. Crescer e Viver's programmes include training, production, and promotion of all aspects of modern circus, and it is considered to be in the vanguard of the renovation of circus aesthetics in Brazil (Fig. 22.2). Junior Perim explains the aims of Crescer e Viver:

'Crescer e Viver is a circus that was born in carnival. In 2000 the Samba School Porto da Pedra chose the 10th anniversary of the Federal Statute of the Child and Adolescent as the theme for their annual carnival parade. I convinced the Samba School to also begin a social project for poor children from local communities that ran for 3 years before a group of us set up a separate, independent NGO. We hold on to the ideal of the Statute of the Child and Adolescent through all our programmes, activities, and interventions. Our overall objective is the emotional development of the young person as a subject. We are not just concerned with the young person's physical development, because if she doesn't have an emotional balance then the young person is not fully healthy and fit. This is fundamental in our work because if you are not able to handle your own emotions they you won't have the equilibrium to achieve the principal aesthetic of the circus language: risk.'

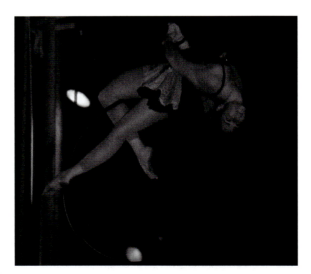

**Fig. 22.2** Participant in a circus project led by Crescer e Viver (Rio de Janeiro, 2013).

'Everything in the circus relates to risk. You give yourself to that risk, showing the ordinary person that you too are ordinary but capable of doing extraordinary things. Without equilibrium you can't submit yourself to risk because you would put your own wellbeing at risk. To help the young person towards that state of necessary balance, we work on body/space and body/object relationships. Above all, we work on the infinite possibilities of the meeting of bodies in the same space with the same collective objective. Nothing can be done in the circus without cooperation between everyone. Even the trapeze artist who flies alone has to trust that someone else will be there to hold the apparatus. You have to learn to trust the other person in the circus ring.'

'I am interested in how what we do is different from the football coach. When we hang a young person upside down by his feet, we turn his world upside down. We open up the symbolic possibility and say: 'Pay attention: you can see the world differently, so now you can begin to create.' The circus is a rich environment in which to produce symbols, to provoke new subjectivities. The young person's body needs this space for subjectivity. At the same time, ideological reflection has to have materiality. It is expressed in a gesture, in a discourse, in a pamphlet, in the materiality of thought. But like the football coach, we have to provide the means by which that physical body is trained and sustained.'

'At a basic level in order to practice, the young person needs calories. She has to eat. Because we work with some of the poorest children from different communities, we take on the responsibility of feeding them while they are with us. We serve about 100 full meals per day, working with a nutritionist that creates a menu dedicated to young people practising physical activities. In addition to the main meal at lunchtime, we also provide snacks between sessions and soup at the end of the afternoon. For many of the children this might be their only food for the day. In addition to the nutritionist and the cooks, we also employ a pedagogic coordinator, a social worker, and a psychologist.'

'Every block of physical training in the curriculum is accompanied by discussions of transverse themes. We deal directly with health issues such as STIs, AIDS, adolescent pregnancies, drugs, alcohol, sexual and racial assault, tuberculosis, domestic violence, etc. The young people themselves usually chose the particular theme they want to cover during that period based on things that are real for them in their lives. The theme is incorporated into the physical circus training, generating meaning and symbols that relate to the discussions before being brought into the public domain through performance.'

'Crescer e Viver has a policy of working in an integrated way with the families of the young people so that we can address as effectively as possible the issues that are going to affect the young person's capacity to benefit most from our activities. On the social circus programme—specifically aimed at young people in situations of risk as defined by government social welfare programmes—we meet the family every 15 days. It's about family support; it's about education; it's about health in the most basic way. One of the most important reasons we want to mark a presence in the home is because of the casual domestic violence that is so much a part of these young people's lives. The mother knocks about the son, the father hits a brother-in-law who beats up his wife, and as far as possible we intervene. Across the years we've seen how our work improves internal family relationships, supporting families to deal with the sort of conflicts that are common in any social nucleus. That intervention in turn makes it possible for the young person to achieve their goals at the circus. Our process is about using circus training as a pedagogic tool to develop social skills, to mobilize a socio-cultural territory that can help these young people structure their own lives, in their own contexts.'

'We are not here to cleanse, discipline, or strengthen young people's bodies. Our aim is to empower young people as subjects in their own lives. There is a philanthropic, hygienist, and deeply prejudiced discourse about the poor that supposes that it is important to occupy them because idleness leads to vice. It is important for us at Crescer e Viver that the young person is always seen as subject-author. The training processes focus on the development of the capacity to author action. They learn within an intensely didactic environment with clear pedagogic methodologies, but our institutional aim is in the training of creative and critical subjects. Our objective is to develop an environment where each of them can develop their own subjectivity with the necessary critical faculties to perceive and interpret the world. As technique, we teach circus skills. As methodology, we open up a continuous process by which young people acquire knowledge and an ongoing desire to relate to new ideas, people, and things. They have to understand the limits that have been put on them if they are to discover how to construct a new subjectivity within a city that now no longer needs to begin and end for them in the same way as when they were born.'

'In order to achieve this aim, it is important that the young person is not just a 'pupil' learning circus skills but is active in every part of the cultural chain of production that makes circus happen. Our organization is built around the social circus project, and many of the young people who began with us at the age of 11 are still with us in that company 10 years later. But we also have a 3-year artistic training programme for those aged 18+. Some of those who have been on the social circus programme will 'graduate' to undertake the formal 3-year training; others will stay working with the social circus. All of them can become part of the professional company for touring circus productions, whether in the cast, technical crew, or production office. Every 2 years we produce the Americas' biggest international circus festival, which in 2014 was hosted across 30 *favelas* producing the kind of transit, circulation, and affective flux that Rio needs to invent a different generation of citizens, who will experiment with the city, swallow it up, absorb it into themselves and re-create Rio as a more human place in which people are effectively and affectively mobile. This means much more than the classic notion of building better public transport systems, but requires that dynamic subjects feel they belong to the city and are empowered to cross from one end of Avenida Brasil to the other. Crescer e Viver provokes young people to find themselves and each other through new transitions and encounters with other social, artistic and political subjects across the city.'

## Conclusions

Flapping on the walls of every arts and community organization that lines the 60 polluted kilometres of Avenida Brasil, there will be a poster about health and wellbeing. Help-lines will be advertised, healthy behaviours promoted, bad behaviours discouraged. Alerts and warnings, encouragements, and incentives are the over-familiar background for the drumming sessions, theatre groups, dance performances, and graffiti workshops. Just as in so many places around the world, the arts are looked to in Brazil as a means of 'effective delivery' of positive health messages and an opportunity for challenging behaviours that have a negative impact on wellbeing. However degraded the environments in which these activities take place, or extreme the contexts in which the young people are living, there are organizations across the city of Rio de Janeiro working on a daily basis to improve the quality and even the chance of life through art.

We asked the directors of just two of those organizations, AfroReggae and Crescer e Viver, to consider the ways in which their own work can be considered within the frame of health and wellbeing. Rather than analysing a wide sample of answers through a survey we were interested in the detail of their responses and were rewarded with testimonies that narrate the transformation on young people's bodies within a trajectory that imagines new citizens, new subjects, new players in the city of Rio de Janeiro. Both AfroReggae and Crescer e Viver fuse the actual wellbeing of the individual with the physical, social, and symbolic 'health' of the city. The artists have joined forces with the epidemiologists and urban planners. A hundred years after Pereira Passos ripped open the streets and Oswaldo Cruz stirred up revolt with his vaccines, the artists from AfroReggae, Crescer e Viver, and so many other groups like them, are the ones who are talking about a revolution.

## References

Global Burden of Armed Violence (2008). *Global Burden of Armed Violence 2008*. Available at: <http://www.genevadeclaration.org/measurability/global-burden-of-armed-violence/global-burden-of-armed-violence-2008.html> (accessed 11 January 2014).

Heritage, P. (2009). *Intense Dreams: Reflections on Brazilian Culture and Performance*. Queen Mary University of London: People's Palace Projects.

Jovchelovitch, S. (2012). *Underground Sociabilities*. Research report. Available at: <http://www.psych.lse.ac.uk/undergroundsociabilities/index.php>

Minayo, M. (2005). Violência: um velho-novo desafio para a atenção à Saúde. *Revista Brasileira de Educação Médica*, **29**, 55–63.

Mir, L. (2004). *Guerra Civil, Estado e Trauma*. São Paulo: Geração Editorial.

Roque, A. (2013). *Epidemia da Indiferença*. Anistia Internacional Brasil. Available at: <https://anistia.org.br/noticias/epidemia-de-indiferenca/>

Soares, L.E. (2006). Segurança pública: presente e futuro. *Estudos Avançados*, **20**, 91–106.

Waiselfisz, J.J. (2013). *Mapa Violência 2013: Homicídios e Juventude no Brasil*. Rio de Janeiro: CEBELA e FLACSO.

Yúdice, G. (2003). *The Expediency of Culture: Uses of Culture in the Global Era*. Durham, NC: Duke University Press.

# CHAPTER 23

# Case study: 'I once was lost but now am found'— music and embodied arts in two American prisons

André de Quadros

## Introduction to music and embodied arts in two American prisons

Every Tuesday for the best part of 3 years from 2012 to 2014, around 20 men from different parts of a Boston prison came together at the appointed time for a 3-hour music session. In similar fashion, every Wednesday a slightly smaller group of women gathered in a Boston women's prison for such an activity. Both of these prison programmes exist under the umbrella of Boston University's Prison Education Program, one of the few programmes worldwide that offers a university degree to incarcerated men and women. I teach in both prisons along with my colleagues Jamie Hillman and Emily Howe.

This chapter describes the music activity in this programme in both prisons, drawing attention to the personal transformations that have taken place and framing these as a consequence of the artistic and pedagogical processes. As evidence of the impact of the programme on the prisoners, I put forward their writings and commentary for review by readers. Using portraiture as a research approach (Lawrence-Lightfoot 2005; Lawrence-Lightfoot and Hoffman Davis 1997), I seek to illuminate the experiences of the incarcerated men and women within the context of a specific pedagogy, based on Boal's (2006) *The Aesthetics of the Oppressed*. Portraiture is

'fundamentally premised on an inductive rather than deductive orientation to research. The purpose of portraiture is not to test previously established theories or hypotheses. Rather, like most qualitative methodologies, the purpose is to explore participants' experiences and the complexities of how meanings are produced within a particular context.'

Gaztambide-Fernandez et al. (2011, p. 4)

Indeed, the arts, particularly in more restrictive contexts, may be easier to represent in arts-focused methodologies (Conquergood 2006; Knowles and Cole 2008).

Although the rights and privileges of incarcerated people to education and the arts are less defined than their right to healthcare, and legislation exists in several countries including in the United States to diminish certain rights such as the right to liberty and suffrage, one can argue, nonetheless, that the health not only of the imprisoned but also of those with whom they interact is greatly enhanced by access to musical participation. As an example, the newly discovered musical passion of one of the incarcerated men has led him to encourage his young son to take up a musical instrument. Another man with a Baltic background, sentenced unconstitutionally as a teenager to life without parole, has found that Baltic music can be a conversation topic with his mother when she visits him.

A holistic concept of health is in keeping with the Alma Ata Declaration (UNICEF 1978) and the preamble to the WHO Constitution in its assertion that 'health, which is a state of complete physical, mental and social wellbeing, and not merely the absence of disease or infirmity, is a fundamental human right' (UNICEF 1978, p. 1) Enough has been written and argued about music and other cultural forms as being central, indeed essential, to wellbeing. Thus, if this centrality makes it a right, then the Alma Ata Declaration prepares the ground for a discussion of whether those in prison can claim access to music as a right rather than as life-enhancement, or as therapy, or as rehabilitation. That music is not valued in prisons, by and large, reinforces the routine exclusion of several basic needs for certain populations—the sick, the poor, the elderly, those with dementia, the mentally ill, and the imprisoned. Even if one could argue that the imprisoned cannot claim music as a right, in view of their diminished rights, one can scarcely argue the same for other sectors of the population. Music, apparently, is an instrument of social exclusion.

The Ottawa Charter for Health Promotion (WHO 1986) goes even further than the Alma Ata Declaration in advocating for education, social justice, and equity, among others, as basic prerequisites for health. The charter defines health as a 'resource for life, not the object of living' (WHO 1986). In this context, quality of life and social equity outcomes, rather than health outcomes, should be the ultimate goal of health promotion (Potvin and McQueen 2008). The Alma Ata Declaration and the Ottawa Charter invite a conceptualization of how the arts, specifically music, might work as a resource for life and essential for health and wellbeing. Incarcerated people can find rich life resources in music (Cohen 2007); my fieldwork in and with prisons, prison music leaders, and ex-convicts in Argentina, Australia, Germany, South Africa, Sweden, and Thailand, and my undertakings first in a Thai prison and now in the Massachusetts prisons seem to demonstrate this.

With the large number of incarcerated men, women, and young people, America ranks at the top of countries for the population, per capita, of those under some kind of supervision in the criminal justice system (Pattillo et al. 2004). With 5% of the world's population, America has 25% of the world's prisoners, and this population by number and proportion shows all signs of increasing, particularly as it applies to African Americans and the poor (Loury 2008; Alexander 2010; Reiman and Leighton 2010; Drucker 2011). Between the years 1980 and 2008, the prison population increased from 500,000 to over 2.3 million. In the same time period, the female prison population increased more than six-fold (Talvi 2007).

If we are to achieve the health of a nation by constituting the health of individual citizens, the health of the millions of incarcerated people needs attention, as this will affect the health of all. The case for music with these neglected populations is indeed very strong for the reasons contained in this chapter and elsewhere in this book.

## Pedagogy, rehabilitation, therapy?

Several colleagues have labelled our work as either 'pedagogy', or 'rehabilitation', or 'therapy'. Readers can come to their own conclusions on this question, but the purpose of this chapter is to demonstrate that the musical activity and interdisciplinary arts work have led to substantial transformations in the lives of the individual members and the groups as a whole, while acknowledging a kinship with all three of these labels and many of the paradigms that belong within them.

It is not for lack of facilities or time that we have chosen to situate our work in a number of participatory paradigms, most particularly the work of Boal (2006), who writes in his seminal *Aesthetics of the Oppressed*, 'All I ask is: let us sing with our own voice, even if it is hoarse, let us dance with our own body, even if it is doddery; let us speak our own speech, even if we are uncertain' (Boal 2006, p. 61). There are no auditions to enter these groups, making this quotation from Boal's work particularly meaningful; participants are encouraged to find security, identity, and comfort in the sound of their own voices even when these voices are clearly weak or tuneless. My colleagues and I have developed an artistic process in contrast with many prison music programmes in that it combines song with bodywork and various kinds of improvised work in other art forms.

To the prisoners, I emphasize that our cave ancestors obtained a survival advantage by being able to communicate through art, through metaphor; they used communal art to bond together, and they used music in ritual, in everyday life, to inspire, to console, and to transmit information (Levitin 2006, 2008). That we are genetically hardwired to make art, not to consume it, compels us to rediscover this aspect of our humanity. It is within this argument that the pedagogy is situated.

For most of the prisoners, men and women, their voices have been dormant and undiscovered, for they are all creatures and victims of the commodification of art and the musical product. In many cases, due to their educational disadvantage and poverty, they have had a limited background in music education. They have become habituated to listening to music on the radio, to consuming theatre on television, and are losing or have lost the ability, if they ever had it, to make art as part of everyday life, to sing, to dance, to write, to paint, to carve, to tell stories, to build narrative. Therefore, our approach seeks to empower them to make art. Essential to this process is to find voice through singing. Our teaching seeks to unlock these latent capacities, and indeed this is the essential aspect of providing opportunities for self-discovery.

Referring back to Boal's quotation, our pedagogy seeks to displace existing notions of beauty that have frequently been created by the digitization and professionalization of art. The only music that the prisoners usually hear is made by professionals, and professionally produced. In our sessions, we follow Boal's principles, '*by discovering their art and, in the act, discovering themselves*; to discover the world, *by discovering their world and, in the act, discovering themselves*, instead of receiving information from the media, TV, radio' (italics in the original; Boal 2006, p. 39).

We could have gone into the prison and taught them the masterworks, we could have got them to sit behind desks and learn to appreciate music, using standard works of music and following the kind of curriculum that many people use in the teaching of non-music students. Or, we could have just opted for active music making as in a choral programme, lining the prisoners up and teaching them songs, teaching them to read music. All these activities would have led to incontestable triumphs. We chose, however, to engage them in participatory music of dialogue, the art-making of dialogue rather than the art-making of monologue. Rather than following instructions in a patriarchal fashion, our work is circular and consensual, engaging people in dialogue through mutual creativity, such as improvising song conversations.

Our brand of participation is particularly anti-authoritarian. Following instructions unquestioningly is an essential aspect of being in prison. Authoritarian music is consistent with the prison ethos. We took an alternative route, one of collaboration and consensus. By working in circles and acknowledging that each one has a story and a unique expressive dimension, we are displacing conventional authority. In our work, we seek to harmonize the mind with the heart, the emotion, and the body, to work in an embodied fashion, to allow the body to express the music. We are encouraging participants to show sensitivity and affirmation in a legitimate manner in our sessions, and surprisingly, through the musical activity, a group spirit has developed that is generally warm, caring, and loving.

The process is designed to generate mutual respect, to show tenderness, and to experience vulnerability. This vulnerability is experienced by legitimizing many of the behaviours that are taboo. As volunteers in the prison, we were advised that eye contact, particularly prolonged eye contact, is likely to send a message of a certain kind. So, what we did was to make a point of it; we asked the men to sing facing each other in pairs and to gaze into each other's eyes. Physical contact does not typically happen between men unless as a violent or sexual act, so we make a point of legitimizing physical contact by holding hands as we sing. Our prison participants have learned that taking risks is essential, but not the risks that they may have been used to; they should take the risks of singing out loud, the risks of touching, the risks of telling themselves in song and art.

A typical session with the men and the women includes starting in a circle, holding hands, and singing and moving together. This opening circle activity instantly creates an egalitarian, inclusive, communal quality, which is preserved throughout the session, which proceeds apace with bodywork, stretching, centring, mindful breathing, and consciousness work, vocalizing, poetry, and imagery. Jamie Hillman, Emily Howe, and I have called this process the 'empowering song approach', an approach rooted in improvised song, poetry, bodywork, movement, and imagery for personal and communal transformation.

## 'I once was lost but now am found' as a theme

In January 2012, my colleagues Hillman and Howe and I settled on a theme that would guide the teaching, that would anchor the song material, and would provide an avenue for the poetry and the visual art. So, it was with this in mind that, in January 2013, we started the 4-month term with a theme taken from a single line of the folk hymn *Amazing Grace*, 'I once was lost, but now am found'. In the sessions, we encouraged participants to write their own poems, to sing their own texts, and to represent their songs visually. In response to this theme, one of the men wrote this poem:

> When I was lost, no one cared to find me.
> When I was in need, no one gave to me.
> When I was poor, no one provided for me.
> When I was sad, no one offered me a shoulder to lean on.
> When I became angry, no one could stop me.
> When I committed my crime, I felt ashamed.
> When I entered prison, time slowly went by.
> When I pursued education, I was given a chance.
> When I began to study, I was inspired.
> When I finally passed the Boston University entry test, I was joyous.
> When I began to take my courses, I was challenged.

> When I graduate, I'll always remember to keep my feet on the ground.
> Because, 'I once was lost, but now am found'

At the end of the term, each participant was asked to produce short group performance pieces and visual artwork. Visual art in these prisons is extremely difficult, given that there is no access to paints and paintbrushes. Prisoners frequently resort to creating makeshift paintbrushes from their own hair, and making paint by dissolving M&M's (American button-shaped candies). On one occasion, we invited a street artist, Sidewalk Sam, to work with us; in a single session, the women created a group mural (see Fig. 23.1).

At the end of the programme, the men and women wrote anonymously with universally positive responses. A selection of these responses follows.

> Inclusion. Normalcy. Freedom.

> This class gives me two hours of peace and joy. It's an escape from the stress and loudness that fills these prison walls.

> This class connects me to the human aspect of myself, giving me the tools needed to face others who perceive me as less human (those outside of this prison).

> This music class has been and continues to bring joy to my life. I laugh every day, every minute, every moment!!

There were several remarkable pivotal moments in these sessions, even when every session was marked with intensity. D is a young Latino man who sat relatively quietly for a whole term. He was unobtrusive and unremarkable in his participation. Then, one day, when we divided the men into small groups to create short improvised performance pieces, D rapped out this poem in the middle of his group's performance. We were all speechless when he finished. Here was that quiet, almost morose young man performing this dramatic poetic text with such intensity. He sat down in silence and then he said, 'That's the first time in my life that people shut up and listened to me'. Here is that touching poem

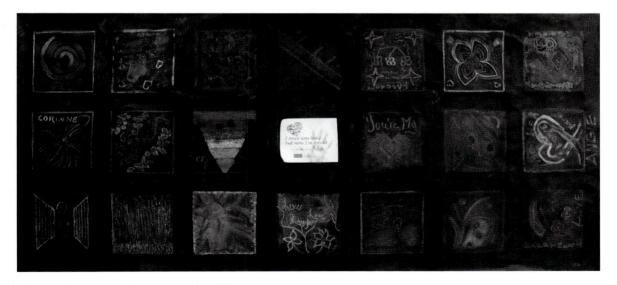

**Fig. 23.1** Mural created at the Framingham women's prison, 2013.

with its compelling rawness and authenticity and with the original spellings and punctuation preserved:

My Adolences
How can one stare deeply into my eyes
and don't see innocence, my adolescence,
taken away from me in hand-cuffs
because of one misstep in my misguided life.

Misread, Misjudged, and Misunderstood
by the blinded, but never nearly once
in my adolescence had anyone listened
or let me explained my misbehavior to an adult
in order to comprehend an adolescence's mind
as to 'why' a child could commit a crime.

Because of one mistake, I'm mislead
and misrepresented by dominions
playing the double standards of the law,
which my family, my future, and my faith
are fading away slowly like dark clouds
covering the sunny sky, and my smiles
turn into frowns, frightening,
and fighting off a dark shadow that isn't mine

Listen to my own tears
pouring and pounding off the concrete floor,
Ripping my heart out for attention
in order for anyone to hear my cries
beyond these barb wires, white walls,
screaming for someone to help
save my adolescence behind these cell doors.

I'm just a child misplaced
in a machine without mercy
and I'm missing my mother warmth
who nurtured me to become
somebody for the future of today's society, yet
my adolescence gone.

Linking these sessions to social inclusion, I requested participants to discuss our work relative to other musical experiences and to their own personal experiences. An abridged version of one of the most striking comments follows:

'Music can be inclusive when it brings people together . . . Yet it can be just as exclusive under lesser intention . . . Music can instil and bring out various emotions . . . for good or for evil . . . Recently in class, I was caught unaware of how deeply I could be caught feeling excluded, yet desiring to be included . . . This experience has opened another inner child wound that has laid dormant and under the surface for many years. All in need of healing . . . I love music, it has become my bridge to the world. A child given up at birth, sexually abused from the age of 6 to 8, dealing with many abandonment and trust issues, fighting to survive and keep the music within alive . . . a wounded child of 52.'

## A closing comment

The public health problems represented by incarceration are both complex and of extreme concern. Regrettably, incarceration is insufficiently evaluated and assessed; major health issues in prisons are frequently disregarded. To point to only one such example, the official statistics show rape of incarcerated men is on a massive, largely undiscussed scale (Beck and Harrison 2006). With these concerns in mind, we need to harness a broad range of society's resources to create non-violent arts-based programmes in prison, not only for the prisoners but also for the people inside and outside the prison with whom they interact while incarcerated and after they are freed. Indeed, in both of the prisons, the participants commented that their involvement in music had tempered their extreme feelings and that they had found ways to understand their past, to come to terms with their current situations, and to face the future with greater optimism and hope.

## References

Alexander, M. (2010). *The New Jim Crow: Mass Incarceration in the Age of Colorblindness*. New York: New Press.

Beck, A.J. and Harrison, P.M. (2006). *Sexual Violence Reported by Correctional Authorities, 2005*. Washington, DC: US Department of Justice, Office of Justice Programs. Available at: <http://purl.access.gpo.gov/gpo/lps80380>.

Boal, A. (2006). *The Aesthetics of the Oppressed* (transl. A. Jackson). New York: Routledge.

Cohen, M.L. (2007). Christopher Small's concept of musicking: toward a theory of choral singing pedagogy in prison contexts. PhD dissertation, University of Kansas.

Conquergood, D. (2006). Rethinking ethnography: towards a critical cultural politics. In: D. Soyini Madison and J. Hamera (eds), *The Sage Handbook of Performance Studies*, pp. 351–366. Thousand Oaks, CA: Sage.

Drucker, E.M. (2011). *A Plague of Prisons: The Epidemiology of Mass Incarceration in America*. New York: New Press.

Gaztambide-Fernandez, R., Cairns, K., Kawashima, Y.L., Menna, L., and VanderDussen, E. (2011). Portraiture as pedagogy: learning research through the exploration of context and methodology. *International Journal of Education and the Arts*, **12**(4).

Knowles, J.G., and Cole, A.L. (eds) (2008). *Handbook of the Arts in Qualitative Research: Perspectives, Methodologies, Examples, and Issues*. Los Angeles: Sage.

Lawrence-Lightfoot, S. (2005). Reflections on portraiture: a dialogue between art and science. *Qualitative Inquiry*, **11**(1), 3–15.

Lawrence-Lightfoot, S. and Hoffman Davis, J. (1997). *The Art and Science of Portraiture*. San Francisco, CA: Jossey-Bass.

Levitin, D.J. (2006). *This is Your Brain on Music: The Science of a Human Obsession*. New York: Dutton.

Levitin, D.J. (2008). *The World in Six Songs: How the Musical Brain Created Human Nature*. New York: Dutton.

Loury, G.C. (2008). *Race, Incarceration, and American Values*. Cambridge, MA: MIT Press.

Pattillo, M.E., Weiman, D.F., and Western B. (2004). *Imprisoning America: the Social Effects of Mass Incarceration*. New York: Russell Sage Foundation.

Potvin, L. and McQueen, D.V. (eds) (2008). *Health Promotion Evaluation Practices in the Americas: Values and Research*. New York: Springer.

Reiman, J.H. and Leighton, P. (2010). *The Rich Get Richer and the Poor Get Prison: A Reader*. Boston, MA: Allyn & Bacon.

Talvi, S. (2007). *Women Behind Bars: The Crisis of Women in the U.S. Prison System*. Emeryville, CA: Seal Press.

UNICEF (1978). *Declaration of Alma Ata*. International Conference on Primary Health Care, Alma-Ata, USSR, 6–12 September 1978. Geneva: World Health Organization. Available at: <http://www.who.int/publications/almaata_declaration_en.pdf>

WHO (1986). *Ottawa Charter for Health Promotion, 1986*. Geneva: World Health Organization. Available at: <http://www.who.int/healthpromotion/conferences/previous/ottawa/en/>

WHO (1946). Preamble to the Constitution of the World Health Organization as adopted by the International Health Conference, New York, 19–22 June, 1946; signed on 22 July 1946 by the representatives of 61 States (*Official Records of the World Health Organization*, no. 2, p. 100) and entered into force on 7 April 1948.

# CHAPTER 24

# Case study: lost—or found?—in translation. The globalization of Venezuela's El Sistema

Andrea Creech, Patricia A. González-Moreno, Lisa Lorenzino, and Grace Waitman

## Introduction to El Sistema in a global setting

During the last few decades El Sistema, Venezuela's national system of youth orchestras and choirs, and Sistema-inspired programmes around the world, have captured the public imagination as well as that of music educators and social policy-makers. El Sistema uses music education as a vehicle for fostering positive changes in health and wellbeing. Access to high-quality and intensive music education, it is thought, cultivates an 'affluence of spirit' that brings enhanced wellbeing to children, their families, and their wider communities (Chang 2007).

The positive outcomes of this global movement (now reaching at least 59 countries), in terms of personal and social wellbeing as well as musical excellence, have been documented through a growing body of formal evaluation and research (Creech et al. 2013). Sistema programmes are founded on holistic principles of cooperative education characterized by trust, support for self-esteem, empathy, team work, commitment, structure, and discipline. Sistema teachers aim to support each child's holistic development, including musical, cognitive, social, and creative domains.

## Background to El Sistema

El Sistema's founder and inspirational leader is Dr José Antonio Abreu, a distinguished economist and musician. Abreu's vision has been to 'solve Venezuela's long-standing poverty issues by blending his expertise in music and social reform' (Mauskapf 2012, p. 202). The initial El Sistema orchestra comprised a group of young professional musicians who played alongside younger music students and acted as teachers and mentors for the aspiring musicians. This principle of peer mentoring and modelling has remained as a core feature of El Sistema (Hollinger 2006). During the early years, Abreu collaborated closely with Juan Martínez, who, in the same year that El Sistema began (1975), founded the Orquesta Sinfónica Infantil de Carora, comprising 103 children aged 8–16 (Carlson 2013). Martínez was deeply influenced by the Chilean music educator and visionary Jorge Peña Hen, whose ideals may be interpreted as antecedents of the El Sistema movement.

Peña Hen had been devoted to inclusive practice in music, had emphasized the powerful potential of learning through ensemble for promoting a strong sense of community, and highlighted the role of music in helping children to overcome disadvantage (Carlson 2008). These ideals, translated into a pedagogy that includes daily contact, learning collectively from the start, and teaching with love, underpinned the development of the Sistema movement.

## El Sistema principles and practices

Sistema programmes regard orchestras and choirs as structures through which social change can be fostered at the level of the individual child, family, and community. Key tenets are inclusivity and accessibility, immersion in music, daily participation in ensembles, strong internal unity as well as outward-facing community connections, holistic development, and lifelong learning (Govias 2011; Marcus 2012).

The 'ensemble' is central; intensive ensemble activities are seen as a rich opportunity for nurturing positive social and individual wellbeing, including citizenship skills, 'respect, equality, sharing, cohesion, team work, and, above all, the enhancement of listening as a major constituent of understanding and cooperation' (Majno 2012, p. 58). Alongside the intensity and frequency of contact, consistency is another key feature (Uy 2012). Programmes offer a constant, dependable social and musical experience, regardless of what may be happening outside of the núcleo (music centre).

The concept of interdependence is key to understanding the positive outcomes that have been noted in connection with El Sistema (Billaux 2011). Interdependence fosters solidarity, responsibility, and self-esteem, in turn supporting social skills, sensitivity, leadership, and cooperative learning and shared goals amongst the children.

The programme at its most successful involves optimal challenge and collaborative learning. Marcus (2009) adds that 'at least part of the reason [for the success of El Sistema] is the unique "high" that upwards of 100 players on a stage get from playing great music together'. Frequent performances create safe opportunities

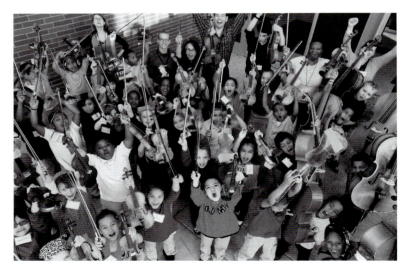

**Fig. 24.1** Group photo—BRAVO Youth Orchestras launched an intensive, El Sistema-inspired music programme at Rosa Parks School, Portland, OR, in 2013. The programme serves nearly 200 students at Portland poorest and most culturally diverse school (95% living in poverty, 18 languages spoken).
Reproduced by kind permission from Kimberly Warner/BRAVO Youth Orchestras. Copyright © 2015 Kimberly Warner/BRAVO Youth Orchestras.

for risk-taking, thus allowing children to acquire many cumulative experiences of success, thereby building self-efficacy and self-esteem, raising aspirations, and fostering aesthetic sensibility (Uy 2012).

The pedagogy within the Sistema ensemble context is structured, focused, and disciplined, the theory being that 'social change comes through the pursuit of musical excellence, with the discipline it demands and the emotional bonds it creates through mutual struggle and celebration' (Govias 2011, p. 22). It is through a deep, positive engagement with music and a shared pursuit of musical excellence that participants in El Sistema develop qualities as responsible, productive citizens (Booth 2011). Through what Booth (2013, p. 3) describes as the 'porous membrane' of the núcleo, the ethos and solidarity that characterize the learning community spreads to the wider community.

Yet, alongside this unified vision, an underpinning facet of El Sistema and its derivatives elsewhere is openness to 'improvisation' with regards to the day to day interpretation of the overarching principles. Govias (2011, p. 23) suggests that this quality may be a sixth key tenet of El Sistema, claiming that the 'genius' of the organization lies in its unfailing commitment to 'identifying and assimilating new best practices' (Fig. 24.1).

## A theoretical framework for understanding how El Sistema might support community health and wellbeing

One framework that helps to understand the link between the Sistema movement and community health and wellbeing is the idea of 'health music(k)ing', developed by Bonde (2011). Bonde (2011, p. 122) outlines four overarching health-related goals that can be supported by music making: (1) the development of communities and values; (2) the shaping and sharing of musical environments; (3) helping individuals; and (4) the formation and development of identity.

The model of 'health music(k)ing' comprises a vertical axis labelled 'mind–body', intersecting with a horizontal axis labelled 'individual–social' (Bonde 2011). Within the mind–social quadrant of the model, music may be seen to provide health affordances that relate to shared emotional, relational, correctional, or affirmative outcomes experienced through making music within a social space. This may link with peer learning and group identity that have been noted in Sistema contexts. The body–social quadrant is concerned with the embodied, yet social, nature of music making. For example, this may refer to the shared 'high' of making (and listening) to music, highlighted by Marcus (2009). The third quadrant, bringing together the individual–body elements of Bonde's model, may be concerned with relaxation, regulation of emotional or physical pain, motor skills, mobility, dexterity, and general fitness. Finally, the individual–mind quadrant refers to the link between music making and cognitive processes (Fig. 24.2).

### El Sistema's link with community health and wellbeing

A review of research and evaluation concerning Sistema programmes worldwide (Creech et al. 2013) revealed widespread reports of positive personal development amongst programme participants. Amongst 85 research and evaluation papers, relating to 44 Sistema programmes around the world, wellbeing and personal development were conceptualized in broad terms, with at least 32 different constructs mentioned (e.g. Esqueda Torres 2004; Uy 2010; Gen 2011; Lewis et al. 2011; Burns and Bewick 2012; Galarce et al. 2012).

### Personal development, health, and wellbeing

Positive benefits such as self-esteem, self-worth, self-confidence, pride, motivation, commitment, social responsibility, positive behaviour, optimism, happiness, and pleasure have consistently been reported by Sistema students, parents, and programme coordinators. These positive benefits have been attributed to musical participation and achievement within a safe and structured environment.

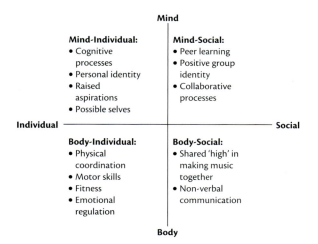

**Fig. 24.2** Health music(k)ing within Sistema contexts.

A specific example where enhanced personal development amongst children in the early years has been linked with a Sistema programme is offered by In Harmony England (Lewis et al. 2011). In England, a key indicator of a 'good level of development' in personal and social education and communication, language, and literacy is a score of 78 points (representing a score of six or more points on each of several assessment scales). At the time of implementation of the In Harmony (Lambeth) programme in 2009 the percentage of Foundation Stage (age 4–5) children in the two core schools achieving 78 points was 29% and 27%, compared with 52% nationally. In 2010 this had increased to 43% and 62%, respectively, compared with 56% nationally. These improvements were consistent within the cohorts, with improvements noted amongst children from the most disadvantaged homes as well as others who were better off. While the improvement may have been in part attributable to cohort effects or to generally rising standards of teaching, headteachers noted that In Harmony played a

contributory role in raising levels of concentration, attention, cooperation skills, pride, and self-esteem amongst Foundation Stage children.

Uy (2010) carried out a cross-cultural comparison of El Sistema in Venezuela and the United States. Participation in El Sistema programmes was found to have had a major positive impact with regard to enhanced academic aspirations amongst the students. Uy illustrated this point with the example of the núcleo of Chacao in El Sistema, where 100% of the students were enrolled in high school, university, or conservatoire, with 40% of these studying music and the others pursuing careers in engineering, medicine, and other subjects. Within the context of underprivileged communities, this, according to Uy (2010, p. 28) was 'astounding'.

Four key factors have been identified that are said to underpin the Venezuelan programme's positive influence on personal development and wellbeing (Chang 2007). First, the núcleos (local or regional music centres) offer a safe environment. Secondly, the programme is characterized by a network of close interpersonal bonds amongst the pupils and teachers. Thirdly, it offers the children a medium through which to acquire cultural capital, and finally the activities themselves are structured in such a way as to nurture self-esteem, taking place within a supportive sphere of activity in which the students can develop skills and take pride in their achievements. Additional explanatory factors include solidarity in pursuing goals, mutual respect of capacity, and cultivation, recognition, and rewarding of excellence (Majno 2013) (Fig. 24.3).

## Community wellbeing

Several studies have explored a potential link between El Sistema and community wellbeing. For example, Venezuelan communities with the highest number of núcleos per capita reported lower school dropout and crime rates (Guevara 2006), and participation in El Sistema reportedly resulted in a significant and positive impact on employment (Sanjuán 2007). Cuesta (2008) reported that for every dollar invested in El Sistema there was a saving of 36 cents compared with an alternative of

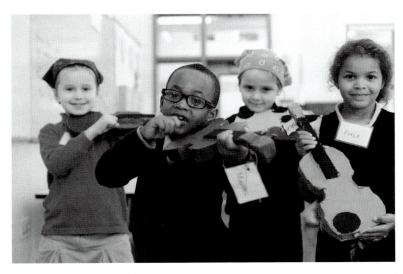

**Fig. 24.3** Paper violins—BRAVO students started the year by building and painting papier mâché violins with help from their families. They used these practice instruments for the first week of the programme before graduating to real violins, violas, and cellos.

additional tuition within public education. Personal narratives have demonstrated how El Sistema has offered an alternative to crime (Ceretti and Cornelli 2013), enabling participants to escape both material and spiritual misery. These findings point to the need for further research that investigates the costs and benefits for community wellbeing.

Outside Venezuela, the extent to which Sistema-inspired programmes have impacted positively on the wellbeing of the communities they serve has been investigated. Some encouraging trends have emerged. For example, when surveyed, 88% of the parents/caregivers of children in Big Noise, Scotland indicated that Big Noise had fostered positive changes in the way that people living in the area thought about their community (GEN 2011). In England between 2008 and 2011 overall rates of anti-social behaviour, domestic burglary, and drug offences decreased in West Everton (where an In Harmony project was located) compared with an overall rise in these crimes within a neighbouring area that did not offer an El Sistema programme (Burns and Berwick 2012).

## The 'transferability' of El Sistema

The question of whether El Sistema can be transplanted to cultural contexts outside Venezuela with similar effect has been discussed extensively. According to Abreu himself, 'a translation to the specificities of each context' is required (Majno 2012, p. 58).

The imperative for a programme of social action through music is perhaps particularly clear within the Venezuelan context where, for example, poverty levels are 'double those in the United States' (Hulting-Cohen 2012, p. 44). In Venezuela, intensive commitment on the part of the young people may represent a very direct and well-understood pathway out of disadvantaged or dangerous environments (Uy 2010)—a pathway that may be neither certain nor salient in all contexts. This may be a significant issue for any attempts to adopt or adapt the approach outside of the Venezuelan context.

Another major challenge is funding. Within the Venezuelan context dependence upon state support has been an 'operational condition from the start' (Majno 2012, p. 59). Sistema-inspired programmes elsewhere have had to develop alternative models that involve partnership working, for example with symphony orchestras, community arts organizations, higher education institutions, conservatoires, social service agencies, and charitable foundations. From an organizational perspective, this may mean that Sistema-inspired programmes have the scope to be driven truly from the grassroots and to be responsive to local community needs, although sustaining a 'unified vision' amongst the wider Sistema network may be problematic.

A further challenge relates to musical genre and context, ensuring that these are relevant and representative of local cultures. For example, a competing discourse identified in relation to Big Noise, Scotland and summarized as 'Venezuela and Scotland' (Allan 2010) focused on the extent to which western classical music needed to be balanced with a recognition and responsiveness to the very rich cultural context of traditional Scottish music.

The notion that the orchestra per se can be conceptualized as an idealized community where positive wellbeing is fostered permeates much discourse on El Sistema (Tunstall 2012). However, the view has also been put forward that the symphony orchestra is not the only musical medium for bringing about personal and social development (Allan 2010). Borchert (2012, p. 59) suggests that the symphony orchestra is 'symbolically representative of the ideals of discipline and productivity'. He cautions that 'discipline' does not necessarily align with 'social inclusion', and that to reduce the complexity of social exclusion to lack of discipline is over-simplistic.

A further challenge of transferability relates to pedagogy. Particularly in programmes that target deeply disadvantaged children, teachers require a wide set of skills in order to nurture the musical, personal, social, cognitive, and creative development of their students. Where Sistema teachers work in partnership with

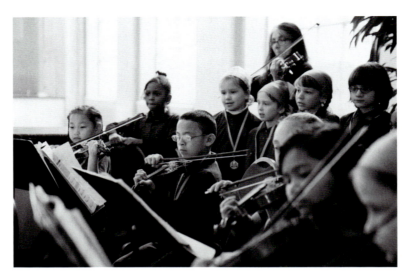

**Fig. 24.4** Performance—BRAVO Rosa Parks String Orchestra and Chorus performed a short programme at the Arlene Schnitzer Concert Hall, home of the Oregon Symphony, less than 3 months after starting music lessons. Regular performance and participation in community events is an important component of the programme.

school classroom teachers, it is important that these are strong partnerships, with shared understandings and practices with regard to behaviour management strategies and wider pedagogical approaches such as differentiation. Thus, a pedagogy that supports links between music-making and wellbeing involves much more than musical expertise, and may, for example, be informed by the field of social pedagogy, which is concerned with holistic education and care (Kyriacou et al. 2009).

Furthermore, although learning through the ensemble is a core principle of El Sistema, the pedagogy that underpins the positive peer learning and teaching noted in El Sistema Venezuela has not yet been clearly articulated or thoroughly investigated within Sistema-inspired contexts. It has been acknowledged that peer learning and teaching may be most effective when students are supported with guidance on strategies and approaches to listening, encouraging and explaining, as well as building trust and respecting boundaries (Kutnick et al. 2008). Given the emphasis on peer learning and its role in supporting personal development within Sistema-inspired programmes, this is an area of teacher development that deserves attention, and where El Sistema and Sistema-inspired programmes may have much to offer the wider music education community.

Notwithstanding these challenges, we have noted that some evidence indicates that El Sistema has been adopted widely and adapted successfully, with consistent reports of positive implications for personal and community wellbeing. Arguably, the power of musical participation is most salient within those contexts that are optimally flexible in approach and responsive to the communities that they serve (Fig. 24.4).

## Summary

There can be little doubt that El Sistema is a remarkable phenomenon, with significant implications for 'arts and health' interventions and programmes. In particular, it may be said that El Sistema offers a powerful model for music programmes with community health and wellbeing aims. Interpreted within the framework proposed by Bonde (2011), El Sistema programmes may support individual wellbeing through intensive musical activities that are holistic, involving cognitive processes, identity, emotional regulation, as well as physical response. Community wellbeing, on the other hand, is supported within the programme through shared joyful musical experiences. Within the wider community, wellbeing is fostered through family engagement and community pride in being a home to valued social spaces for music making. There are encouraging signs that in the longer term communities may benefit from the raised aspirations and positive social values that are nurtured within Sistema programmes.

# References

Allan, J. (2010). Arts and the inclusive imagination: Socially engaged arts practices and Sistema Scotland. *Journal of Social Inclusion*, **1**, 111–122.

Billaux, N. (2011). New directions for classical music in Venezuela. Masters Thesis, Hochschule für Musik, Freiburg.

Bonde, L.O. (2011). Health music(k)ing—music therapy or music and health? A model, eight empirical examples and some personal reflections. *Music and Arts in Action*, **3**, 120–140.

Booth, E. (2011). El Sistema's open secrets. *Teaching Artist Journal*, **9**, 16–25.

Booth, E. (2013). Fundamental elements of Venezuela's El Sistema which inform and guide El Sistema-inspired programs. Unpublished. Available at: <http://www.laphil.com/sites/default/files/media/pdfs/shared/education/yola/el_sis_fundamentals_jan_2013.pdf>

Borchert, G. (2012). El Sistema: a subjectivity of time discipline. In: E. Araujo and E. Duque (eds), *Os Tempos Sociais e o Mundo Contemporaneo: Um Debate Para as Ciencias Socias e Humanas*, pp. 59–79. Universidade do Minho: Centro de Estudos de Comunicacao e Sociedade/Centro de Investigacao em Ciencias Sociais.

Burns, S. and Bewick, P. (2012). *In Harmony Liverpool—Interim Report: Year Three*. Liverpool: In Harmony Liverpool.

Carlson, A. (2008). Inundating the country with music: Jorge Peña Hen, music education and democracy in Chile. Honors Thesis, Department of History, Weinberg College of Arts and Sciences, Northwestern University, Evanston, IL.

Carlson, A. (2013). The story of Carora: the origins of El Sistema. Unpublished manuscript, University of Colorado.

Ceretti, A. and Cornelli, R. (2013). *Cinque Riflessioni su Criminalita, Societa e Politica*. Milan: Feltrinelli.

Chang, J.D. (2007). Orchestrating an affluence of spirit: addressing self-esteem in impoverished Venezuelan children through music education. BA Dissertation, Harvard University.

Creech, A., González-Moreno, P.A., Lorenzino, L., and Waitman, G. (2013). *El Sistema and Sistema-inspired Programmes: A Literature Review*. London: Institute of Education, for Sistema Global. Available at <http://sistemaglobal.org/litreview/>.

Cuesta, J. (2008). Music to my ears: the (many) socioeconomic benefits of music training programmes. *Applied Economics Letters*, **18**, 915–918.

Esqueda Torres, L. (2004). *Ejecución de la Fase 3 del Plan de Seguimiento y Evaluación de Impacto del Sistema Nacional de Orquestas de Venezuela: Informe Final*. Mérida, Venezuela: Centro de Investigaciones Psicológicas—Universidad de Los Andes.

Galarce, E., Berardi, L., and Sanchez, B. (2012). *OASIS, OAS Orchestra Programme for Youth at Risk in the Caribbean—Music for Social Change: Final Report*. Washington, DC: Organization of American States.

GEN (2011). *Evaluation of Big Noise, Sistema Scotland*. Edinburgh: Scottish Government Social Research.

Govias, J. (2011). The five fundamentals of El Sistema. *The Canadian Music Educator*, **Fall**, 21–23.

Guevara, J.C. (2006). Diseño y Estimación de Indicadores para la Relación Costo–beneficio del Sistema Nacional de Orquestas. Indicadores Costo–beneficio BID/SNOJIV. Caracas, Venezuela.

Hollinger, D.M. (2006). Instrument of social reform: a case study of the Venezuelan system of youth orchestras. DMus Arts Thesis, Arizona State University, Tempe.

Hulting-Cohen, J. (2012). Diffusion, adoption and adaptation: El Sistema in the United States. BA Organizational Studies Dissertation, University of Michigan, Ann Arbor.

Kutnick, P., Ota, C., and Berdondini, L. (2008). Improving the effects of group working in classrooms with young school-aged children: facilitating attainment, interaction and classroom activity. *Learning and Instruction*, **18**, 83–95.

Kyriacou, C., Tollisen-Ellingsen, I., Stephens, P., and Sundaram, V. (2009). Social pedagogy and the teacher: England and Norway compared. *Pedagogy, Culture and Society*, **17**, 75–87.

Lewis, K., Demie, F., and Rogers, L. (2011). *In Harmony Lambeth: An Evaluation*. London: Lambeth Children and Young People's Service with the Institute of Education, University of London.

Majno, M. (2012). From the model of El Sistema in Venezuela to current applications. *Annals of the New York Academy of Sciences*, **1252**, 56–64.

Majno, M. (2013). Educazione musicale, integrazione, e apprendimento sociale. In: G. Avanzini, T. Longo, M. Majno, S. Malavasi, and D. Martinelli (eds), *Fiologenesi e Ontogenesi Della Musica*, pp. 131–144. Milan: FrancoAngeli (in collaboration with the G. E. Ghirardi Foundation).

Marcus, M. (2009). From street to stage. *Guardian*, 9 April. Available at: <http://www.theguardian.com/music/2009/apr/04/simon-bolivar-youth-orchestra>

Marcus, M. (2012). Sistema Europe membership and values: an in-progress document describing core values, principles and methodology for Sistema Europe members. 18 July. Available at: <http://marshallmarcus.wordpress.com/sistema-europe-membership-values-principles-and-methodology/>

Mauskapf, M.G. (2012). Enduring crisis, ensuring survival: artistry, economics and the American Symphony Orchestra. PhD Thesis, University of Michigan, Ann Arbor.

Sanjuán, A.M. (2007). *Línea de Base del Programa de Apoyo al Centro de Acción Social por la Música Etapa II: Informe Final (Borrador Preliminar)*. Caracas, Venezuela.

Tunstall, T. (2012). *Changing Lives: Gustavo Dudamel, El Sistema, and the Transformative Power of Music*. New York: Norton.

Uy, M. (2010). Positive behavioral and academic outcomes in students participating in two after school music programs: The Harmony Project and El Sistema. Unpublished manuscript. Berkley's College of Letters and Sciences, University of California.

Uy, M. (2012). Venezuela's national music education programme El Sistema: its interactions with society and its participants' engagement in praxis. *Music and Arts in Action*, **4**, 5–21.

# PART 3

# Creative arts and public health across the life-course

25 **Creativity and promoting wellbeing in children and young people through education** 201
Jonathan Barnes

26 **The value of music for public health** 211
Gunter Kreutz

27 **Addressing the needs of seriously disadvantaged children through the arts: the work of Kids Company** 219
Camila Batmanghelidjh

28 **The power of dance to transform the lives of disadvantaged youth** 227
Pauline Gladstone-Barrett and Victoria Hunter

29 **The arts and older people: a global perspective** 235
Trish Vella-Burrows

30 **Case study: engaging older people in creative thinking—the Active Energy project** 245
Loraine Leeson

31 **Group singing as a public health resource** 251
Stephen Clift, Grenville Hancox, Ian Morrison, Matthew Shipton, Sonia Page, Ann Skingley, and Trish Vella-Burrows

32 **Intergenerational music-making: a vehicle for active ageing for children and older people** 259
Maria Varvarigou, Susan Hallam, Andrea Creech, and Hilary McQueen

# CHAPTER 25

# Creativity and promoting wellbeing in children and young people through education

Jonathan Barnes

## Introduction to creativity and wellbeing in children and young people

Creativity is a fundamental human attribute. The limitless range of contexts in which we can think of, act out, make, or talk through new, imaginative, and valued ideas, marks us out from other creative creatures. Human creativity, both good and evil, shows no signs of diminishing in a globalized and increasingly technological twenty-first century despite the pressures of standardization.

This chapter specifically considers creativity and its relationship to wellbeing in children. Examples will be confined to educational contexts and the arts alone, though creative projects across *all* subjects can have a powerful positive impact upon social and psychological health. The discussion will examine this claim.

## Creativity

Creativity may be defined as: 'Imaginative activity fashioned so as to produce outcomes that are both original and of value' (NACCCE 1999). Creative activities can be mental/intellectual, social, practical, physical, or spiritual. The product may be unintended, such as play, a changed relationship, or different understanding. It might be purposeful, a thing, an idea, or a solution to a problem. The originality and value inherent in creativity can be personal, social, institutional, cultural, or global. Creativity is part of the daily experience of almost all human beings, we can be creative individually or collaboratively (John-Steiner 2006), and enhanced and developed by teaching (Barnes and Scoffham 2007; Robinson 2010).

Two terms, *creative teaching* and *creative learning*, will be used throughout. Creative teaching includes the intention to promote creativity in children as well as imaginative and responsive approaches to pedagogy itself. Creative teachers do not always promote creative learning. Creative learning is characterized by imaginative connection-making and original thinking. It depends on the learner's agreement to employ and extend their inherent creative strengths. It is argued that creative learning deepens thinking and broadens the capacity to relate, enjoy, and find fulfilment (Roberts 2006).

Creativity is humanizing. Awareness of our own creativity and involvement in joint creative activity can feel highly meaningful (Csikszentmihalyi 2002). The case studies in this chapter will show how creative involvement has built individual and collective identity, developed self-acceptance, environmental mastery, positive relations with others, autonomy, and purpose in life—factors commonly understood to generate the sense of personal wellbeing (Ryff 1989). However, *what* we accept in ourselves, or what constitutes 'mastery', 'positive', or 'purpose,' requires the application of values (not just value) to creativity. Creativity can be evilly applied. The sense of wellbeing can be wholly self-centred and be sought at the expense of others. Additionally we know that psychological and social health are unevenly distributed (Marmot 2010), therefore discussions linking creativity with health and wellbeing must first be conscious of a values context.

## Values and wellbeing

Values are central to understanding wellbeing. A value is 'a deeply held belief that acts as a ... fundamental guide to action ... spur[ring] us forward, givi[ng] a sense of direction and defin[ing] a destination' (Booth 2010). Personal and familial health may be one of the few universally agreed values. *Wellbeing* is a more contested concept. For the purposes of this chapter wellbeing has both social and personal aspects and involves:

- the acceptance of a self, sensitive to other's wellbeing
- a sense of environmental control, careful of its sustainability
- generous and respectful social relations
- a feeling of autonomy that does not impinge on the happiness of others, and
- a sense of purpose that is both inclusive and just

Other values underpinning this chapter fall under the heading '*inclusive values*'—a framework of linked values that support inclusive behaviour: for example shared concepts of beauty, compassion, community, equity, joy, participation, respect for diversity, social justice, sustainability and truth (Booth 2012). Across the world such values are often claimed as essential in building successful learning communities and individual happiness (Booth and Ainscow 2011).

## Children's health and wellbeing

Csikszentmihalyi (2002) suggests that the majority of prolonged happy, or 'flow', experiences occur when we are involved in creative or physically engaging activities. Other studies have demonstrated similar connections between wellbeing and creative activity, but most use adult respondents (Fredrickson 2009). Although this book summarizes current knowledge on arts and health, this chapter illustrates the benefits for health and wellbeing of creative teaching and learning in schools. It builds on proposals first outlined in 2008 (Hope et al. 2008) and extended in 2012 (Barnes 2013).

Child health and wellbeing are global issues and a significant focus of United Nations (UN) research, reports, and guidance (e.g. WHO 2012). Hopes for children's security, freedom from exploitation, personal happiness, and other aspects of wellbeing have guided policy since the Convention on the Rights of the Child (CRC) (UN 1989). National governments, non-governmental organizations (NGOs), and the world's press have followed suit, taking the health and wellbeing of the under 21s up the agenda. A worrying story of health inequalities among children has emerged from this focus. Poverty universally, unequally, and negatively affects the health and wellbeing of all young people, and some of the richest nations tolerate high degrees of child poverty and scandalously poor levels of child health and wellbeing (UNICEF 2013).

## Healthy child development

Child development is a complex interaction of environmental, cognitive, motor, social, emotional, and language factors. Piaget's work in the mid twentieth century that focused on a stage theory of development continues to influence western descriptions of healthy development. More recent research and a greater consciousness of the roles of culture and socio-economic status have widened the scope of healthy child development. The Marmot Report from the United Kingdom claims, for instance:

> '... early cognitive ability is strongly associated with later educational success, income and better health. The early years are also important for the development of non-cognitive skills such as application, self-regulation and empathy. These are the emotional and social capabilities that enable children to make and sustain positive relationships and succeed both at school and in later life.'
>
> Marmot (2010, p. 62)

## Culture and development

Culture is 'the behaviours, artefacts and beliefs [that] define social identity . . .' (Riqueime and Rosas 2014, p. 233). Societies contain many cultures recognizable by common attitudes towards child rearing, gender, sexuality, religion, language, eating behaviours and preferences, celebrations, relationships, play, work, education, and creativity. Culture, plus individual life stories and differences in social and physical environments mean that every brain and mind develop differently. New understandings of illness and health increasingly recognize these cultural and environmental variables.

The 'new science of learning' (Claxton and Lucas 2010) casts doubt on some of Piaget's conclusions. Educational neuroscience suggests that learning is an emotionally motivated phenomenon (Damasio and Immordino-Yang 2007), that joy is the optimum condition for learning (Damasio 2003), and that social, sensory, and multimodal learning environments are all involved (Goswami and Bryant 2007). Neuroimaging indicates that brain areas controlling the understanding of consequences and forward planning only become fully matured at the age of 22 or 23 years (Geidd et. al. 1999), though this may vary by culture.

Intelligence is learnable not fixed (Shayer and Adey 2002). Culture, wealth, and the sense of personal control influence learning and progress much more than Piaget imagined. Children may operate at three or four developmental levels simultaneously. Descriptions of 'normal' child development must therefore be a qualified, and conclusions or solutions tentative and partial.

## Assessing development

Many children do not experience good development by any cultural measure. These children may be concentrated in areas of general deprivation, but poor development is not simply a 'developing world' issue—a UK government report estimated that 47% of British children 'do not achieve a good level of development' (Marmot 2010).

## Intellectual health and wellbeing

Learning may depend on emotional engagement but it also involves the conscious mind. Perkins summarized his work on children's learning in the memorable phrase 'Learning is a consequence of thinking' (Perkins 1992, p. 12). Nurturing thinking involves progressively broadening mental connections between self and the environment, emotion and logic, language and feeling, imagination and fact, and the accommodation of diverse mindsets, materials, and people—the very stuff of creativity. Connection-making can, however, be inhibited by social, psychological, and physical barriers and schools are charged with overcoming these. The ethos of the school may therefore be a crucial factor.

Recent work on positivity suggests that dominant mind-sets have powerful effects on individuals. Positive attitudes, constructive, affirmative, and optimistic thoughts, words, and behaviours appear to engender enhanced physical, intellectual, social, and mental capacities, including creativity (Fredrickson 2009). This research has implications for schools. How a child perceives school life is likely to have significant impact on attainment (see Murphy and Weinhardt 2013).

Curricula too can generate intellectual health. Improved thinking involves increased breadth and depth, the opportunity to make new connections, and personal 'buy in' from the learner. When schools apply agreed values, provide stimulating, personally relevant curricula, real opportunities to use and act on imagination, and genuine challenges then intellect thrives (see Wrigley et al. 2011). Such schools are often labelled, 'creative schools' (Jeffrey and Woods 2003).

## Psychological health and wellbeing

A culturally acceptable sense of self influences perceptions of psychological health. Self-consciousness seems to appear between 18 months and 2 years of age when social play usually starts.

Typically children also begin to *pretend* from this age, demonstrating they can hold two realities about themselves simultaneously (Greenfield 2011).

Outward indicators of psychological health are culturally variable. Eye contact, encouraged in some cultures, is avoided in others; submissive behaviour among elders is seen as weakness in some but strength in others. From the age of 2 social/cultural concepts like community, gender/status roles, empathy, jealousy, contempt, or generosity also begin to develop. So too does the sense of the *unique* self as children recognize the originality of their creations. Mature understandings of self in some cultural settings also involve aspects of creative thought: self-criticality, awareness of contradictions, a sense of the absurd, the ability to objectify, see deeper meanings, and symbolize values.

Psychological development shows in increasing self-control and understanding of emotions. Collaborative creative involvement has been shown in western contexts to enhance what has become known as 'emotional intelligence' (Goleman 1996), though other cultures may not interpret creative thinking in the same way (Craft 2005).

## Social health in children

Two-year-olds use language to make things happen. Playing socially, children refer to other people and objects and request them to do or provide things (Bruner 1983). Who to play with, how to make requests, what is and is not appropriate to say or have, become internalized from this age. By 4 years children begin to justify their requests, negotiate, and challenge refusals from others. Children are aware of social rules and how successfully to get their needs addressed. They modify speech, facial expressions, and body language according to the age and status of the other. Between 4 and 7 they learn to take and give turns, develop 'social emotions' like embarrassment, guilt, and shame and listen to other's views or stories. They have their own stories and opinions too (see Westby 2014). Such elements form the raw materials of 'social creativity', the ability to make, mend, develop, and change relationships.

## Speech, language, and communication health in children and young people

Speech and language are socially developed. Progress shows in changes in speech, language, and communication. Children appear ready to understand and collect a useful vocabulary from about 1 year of age when their first word is uttered. Culture influences the development of language: some favour short, direct utterances, some use convoluted sentences to communicate with even very young children, but by the age of 4 the average child has gathered hundreds of words including some for complex emotions. For example, at 4 years 55% of American children can name and recognize basic emotions such as happiness, sadness, fear, and anger when prompted by pictures of facial expressions, by the following year this figure rises to 75%.

By 18 years an English-speaking college student may have accumulated between 10,000 and 17,000 words (Cervatiuc 2008). However, environment affects the collection or use of vocabularies. Various barriers to communication, such as mutism, shyness, stammers, or lack of confidence may develop for personal, social, cultural, physical, or pathological reasons. Increasingly, authorities see children's healthy development as dependent on healthy progress in speech, language, and communication.

## A child's right to healthy development with wellbeing

The descriptions we have given highlight some aspects of the positively developing child. While judgements of poor development must guard against 'cultural imperialism', it is clear that, wherever the child is, good development is adversely affected by poverty, abuse, illness, or a risky lifestyle. Research has shown such barriers are often interrelated, and while poor development can result from an accident of genetic inheritance, there is growing evidence that genetic predispositions can be activated in certain social/environmental conditions (Marmot 2010).

The UN has helped us move closer towards cross-cultural definitions of child wellbeing. The CRC establishes that wellbeing involves having a name, living with and being loved by a family, having an education, a language, play, and security, and being free from bondage (UN 1989). The CRC itemized a universal minimum and these rights have since guided many international conventions and studies on children's wellbeing (e.g. OECD 2009). Subsequent UN conventions and goals imply that *within a sustainable physical and social environment*, children's social and psychological health and wellbeing involves:

- living in an atmosphere of 'happiness, love and understanding' (CRC preamble)

- speech, language, and communication skills, that help get the most out of education

- confidence to express views about and participate in educational and cultural life

- emotional security and self-regulation

- empathy, fairness, and an understanding of the needs and emotions of others so that schools feel good and safe places

- opportunities to discover, value, and develop their own, mental and physical strengths, and abilities

(see United Nations 1989, CRC articles 12,13,14,15, 28, and 29).

## Creative arts education addresses barriers to healthy development

Education ideally widens access to the principles of the CRC, offering a second chance to those whose development is threatened. Despite a worldwide decline in arts provision, the arts continue to be championed in attempts to address wellbeing (Arts Council England 2007; PCAH 2010). The transformative power of the arts is illustrated by the story of Ishmael Beah, an ex-child soldier from Sierra Leone, now a UNICEF advocate. He describes his rehabilitation through the sensitive use of rap and hip-hop music (Beah 2007) in an education centre. Beah argues that music can engender change in others:

'... A lot of young people are more willing to listen to rap artists or musicians ..... hip hop and any musical form that's popular can definitely, if it's done well, be used creatively to talk about social issues.'
African Magazine (2007)

Across the world it is clear that multidisciplinary teams must come together to address such wellbeing issues (e.g. Royal Government of Bhutan 2012). Education authorities commonly recommend that teachers, therapists, and the community should work together to address children's wellbeing. The following case studies involve teachers, health professionals, arts practitioners, and children themselves working together towards intellectual, psychological, and social wellbeing.

## Case study 1: addressing speech language and communication needs through creativity—the Speech Bubbles programme

Good social, intellectual, and mental health rests on healthy communication. A recent Canadian report on child mental health stated:

'Positive mental health outcomes are associated with environments that are supportive, and with good communication with adults and peers in those environments.'

Canada Public Health Agency (2012)

The speech, language, and communication needs (SLCN) of children have become a priority for education authorities around the world. Good communication—the ability to understand others non-verbally and verbally, to make oneself understood, and to understand precise meanings of words—is fundamental to progress in learning. SLCN are a common problem; in London, for example, up to 50% of children face some kind of treatable communication difficulty (I CAN 2006).

Speech difficulties range from stammering and stuttering, through physical and mental processing barriers, to difficulties in word and sentence formation. Language barriers may involve not understanding or speaking the host community language or result from immature, incomplete learning. Reductions in funding for the external agencies that support young children with such problems have seriously declined since 2008 and schools and education authorities have become increasingly interested in low-cost, high-impact programmes that address SLCN.

'Speech Bubbles' is a drama-based programme designed by The London Bubble Theatre Company to support speech, language, and communication in young children displaying significant difficulties. Groups of ten 6- or 7-year-olds with SLCN

**Table 25.1** The Speech Bubbles process in the words of child participants

| Speech Bubbles activity | . . ..In children's words |
|---|---|
| Ten children plus teaching assistant arrive to meet the facilitator | We just come straight in and make a circle |
| Good morning/hello game: everyone walks across the circle and greets another | 'Hello Sadie', I say and she says, 'Hello Ismail' |
| Chanting values: with hand actions | In speech bubbles we do good listening, we take turns, and we are kind to each other. |
| Name in bucket game: everyone projects their name into an imaginary bucket in the centre of the circle | . . . it's not a real bucket it's a pretend bucket<br>We throw our names in the bucket loud, quietly and silly<br>. . . sometimes you can do it in a funny way—Jaaaaaaaaanel |
| Bubbles game: everyone blows an invisible bubble and carefully steps inside, cleans the walls so they can see and then floats up | They blow the bubble and the bubbles start getting bigger and bigger—they are floating around<br>If they touch each other you'll go inside and they'll just pop |
| Preparatory exercises 'soundscapes': everyone practises key characters, events or scenes from the day's story | They making Stirling's story and my one, they're pretending there was snow on the floor, they carefully walked and then they fall down . . .<br>That's the sound of swords crashing together, not snakes |
| Marking out the story square: practitioner makes a rectangular space with tape where the story will be acted out | . . . its where we do our acting in<br>. . . he [Adam the theatre practitioner] was putting the story square on the floor<br>People act out their characters |
| Storytelling and acting: practitioner slowly reads out the day's story, verbatim. Individuals or groups are called to act parts and scenery | Once . . . there lived a king and a princess but the queen did not come back until it was December or November<br>The queen did come from Africa and her grandmother died that's why she's gone to Africa<br>And the queen had forgotten a thing that was really important, she had forgotten her phone |
| Whoosh! Instruction mid-performance for the players to leave the story square and a new group enter | When Adam says 'whoooosh!' then we've got to get out of the square and sit down |
| 'Washing off' characters | They're washing all the dirt—the characters off. They were pretending to have a shower |
| Hedgehog feedback | Then we say to the hedgehog what do we enjoy today |
| Telling next week's story: two children stay and tell their story to facilitator who writes exactly what they say | We take turns, . . . . Adam has our names in his book and after we make all of it up, we actually act what we told the last day, whatever we say they write it down |
| Teaching assistants and facilitators assess each child for developments in, turn taking, listening, acting and kindness | |

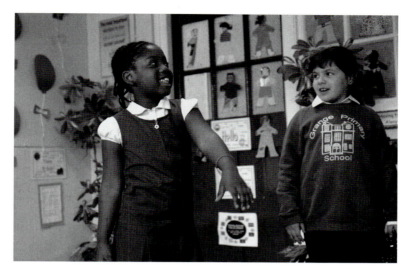

**Fig. 25.1** Speech Bubbles—developing good communication though drama.
Reproduced by kind permission of London Bubble Theatre. Copyright © 2015 London Bubble Theatre.

from communities in London and Manchester attend weekly sessions with a theatre practitioner throughout the year. Each session follows a similar format—a story previously dictated by one child is enacted by the whole group after a period of rehearsal.

Theatre practitioners lead the children towards creative learning by constructing sessions that feel secure, predictable, and personalized. Individual children dictate progressively more creative stories and the group makes increasingly creative dramatic responses to them. Participating children rapidly and generally become more confident, articulate, and collaborative. The process is shown in Table 25.1.

The impact on children's speech, language, and communication skills is rapid—often measurable after three or four sessions. Improvements in confidence (see Fig. 25.1) and speaking out are sustained and transfer to the mainstream classroom for between 70 and 85% of referred children. The effect on social and psychological health is evidenced through standardized measures of wellbeing and involvement (Laevers 1994a,b) but also in significantly fewer behavioural difficulties, better attendance, improved teacher assessments and predictions in reading, writing, speaking, and listening, and markedly improved happiness. The teaching assistants also consistently report heightened job satisfaction and commitment to promoting creative learning (Barnes 2013b).

### Case study 2: tackling deprivation with creativity—the Haringey Nursery Schools Consortium Lullaby Project

In Tottenham, in the London Borough of Haringey, 88% of the population live in areas classified as being within the poorest 20% in the United Kingdom. Life expectancy for men is almost 10 years lower than in the more affluent parts of London and the population is significantly younger, more ethnically diverse, has poorer health and housing, lower incomes, and is subjected to more crime than London averages (Haringey Council 2012a)

Such conditions have a strong impact on the very young. The adults living with the toddlers in this part of London have higher rates of mental illness, suffer more asthma and other lung problems, and have more cancers, heart disease, and strokes than those in most other parts of the city. Children's birth weight tends to be lower and they are more likely to visit accident and emergency centres. Large percentages show developmental delays, SLCN, or are described as 'unready for school'. This 'unreadiness' presents as lack of confidence, limited use of language, behavioural difficulties, and a wide range of social and other immaturities.

The Youth Music Lullaby Project was designed to address barriers to the wellbeing of 2- and 3-year-olds in Tottenham. Songwriter/singer Angeline Conaghan works with families to create bespoke lullabies, encapsulating all that is special and personal about an individual child (see Nursery World 2013).

Angeline first meets the child's parent/carer(s), and using props and photographs encourages them to talk about their child: her first words, funny phrases, what she loves doing, pets, favourite toys, favourite relatives, holidays, and activities. She also asks if there is anything the carer really wants to say to their child through the song. Conversations are positive, warm, and follow the lead of the carer. Details are captured on a large 'spider diagram' during the conversation. Angeline next composes a song with repeated chorus and culturally sensitive nuances, capturing as much of the conversation as possible. Pronunciations are checked as the new song is sung through to the carer. Finally the completed song is sung with guitar accompaniment to the child, carers, key worker, and other children (see Fig. 25.2). The lullaby is recorded, burned onto discs, and given to the family and children's centre. Many parents make multiple copies for home computers and send them to relatives and friends.

This highly personalized process generates profound changes in participating children and families. Adult responses are often emotional. One grandparent said, 'If had a song like this when I was a kid, it would have changed my life.' Carers frequently cry as they hear the song that expresses the identity and uniqueness of their child. The children are initially nonplussed at how the singer knows so much about them, but on second hearing they often display the physical, facial, and relational signs of confidence. They dance, smile, and beat time to the music when it is played to their

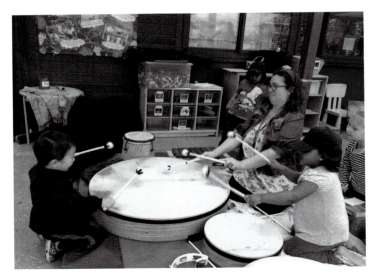

**Fig. 25.2** Angeline playing children to security and confidence.
Reproduced by kind permission of Angeline Conaghan. Copyright © 2015 Angeline Conaghan.

class. Teachers, key workers, and helpers sing the catchy choruses or play individual songs throughout the week, expressing their own pleasure in the songs and remarking on the children's positive responses.

Over a year Angeline has composed some 80 songs. The impact on individuals, centre staff, carers, observers, and children was monitored and recorded by parents/carers, key workers, and researchers. Evidence from videos, observations, written evaluations, and interviews was scrutinized and suggested that children's wellbeing showed itself in:

◆ increased involvement

◆ greater confidence

◆ calmer transitions between classes/families/life events

◆ increased resilience

◆ improved relations with others (including carers)

◆ More fluent and confident speech

◆ more confident communication

◆ improved attendance

Positive interactions (child/child; child/carer; carer/centre) increased. The warm relationship between composer and carer was a catalyst in several case studies to improved trust and collaboration with the children's centre. Parallel musical initiatives such as parent/staff development sessions and the sharing of traditional songs were successfully launched at the centres and created what many reported as an improved atmosphere of positivity.

The songs have become treasured family possessions. Parents report that attachment, relationships, and behaviour have improved since the songs became part of family life—one parent calling the songs her 'get out of jail free card'. Children see them as important records too. One asking that new adoptive parents' names replaced those of former foster carers in her song, another that her song was copied for each of the seven cousins mentioned in the lyrics.

By focusing on personal and family identity through creativity this project centrally addresses local aims for health and wellbeing to:

'. . . reduce health inequalities through working with communities and residents to improve opportunities for adults and children to enjoy a healthy, safe and fulfilling life.'

Haringey (2012b)

### Case study 3: constructing cultural identity through the arts—the Usinga World Centre for Dance and Music, Bagamoyo, Tanzania

Among the ruins of an old slaving post on Tanzania's coast, dancer–choreographer John Mponda, a college lecturer, has established a training centre for rescued street children aged 11–18 years. These homeless and vulnerable youngsters, often far from the villages, families, and schools of their early childhood, occupy a risky culture of petty crime and begging. The Usinga centre, attached to the International School of Art in Bagamoyo, uses traditional Tanzanian dance/drama, drumming, song, visual arts, and craft to unite young people with little sense of cultural identity in what it calls a spirit of 'peace, love, respect and harmony'. Founded in 1996, this registered NGO is an integrated and self-sustaining community aiming to reintegrate into Tanzanian society children damaged through poverty, neglect, illness, or abuse. They fund themselves

'. . . through a focus on [ . . . ] gardens for food production and renewable energy systems, and a variety of commercial activities such as the sale of art and handicraft products made by students, along with courses offered for visitors, performances and social activities in the community.'

Usinga (2013)

Through the arts, the centre works to develop group identity and the skills and attitudes that will help its graduates find jobs and a settled life in Tanzania's burgeoning towns.

Many projects in the developing world use drama, arts, or music to communicate particular messages (e.g. the International

Labour Organization's SCREAM programme, <http://www.ilo.org/ipec/campaignandadvocacy/scream/lang--en/index.htm>). The Usinga centre is different. Indigenous arts—music, drama, and dance—have become central to its life and the lives of the staff and young people there. Authentic and creative engagement in these culturally relevant arts quickly generates group and cultural identity among the majority of young students. Dance and drama support participants in expressing and controlling feelings of anger, jealousy, fear, sadness, and joy while also safely encountering them in others—building empathy, team spirit, trust, and responsibility through creative learning. Observations also record the body and facial language of pride and self-confidence during and after impromptu performances and within sessions. The effects of such projects are rarely formally researched, but the leaders of the Usinga centre, its young graduates, and their frequent visitors from schools in Dar es Salaam are confident that they provide social/personal rehabilitation, security, and a route towards a livelihood for the majority of their young people.

### Case study 4: addressing social isolation through drumming—the Art Talks project, Pune, India

Art Talks in Pune, India was established to use group music-making to address the needs of children suffering from a rage of diagnosed barriers to learning. Autism, dyslexia, dyspraxia, and attention deficit hyperactivity disorder (ADHD) are being identified in growing numbers of children throughout India. One 7-year-old with epilepsy and ADHD was referred for 40 sessions of shared rhythmic drumming, song, and other musical activities. Her parents and teachers had reported high degrees of social isolation brought on by restlessness, a very short attention span, and a poor memory. Her educational progress was painfully slow, separating her from other members of her class. After six Art Talks drumming sessions she was able to remember Djembe rhythms from the previous week, paid greater attention, and could easily relate to others in the session. Her growing confidence showed in the ways she went out of her way to be helpful without being asked. Venkit, her mentor, noted:

'. . . since the drums fell short, we used small buckets (inverted) that were originally from the sand pit . . . some sand fell in the class area. I noticed this and thought I would clean it up post class. Aabhi was sitting next to me. I looked down at the close of the session and noticed it was all spick and span . . . Aabhi had cleaned it all up. This was also the day that she was particularly more attentive and calm.'
V. Venkit (personal communication, 23 September 2013)

The next six sessions were planned to involve the use of stories, rhythmic drumming, and song to build confidence further and reduce dependence on her mentor.

### Case study 5: tackling lack of engagement through creative teaching—Teach for Malaysia

Malaysia, like many rapidly developing economies, faces negative as well as positive change. Secondary schools in the deprived areas of its cities and rural areas confront challenges once only associated with the west, involving apathy, antagonism, alcohol, and violence. The government has instituted a Teach for Malaysia scheme (<http://www.teachformalaysia.org>) to attract the very best graduates to work in these poorer areas and lead change by creating challenging and collaborative experiences, possibilities, and excellence for young people. The TFM course includes a module on creative teaching and learning. Some teachers like Liew Suet Li use creative teaching ideas to generate creative learning in the English language. Her story captures a personalized, emotionally powerful, and creative approach to writing that generated sustained involvement in previously unengaged pupils. Creativity clearly had as much positive impact on Suet Li as upon the young people in her care (see Box 25.1).

---

**Box 25.1** 'I have a dream that one day . . . '

My journey as a teacher is a massive roller-coaster experience. Some days I feel like I'm wasting my time with these kids, but some days I truly feel so contented that I feel like I can do this forever. Thankfully, today is one of those days that trumps a million of the other bad days.

I taught my Form 3 class about Martin Luther King [MLK] a few days ago and told them about his 'I have a dream' speech. I was supposed to move along the syllabus since I have to finish it by July but decided instead to take both periods today to get them to learn more about MLK instead. I had watched his speech again the night before and got goosebumps all over, and thought I could inspire my kids with it as well.

In class, I wrote out quotes from his speech and pasted them all over the room. I briefly spoke about what some of those quotes meant and the kids got more and more excited about MLK. I think listening to stories beat doing more grammar exercises and writing boring essays anytime!

I have a dream that one day, little black boys and black girls will beable to join hands with little white boys and white girls and walktogether as brothers and sisters.

I spoke about how bad slavery was in America and how African Americans couldn't even board the same bus or use the same toilet or the same water fountains as whites. The kids were appalled and got riled up about it. They couldn't believe how bad racism can get and we discussed the importance of civil rights and equality.

We then read out my favourite MLK quote:

I have a dream that one day, we will live in a nation where we will not be judged by the colour of our skin but by the content of our character.

Before we watched the speech, I got the kids to write out their own dreams. They could write about anything they want, as long as those dreams are big enough that they seem impossible.

*(continued)*

---

**Box 25.1** Continued

Then they pasted their dreams next to their tracker and we watched the speech together. They watched a few minutes of it, noisily commented on everything, but many could not understand everything he said . . .. after the video ended, I asked if they would like to hear my dream now.

I have a dream that one day, all 31 of you will be sitting in your university dorm room one day and will remember this moment. Then, you will go on YouTube to rewatch this speech but this time, this time you'll be able to understand every word in MLK's speech and will be inspired by those words as well. I have a dream that one day, you too will fight for something you believe in, just like MLK fought for his own rights.

I choked midway while saying that because I was so emotional about it, so emotional about the thought of my kids achieving that dream. The class was silent for a while, and one boy quietly said, 'Teacher, I want that dream to come true too.'
While they worked on their work after that, I read all their Post-Its in awe:

I have a dream that one day, people who are stupid like me can be geniuses too.
I have a dream that one day, I will fight for poor people like me and help change their fate forever.
I have a dream that one day, everyone in this class will own expensive cars like Ferrari, Porsche, Audi, McLaren . . . [He listed down 10 different cars; obviously written by a boy!]
I have a dream that one day, my village will be proud of me and will not look down on me or my family for being poor anymore.
I have a dream that one day, Malaysia will be the best country in the world.
I have a dream that one day, everyone in this class will be astronauts and we can live on the moon together.

One after another, big dreams, wonderful dreams, inspiring dreams.
. . . thinking back at this moment [ . . . ] I realized that I don't know if I will ever feel such a strong rewarding and fulfilling feeling again. You know how people use the term 'once in a lifetime'? Why go bungee jumping, why go climb Mount Everest, why do a million other things when you can change lives, once in your lifetime? When you can get kids to dream big, to want to achieve more, to want to succeed, once in your lifetime.

## Conclusions: messages for education

The language of positivity binds the research, case studies, and reflections we have described. This language is common in the discourse about creativity within education, yet education policy may seem to be moving away from such humanizing concepts. As competition, comparison, testing, and the language of business and the marketplace dominate education decisions, schools face a dilemma: how to address personal and societal needs. Creative practitioners argue that creative teaching and creative learning provide the answer. Creativity in education has been argued to promote the humanizing qualities that build identity and confidence, motivation, and empathy in individuals and trust, friendship, hope, and collaboration in communities (e.g. PCAH 2011).

The case studies also illustrate ways in which *adult* teachers and mentors shared creative experiences with children and discovered personal meaning and fulfilment. Creativity in education—mind-changing, identity-forming, idea-generating, and fun for all—can create healthy, caring, and hopeful communities.

# References

African Magazine (2007). Five questions for Ishmael Beah. *The African Magazine*, 18 June. Available at: <http://www.africanmag.com/FORUM-464-design004> (accessed 4 October 2013).

Barnes, J. (2013a). What sustains a fulfilling life in education? *Journal of Education and Training Studies*, **1**(2), 74–88.

Barnes, J. (2013b). Drama to promote personal and social wellbeing in 6 and 7 year olds with communication difficulties: the Speech Bubbles Project, *Perspectives in Public Health*, **134**, 101–109.

Barnes, J. and Scoffham, S. (2007). Memorandum to Commons Select Committee. Available at: <http://www.publications.parliament.uk/pa/cm200607/cmselect/cmeduski/memo/creativepartnerships/uc2002.htm> (accessed 4 October 2013).

Beah, I. (2007). Memoirs of a boy soldier. NPR radio interview, 21 February. Available at: <http://www.npr.org/templates/story/story.php?storyId=7519542> (Accessed 4 October 2013).

Booth, T. (2010). Keynote address at Project Kinderwelten, Berlin, July, 2010. Available at: <http://www.kinderwelten.net/pdf/tagung2010/07_tony_booth_keynote_engl.pdf> (accessed 4 October 2013).

Botth, T. (2012). Responding to 21st century imperatives: a new index for inclusion, *Enabling Education Review*. Available at: <http://www.eenet.org.uk/resources/eenet_newsletter/eer1/page20.php> (accessed 2 March 2015).

Booth, T. and Ainscow, M. (2011). *Index for Inclusion: Developing Learning and Participation in Schools*, 2nd edn. Bristol: Centre for Studies in Inclusive Education.

Bruner, J. (1983). *Child's Talk*. New York: Norton.

Canada, Public Health Agency (2012). *The Health of Canada's Young People: A Mental Health Focus*. Available at: <http://www.phac-aspc.gc.ca/hp-ps/dca-dea/publications/health-young-people-sa nte-jeunes-canadiens/index-eng.php> (accessed 4 October 2013).

Cervatiuc, A. (2008). ESL vocabulary and acquisition. *The Internet TESL Journal*. Available at: <http://iteslj.org/articles/cervatiuc-vocabularyacquisition.html> (accessed 4 October 2013).

Claxton, G. and Lucas, B. (2010). *New Kinds of Smart: How the Science of Learnable Intelligence is Changing Education*. Milton Keynes: Open University Press.

Craft, A. (2005). *Creativity in Schools: Tensions and Dilemmas*. London: Routledge.

Csikszentmihalyi, M. (2002). *Flow: The Classic Work on How to Achieve Happiness*. New York: Ebury Press.

Damasio, A. (2003). *Looking for Spinoza: Joy, Sorrow and the Feeling Brain*. Orlando, FL: Harcourt.

Damasio, A. and Immordino-Yang, M. (2007). We feel therefore we learn: the relevance of affective and social neuroscience to education. *Brain, Mind and Education*, **1**, 3–10.

Fredrickson, B. (2009). *Positivity*, New York: Crown.

Goleman, D. (1996) *Emotional Intelligence*. London: Bloomsbury.

Goswami, U. and Bryant, P. (2007). Children's cognitive development and learning. *Primary Review Research Briefings 2/1*. Cambridge: University of Cambridge Faculty of Education.

Greenfield, S. (2011). *You and Me: The Neuroscience of Identity*. London: Notting Hill Editions.

Haringey Council (2012a). Ward profiles. Available at: <http://www.haringey.gov.uk/council-and-democracy/about-council/facts-and-figures/ward-profiles> (accessed 4 October 2013).

Haringey Council (2012b). *Health and Wellbeing Strategy (2012–15): A Healthier* Haringey. Available at: <http://www.haringey.gov.uk/social-care-and-health/health/health-and-wellbeing-strategy> (accessed 4 October 2013).

Hope, G., Barnes, J., and Scoffham, S. (2008). A conversation about creative learning. In: C. Craft, P. Burnard, and T. Cremin (eds) *Documenting Creative Learning*, pp. 125–133. Stoke on Trent: Trentham Books.

I CAN (2006). *The Cost to the Nation of Children's Poor Communication*. Available at: <http://www.ican.org.uk/~/media/Ican2/Whats%20 the%20Issue/Evidence/2%20The%20Cost%20to%20the%20 Nation%20of%20Children%20s%20Poor%20Communication%20 pdf.ashx> (accessed 4 October 2013).

Jeffrey, B. and Woods, P. (2003). *The Creative School*. London: Routledge.

John-Steiner, V. (2006). *Creative Collaboration*. Cambridge: Cambridge University Press.

Laevers, F. (ed.) (1994a). *Defining and Assessing Quality in Early Childhood Education*. Leuven: Leuven University Press.

Laevers, F. (1994b). *The Leuven Involvement Scale for Young Children, LIS-YC, Manual*. Leuven: Centre for Experiential Education.

Marmot, M. (2010). *Fair Society: Healthy Lives* [report to UK Government]. Available at: <http://www.instituteofhealthequity.org/projects/fair-society-healthy-lives-the-marmot-review> (accessed 4 October 2013).

NACCCE (National Advisory Committee on Creative and Cultural Education) (1999). *All Our Futures: Creativity, Culture and Education*. London: DfEE.

Murphy, R. and Weinhardt, F. (2013) The importance of rank position. *CEP Discussion Paper No. 1241*. Available at: <http://cep.lse.ac.uk/pubs/download/dp1241.pdf> (accessed 4 October 2013).

Nursery World (2013). Learning and development: music—your song. Available at: <http://www.nurseryworld.co.uk/nursery-world/feature/1097781/learning-development-music-song> (accessed 4 October 2013).

OECD (Organisation for Economic Cooperation and Development) (2009). *Doing Better for Children*. Paris: OECD.

PCAH (President's Committee on the Arts and Humanities) (2011). *Reinvesting in Arts Education. Winning America's Future through Creative Schools*. Available at: <http://pcah.gov/sites/default/files/pcah_reinvesting_4web_0.pdf> (accessed 4 October 2013).

Perkins, D. (1992) *Smart Schools*, New York: The Free Press.

Riqueime, L. and Rosas, J. (2014). Multicultural perspective: the road to cultural competence. In: N. Singleton and B. Shulman (eds), *Language Development; Foundations, Processes and Clinical Applications*, 2nd edn, pp. 349–378. Burlington, MA: Jones and Bartlett.

Roberts, P. (2006) *Nurturing Creativity in Young People: A Report to Government to Inform Future Policy*. London: Department of Culture, Media and Sport.

Robinson, K (2010). *The Element: How Finding Your Passion Changes Everything*, London: Penguin.

Royal Government of Bhutan (2012). *The Report of the High-Level Meeting on Wellbeing and Happiness: Defining a New Economic Paradigm*. New York: The Permanent Mission of the Kingdom of Bhutan to the United Nations. Available at: <https://sustainabledevelopment.un.org/content/documents/617bhutanreport_web_f.pdf >

Ryff, C. (1989). Happiness is everything or is it? Explorations on the meaning of psychological wellbeing. *Journal of Personality Social Psychology*, **57**, 1069–1081.

Shayer, M. and Adey, P. (2002) *Learning Intelligence: Cognitive Acceleration Across the Curriculum From 5–15 years*. Buckingham: Open University Press.

United Nations (1989). A summary of the United Nations Convention on the Rights of the Child [CRC]. Available at: <http://childrenandyouthprogramme.info/pdfs/pdfs_uncrc/uncrc_summary_version.pdf> (accessed 4 October 2013).

UNICEF (2011) *Report: Child Wellbeing in the UK, Spain and Sweden*. Available at: <http://www.unicef.org.uk/latest/publications/ipsos-mori-child-wellbeing/> (accessed 4 October 2013).

UNICEF (2013) Child wellbeing in rich countries. A comparative overview. *Innocenti Report Card 11*. Florence: UNICER Office of Research. Available at: <http://www.unicef.org.uk/images/campaigns/final_rc11-eng-lores-fnl2.pdf> (accessed 4 October 2013).

Usinga (2013). Usinga, World Centre for Dance and Music. Available at: <http://www.emmasworld.net/usinga.swf> (accessed 4 October 2013).

Westby. C. (2014). Social-emotional bases of pragmatic and communication development. In: N. Singleton and B. Shulman (eds), *Language Development: Foundations, Processes and Clinical Applications*, 2nd edn, pp. 135–176. Burlington, MA: Jones and Bartlett.

WHO (2012). *Health Behaviour of School Aged Children Report*. Available at: http://www.euro.who.int/__data/assets/pdf_file/0003/163857/Social-determinants-of-health-and-wellbeing-among-young-people.pdf [Accessed 4 Oct 2013].

Wrigley, T., Thomson, P., and Lingard, R. (2011). *Changing Schools: Alternative Ways to Make a World of Difference*. London: Routledge.

# CHAPTER 26

# The value of music for public health

## Gunter Kreutz

## Cultural participation and public health

Developed countries are characterized by affluence and wealth as well as by continued advancement in medical science and, in principle, the provision of high standards in medical care for each individual, irrespective of his or her socio-economic status. However, public health appears to be compromised to some extent by various individual behaviours including a poor diet, drug and alcohol abuse, or lack of physical exercise. The World Health Organization (WHO), for example, has identified a need for global strategies to promote healthy diets and physical exercise (WHO 2013). However, additional challenges to the health systems arise as standard treatment alone, namely surgery and pharmaceutical therapies, can only be effective if adjuvant therapies are used to harness individual resources to alleviate side effects from both illness and treatment. In short, health, as stated in the well-known WHO definition, is based on individual physical, psychological, physical, and social wellbeing. Therefore, enhancing an individual's quality of life is crucially dependent on preventing illness and promoting health.

Epidemiological research is concerned with the risks associated with life conditions and lifestyles, with a tendency to emphasize negative health effects, but some attention has been given to those aspects of life and activities which have positive benefits. Bygren et al. (2009), for example, investigated the health consequences of cultural activities in a Swedish cohort. The authors found that those rarely attending cultural events (e.g. cinema, theatre, live music shows, or art galleries) showed a three-fold increased risk of death from cancer compared with those who participated in cultural activities more regularly. Importantly, this effect was present in the urban population but not the rural population. In another epidemiological study, Cuypers et al. (2012) focused on the relationship between both receptive and creative cultural activities on the one hand, and subjective measures of perceived health and other psychological variables on the other. The findings were complex, suggesting perceived health benefits for men who engage regularly in receptive cultural activities. Such general associations between cultural participation and objective and subjective outcome measures notwithstanding, public health epidemiology to date has failed to more directly investigate the effects of the arts and culture in general (Clift et al. 2010c) as

well as the role of musical behaviours in particular (Theorell and Kreutz 2012).

## Why is music important to public health?

People around the globe are musically active throughout their lives. Indeed, musical activities are universal in human culture and behaviour (Nettl 1956). Babies are born with neural networks to process musical rhythms efficiently (Winkler et al. 2009), pre-school children reveal enhanced empathy and cooperation when joining in synchronous musical behaviours (Kirschner and Tomasello 2010), adult amateur choristers (Clift and Hancox 2001; Clift 2012a) and dancers (Quiroga et al. 2011) show similar psychological benefits as a result of their engagement, and even individuals suffering from dementia preserve musical memories and singing as opposed to speaking capabilities as part of the semantic code that is still accessible in the process of cognitive decline (Davidson and Fedele 2011). These heterogeneous examples all suggest that music may function as a social, emotional, and cognitive resource across the life span (MacDonald et al. 2012).

There is little doubt that the basic musical abilities necessary for dancing and singing as well as for learning to play a musical instrument to a certain level of proficiency exist in the majority of the general population. For example, tone deafness, which is described mainly as a pitch-processing disorder (Albouy et al. 2013), is present in only a fraction of the individuals who characterize themselves as non-musical or as poor singers (Wise and Sloboda 2008). Clearly, there is substantial potential for music to be drawn upon in the context of public health interventions that to date has only been explored in a limited way (e.g. Cohen et al. 2007).

## What is music? And what are musical activities?

To most people, the nature of music reveals itself in personal experiences. Although only a very few people invent or compose music, aesthetic experiences are nevertheless associated with a range of creative processes, for example in singing, dancing, or playing musical instruments. Even listening to music cannot be equated just with passive consumption if an active mind is engaged.

Therefore, musical activities need to be acknowledged as essential personal needs rather than merely distracting or leisure time behaviours. Instead of an authoritative prescription of what music, as well as any associated musical behaviours, should be, music is seen rather as an emerging property of people's interactions with their own minds and bodies. These interactions, of course, also entail extending those natural musical behaviours by the use of instruments as well as developing interpretations, revisions, or creating entirely new musical materials through improvisation. From this point of view, a baby responding with movements to rhythmic stimulation, someone singing under the shower, or a group of adults playing the claves while chanting and swaying their bodies rhythmically in synchrony all suggest musical activity.

Having said that, it is still possible and necessary to differentiate musical from non-musical or concomitant activities in some way. In fact, experimental approaches rely on defining conditions to differentiate the respective influences of musical on specific outcome measures in comparison with other behaviours. Importantly, these may well share aspects with musical activities. For example, having people sit in a room and talk to each other might engage social processes that are somewhat similar but not equal to singing or playing music together.

It is common in the literature to distinguish between listening to music on the one hand and more active musical behaviours such as singing, dancing, and playing a musical instrument on the other. This distinction is difficult for several reasons. One is that listening to music also involves a range of brain activities and therefore cannot be characterized by mere exposure to a class of sound that needs to be distinguished from speech and environmental noise. A second reason is that musical activities generally involve listening to music. Even individuals who are hard of hearing may experience music by means of vibrations that may evoke responses like dancing or playing along that are in many ways similar to listening with intact hearing. A third reason why music listening (and for that matter even imagining music) should be qualified as an activity is because there is no certainty whether and how the psychophysiological feedback of music experiences differ in performers and listeners beyond the perceptual-motor processes that are necessary to perform music (Altenmüller et al. 2006).

## Music experience and/as therapy

Musical practice is leisure, education, and therapy in one. These domains naturally afford some fundamental similarities and distinctions with respect to their philosophies, settings, target populations, contexts, and prospective achievements, particularly with respect to the latter two. Ideally, the primary goal of music education and learning is to enable practitioners to perceive music in its own right without consideration of a particular goal or purpose. By contrast, when music is applied as a central element in therapeutic interventions, then the musical activities and sharing between patient and therapist are thought to support some therapeutic process.

In theory there is a categorical distinction between healthy individuals who learn to play music to increase their musical proficiency and individuals who are in treatment for some kind

of physical or psychological disorder. From a public health point of view, however, this distinction may be questioned. For example, the so-called salutogenic approach (Antonovsky 1987) places health and illness at the extreme ends of a continuum. Therefore, from the perspective of an individual in good health performing music there may well be preventative value in such an activity, and there is empirical evidence to support this. From the perspective of an individual in poor health, however, there may be still a need for aesthetic expression and the activation of positive emotions in the presence of even a life-threatening condition (Conrad et al. 2007).

In sum, not only is the dichotomy between health and illness to be questioned, depending on the underlying health model, there is also a need to consider notions such as aesthetic, emotional, pedagogical, therapeutic, and preventative values in a more holistic fashion, emphasizing individual needs for engaging in music in general and its importance in response to global health inequalities (Clift et al. 2012b) in particular.

## Measuring the value of music for individual health

How can the effects of musical activities on individual health be measured? Leaving aside qualitative approaches, which rely on self-reports such as verbal or visual materials by individuals, numerous studies have used quantitative measures in order to objectify music-induced changes, usually at a group level in specific populations.

Clearly, to produce evidence suggesting that a given musical activity causes positive health outcomes is highly challenging. Despite the frequent claim that music acts like a psychoactive substance or drug it cannot be studied under the regime of a double-blinded, placebo-controlled methodology, which is standard for the approval of pharmaceuticals in healthcare. Because all individuals in our society are exposed to music throughout their lives, it is neither feasible nor desirable to remove music from an individual's life. For similar reasons, it would be unethical to raise children without music in order to assess the consequences of lack of music stimulation.

One further reason why evidence for the effects of music is difficult to specify is context. Musical behaviours are so intertwined with other everyday activities that it is even difficult to tease out any single element of these that is uniquely evoked by music. For example attending a concert shares numerous similarities and differences with watching television, attending a soccer game in a stadium, or drinking wine with some friends. Instead of controlling each and every variable characterizing situation and context of these behaviours, a more pragmatic strategy might be to accept that the context variables of a musical activity contribute to its potential health effects. Systematic differences from other behaviours may nevertheless be successfully studied by carefully designed experiments.

Beyond these limitations it is important to consider that studies on music-induced health effects need to be grounded methodologically in a different way from, for example, the application of a medication. This does not preclude the possibility of comparing the effects of music with pharmaceutical medication (Bringman et al. 2009), but is important to note that while the medication can be controlled for delivery as a novel stimulus or as a placebo neither aspect can be represented by music stimulation.

## Modelling the value of music for individual health

Most authors agree that studying the effects of music interventions and identifying the mechanisms which generate or modulate such effects are of similar importance. However, there are currently few models of music-induced health outcomes which might provide a basis for systematically studying the effects and underlying mechanisms. The development of such models is important with respect to the heterogeneous practices and the scattered literature, which is perceived as an obstacle to theory-building.

Västfjäll et al. (2012, p. 109), for example, characterize the effects of listening to music in a theoretical model that accommodates to the influences of the situation and context on health effects. According to these authors, music is primarily seen as a stimulus eliciting emotions (Juslin and Sloboda 2010). Recent studies have shown that perceived emotions in music can be predicted by physiological responses by means of both linear and non-linear relationships (Russo et al. 2013). The important point is that a relatively small variation in musical stimulation and the respective emotional content may have a smaller or larger leveraging effect on physiological responses, and vice versa.

One disadvantage of Västfjäll et al.'s model as well as others (e.g. Koelsch 2011, Fig. 1), however, is the neglect of musical behaviours other than listening. Arguably, given intact hearing, listening is present in all these behaviours. However, it is clear that playing music, singing, or dancing, may have substantially different effects compared with listening alone.

Figure 26.1 depicts a simple model of the relationship between musical behaviours on the one hand and clinical and non-clinical outcome measures on the other. It shows that instead of a direct path between musical behaviours and outcomes, some activation of health-related psychosomatic functions occurs. Also, instead of claiming that music can cure illness, the model predicts improvements in more general terms only.

The proposed model requires specifications for each of its components in order to assess the effects of a given musical intervention. For example, the activation of health-related psychosomatic systems is often represented as dependent or outcome measures, whereas independent factors may be derived, for example, from

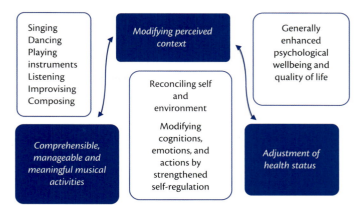

**Fig. 26.2** Contextual model of the beneficial effects of musical activities on wellbeing and quality of life.

comparisons between musical and non-musical behaviours and/or characteristics of the targeted populations. However, the context of intervention, such as the characteristics of where and how the musical intervention is delivered, remains implicit within this model.

Figure 26.2 suggests a relationship between musical behaviours and psychological wellbeing that is mediated by perceived context. The model is inspired by Antonovsky's idea of salutogenesis by suggesting that those musical behaviours in the top left corner of the model must be perceived as comprehensible, manageable, and meaningful by an individual in order to have any consequences for wellbeing and health. Therefore, psychosomatic changes resulting from musical experiences are inextricably linked to context variables. The important point is that modifications of self-related variables occur, enabling the activation of individual resources and the (positive) adjustment of health status. As a consequence, according to the contextual model, engagement in music may have positive health outcomes irrespective of the proof of any causal relationships between specific elements of musical behaviours and a direct and measurable impact on psychosomatic systems and functions. It appears entirely sufficient if such musical behaviours in combination with context variables evoke self-regulatory processes at conscious and/or subconscious levels.

The models presented so far suggest that musical behaviours have health consequences only in general terms. They were designed to highlight conceptual as well as methodological aspects of this rather complex relationship in a simplified way. However, they may well be used to predict specific health outcomes in rigorous investigations. For example, the various forms of psychophysiological feedback arising from a musical activity as well as its social context may well be disentangled in carefully designed studies (e.g. Quiroga et al. 2009). Thus musical behaviours can be systematically studied in comparison with other types of behaviours in order to see how individuals can maximally benefit from engaging in music.

## Psychoneuroendocrinology of musical behaviours

Psychoneuroendocrinology (PNE) is a relatively new area of health research. Traditionally, it has been associated primarily

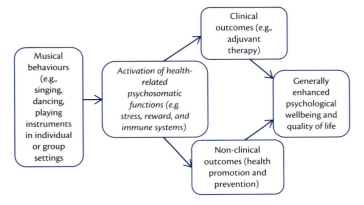

**Fig. 26.1** Psychophysiological (causal) model of the relationship between musical behaviours and psychological wellbeing.

with studies addressing maladaptive consequences of stress, and less so with more positive psychological influences on our lives (see Kreutz et al. 2012 for more details). Singing and dancing as well as playing a musical instrument are suggested to have beneficial effects, with some emphasis on stress reduction and relaxation (McDonald et al. 2012). These effects occur particularly, but not exclusively, at amateur levels. This means that the psychophysical demands that arise from musical behaviours appear limited. Playing music is rather safe and bears little risk, and many individuals with poor health may benefit from music in various ways. By contrast, research in the field of music medicine has focused primarily on music-related health problems in professional musicians (e.g. Ginsborg et al. 2012). Of course, performing music professionally does not preclude there being positive health effects. Beck and co-workers, for example, found similar increases of secretory immunoglobulin A in studies including amateur (Beck et al. 2000) and professional singers (Beck et al. 2006). Similarly, Grape et al. (2003) observed favourable endocrine responses in both amateur and professional singers during a singing lesson. However, these positive changes only extended to psychological levels in the amateur participants.

Both Koelsch and Stegemann (2012) and Västfjäll et al. (2012) suggest in their models that listening to music may elicit (positive) affect through the activation of mid-brain structures (Blood and Zatorre 2001; Zatorre and Salimpoor 2013). These regions contain brain circuits that are crucial for processing emotions (LeDoux 1996). Therefore, their models specifically predict music-induced modulations of endocrine functions, as evidenced in a growing body of literature (for recent reviews see Quiroga et al. 2011; Kreutz et al. 2012; Chanda and Levitin 2013).

## The specific value of different musical activities

### Listening to music

Listening to music is far more widespread than active playing of music on instruments. Humans love to listen to music, either by using audio devices or by attending concerts as a leisure activity. Therefore, each individual normally develops implicit musical knowledge to make sense of music. Indeed, musical skills are initially acquired during exposure to music early on in life, before and after birth. Their development may extend through life-long learning and practice within both formal and informal settings to older age.

Listening to music very often gives rise to (inner as well as overt) movement, dancing, and singing. Therefore, listening to music is different from, for example, listening to speech, environmental noise, or being exposed to silence. One main reason for the substantial affinity to music may be that music listening evokes feelings of reward and pleasure. Some of these positive emotions may be so strong that they resemble feelings of profound satisfaction. Neurobiological responses, in fact, are similar to the experience of tasty food or sex (Blood and Zatorre 2001). Music is powerful, at least in part, because of the associations and memories it evokes.

A seminal review by Bartlett (1996), who summarized roughly a century of research into psychophysiological responses to music, concluded with respect to cardiovascular measures (e.g. heart rate, systolic and diastolic blood pressure) that there existed little evidence of any specific effects of music on any of these measures.

Recently, however, this picture of non-specific psychophysiological responses to music has been questioned (Trappe 2012). Bernardi et al. (2006, 2009), for example, investigated cardiovascular responses in several experiments. In one study, a group of healthy individuals listened to selected pieces of classical vocal (e.g. Puccini's *Turandot*) and instrumental music (the *Adagio* from Beethoven's Ninth Symphony). Irrespective of the participants' individual musical proficiency, significant relationships between musical crescendi (the swelling of loudness over a period of several seconds) and cardiorespiratory measures including skin vasoconstriction and blood pressure were noted (Bernardi et al. 2009). In a related study, similar autonomic responses occurred in different participants listening to the same music. Again, temporal aspects of the music, such as the loudness profile in selected classical arias as well as the overall tempo of the music, correlated with cardiorespiratory activity. It appears that, to an extent, the cardiovascular system tracks the musical profile and responds to both sudden and slower continuous changes in characteristic ways (Bernardi et al. 2006). Importantly, silence following either slow or fast music had the greatest effect on cardiovascular relaxation compared with all the musical stimuli used in that experiment.

Taken together, these studies suggest that specific patterns of change in tempo and loudness can regulate the cardiorespiratory functions in rather positive ways by inducing relaxation. Thus music may be purposefully chosen to influence the antagonistic activities of processes controlling heart rate on the one hand, and vasoconstriction (and blood pressure levels) on the other.

Finally, the psychologically and physiologically positive effects of listening to music have been observed in numerous health settings, including pain and stress management (Bernatzky et al. 2011) and enhancing relaxation during medical procedures (Spintge 2012). Listening to music is provided as a safe adjuvant intervention with no known side effects. Delivering selected music to patients undergoing surgery may have effects that are equal to or even superior to standard medication (Bringman et al. 2009; Nilsson 2009). As a consequence, details of the patient's musical preferences and the availability of appropriate devices for delivery of music could become a valuable part of any medical treatment (Spintge 2012).

### Singing

Singing lessons in combination with vocal exercises have also been implicated in the promotion of vocal health. For example, Gütay and Kreutz (2011) investigated two cohorts of fifth-graders (age 10–11 years) within a controlled longitudinal study design. One group of children received vocal training in small groups each week over the entire school year while the other group served as controls. The control group also had music lessons which included singing. Each child underwent a series of tests including measurement of the pitch and dynamic ranges of the voice. The acoustic flexibility of the voice contains quantitative information about its quality and health status, the so-called dysphonia severity index (DSI). The DSI often complements laryngoscopy. Results showed that vocal performance was similar for all children at baseline. However, at the end of the school year those children who received singing lessons showed an average improvement of about six to seven semitones (about half an octave) as well as an increase of about 7 dB in the sound pressure level (10 dB would mean a doubling of perceived loudness). The control children showed no improvement at all. Therefore, singing lessons might contribute to promotion of vocal health.

The values of singing may well extend beyond vocal health to the promotion of general mental and physical health (Clift 2012a; Clift et al. 2010a,b, Chapter 31 this volume). They include, for example, perceived psychological benefits (Unwin et al. 2002) as well as enhanced local immune responses (Kreutz et al. 2004) in singers. These benefits, however, may well extend beyond immediate feedback to the person singing; in specific health settings they may improve the quality of carer–patient relationships (Bannan and Montgomery Smith 2008).

Many facets of the potential health benefits of singing may well extend from non-clinical to clinical contexts. For example, one study targeting an amateur choir whose members were homeless men suggested significant improvements in wellbeing and quality of life in some individuals (Bailey and Davidson 2002). The experience of flow during singing, the increase in self-esteem from public performance, as well as group participation and individual mental engagement, all suggest that singing together may be beneficial. Therefore, it may not be one single component or factor that facilitates health benefits. Instead a rather complex pattern of mutually reinforcing influences could lead to positive effects.

## Dancing

Dancing is obviously a more physical form of interpreting and performing music than singing. Despite the human affinity for dancing across the life span from infancy to older age, dance appears to be less prominent in education compared with singing, which perhaps could indicate its undervaluation. However, dance is equally a subdomain of music as well as of sport and physical exercise. It can be performed, in principle, in the absence of sound, but usually involves the presence of music. Thus physical and aerobic qualities in human movement are the main characteristics of dance. The ease and flexibility with which humans are able to dance in coordination with musical beats, and with other individuals in partnered or group dance, is unique and is found in no other animal species.

Recent systematic and controlled studies suggest significant effects of dance/movement therapies to alleviate problems related to neurological disorders including Parkinson's disease (Earhart 2009; Duncan and Earhart 2012) and multiple sclerosis (Salgado and de Paula Vasconcelos 2010; Hackney and Earhart 2009ab). Dance has also been identified in one study as reducing the risk of dementia (Verghese et al. 2003), although similar to many observations in this area of research replication is needed to ascertain such findings. Research into the psychological benefits of dancing in non-clinical contexts is not as advanced as research on singing, but the two activities share many characteristics in terms of perceived health benefits (Quiroga et al. 2010). People often respond to singing or dancing with perceived stress reduction as well as enhanced relaxation. In addition, both domains play a role in communal health promotion because the wide range of styles offers the potential to accommodate varying individual preferences. Finally, listening to music and dancing appear to interact at endocrine levels. For example, Quiroga et al. (2009) found that significant reductions in the stress hormone cortisol could be attributed to the presence of music during the performance of dance movements with or without a partner.

## Playing a musical instrument

Millions of children around the world learn to play a musical instrument for a number of years. However, the opportunity of learning to play an instrument appears most vulnerable to socio-economic influences, even in developed countries. Clearly, only a few children who play music begin a career as a professional musician in later life, which leaves the vast majority of players as amateur musicians who nevertheless carry on playing throughout their lives. Some individuals start learning an instrument as adults or even in older age. This suggests that the capacity to learn music is less restricted to critical periods than, for example, the acquisition of the first language.

Learning to play a musical instrument is believed to have long-lasting consequences for the development of the brain and cognitive capacities. For example, there is growing evidence from the field of musical neuroscience which suggests that music training may alter the brain at different levels and lead to structural as well as functional modifications within and beyond the musical domain. Randomized controlled studies in this domain are rare, but at least one has shown that music training over the course of 1 year enhances IQ by about four points, which is a relatively small but significant effect (Schellenberg 2004). Further work has identified enhanced capacities of auditory perception and cognition in 8- to 9-year-olds receiving instrumental lessons at school in small groups (Roden et al. 2012). In sum, this research suggests that learning to play a musical instrument may well contribute to a cognitive reserve preventing or delaying decline in older age (Hall et al. 2009).

## Conclusions

Music has long been implicated as an adjuvant psychotherapy to promote mental health, specifically alleviating communicative and behavioural disorders that very often comprise elements of emotional disturbances. However, engaging in musical activities may also have broader implications for public health. A growing number of initiatives and practices, some of which are documented in this book, suggest that music education has a key role in health promotion. To the extent that musical learning can provide individuals with strategies for coping with stress and enhancing relaxation, for example, it is likely that routines like playing music in ensembles, or in private, as well as other musical activities that are performed on a regular basis, may aid to regulate emotions and guard individuals against disturbances or life-events which could otherwise lead to the onset of mental or physical health problems. Although at the moment it appears difficult to demonstrate the protective effects of musical behaviours by objective measures, there exist at least initial findings which suggest a role for music in health promotion.

The preliminary models suggested in this chapter both overlap and complement each other. Clearly, this area of research is still in need of further systematic exploration before more comprehensive models can be formulated. Such models should account, for example, for feedback to musically engaged individuals as well as for short- and long-term benefits for wellbeing and health. The question of causal association between specific musical elements and health outcomes cannot be answered for ethical and methodological reasons. However, it seems relevant and important to continue to research the potential relevance of music in all its forms for health and wellbeing in communities and healthcare settings.

## References

Albouy, P., Mattout, J., Bouet, R., et al. (2013). Impaired pitch perception and memory in congenital amusia: the deficit starts in the auditory cortex. *Brain*, **136**, 1639–1661.

Altenmüller, E., Wiesendanger, M., and Kesselring, J. (eds) (2006). *Music, Motor Control and the Brain*. Oxford: Oxford University Press.

Antonovsky, A. (1987). *Unravelling the Mystery of Health*. San Francisco: Jossey-Bass.

Bailey, B.A. and Davidson, J.W. (2002). Adaptive characteristics of group singing: perceptions from members of a choir for homeless men. *Musicae Scientiae*, **VI**, 221–256.

Bannan, N. and Montgomery-Smith, C. (2008). 'Singing for the brain': reflections on the human capacity for music arising from a pilot study of group singing. *Journal of the Royal Society for the Promotion of Health*, **128**, 73–78.

Bartlett, D. (1996). Physiological responses to music and sound stimuli. In: D.A. Hodges (ed.), *Handbook of Music Psychology*, 2nd edn, pp. 343–385. Lawrence, KS: National Association for Music Therapy.

Beck, R.J., Cesario, T.C., Yousefi, A., and Enamoto, H. (2000). Choral singing, performance perception, and immune system changes in salivary immunoglobulin A and cortisol. *Music Perception*, **18**, 87–106.

Beck, R.J., Gottfried, T.L., Hall, D.J., Cisler, C.A., and Bozeman, K.W. (2006). Supporting the health of college solo singers: the relationship of positive emotions and stress to changes in salivary IgA and cortisol during singing. *Journal for Learning through the Arts*, **2**(1). Available at: <http://www.escholarship.org/uc/item/003791w4> (accessed 30 August 2013).

Bernardi, L., Porta, C., and Sleight, P. (2006). Cardiovascular, cerebrovascular, and respiratory changes induced by different types of music in musicians and non-musicians: the importance of silence. *Heart*, **92**, 445–452.

Bernardi, L., Porta, C., Casucci, G., et al. (2009). Dynamic interactions between musical, cardiovascular, and cerebral rhythms in humans. *Circulation*, **119**, 3171–3180.

Bernatzky, G., Presch, M., Anderson, M., and Panksepp, J. (2011). Emotional foundations of music as a non-pharmacological pain management tool in modern medicine. *Neuroscience and Biobehavioral Reviews*, **35**, 1989–1999.

Blood, A.J. and Zatorre, R.J. (2001). Intensely pleasurable responses to music correlate with activity in brain regions implicated in reward and emotion. *Proceedings of the National Academy of Sciences of the United States of America*, **98**, 11818–11823.

Bringman, H., Giesecke, K., Thorne, A., and Bringman, S. (2009). Relaxing music as pre-medication before surgery: a randomised controlled trial. *Acta Anaesthesiologica Scandinavica*, **53**, 759–764.

Bygren, L.-O., Johansson, S.-E., Konlaan, B.B., Grjibovski, A.M., Wilkinson, A.V., and Sjöström, M. (2009). Attending cultural events and cancer mortality: a Swedish cohort study. *Arts & Health: An International Journal for Research Policy and Practice*, **1**, 64–73.

Clift, S. (2012a). Singing, wellbeing and health. In: R. MacDonald, G. Kreutz, and L. Mitchell (eds) *Music, Health, and Wellbeing*, pp. 113–124. Oxford: Oxford University Press.

Clift, S. (2012b). Creative arts as a public health resource: moving from practice-based research to evidence-based practice'. *Perspectives in Public Health*, **132**, 120–127.

Clift, S. and Hancox, G. (2010). The significance of choral singing for sustaining psychological wellbeing: findings from a survey of choristers in England, Australia and Germany. *Music Performance Research*, **3**, 79–96.

Clift, S. and Hancox, G. (2001). The perceived benefits of singing: findings from preliminary surveys of a university college choral society. *Journal of the Royal Society for the Promotion of Health*, **121**, 248–256.

Clift, S., Nicols, J., Raisbeck, M., Whitmore, C., and Morrison, I. (2010a). Group singing, wellbeing and health: a systematic review, *The UNESCO Journal*, **2**, 1–25.

Clift, S., Hancox, G., Morrison, I., Hess, B., Kreutz, G., and Stewart, D. (2010b). Choral singing and psychological wellbeing: quantitative and qualitative findings from English choirs in a cross-national survey. *Journal of Applied Arts and Health*, **1**, 19–34.

Clift, S., Camic, P., and Daykin, N. (2010c). The arts and global health inequities. *Arts & Health: An International Journal for Research Policy and Practice*, **2**, 3–7.

Chanda, M.L. and Levitin, D.J. (2013). The neurochemistry of music. *Trends in Cognitive Sciences*, **17**, 179–193.

Cohen, G.D., Perlstein, S., Chapline, J., Kelly, J., Firth, K.M., and Simmens, S. (2007). The impact of professionally conducted cultural programs on the physical health, mental health and social functioning of older adults—2-year result. *Journal of Aging, Humanities and the Arts*, **1**, 5–22.

Conrad, C. Niess, H., Jauch, K.-W., Bruns, C.J., Hartl, W.H., and Welker, L. (2007). Overture for growth hormone: requiem for interleukin-6? *Critical Care Medicine*, **35**, 2709–2713.

Cuypers, K., Krokstad, S., Holmen, T.L., Knudtsen, M.S., Bygren, L.-O., and Holmen, J. (2012). Patterns of receptive and creative cultural activities and their association with perceived health, anxiety, depression and satisfaction with life among adults: the HUNT study, Norway. *Journal of Epidemiology and Community Health*, **66**, 698–703.

Davidson, J.W. and Fedele, J. (2011). Investigating group singing activity with people with dementia and their caregivers: problems and positive prospects, *Musicae Scientiae*, **15**, 402–422.

Duncan, R.P. and Earhart, G.M. (2012). Randomized controlled trial of community-based dancing to modify disease progression in Parkinson disease. *Neurorehabilitation and Neural Repair*, **26**, 132–143.

Earhart, G.M. (2009). Dance as therapy for individuals with Parkinson disease. *European Journal of Physical and Rehabilitation Medicine*, **45**, 231–238.

Ginsborg, J., Spahn, C., and Williamon, A. (2012). Health promotion in higher music education. In: R. MacDonald, G. Kreutz, and L. Mitchell (eds), *Music, Health, and Wellbeing*, pp. 356–366. Oxford: Oxford University Press.

Grape, C., Sandgren, M., Hansson, L.O., Ericson, M., and Theorell, T. (2003). Does singing promote wellbeing? An empirical study of professional and amateur singers during a singing lesson. *Integrative Physiological and Behavioral Science*, **38**, 65–74.

Gütay, W. and Kreutz, G. (2011). Entwicklung der Singstimme von Kindern in Chorklassen: Eine medizinisch-physikalische Längsschnittuntersuchung von Stimmleistungsparametern [Development of the singing voice in children: a medical–physical longitudinal study of vocal performance]. In: B. Schwarz, P. Nenniger, and R.S. Jäger (eds), pp. 155–163. *Erziehungswissenschaftliche Forschung—nachhaltige Bildung*. Landau: Verlag Empirische Pädagogik.

Hackney, M.E. and Earhart, G.M. (2009a). Effects of dance on movement control in Parkinson's disease: a comparison of Argentine tango and American ballroom. *Journal of Rehabilitation Medicine*, **41**, 475–481.

Hackney, M.E. and Earhart, G.M. (2009b). Short duration, intensive tango dancing for Parkinson disease: an uncontrolled pilot study. *Complementary Therapies in Medicine*, **17**, 203–207.

Hall, C.B., Lipton, R.B., Sliwinski, M., Katz, M.J., Derby, C.A., and Verghese, J. (2009). Cognitive activities delay onset of memory decline in persons who develop dementia. *Neurology*, **73**, 356–361.

Juslin, P.N. and Sloboda, J.A. (eds) (2010). *Handbook of Music and Emotion: Theory, Research, Applications*. New York: Oxford University Press.

Kirschner, S. and Tomasello, M. (2010). Joint music making promotes prosocial behaviour in 4-year-old children. *Evolution of Human Behavior*, **31**, 354–364.

Koelsch, S. (2011). Towards a neural basis of music perception—a review and updated model. *Frontiers in Psychology*, **2**, 110, doi: 10.3389/fpsyg.2011.00110.

Koelsch, S. and Stegemeier, T. (2012). The brain and positive biological effects in healthy and clinical populations. In: R. MacDonald, G. Kreutz, and L. Mitchell (eds). *Music, Health, and Wellbeing*, pp. 113–124. Oxford: Oxford University Press.

Kreutz, G., Bongard, S., Grebe, D., Rohrmann, S., and Hodapp, V. (2004). Effects of choir singing or listening on secretory IgA, cortisol, and emotional state. *Journal of Behavioral Medicine*, **27**, 623–634.

Kreutz, G., Quiroga Murcia, C., and Bongard, S. (2012). Psychoneuroendocrine research on music and health. An overview. In: R. MacDonald, G. Kreutz, and L. Mitchell (eds), pp. 457–476. *Music, Health, and Wellbeing*. Oxford: Oxford University Press.

LeDoux, J. (1996). *The Emotional Brain: The Mysterious Underpinnings of Emotional Life*. New York: Simon and Schuster.

MacDonald, M., Kreutz, G., and Mitchell, L. (2012). What is music, health and wellbeing and why is it important? In: R. MacDonald, G. Kreutz, and L. Mitchell (eds), pp. 3–11. *Music, Health, and Wellbeing*. Oxford: Oxford University Press.

Nettl, B. (1956). *Music in Primitive Culture*. Cambridge, MA: Harvard University Press.

Nilsson, U. (2009). The effect of music intervention in stress response to cardiac surgery in a randomized clinical trial. *Heart and Lung*, **38**, 201–207.

Quiroga Murcia, C., Bongard, S., and Kreutz, G. (2009). Emotional and neurohumoral responses to dancing tango Argentino: the effects of music and partner. *Music and Medicine*, **1**, 14–21.

Quiroga Murcia, C., Kreutz, G., Clift, S., and Bongard, S. (2010). Shall we dance? An exploration of the perceived benefits of dancing on wellbeing. *Arts & Health: An International Journal for Research, Policy and Practice*, **2**, 149–163.

Quiroga Murcia, C., Kreutz, G., and Bongard, S. (2011). Endocrine und immunologische Wirkungen von Musik [Endocrine and immunologic effects of music]. In: Schubert, C. (ed.), *Psychoneuroimmunologie und Psychotherapie*, pp. 248–262. Stuttgart: Schattauer.

Roden, I., Kreutz, G., and Bongard, S. (2012). Effects of a school-based instrumental music program on verbal and visual memory in primary school children: a longitudinal study. *Frontiers in Psychology*, **3**, 572, doi: 10.3389/fpsyg.2012.00572.

Russo, F.A., Vempala, N.N., and Sandstrom G.M. (2013). Predicting musically induced emotions from physiological inputs: linear and neural network models. *Frontiers in Psychology*, **4**, 468, doi: 10.3389/fpsyg.2013.00468.

Salgado, R. and de Paula Vasconcelos, L. (2010). The use of dance in the rehabilitation of a patient with multiple sclerosis. *American Journal of Dance Therapy*, **32**, 53–63.

Schellenberg, E.G. (2004). Music lessons enhance IQ. *Psychological Science*, **15**, 511–514.

Spintge, R. (2012). Clinical use of music in operating theatres. In: R. MacDonald, G. Kreutz, and L. Mitchell (eds), *Music, Health, and Wellbeing*, pp. 276–288. Oxford: Oxford University Press.

Theorell, T. and Kreutz, G. (2012). Ep idemiological studies of the relationship between musical experiences and public health. In: R. MacDonald, G. Kreutz, and L. Mitchell (eds). *Music, Health and Wellbeing*, pp. 424–435. Oxford: Oxford University Press.

Trappe, H.J. (2012). The effect of music on human physiology and pathophysiology. *Music and Medicine*, **4**, 100–105.

Unwin, M.M., Kenny, D.T., and Davis, P.J. (2002). The effects of group singing on mood. *Psychology of Music*, **30**, 175–185.

Västfjäll, D., Juslin, P.N., and Hartig, T. (2012). Music, subjective wellbeing, and health: the role of everyday emotions. In: R. MacDonald, G. Kreutz, and L. Mitchell (eds). *Music, Health, and Wellbeing*, pp. 405–423. Oxford: Oxford University Press.

Verghese, J., Lipton, R.B., Katz, M.J., et al. (2003). Leisure activities and the risk of dementia in the elderly. *New England Journal of Medicine*, **348**, 2508–2516.

Winkler, I., Háden, G.P., Ladinig, O., Sziller, I., and Honing, H. (2009). Newborn infants detect the beat in music. *Proceedings of the National Academy of Sciences of the United States of America*, **106**, 2468–2471.

Wise, K.J. and Sloboda, J.A. (2008). Establishing an empirical profile of self-defined 'tone deafness': perception, singing performance and self-assessment, *Musicae Scientiae*, **12**, 3–26.

WHO (2013). *Global Strategy on Diet, Physical Activity and Health*. Available at: <http://www.who.int/dietphysicalactivity/goals/en/index.html> (accessed 28 December 2013).

Zatorre, R.J. and Salimpoor, V.N. (2013). From perception to pleasure: music and its neural substrates. *Proceedings of the National Academy of Sciences USA*, **110**(Suppl. 2), 10430–10437.

# CHAPTER 27

# Addressing the needs of seriously disadvantaged children through the arts: the work of Kids Company

Camila Batmanghelidjh

## Introduction

Adam is starving. He draws pictures of food and then swallows the piece of paper. He's 5 years old. Susan was 12 when she ran away from home because her stepfather was abusing her. As an 18-year-old, she looks back on her life creating an installation which shows her experiences of surviving her childhood on the streets: the sandpit she slept in for warmth; the bin liners she scavenged in for food; the buses she rode on to keep safe in the dark. Henry makes a chair exploring the oppression of disadvantaged children through the symbolisms of Nazi Germany.

These three young people are members of Kids Company; a charity founded in 1996, supporting some 36,000 children, young people, and vulnerable adults, many of whom have endured chronic childhood maltreatment (see Box 27.1).

At Kids Company, staff made up of social workers, mental health specialists, teachers, artists, and performers work together to enable traumatized children to regain mastery over their trauma. Ninety-seven per cent of the client group self-refer, hearing about Kids Company services in their schools and on the streets. Once they come to our premises they are greeted with an environment full of colour and welcome. In fact, independent research shows that the children become attached to the fabric of the building and its routines before they make investments in the workers (Lemma 2010).

Kids Company's street-level centres are open 5–7 days a week, from early morning until evening. Kids Company offers opportunities to children and young people to engage in a wide range of creative activities including music, fashion (the young people have developed their own fashion brand, Bare Thread, which has been stocked in department stores such as Liberty and Selfridges), and film-making. All the centres have art rooms which are staffed with therapists, artists, and arts therapists who are all supervised once a week by a senior clinician. Children can drop in to these art rooms and engage in work. Over the last 17 years we have acquired an understanding of the type of journey traumatized children take through their art. In this chapter I hope to share some of the significant aspects of the children's relationship with artistic expression.

## The children served by Kids Company

Many of the clients of Kids Company are recognized as being profoundly traumatized. They endure a toxic combination of childhood maltreatment and environmental adversity. An independent evaluation carried out by a research team at University College London demonstrated that of those children assessed and attending our street-level centres one in five had been shot at and/or stabbed in their lifetime, with 50% of the children witnessing shootings and stabbings within the last year. This group ($n = 105$) of children had experienced levels of sexual abuse 13 times higher than a control group ($n = 108$) recruited from inner city London and matched for age and socio-demographic status, with accumulative trauma being at 11.5 times greater than in the controls (data collected as part of Cecil et al. 2014).

Many of the children are excluded from school. They have complex mental health problems, specific learning difficulties, and language-processing challenges. Many are on the autistic spectrum and all are negatively affected by poverty. A survey of 200 home visits involving children aged under 14 demonstrated that a third of the children didn't have a bed to sleep on, with one in four having no chairs or tables. Fifty-eight per cent of the parental group suffered from illnesses, including cancer and mental health difficulties, with only 2% of the children living with both parents (Kids Company 2012).

Our neurophysiological research project with the Anna Freud Centre, led by Professor Pasco Fearon, provided the first preliminary evidence of the effects of Kids Company's intervention in reversing the negative consequences of childhood adversity for children attending Kids Company. This project was a world first in collaborative, clinically focused neuroscientific research. This project measured adolescents' pre-conscious response to emotional stimuli. Three groups participated: a control group of healthy, typically developing children, a group of children new

---

**Box 27.1**  The history of Kids Company

Eighteen years ago, supporting a handful of neglected and vulnerable children and young people under the Arches in Waterloo, Camila Batmanghelidjh recognized the urgent need to provide these children with the crucial support they were not receiving elsewhere.

Five years later, in 1996, she established Kids Company which opened its doors to some 400 profoundly disturbed children and young people. The charity now supports 36,000 inner-city children across London and Bristol; 18,000 of these are intensively supported with therapeutic and social interventions. Kids Company operates through four street-level centres, four alternative education centres, and two therapeutic centres across London and Bristol. It also offers therapeutic and social work services in over 40 schools.

Uniquely, Kids Company works on a self-referral basis, meaning that typically hard-to-reach children are able to access support themselves, rather than relying on a carer to seek help for them. The intention is to 'return to children their childhood', facilitated by practical and emotional guidance, as well as much-needed love and comfort. By fostering a sense of emotional interconnectedness, the organization empowers children who have been disenfranchised, offering them a sense of self that may previously have been absent. Currently, Kids Company is working as a catalyst for a marked change in government policy and practice in relation to young offenders.

---

**Box 27.2**  Indicators of the success of Kids Company

Independent evaluation of Kids Company clients by Queen Mary University of London (Gaskell 2008) has shown that of those assessed:

- 94% reduced their substance misuse
- 89% of our young people improved their anger management
- 97% of our children find Kids Company's services to be effective in supporting their needs

**Higher education**

In 2013, Kids Company was able to compile a comprehensive summary of its provision and impact on the lives of the young people as part of their report to the Department for Education (Kids Company 2013). The needs of a select group of the most at-risk clients (the 'Legit Living' group of 750 children and young people) were closely monitored, along with the impact of the interventions and support that Kids Company provided. Of the Legit Living kids, 96% of those aged under 16 were helped to either return to education or sustain themselves within it through additional support from Kids Company. Ninety-five per cent of young people over 16 were supported into further or higher education, to secure apprenticeships, short courses, work experience, and employment.

The results of Kids Company's interventions were:

- 86% (of relevant age) engaged in work experience
- 91% were reintegrated into education
- 81% achieved academically

---

to Kids Company, and a group who had been at Kids Company for an average of 1.5 years. Significant differences were found in the group new to Kids Company. Their pre-conscious emotional response to negative stimuli was almost non-existent compared with the control group. Such hypo-activation is an indication of chronic exposure to adversity and is maladaptive in that it can inhibit the normal interactional processes that are important in forming and maintaining healthy relationships. The third group who had all been supported by key workers from Kids Company for an average of 1.5 years showed a level of pre-conscious emotional response that was almost the same as the control groups (Fearon et al. 2013, pre-press preliminary findings).

Kids Company is committed to the careful evaluation of its services and the promotion of basic research into the damaging effects of early childhood neglect and abuse (see Box 27.2).

## Reaching children through art

When children are catastrophically consumed by complex trauma involving deficiencies in attachment and depletions in material resources they already present with fragilities which can be devastated by abuse. Devastated children have an idiosyncratic relationship with the creative task: faced with a blank piece of paper, they experience the demand of a creative opportunity more as a persecution than a source of joy. In the art room the child often feels furious when asked to be creative, or profoundly empty, unable to draw out an image or engage in a communication.

For children like this there is a need for a starting point. The arts facilitator goes to meet the child on the page by maybe drawing a line and then helping the child to develop it, or by using collage,

which involves the rearrangements of objects as opposed to their primary creation. It is as if the child is being invited onto the page with the promise that there won't be abandonment or the demand to produce a personally creative expression on their own. As children grow in confidence and begin to feel safe in the art room, reassured by the compassionate and thoughtful presence of the arts facilitator, they gradually attempt to venture into more personalized creative communications. These tend to have a concrete likeness to the trauma they may be grappling with, as reflected in Fig. 27.1, 'The Pink Room'. It is not uncommon in phase two of the creative evolution to see children disclose traumatic events through visual images: sexually abused children will make clay penises, those who have had encounters with firearms will draw the weapon in great detail and, in doing so, the object of their terror is made manifest, almost like a carbon copy telling a story, recreating the weaponry of trauma in the art room.

These concrete presentations are the child's attempt to check the worker's tolerance and sensitivity. If the worker is over-shocked the child will feel they are incapable of receiving the traumatic encounter. On the other hand, if the worker is under-reactive, the child will feel unsafe as the magnitude of their experience is not recognized. So the reaction of arts facilitators to these concrete manifestations of traumatic encounters is an important prerequisite for allowing the emotional reactions that are not yet delivered to be made visible. Arts facilitators need to establish a dialogue in which they acknowledge that something important is being

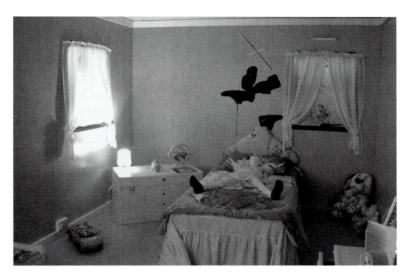

**Fig. 27.1** 'The Pink Room' was made by a group of children who had been sexually abused. The mobile symbolizes how the innocence of childhood was prematurely jeopardized by the men who raped them. From the Kids Company exhibition Shrinking Childhood at Tate Modern, 2004.
Reproduced by kind permission of Camila Batmanghelidjh. Copyright © 2015 Camila Batmanghelidjh.

communicated. They have to be honest about its impact on them, and in being appropriately and genuinely emotional they give the child permission to come through with their reactions, knowing that the discourse of emotions is possible within the art room.

Once children feel safe they move on to represent the ferociousness of their emotional reactions in the trauma narrative. The sexually abused child may scribble spirals on the page showing the sensations of being penetrated. The child who is being attacked with a firearm will spill the red paint all over the page and over themselves to communicate the impact of their head being cracked open with the butt of the gun. These expressions are often repetitive, trance-like, and visceral, as the body mimics the linear movement generated on the page. Children can feel out of control, their upset can spill into the art room where they may engage in fights with other kids, destroy pieces of work—their own and others—and generally vacillate between defensive hyperactivity or despairing apathy.

This phase of making the trauma visible tends to be repetitive, as the child has the compulsion to grapple with the material. The arts facilitator needs to travel the tightrope between allowing the work and yet maintaining the boundaries so that the child doesn't feel overwhelmed by the repetition. On a neurophysiological level this evacuation phase has the impact of shifting the traumatic memory and the tension that it has generated within the limbic system and allowing a release of the stress. Traumatized children harbour very concrete memories of events which are triggered through delivering a repetition where, once again, the child is re-traumatized through a re-experiencing of the assaults. Children can become very disorientated as the boundaries between now and the traumatic events of the past are eroded and the child is simultaneously enacting and re-experiencing traumatic events in which the whole of the art room is perceived in the context of protagonists. Children describe seeing the features of their persecutors on the faces of the arts facilitators. They may experience bodily sensations, smells, and even have auditory hallucinations. Within minutes the art room can erupt, driven by the frenzy of one child which can vicariously spread to other children who are simultaneously drawn into the acting out. Therefore it's imperative to have high staff levels so that at times like this children can be given intensive one-to-one support and assisted to regain equilibrium. No matter what the damage in the room, it's important not to engage in using punitive sanctions but to focus on reparation once the potency of the emotions that have been exchanged are acknowledged and the child is reassured.

The visceral acting out phase of traumatic memories gives way to symbolic representations. The child stops manifesting the objects of their traumatic experiences so concretely and they move on to symbolization, transforming everyday material into representations of protagonists in the trauma drama. They may abstract objects, disguise them, hide them, or substitute them. The trauma is there, but it's been manipulated; it's malleable and the child makes a shift from being possessed and persecuted by it to gaining mastery over it by transforming it visually, as demonstrated in Fig. 27.2, 'Mr Googly Woogly'.

Subtleties develop, children become pensive and reflective and they begin to look back on traumatic events rather than be overcome by them. Their art acquires a poetry as it becomes more archetypal in its representation.

## Moving on from art as therapy

It is at this juncture that traumatized children often make a choice as to whether they would like to go on to pursue art as a potential career or a political commentary. Those who pursue the arts as a hobby or a vocation begin to widen their artistic language, showing an interest in other artists assimilating other people's works, and developing an artistic dialogue with a viewing public in mind. The private visceral repetition of personal trauma gives way to a more universal artistic language which is more commonly shared and which, intrinsically, has an audience in mind. These children and young people develop a powerful socio-political artistic language where they use their childhood traumas to explore issues of social justice and universal emotions and engage in camaraderie with the dispossessed using their artistic talents. Their work is

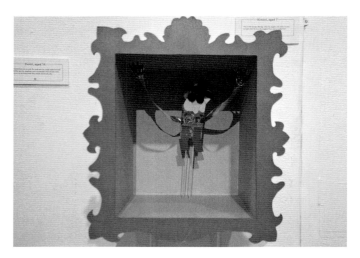

**Fig. 27.2** 'Mr Googly Woogly. When he wiggles his arms no one can get close to him. He wiggles them about really fast', by Kimoni, aged 7. Displayed at the Kids Company's Safe in Our Hands exhibition at the Morley Gallery, 2011.
Reproduced by kind permission of Camila Batmanghelidjh. Copyright © 2015 Camila Batmanghelidjh.

often very powerful because it's delivered at the cusp of private/public tension where deep personal material is universally shared and acknowledged but without it being in the service of processing personal traumatic events.

However, the legacy of damage caused by overwhelming childhood adversity continues to colour the young person's relationship with the arts as a career. These young people have had their sense of personal cohesion prematurely ruptured. They rarely feel solidly glued together. They describe their sense of self as being immensely fragile. Consequently, they tend to experience themselves being at the mercy of personal, emotional storms. Often their moods and energy states fluctuate dramatically and rapidly. When there is a need for consistent engagement with work opportunities or the delivery of artistic projects, the volatility of their emotional state presents them with difficulties in maintaining consistency. If a project is not going well, or the young person feels criticized, they tend to descend into a dark despair from which they often cannot emerge without professional support.

It is in this context that the developmentally traumatized young person requires an on-going 'secure base', both emotionally and practically. The purpose of the secure base is to function like a regulating parental figure, as many of these young people have had disturbed attachment figures. The ability to regulate their own emotions and energy is not so available to them due to vulnerabilities in their frontal lobes where the mechanisms of personal management are thought to be located. In effect, the 'secure base' needs to function like the young person's frontal lobe—the outsider-carer/parental substitute doing the caring and the regulating which the young person cannot do themselves on their own. Over a period of time, as young people continue to receive this type of support, they will be able to tolerate artistic disappointments without being shattered by them. They will also begin to believe in the notions of incubation where the artistic task is being unconsciously processed but is not yet available for realization.

Periods when creative material is blocked terrify the traumatized artist because they feel that, potentially, the only lifeline they

have to pro-social functioning in mainstream society is going to be denied them. Praise and acknowledgement presents its own challenges for young artists who have had chronic childhood adversity. These individuals have a complex relationship with shame. During the abuse they have been catastrophically over-powered and subjected to the perverse intentions of a perpetrator who, in denying them dignity, has rendered them a victim. These children have an exquisite and intrinsic, almost visceral, understanding of how quickly dignity and power can be taken away by someone who may exercise greater force. When they are at the receiving end of criticism, they can almost experience the critical narrative as if it is the abusive encounter repeated. Some of them go as far as fearing and despising the scrutiny of an onlooker because they have developed an idiosyncratic relationship to the human eye. When they've been looked at as a child, the onlooker has made a decision to reject them or to harm them. Therefore, every opportunity for scrutiny presents with an enormous potential for risk to personal safety.

Critical appraisal of their work can feel reminiscent of the initial stages of harm: young people can either despair so much that they want to give up continuing with the creative task entirely or they cannot bear the similarity they perceive between being criticized and being abused. Since they hate the power residing with the critic, as if the abuser is commanding the space, what they do is try and gain mastery over the critical moment: they become defensive, aggressive, and even destructive to the art piece they have created so that they get to do the abusing rather than, as they see it, become the victim of the critic/abuser.

Therefore, in order to give them critical feedback, it is very important for the critic to first acknowledge the artist's gifts and talents and, in doing so, maintain their dignity, and to allow a differentiation between constructive feedback versus critical appraisal which may be confused by the young person as mimicking the degrading moment of abusive assault. For art facilitators to be able to negotiate the complex tightrope of encouraging genuine artistic excellence in young people who want to take up the arts as a career they need to understand the tightrope between critical appraisal and unwittingly re-traumatizing the young person.

At Kids Company a team of art therapists and psychotherapists is available to assist workers as they negotiate the young artists' emotional landmines on a daily basis. Fundamentally, the primary assault of chronic childhood maltreatment impedes the young artist's sense of belief that their achievements are real and valid. Young people describe feelings of profound terror whenever they do well because they believe that their achievements will not have longevity. They expect persecutory and sinister events to randomly interfere with their creative gains just as the perpetrator of their childhood maltreatment interrupted their childhood stability.

The fragility of these artists' sense of self can also mean that they disassociate all too easily. Often these children would have resorted to out of body and mind strategies in order to be able to endure the harm they were being subjected to.

The capacity to absent the self, as a form of defence, is paradoxically what attacks their sense of stability: If they, in their minds, can choose to be present or not then any good that happens can equally be a delusion. Consequently, these young artists seek reassurance, wanting to confirm that those around them did genuinely like their work and actually 'saw it', as if the artist themselves

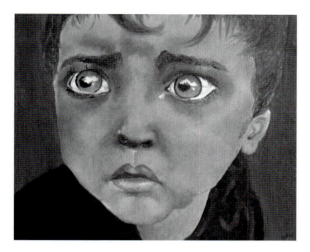

**Fig. 27.3** Child Waiting by Natalie Murphy aged 24. This painting was intended to capture the complexity of abandonment from the perspective of a child. Confusion, fear, and grief—all consequences of loss.
Reproduced by kind permission of Camila Batmanghelidjh. Copyright © 2015 Camila Batmanghelidjh.

doesn't have the confidence to believe they alone created the work; that it was genuinely their own.

When sources of praise and acknowledgement are not available, the artist can experience a catastrophic crisis of abandonment where they feel their mind is playing tricks on them. Maybe they don't exist, maybe the artwork doesn't exist—all because there is no outsider telling them that they are seeing the work and they're valuing it.

Even though the erosion of boundaries between now and then, existence and non-existence, can present as assaults on the integration of the self, the gift from such fragility is also the artist's ability to cross boundaries and draw from seemingly disparate fields, commonalities that get beautifully communicated through the art. It is in this context that traumatized children often go on to produce

awe-inspiring works with subtle, nuanced, and poetic observations about life. The dichotomy between the young people's substantial talent and their exquisite emotional fragility makes for a complex presentation and management of artistic life as a career (Fig. 27.3).

The other factor that often has an impact on these young people is their poor physical health. Prolonged childhood adversity produces chronic terror which in turn heightens the stress response. Relentless exposure to toxic stress results in physiological dysregulation which can manifest as immune or metabolic disorders. So these young artists tend to require assistance with on-going medical issues. A combination of poor care in childhood and the volatility of their mood, as well as creative states, means that as individuals, they can experience themselves as being at the mercy of their own unpredictable bodily states. They may have poor sleep, a fluctuating appetite, and be attracted to substances as a way of regulating themselves.

## Young people's artwork to raise awareness

In 2012 the arts programme at Kids Company was honoured by the Royal Society for Public Health with an award for 'innovative and outstanding contributions to the field of arts and health practice with children and young people'.

Kids Company has produced a number of exhibitions to critical and public acclaim. These exhibitions have been a profound depiction of the challenges the young people face. In 2005 we created Shrinking Childhoods, at the Tate Modern, demonstrating daily life dominated by violence and poverty, such as in Fig. 27.4 'My Emotions', and in 2007 Demons and Angels at Shoreditch Town Hall.

In 2010 we worked with our children to create Shoebox Living, in which children were asked to re-create their home in a shoe box and give a short description; the results providing a snapshot of the lives of children in urban Britain. It toured government departments and was then showcased at the Haunch of Venison and the Saatchi Gallery. More recently, in 2012, 1049 children and young people contributed to our exhibition Childhood—The Real

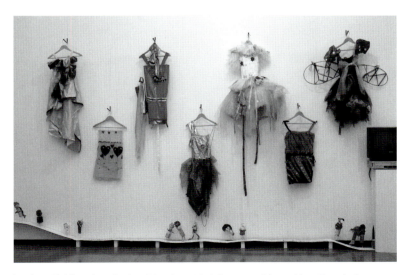

**Fig. 27.4** Kids Company exhibition Shrinking Childhoods at the Royal Academy, 2012. Fourteen girls aged 8 to 13 each chose an emotion which they felt resonated with them and designed a dress to express this.
Reproduced by kind permission of Camila Batmanghelidjh. Copyright © 2015 Camila Batmanghelidjh.

Event at the Royal Academy of Arts which earned five-star reviews and received national attention. In 2013, our children and young people featured their work in a second exhibition at the Royal Academy, Holding Up Childhood which explored themes of family and belonging.

## Summing up

In summary, if a child makes the transition from grappling with personal trauma using the arts to the arts as a career, the legacy of child abuse continues to influence not only the artwork but also the artist's relationship to the arts world. The resilience-giving factor, for both the child who is exploring therapeutically using the arts and the young person who moves on to be an artist, is the availability of a secure base in which the arts facilitator/parental figure functions as a regulator of emotion and energy, as a translator of other people's intentions, and as a source of hope. Many victimized children need to regain access to the hero within themselves. Human beings have a need to believe that they have mastery over their lives. We all depend on a delusion of order, an assumption that everything will be OK. Traumatized children see through this delusion prematurely because they know that their achievements can be destroyed by the cruel intention of another human being at any given moment. For the maltreated child to feel motivated about their future, they therefore need to tune into the ability to be heroic, to experience moments of exceptional excellence or a sense of personal agency. Hopelessness is a painful reality for maltreated children; it follows them like a dark shadow and demotivates them. They need a lot more encouragement to stay on task and cope with frustrations.

Many of the young artists we come across at Kids Company are immensely brave, but their ability to remain heroic despite their devastation is only made possible if, at times of personal collapse, they can turn to someone they trust for help to be glued back together.

Children who do not decide to use the arts as a career often disengage from the art room where they feel they have completed their trauma-processing journey and they almost don't see the point of engaging in the creative process any further. However, interestingly, they periodically come back to the art room almost as if to touch base with the arts facilitators in whose minds they feel a more fragile part of themselves is held safe. It's interesting to see that returns to the art room either bring the child in a more regressed state, as if they want to be nurtured again by the arts worker, or in a more removed state, where they adopt a protective skin and then run a commentary on the fact that the other children are producing artistic material but they don't have a need or the ability to do so. It's as if the child has come back into the room to confirm that they have left it and left the trauma behind in it.

Working artistically with traumatized children is an exciting privilege with profound implications for the child as well as the arts facilitator. Creativity generates an immediate bond which bypasses language and boundaries. The intensity and intimacy of the contact requires a disciplined and thoughtful approach which negotiates permission to be free with the safety of having boundaries. To achieve the required equilibrium, workers need to be psychologically and practically supported so that they enter the art encounter with an open heart and mind. If workers are under-resourced they use defences to protect themselves against the fallout of the child's disturbance. Once traumatized children sense self-protection in workers they lose faith in the ability of the arts facilitator to manage the magnitude of their pain. Withdrawal becomes both the worker's and the child's strategy for survival, and in non-engagement the creative process is murdered.

Every moment in the art room is a psychological treasure, promoting growth in workers and children alike. It's not an easy journey but you'll never forget it.

## References

Cecil, C.A., Viding, E., Barker, E.D., Guiney, J., and McCrory, E.J. (2014). Double disadvantage: the influence of childhood maltreatment and community violence exposure on adolescent mental health. *Journal of Child Psychology and Psychiatry*, **55**, 839–848.

Fearon, P., Pincham, H., and Bryce, D. (2013). A community-based study of neuro-cognitive and endocrine mechanisms associated with behavioural change in children with conduct problems who are offered services by Kids Company. Pre-press preliminary findings.

Gaskell, C. (2008). *Kids Company Helps with the Whole Problem*. London: Kids Company.

Kids Company (2012). *Kids Company: The Flourish Report*. London: Kids Company.

Kids Company (2013). *Improving Outcomes for Children, Young People and Families 2011–2013, for the Department for Education*. London: Kids Company.

Lemma, A. (2010). The power of relationship: a study of key-working as an intervention with traumatized young people. *Journal of Social Work Practice*, **24**, 409–427.

# CHAPTER 28

# The power of dance to transform the lives of disadvantaged youth

Pauline Gladstone-Barrett and Victoria Hunter

## Introduction to dance in mental health and wellbeing

This chapter focuses on the work of Dance United, a national dance charity operating in the United Kingdom in the field of dance and social concern. It provides an overview of Dance United's ethos and approach and explores how the company is adapting and applying its methodology within the context of the mental healthcare field. The chapter presents an outline of a case study: a dance and mental health trial that took place in south London in November and December 2013. Throughout the chapter the images are of the young people in this project performing (Fig. 28.1).

## Background

Applied contemporary dance practice is rapidly expanding in the United Kingdom in line with the growth of the arts in health and social inclusion sector. Over the last 10 years in particular, dance-based interventions within a range of social and healthcare contexts have increased and the social, physical, and psychological benefits of participation in dance have become widely acknowledged (see Box 28.1).

The potentially transformational and life-enhancing properties of dance have received increased attention in the United Kingdom in recent years. A 2012 report commissioned by Dance Exchange and the Department of Health, West Midlands, England, observes:

'Dance is a form of cultural expression that is uniquely placed to achieve health and wellbeing outcomes. At best it combines physical activity, social interaction, creative and emotional expression. All these elements have independent evidence bases showing their potential to improve health and wellbeing. In dance these elements are brought together in a holistic experience that provides pleasure to participants.'

Burkhardt and Rhodes (2012, p. 4)

Dance United is the leading UK dance organization in this field with an international reputation for creating quality contemporary dance training and performance projects with disadvantaged and marginalized individuals and communities and for marrying artistic excellence with social concern in cross-sector collaborations that develop new ways of thinking.

For over a decade the company has demonstrated that intensive interventions modelled on professional dance training can transform the lives of people living in challenging circumstances, such as Ethiopian street children, young people from across the political divides in Berlin and Belfast, and in a range of contexts from across the UK: women in prison, young people in the youth justice system, young people involved with gangs, and those who are not in education, training, or work. Dance United has developed and accredited a core methodology and adapted it for all these situations.

The company is best known in England for its award-winning 2- or 3-month full-time 'academy' programme for young people experiencing multiple challenges and deficits in their lives, such as exclusion from education, homelessness, criminality, addiction, and sexual exploitation. The academy model was piloted in Bradford in 2006 and replicated in London and Hampshire in 2010.

Currently these three academies support around 150 young people every year to overcome their resistance to learning, leave behind destructive behaviour, increase self-efficacy, appreciate their potential, and create realizable goals in education, training, and work. Upon completing the course, 98% of participants gain a National Open College Network qualification at levels 1 or 2, and around 80% go on to live pro-social lives and sustain places at college, in apprenticeships, or work pursuing all manner of subject areas and careers. For these young people, dance has been a means to an end. A third continue dancing as a leisure activity by joining one of Dance United's three regional performance companies and around 10% progress to professional dance training (Miles and Strauss 2008).

Dance United works with people who have never danced before and they are encouraged to go beyond self-limiting beliefs in a tightly focused, highly structured, unerringly consistent and supportive process which is profoundly catalytic. They train every day in contemporary dance, and learn pieces created by leading choreographers and then perform them. This experience provides a powerful metaphor for what else they could go on to achieve in life.

This immersive model offers a holistic dance intervention as it addresses the participants' physical, emotional, and social skills through their daily participation in class and interaction with

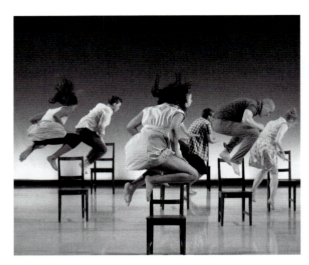

**Fig. 28.1** Dance United repertory piece 'Inbetween' in performance. Choreographed by Carly Annable-Coop and Helen Linsell.
Reproduced by kind permission of Dance United. Copyright © 2015 Dance United.

their peers, dance tutors, and pastoral staff. Through this process the individual's intersubjective and interpersonal skills are significantly developed through physical interactions with others involving touch, spatial partnering, lifting, and weight-bearing tasks and through verbal interactions in which instructions and feedback on others' performance and choreographic work are expressed.

The approach presents a series of challenges for the young people who enter into the programme. These include practical and pragmatic challenges such as turning up on time, abiding by studio discipline, and setting goals alongside the physical demands of developing fitness, flexibility, and stamina. Beyond these very obvious challenges lie a series of more subtly nuanced demands that are specific to the dance genre itself; one of these elements is the challenge of stillness. Finding stillness plays a major role; retreating from external stimuli and focusing 'in' on oneself in order to find a basis from which to begin moving in a controlled manner is a process that many participants find particularly daunting and demanding. This generally involves a process of reckoning and reflection because it requires the individual to be 'here' and consciously engaged in the present moment.

---

**Box 28.1** Examples of UK dance for health and wellbeing initiatives

Dance for Parkinson's Network, including work with the English National Ballet: <http://www.danceforparkinsonsuk.org/>

Merseyside Dance—work with the Alzheimer's Society: <http://www.mdi.org.uk/take-part/health/alzheimers>

Dance Action Zone Leeds—dance and obesity in young people: <http://www.dazl.org.uk/>

---

For many young people whose lives may be particularly chaotic and conflicted, retreating from socio-cultural reality and attending to themselves in a present manner requires considerable effort and practice. The performance of controlled actions either within a solo or group dance situation requires the participants to be responsible for their actions in a particular manner: poised, resisting any temptation to fidget, and ready to move, sometimes leading sometimes following. Through this responsibility and corporeal attunement comes a form of awareness of both themselves and others; an awareness of shared space and shared responsibility for the body's movement in and around the dance/stage space.

## Why dance?

From 2006 to 2008, Dr Andrew Miles and Paul Strauss from the Centre for Research on Sociocultural Change at the University of Manchester evaluated the impact of Dance United's methodology on six cohorts of vulnerable and volatile young people who attended the Bradford pilot during that period. The main focus of the research was whether this particular pedagogy could bring about positive shifts in these young people's lives and, if so, why and how it worked (Miles and Strauss 2008).

From this evaluation there is convincing evidence that this intensive methodology successfully engages a constituency that is largely alienated from formal learning and facilitates measurable increases in confidence, self-awareness, communication, coping skills, flexible thinking, and self-control. Miles and Strauss found that:

◆ dance makes a major positive impact on participants' attitudes and behaviour,

◆ young people are less likely to offend/re-offend than their peers, and

◆ participants have much higher than expected rates of transfer into education, training, and employment; experience improved personal and family relationships; and adopt pro-social lifestyles.

To explain why and how dance works their findings were organized under six headings:

◆ focus

◆ embodied confidence

◆ independent, cooperative and non-verbal learning interactions

◆ teamwork and group identification

◆ emotional engagement

◆ inspiration and aspiration

Focus emerged as a pivotal concept that could not be reduced to an everyday synonym such as 'concentration', but rather encapsulated an approach to bearing and behaviour which stressed the importance of dance as a mental as well as a physical discipline. Focus is an essential foundation for clear thinking, perspective taking, and considered decision-making (Fig. 28.2).

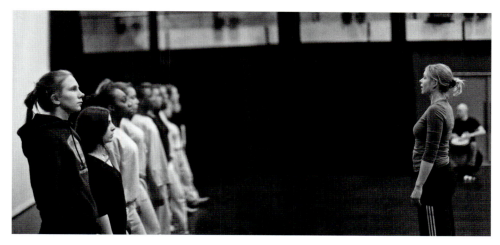

**Fig. 28.2** Dance United Academy dancers focusing for performance. Led by dance director Carly Annable-Coop.
Reproduced by kind permission of Dance United. Copyright © 2015 Dance United.

Embodied confidence was a phrase coined to describe the generally observed improvements in participants' abilities to self-present, such as making eye contact; positive body language, improved posture, listening and asking questions, and displaying a 'can do' attitude. The predictable and oft-repeated claim of 'improved confidence' as an outcome of interventions was refined by the addition of the term 'embodied' to offer a more precise account of the types of changes presented.

Crucially, the report expressed confidence in the bodily techniques employed. The contention was that learning bodily techniques is at least as important as self-reflection or abstract thought in improving one's 'confidence'. The experience of putting together and performing a dance piece led to significant enhancements in

performative self-presentation skills, such as talking in front of the group and interacting with others. Dance was experienced as a physical activity that literally transported participants into a different mindset. For many, embodied confidence was experienced as a 'bodily (re-) awakening' and an emerging sense of physical wellbeing marked by feelings of happiness, increased energy levels, positive outlook, and improvements to body image, including losing weight.

Improvements to the individuals' embodied confidence and their experience of 'independent and cooperative learning interactions' fed and informed a broader process of team-work and group identification as 'a dance company' that was achieved for the most part non-verbally.

One of the key dynamics of the method is its capacity to sponsor or reawaken ambition. The motivation and confidence building associated with personal achievement and public performance in the context of a mutually supportive group gave many participants a new sense of purpose and the belief that they could achieve beyond their current circumstances.

By 2012, having established replications of the academies in London and Hampshire, Dance United was ready to explore a new application of its methodology (Fig. 28.3).

## Contemporary dance in a mental health setting

High rates of mental health issues are encountered within the constituencies the company had focused on to date, so a logical next step was to test the efficacy of a dance-based intervention in a mental health setting with the ambition of developing a teaching model and choreography suited to this context.

In October 2012 senior personnel from a biomedical research institution, the Institute of Psychiatry at King's College, London (IoP), and a front-line clinical team, the South London and Maudsley National Health Service (NHS) Foundation Trust (SLaM), attended The Place in London and watched Dance United's Academy

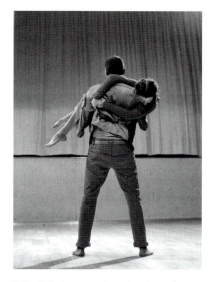

**Fig. 28.3** Dance United's Seabreeze project, duet in performance. Choreographed by Dam Van Huynh.
Reproduced by kind permission of Dance United. Copyright © 2015 Dance United.

beneficiaries performing on stage. Having witnessed the power of dance as an intervention, a research context started to emerge: a unique collaboration between Dance United, the IoP, SLaM, and two voluntary organizations (Bipolar UK and Rethink Mental Illness) that aimed to break new ground artistically and medically.

## The need

The partners wanted to test an intervention for young adults aged 18–35 living in south London who were in the early stages of diagnosis and treatment of schizophrenia, bipolar disorder, and other mental health conditions. The typical profiles included those who had sought help for psychological problems, with impairment in psychosocial functioning and specific signs and symptoms indicating high risk of bipolar disorder and those with an early diagnosis of schizophrenia, experiencing psychosis, or being treated by their GP for depression/anxiety.

The health partners identified three key problems experienced by these young adults:

* they often feel isolated and struggle with interpersonal relationships
* they struggle with their bodily awareness and physical fitness and this has a negative impact on their overall levels of confidence, and
* they find it hard to get up in the morning and to maintain energy and optimism, with a liability to over-focus on their condition and worry about the future

The broader health ambitions were threefold:

1. To reduce the stigma associated with accessing mental health services and to consequently reduce the co-morbidity of delayed diagnosis (over 80% of bipolar symptoms, for example, are detectable by the age of 35). Co-morbidity is a big issue for this particular client group, often resulting from poor social networks and family relationships, drug and alcohol addiction, psychosis and general developmental difficulties, and, sometimes, involvement in the criminal justice system and gang membership (Coid et al. 2013).

2. To illuminate the fact that modern medications for these conditions do not impair movement functions. Rather, people in treatment can carry on living with normal physical mobility and their capacity to dance clearly demonstrated this point.

3. To draw attention to recent radical changes in the model for delivery of care from clinical management to holistic recovery; a combination of rounded assessment and active focused intervention with the language of pushing boundaries, positive risk-taking and personal aspirations.

## The approach

Dance movement psychotherapy and mindful movement practice are both used within the UK NHS. The company found it helpful to spend time with specialists from these two disciplines working within SLaM to clarify commonalities and distinctions. Dance United's process aimed to improve participants' overall mental wellbeing from a number of angles through active engagement with professional contemporary dance.

At the heart of the trial was a 4-week full-time dance-based intervention in which participants, recruited by their clinical workers, learnt how to dance and then rehearsed and performed an original dance work to invited audiences. They also engaged in trust-building and team-building exercises and shared healthy lunches.

The 15-minute dance piece 'Seabreeze' was created in a choreographic laboratory by Dance United's associate artist, Dam Van Huynh, and two of the company's most experienced dance directors, Ellen Steinmuller and Carly Annable-Coop. Van Huynh is highly regarded for his research work in contemporary dance in the United States, Hong Kong, and Europe, and takes a distinctive three-dimensional view of how a person trains, looks, feels, and digests movement through his or her own body (Fig. 28.4).

## The challenges

Because the participants were NHS patients there were a number of safeguarding issues that fell under the heading of the 'do no

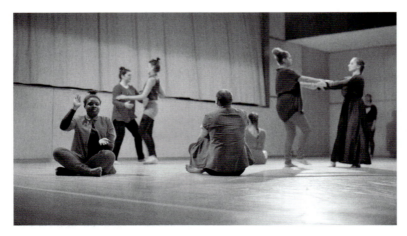

**Fig. 28.4** Dance United's Seabreeze project, dancers in performance. Choreographed by Dam Van Huynh.
Reproduced by kind permission of Dance United. Copyright © 2015 Dance United.

harm' principle, and the referral partners therefore retained overall responsibility for their clients. In preparation for the project, the clinicians and the dance team exchanged skills and knowledge; the former experienced dance first-hand and discovered from within how the process brings about embodied shifts, the latter learnt about models of treatment, medication, duty of care, treatment environments, and the ethics surrounding the collection and use of data.

There were some concerns expressed by the clinical collaborators that working in a highly disciplined art form might be experienced as stressful, so the dance team modified their facilitation style to be gently persuasive rather than driven; the language of pressure, push, and urgency gave way to a softer style, albeit harnessing creative energy and tension and working with high artistic and production values. Four 'role models' drawn from backgrounds such as post-graduate dance and psychology were trained and embedded in the group to help maintain focus and energy. There were also some concerns that people with these profiles could find it very challenging to get up every day to attend an intensive project and might not want to be brought together as a group (which they often seek to avoid because of the associated stigma). This did not prove the case.

Eighteen clients started the trial and 16 completed it, performing three times at the Jerwood Space in London in December 2013 to invited audiences that included clinical staff, families, funders, and academics. It was a huge success.

## Measuring change

A theory of change was created to articulate how the activities and their key qualities could lead to a number of measurable intermediate outcomes to establish whether progress had been made towards the overarching goals: positive functioning, positive affect, and greater satisfaction in interpersonal relationships.

Seven intermediate outcomes were identified:

◆ communication skills—communicating effectively when interacting during classes and rehearsals

◆ stillness and bodily control—showing observable moments of stillness, bodily control, and mastery of movement

◆ resilience—having energy for and commitment to the dance project and overcoming challenges and obstacles along the way

◆ level of trust in others—trusting and being trusted when executing paired and group movements such as lifts and holds.

◆ level of optimism—believing in their capacity to achieve a high-quality dance performance

◆ working as part of a team—negotiating group solutions to dance challenges that require cooperation and timing

◆ symbolic expression—expressing ideas and feelings symbolically through dance movement

The IoP played a key role in assessing the efficacy of the intervention. Evaluation tools included the Warwick Edinburgh Mental Wellbeing Scale which is used extensively in the NHS to measure change and involved participants self-scoring at the beginning, middle, and end of the intervention.

The group moved (overall) from below average wellbeing (levels similar to people describing their health status as poor) to achieving normal levels of wellbeing (above the norm for this population). The average score for the general population as a whole is just under 51. The participants started below this (mid 40s) and had a 10-point increase to a final score of 53.9. For context, a recent evaluation of a range of 3-month group exercise projects in mental health found an average increase of three points from 43 at baseline to 46. The baseline in the Dance United group was similar to that of people taking part in this study, and the increase of 10 points looks very impressive in that context. On an individual level, 13 of those who completed the trial improved in respect of the seven intermediate outcomes.

The assessment of 'symbolic expression', involved systematic observation of each individual's movement qualities and dynamics using Laban Movement Analysis which 'is increasingly recognized world-wide in the fields of dance movement therapy and in the performing arts as a common language for communication about movement' (Bloom, 2006). All 16 had developed and expanded their range of movement dynamics.

Participants were also assessed for aspects of their performance under the headings of flow, weight, space, and time, and showed improvements in all areas. Flow conveys varying attitudes towards the continuity and control with which a motion is performed, either 'free' or 'bound', and is frequently related to feelings. Weight involves varying attitudes towards physically exerting force and using one's weight to have an intentional impact on the environment, either 'light' or 'strong'; it is generally related to sensing and the physical attitude of intention. Space describes different ways of attending to the environment and orientating one's motions in space, either indirectly or directly; it is associated with inner impulses related to attention and is related to thinking processes. Time describes the pace contained in the movement, either 'sustained' or 'sudden'; it is related to intuition and decision-making processes.

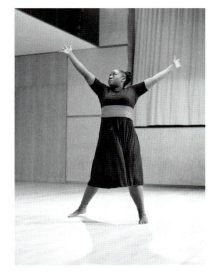

**Fig. 28.5** Dance United's Seabreeze project, solo in performance. Choreographed by Dam Van Huynh.

## The next steps for Dance United

The encouraging early results from the evaluation of dance for young people affected by mental health challenges have galvanized Dance United and the IoP to pursue a longer-term research programme.

The IoP is interested in putting together a small pilot study to thoroughly evaluate short-term impact in which where people are randomized between starting in the next group or waiting for the one after next. Additional measures would be used such as the General Health Questionnaire, and the assessment of symptoms of mental distress.

The current trial completers have the opportunity to carry on learning dance by attending a weekly performance company in south London. A 15-minute broadcast-quality film was made to advocate for the potential of this work within the field of mental health care services.

Dance United's long-term ambition is to build a strong bridge between the worlds of professional contemporary dance and mental healthcare with a repertoire of outstanding dance suited to this context and sufficient dance facilitators and choreographers trained to deliver this work (Fig. 28.5).

## References

Bloom, K. (2006). *The Embodied Self: Movement and Psychoanalysis*. London: Karnac.

Burkhardt, J. and Rhodes, J. (eds) (2012). *Danceactive: Commissioning Dance for Health and Wellbeing*. Available from: <http://www.dancexchange.org.uk/uploads/participate/Commissioning_Doc_Jan_Burkhardt_V6Final1V3.pdf> (accessed 16 March 2014).

Coid, J.W., Ullrich, S., Keers, R., et al. (2013). Gang membership, violence, and psychiatric morbidity, *American Journal of Psychiatry*, **170**, 985–993.

Miles, A. and Strauss, P. (2008). *The Academy: A Report on Outcomes for Participants June 2006–June 2008*. ESRC Centre for Research on Socio-Cultural Change, University of Manchester. Available at: <http://www.dance-united.com/system/files/media/resource/files/two_year_%20academy%20report.pdf>

# CHAPTER 29

# The arts and older people: a global perspective

Trish Vella-Burrows

## Participatory arts in a changing social and political world

In the twenty-first century, long life, health, happiness, liberty, fraternity, equality, power, wealth, wisdom, virtue, and morality are variously prioritized as quests for a good life in societies across the world (Prescott-Allen 2001). There is much historical and present-day evidence to show how human beings use the arts to variably identify, embody, express, celebrate, navigate, maintain, and communicate elements of positive living within the context of their cultural values, beliefs, and practices.

As social and political tides ebb and flow, opportunities to explore and express positive living through the arts have changed. Community-inclusive arts practices that were once widely embedded into the everyday routines of now developed countries through, for example, celebratory and rites-of-passage traditions, now share a place with the worldwide phenomenon of consumer arts and the manufacture of socially and politically motivated opportunities for individuals and communities to participate actively in the arts.

This chapter focuses on older people as active participants in art. It discusses issues of motivation and opportunity, and the relationship between arts and health and wellbeing in the context of an unprecedented rise of the world's older populations over the next 50 years.

## Global demographics: older people in developing and developed countries

Demographic predicators at the beginning of the twenty-first century suggest a tripling between 2000 and 2050 of the global population aged 60 and above, from 600 million to an estimated 2 billion across developed and developing countries (UN 2002). The highest increase in numbers of people aged 65 and above is expected in India and China; in India the number will increase by nearly 280% between 2011 and 2050 (UN 2002). Alongside these demographic projections there are implications for a worrying correlation with age-related ill-health and the subsequent burden on state welfare systems as well as workforce capacity arising from a reversal of the ratio of older to younger people (NIA et al. 2011) (Fig. 29.1).

## Building cultural and social capital

National and international organizations such as the World Health Organization (WHO; Ageing and Life Course), the Centre for Policy on Ageing (England), the Age Institute (Finland), the Institute of Older Persons and Social Services (Spain), the Stockholm Gerontology Research Center (Sweden), the National Council on Ageing and Older People (Ireland), the China Research Center on Aging, the National Council on Aging (United States), the Department of Health and Ageing (Australia), and the International Longevity Centre (India) are driving research and strategic policies in their countries or domains that aim to divert a widespread crisis, commonly referred to as the 'grey tsunami'.

Central to emerging policies is the economic status of a country, as calculated by its gross national income (GNI) (International Statistical Institute 2013). Developmental progress is widely measured by the human development index (HDI) which uses three indicator domains: income, education, and health (UNDP 2013). Linked to these domains are the concepts of *cultural* and *social capital*.

In the twenty-first century the term *cultural capital* is synonymous with community, family, social norms, values, tastes, and preferences (e.g. Yosso 2005; Winkler-Wagner 2010). The relationship between *cultural* and *social capital* and health and wellbeing is evident in the literature on participatory arts. For example, a report for the Chicago Center for the Arts Policy, acknowledges:

> '[Community-based arts] helps to build individual and community assets by fostering social inclinations and skills critical to civic renewal.'
>
> Wali et al. (2002, p. x)

The report highlights activities such as community theatre, drama and community singing groups, writing poetry, portrait-painting, and other less formally organized activities such as cooking and crafts that generally fall outside the commercial world of consumer art and side-step its historical dominance by art-elitism (Bishop 2012). Over half (51%) of the art-generating participants surveyed for this report were aged 50 and above. Similarly, a national survey conducted in 2008 in the United States found that nearly one-third of 18,000 surveyed citizens who had created or performed a work of art over the previous year were aged 55 and above (National Endowment for the Arts 2009).

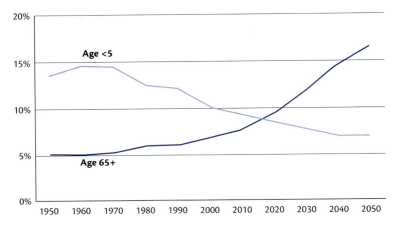

**Fig. 29.1** Ratio shifts between older people and the young globally between 1950 and 2050.
Reproduced with permission from the National Institute on Aging (NIA), National Institute of Health (NIH), and the World Health Organization (WHO), 2011, *Global Health and Ageing.*
Available online at: <http://www.who.int/ageing/publications/global_health/en/>. Copyright © 2011 NIA (NIH)/WHO.

## Participatory arts, health and wellbeing in later life

The apparent appeal of participation in the arts among older people indicates the likelihood of an associated self-regulation of wellbeing. Such self-supporting actions are crucially important in view of the ageing world population and the potential for age-related disadvantages such as ill-health, social exclusion (Greaves and Farbus 2006; Cutler 2009), and, as specifically focused on by the UK-wide End to Loneliness campaign, loneliness and isolation.

For the last two decades, research evidence on the health impact of cultural engagement, creative endeavour and productivity, and aesthetic appreciation has gathered momentum. This growth is based on a better understanding between these elements and evolving definitions of health and wellbeing (e.g. Department of Health 2007; Stickley and Duncan 2007; White 2009; Clift et al. 2009; Bungay and Clift 2012; Clift 2012; Swindells et al. 2013).

Emerging concepts of health and wellbeing support their dynamic nature and highlight the multiple factors that underpin judgements of health. Definitions of good health have shifted from the 'absence of disease' (WHO 1946) to 'positive social and personal resources, as well as physical capacities' (WHO 1986, p. 1), and more recently health has been defined as the ability to engage in 'activity and participation' (WHO 2001, p. 3).

Alongside concern with the nature of health sits the scrutiny of wellbeing, and moreover, mechanisms and pathways that lead to a state of wellbeing. Identified enablers of wellbeing include 'leading a life of purpose' (Ryff and Singer 1998, pp. 7–8) and 'creativity and cultural expression and meaningful connections to others in our social world' (Hasselkus 2011, p. xii). Related to these are the pursuits of 'personal growth', 'noticing things', 'maintaining learning', and 'giving', each of which, according to Aked et al. (2008), is central to the maintenance of wellbeing.

Terms such as *happiness* (Bormans 2011), *healthfulness* (Seedhouse 1997), *flourishing* (Seligman 2011), and *wellness* (e.g. Beaumont 2011) have been adopted in an attempt to define a sense of holistic wellbeing that underpins a good life. While slow, there is emerging in England a renewed momentum to generate

evidence-based pathways to promote such wellbeing through wellness-focused services (Beaumont 2011). On a more global level, the WHO's Active Ageing Policy Framework suggests that healthy ageing services should:

> 'Enable individuals to continue to work according to their capacities and preferences as they grow older, and to prevent or delay disabilities and chronic diseases that are costly to individuals, families and the health care system.'

(WHO 2002, p. 9)

This changing philosophical approach to health and wellbeing sits alongside growing evidence for a positive relationship between participatory arts and good quality of life in older age (e.g. Cohen 2006; Cutler 2009; Organ 2013). Established academic research centres, for example the Sidney De Haan Research Centre for Arts and Health (Canterbury Christ Church University), Arts for Health (Manchester Metropolitan University), the Centre for Clinical and Health Services Research (University of the West of England), and the Winchester Centre for Research into the Arts as Wellbeing (University of Winchester), are each contributing to a greater understanding of the role of the arts in this context. Their work and the continued work of advocates and campaigners for the arts and health movement, such as the National Alliance for Arts, Health and Wellbeing (England) is propelling forward an argument for reorienting mainstream health promotion services to include the widespread prescription of participatory arts (e.g. Bungay and Clift 2010).

The likely motivation for bringing participatory arts into the mainstream will have at its core the need to offset overbearing reliance on state welfare systems in the future. This brings to the fore questions about efficacy; could the widespread mobilization of participatory arts help to quell the worst-case consequences of a global 'grey tsunami'?

## Evidence, opportunities, and challenges

Today, the terms 'arts' and 'culture' are often used interchangeably with 'creativity' to define a spectrum of activities that nurture the human imperative or, arguably, 'biological necessity' for creative employment (Dissanayake 1992; White 2009). Csikszentmihalyi

(1999) defines creativity simply as, 'the ability to add something new to the culture'. Other discussions emphasize the importance of an individuals' ability to draw from the entire range of their experiences in order to respond creatively and positively to new challenges. This is expressed well by Seltzer and Bentley (1999):

> 'It is about equipping people with the skills they need to live full lives; the ability to respond creatively and confidently to changing situations and unfamiliar demands, to solve the problems and challenges they face at home, in education, at work, to make a positive contribution to the life of their communities.'
>
> Seltzer and Bentley (1999, p. 9)

Opportunities for a life-long creative continuum may link to a cyclical process in which creative thinking supports management of, and resilience to, age-related stressors. It may also engender a sense of individuality, community, cultural identity and value, and personal and community growth (e.g. Cohen 2000, 2006; Flood and Phillips 2007). Combining these factors with the common retention of creative will in later life, the use of participatory arts as a mechanism to support individual health and wellbeing and cultural vitality may appear cut and dried. Yet a raft of compounding factors has led to a dichotomy that separates art from everyday practices. These factors include: widespread social mobility, which has disturbed the traditions of family groups and mono-ethnic communities; the global saturation of commercial culture circumventing the arts world; the media-driven, constructed judgements that favour finely tuned elite art products over and above everyday arts and crafts; the growing association between the arts and popular cults of individuality and celebrity; and the widespread marginalization of the arts in education systems. These phenomena, the momentum of which has gathered variably over decades across an increasing number of cultures, have had a significant impact not only on how, when, and where the people practice art, but also on the value assigned to the resulting products.

Alongside the compartmentalization of participatory arts, changing social cultures, youth- and market-driven dominance, digital information technology, media preoccupation with young people, and ageist attitudes have all contributed to the decentralization of older people from the communities to which they belong (Cuddy and Fiske 2002). The consequences of these combined social and political forces simultaneously jeopardize: (1) the common-place practice of everyday participatory arts, which were once well established vehicles for supporting individual, community, and societal wellbeing; and (2) the level at which older people can make a meaningful contribution to their communities, which has hitherto centred on protection of younger generations and conveyance and transfer of skill and cultural heritage. The extent to which re-engagement with participatory arts in older age might reverse these factors, and, moreover, contribute to facilitating perceptions of a good life, depends largely upon a country's strategic targets and economic state, and perceptions of value at a government, community, and individual level.

The following sections report on two participatory art initiatives and two research projects that collectively represent seven national perspectives of the value of participatory arts programmes that aim to promote *healthfulness, flourishing,* and *wellness* in older age.

## Case study 1. India: 'Dance for PD' (Parkinson's disease), Pune

This case study highlights the PD-related work of internationally renowned contemporary dance teacher, choreographer, and founder of the Centre of Contemporary Dance (HCCD), Hrishikesh Pawar. Together with movement-based training specialist Maithily Bhupatkar, Pawar delivers the Dance for PD programme in Pune, India in affiliation with the Mark Morris Dance Group (MMDG) in New York (see <http://danceforparkinsons.org>).

The national context of Pawar's and Bhupatkar's work is one of health inequalities that can severely inhibit a good life for older people. An estimated 100 million people of the Indian population of 1.27 billion are aged over 50. Of this number, 73% are non-literate and dependent on physical labour (HelpAge India 2013). Over one-third live below the poverty line and fewer than 10% have healthcare insurance. By 2050 there will be an estimated 323 million older people living in India. In addition to an unprecedented growth in the number of people aged 80 or more, the ongoing trajectory of social change, which includes more older people living with a spouse or alone rather than with their extended families, highlights the need to sustain a healthy and independent life for as long as possible. Yet currently around half of the older population have multiple chronic diseases and around 13% are affected negatively by a disease burden leading to disability adjusted life-years (DALYs; a measure of overall disease burden, expressed as the number of years lost due to ill-health, disability, or early death) (Population Reference Bureau 2011).

One globally prevalent, long-term health condition that can induce a significant disease burden is PD. According to estimates, in 2008 around 8% of the global total of people with PD lived in India. The growing body of Parkinson's-centred research emphasizes the need to address the complex spectrum of physical, mental, and social challenges associated with the condition. Some of this work centres on the benefits of various types of dance and movement (e.g. Hackney and Earhart 2010; Houston and McGill 2011).

As artistic director and programme manager, respectively, Pawar and Bhupatkar are passionately committed to dance as a medium for positive change. Their interest in people with PD arose initially through the work of the MMDG's Dance for PD programme in New York. In response to the MMDG's mission to train, nurture, and certify qualified teachers in their Dance for PD approach, Bhupatkar spent a month in New York absorbing their working model (Fig. 29.2).

In conversation with the author of this chapter, Pawar reported that planning the initiative in Pune was fraught with cultural, organizational, and financial challenges. However, in partnership with Pune-based support group Parkinson Mitra Mandal, and with initial space for the classes and medical advice provided by the Sancheti Institute for Orthopaedics and Rehabilitation (SIOR), the Pune programme is now thriving. The classes, which are run three times a week in a venue currently sponsored by a participating patient, are free to participants. The content of the classes is grounded in Pawar's diverse training and professional expertise, through which he overcame cultural tensions, and the MMDG training undertaken by Bhupatkar. It uniquely fuses Indian classical dance movements with contemporary dance. Evidence on the

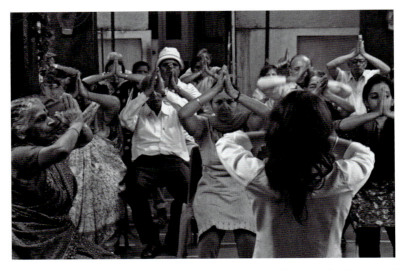

**Fig. 29.2** Maithily Bhupatkar, who attended the Mark Morris Dance Group training in Brooklyn, leads her Dance for PD group in Pune.
Reproduce by kind permission of Maithily Bhupatkar. Copyright © 2015 Maithily Bhupatkar.

positive value of the programme is recorded in a series of short films (see Hrishikesh Centre of Contemporary Dance 2011a,b). The following comments by Dance for PD participants, taken from the films, highlight the initiative's benefit:

'I would get scared to go out of the house but now I don't. I got confidence because of this class. It's very inspiring to me. I feel happy and enthusiastic.'

Hrishikesh Centre of Contemporary Dance (2011a)

Dr Parag Sancheti, Chairman of the Sancheti Institute also comments:

'The movement of the joints tends to reduce the tremors . . . their movements have become faster and also their drug requirement has reduced . . . . dance definitely something that one should look at more closely when treating patients with Parkinsonism'

Hrishikesh Centre of Contemporary Dance (2011b)

## Case study 2. Northern Ireland: 'Strengthening the voice of older people through the arts'—the Arts and Older People Programme

This case report focuses on arts-based programmes for older people in Northern Ireland that aim to support a good and independent life as people age.

At the beginning of 2013, Northern Ireland's Belfast-based charity Engage with Age (EWA), together with multiple agencies concerned with the health and social welfare of older people, launched the initiative Hubs for Older People's Engagement (HOPE). The aim of HOPE is to tackle social isolation among older people by providing regular opportunities for engagement in enjoyable, creative activities in socially supportive settings. These aims mirror those of other initiatives, such as Arts Council Northern Ireland's (ACNI) national Arts and Older People Programme (AOPP) 2013–16. That programme grew from a previous AOPP, the subject of this case report, an evaluation of which (ACNI 2013) showed the potential for arts engagement to

contribute to the strategic management of a changing population profile in Northern Ireland.

Between 2012 and 2025 it is estimated that the number of people aged 85 or more will rise from 32,700 to 57,700. This equates to an 83% increase (NISRA 2013). A ratio shift in favour of older people in the future stems not only from this longevity trend but also from the greater number of younger than older people emigrating ( NISRA 2013). As might be expected, older people are the heaviest users of health and social care services in Northern Ireland. Expenditure on this age group is being driven by long-term conditions such as heart failure, stroke, diabetes, and dementia (Public Health Agency 2012). In addition, mental ill-health currently affects one in five people aged 65 or more. Such data are shaping strategic policy on older people's services, the principal vision of which is a flourishing, independent older population (e.g. Campbell 2010).

The notion of employing the arts at a strategic level to effect a good life for Northern Ireland's older people is not new. In 2005, for example, the government's Ageing in an Inclusive Society strategy stated that 'participation in culture, arts and leisure activities can enhance the quality of older persons' lives' (OMDFM 2005). In 2012, the Director of Public Health emphasized the benefits of creative arts programmes to off-set the effects loneliness and social isolation (Public Health Agency 2012), and the older people's charity Age NI stated a vision for arts engagement to 'create a world in which older people flourish' (Age NI 2012).

For over a decade the ACNI has contributed significantly to an understanding of the role of the arts in older people's issues. A key objective in ACNI's arts and health policy of 2007 was to develop a strategic approach towards the inclusion of older people in arts engagement. To this end, the organization went on to publish an Arts and Older People Strategy 2010–13, and subsequently jointly funded the £700,000, multicollaborative AOPP 2010–13 with the private foundation The Atlantic Philanthropies. The 3-year programme provided 50 sustained arts projects to over 6000 older people in two stages. The first stage involved performing and visual arts and crafts projects, some of which were showcased at the

**Table 29.1** Impact of the Arts for Older People Project (AOPP) (Arts Council of Northern Ireland)

| Poor quality of life indicators | Improvements in quality of life post-AOPP |
| --- | --- |
| Isolation and loneliness | 4% reduction in proportion of participants reporting a lack of companionship |
| | 5% reduction in proportion feeling isolated |
| | 4% reduction in proportion feeling 'left out' |
| Social exclusion | 77% of participants overall reported that they had developed good friendships |
| | 67% engaging in cross-community projects felt they had developed good friendships |
| | 81% engaging in cross-cultural projects felt they had developed good friendships |
| Health/dementia | Increase of 1.3 points overall on WEMWBS |
| | 74% had an increased or stable score on WEMWBS |
| | 4% increase in mental health |
| | 3.5% increase in enjoyment in life |
| | 2% increase in physical health plus anecdotal evidence of reduced joint pain, improved mobility/breathing |
| | 94% of artists perceived that participants were highly engaged |
| | 69% of artists reported that participants' concentration had improved |
| | 78% of artists reported improved listening among participants |
| | 77% of artists reported improved confidence among participants |
| | 75% of artists reported improved self-esteem among participants |
| Poverty | 26% increase in participants living in NRAs |
| | 51% reduction in reported barriers to arts engagement by those living in NRAs |
| Limited capacity to positively affect older people's issues | 75% of participants felt better able to express themselves |
| | 78% reported an increased knowledge of social issues |
| | 83% tried/learned new things |
| | 72% surprised themselves and others by what they could do |
| | 76% had more confidence to try different things |
| | 84% felt good about what they have achieved |

WEMWBS, Warwick–Edinburgh Mental Wellbeing Scale; NRA,

Source: data from Arts Council of Northern Ireland (ACNI), 2013, *Evaluation of the Arts and Older People Programme Final Report*. Compiled for Arts Council Northern Ireland by Wallace Consulting. Copyright © 2013 Arts Council of Northern Ireland.

week-long Celebration of Age event. The second stage was delivered in partnership with arts in healthcare specialist charity Arts Care to older people living in or attending health and/or social care settings (ACNI 2013).

The motivational bases for AOPP 2010–13 aligned fundamentally with the key challenges for older people in Northern Ireland; isolation and loneliness, social exclusion, health/dementia, poverty, and strengthening the voice of older people. Evaluation tools used to assess the impact on these issues included: pre/post-participant surveys, including the three-point Loneliness Scale (Hughes et al. 2004) and the seven-point Warwick–Edinburgh Mental Wellbeing Scale completed by programme attendees, and a post-programme survey completed by artists. The outcomes of the evaluation are shown in Table 29.1.

A community artist engaged in AOPP 2010–13 observed:

'It was all the more rewarding to see the rise in self-esteem [among participants] and the sense of pride and achievement on completion of projects.'

Age of Creativity (2012)

The evaluation report highlights the potential role of community-based creative activities to support a good life as people age, and importantly reveals some remaining challenges, such

as raising engagement among people aged 80 or more. These findings have informed the ACNI's future plans for arts development and underpinned the follow-on AOPP 2013–16, which aims to further strengthen the voices of Northern Ireland's older people and to promote flourishing and independence as they age.

## Case study 3. The United States: creating environments in which older people can thrive

This case study highlights the work of American psychiatrist Dr Gene Cohen (1944–2009), who, on the announcement of his untimely death in 2009, was referred to in the *Washington Post* as 'The psychiatrist who broke ground in geriatrics' (Sullivan 2009). That newspaper also quoted a colleague who said that Cohen had 'Singlehandedly . . . changed the image of aging from one of senescence [weakness] to a period of creativity' (Sullivan 2009).

Over the last two decades of Cohen's life, demographic predictions had increasingly urged strategic action to halt the threatening potential of a 'grey tsunami'. In line with the rest of the world, the growth in the number and proportion of older people in the United States is currently unprecedented. The rapid change is being driven by increasing longevity with many people living into their

70s, 80s, and beyond, and the post-Second World War baby boomers beginning to reach older age (NCCDPHP 2013). By 2030, when the last cohort of boomers reaches 65, one in five Americans, around 72 million, will be classified as 'older', and from 2011 to 2050 the number of people aged 65 or over is anticipated to double from 41.4 million to nearly 89 million (Administration on Aging 2012; NCCDPHP 2013). Healthcare costs for this population of people, two out of three of whom have multiple chronic diseases and degenerative conditions, currently account for 66% of the US healthcare budget, and this is set to rise incrementally in the future (NCCDPHP 2013).

Against this backdrop of predicated burden, Cohen dedicated much of his professional life to challenging mind-sets around ageing. In his early career, macro- and microcultures still accepted as reality the biomedical, age-related inevitability of slow cell death, but Cohen describes a sea change in thinking around ageing which began to emerge during the 1970s. The idea that decline in older age is not inevitable but rather modifiable began to take hold. The titles of his later published books, *The Creative Age: Awakening Human Potential in the Second Half of Life* (Cohen 2000) and *The Mature Mind: The Positive Power of the Aging Brain* (Cohen 2006), are testament to Cohen's passionate commitment to contesting engrained beliefs about ageing which, up to the last quarter of the twentieth century, had no scientific grounding.

Cohen embraced human creativity as key to inner growth, to strengthen morale, to contribute to physical health, to enrich relationships, and to create powerful legacies for future generations (e.g. Cohen 2000, 2009). He contextualized these benefits within gerontology research and its emphasis on the importance of a sense of control and meaningful social engagement, and psychoneuroimmunology that indicates related protection by the immune system. Cohen also raised the centrality of neuroscience and the relatively new understanding of brain plasticity, which, regardless of age, enables the formation of new pathways when the brain is challenged through creative activity (e.g. Kramer et al. 2004).

In 2006, Cohen first reported the findings of a longitudinal study, the Creativity and Aging Study (Cohen et al. 2006). A sample of 300 people aged 65 or more who were living in New York, San Francisco, or Washington DC took part in an intervention/control group design study to investigate the impact of an intensive cultural programme. The intervention group attended weekly, professionally led, community-based classes of literary, performing, and/or visual arts for 18 months (over a period of 2 years). They also continued with creative work at home between classes and attended regular concerts, exhibitions, or other cultural events. The control group were actively engaged in non-art community activities. The tools used to measure impact were: (1) a general health questionnaire; (2) the short-form Geriatric Depression Scale; (3) the UCLA Loneliness Scale; (4) the Philadelphia Geriatric Center Morale Scale; and (5) a detailed assessment of socialization activities.

The results of Cohen's study show strikingly positive benefits in the intervention groups compared with the control groups. For example, the intervention groups reported a greater increase in overall physical health after the first year and a stabilization of physical health after the second year. The improvements manifested as fewer visits to a doctor, a decrease in prescription and over-the-counter medication, and fewer falls. Findings on mental health (morale, depression, and loneliness) showed a similar

pattern, with the intervention group reporting a greater positive impact than the control group.

Cohen concluded that the trends for health improvement and stabilization associated with regular and sustained engagement in community-based cultural programmes ' . . . point to true health promotion and disease prevention effects' (Cohen 2009, p. 59). These effects underline Cohen's career-long mission to reverse preconceptions of inevitable decline in older age and offer tangible hope for a managing a prolonged good life.

## Case study 4. Barbados, England, Italy, and Sweden: music in the care of older people living with dementia—a cross-national study of staff perspectives

This case report highlights the findings of a study that compared the perceptions, attitudes, and behaviours of a sample of dementia-care staff working across England, Sweden, Italy, and Barbados towards the use of music in their care setting. The four countries were chosen because of the author's existing links in each with researchers/health professionals working in similar fields to her own. The countries also represent variable GNI rankings and were assumed to provide a relatively wide spectrum of care models. This study was enabled through a Finzi Trust Scholarship awarded to the author in 2009.

### Background

Currently around 30–50% of people with dementia in high-income countries and around 6% in middle- to low-income countries live in some form of continuing care establishment (CCE) (Prince et al. 2013). A likely consequence of rising incidence of dementia across the world in future years will be a growing need for specialist, sustainable models of care for this condition.

Table 29.2 compares the proportion of older people in the three European countries (England 16.9%, Italy 20.5%, and Sweden 20.2%) and in Barbados (10%). The estimated proportion of people with dementia (aged 60 and above) in England, Italy, and Sweden are very similar, and the most recent figures available from Barbados (in 2007) indicate a lower percentage (1.2%; this is against a backdrop of only very recent

**Table 29.2** Percentage of older people and estimated numbers with dementia in Barbados, England, Italy, and Sweden

| Country | % of population aged ≥65[a] | % of people aged ≥60 with dementia[b] |
|---|---|---|
| Barbados | 10.0[c] | 1.2 |
| England | 16.9 | 6.25 |
| Italy | 20.5 | 6.5 |
| Sweden | 20.2 | 6.34 |

[a] From Index Mundi (undated) and ONS (2012).

[b] From Wimo et al. (2010).

[c] 2007 estimates, kindly provided by Pamelia Brereton, President of Barbados Alzheimer's Association.

Source: data from Wimo, A., Winblad, B. and Jonsson, L. (2010). The worldwide societal costs of dementia: estimates for 2009. *Alzheimer's and Dementia*, **6**, 98–103.

epidemiological attention given to gathering a true picture of incidence in that country).

Across Europe a host of public and charitable agencies continue to campaign for a better quality of life for people living in CCEs (see Bowers et al. 2009; Equality and Human Right Commission 2011; Owen et al. 2012; NICE 2013; Quince 2013). Issues of professional development for staff are frequently highlighted as important, with training to affect creative, person-centred interactions high on the agenda (e.g. Prince et al. 2013). Such interactions might include care staff and residents exploring creative arts together. However, to date only a very small body of research exists on staff perceptions and attitudes to involvement in creative activities at their place of work (e.g. Sung et al. 2011; Vella-Burrows 2011).

## Method

Using a multimethod design, data were collected by the author between July 2009 and January 2010 using a closed questionnaire, focus group discussions, and face-to-face interviews. The Statistical Package for Social Science (SPSS) version 15 data program and a thematic analysis were used to analyse the data.

## Summary of findings

Ninety-five members of staff took part across 19 care settings (Sweden, n = 3; UK, n = 5; Italy, n = 5 each; Barbados, n = 6). The proportions of overseas staff (not indigenous to their country of employment) were: Barbados, around a fifth; Sweden, around a third; England and Italy, more than a half. In order of prevalence, overseas staff originated from the Philippines, Thailand, North Africa, South Africa, Eritrea, Sierra Leone, Peru, and India.

## Staff perceptions, attitudes, and behaviours

A variety of micro- (individual/family/households), meso- (communities/organizations) and macro- (societal/national) cultural factors appeared to influence staff perceptions, attitudes, and behaviours.

◆ Microcultural factors:

• experiences of music in early/family life—a tendency for higher levels of family-based singing among staff from overseas and in Barbados;

• perceptions of self-assessed musical/singing skills—very few staff from any background reported high levels of skill;

• personal confidence to engage in music/singing activities in and out of work—more staff reported enjoying singing outside work (e.g. karaoke) than at work.

◆ Mesocultural factors:

• the effect on staff of music-teaching pedagogy at school—more staff from Sweden were spurred by positive experiences and more in England and Italy were deterred by negative experiences;

• models of care in care settings which showed a spectrum of clinical to quasi-family home—clinically orientated settings were highest in Italy and lowest in Barbados;

• management priorities and practice/training policies of the care settings—aspirations towards person-centred care

observed across all settings, formal focus in European settings, informal in Barbados.

◆ Macrocultural factors:

• national curriculum compartmentalization of music in schools—high levels of formal music training at primary and secondary levels among staff from the Philippines and South Africa, low levels at secondary school among all others;

• national level of organized community music/singing activities—highest town-wide community singing and choirs in Sweden, lowest in Barbados;

• national level of informal, family-orientated music-making/ singing—highest among staff from overseas and Barbados;

• national policy on training dementia care staff—highest clinical/person-centred orientation in European countries, but training not yet formalized in Barbados.

Although these distinct factors were identified by staff as influential, their behaviours were driven largely by a fusion of factors. For example, staff who in childhood enjoyed singing/music-making with their families, and/or who reported feeling at ease with singing out of work, were not necessarily uninhibited enough to sing at work. Impeding factors centred largely on context: perceptions of professional role and the perceived need to maintain a clinical approach to avoid management/colleague disapproval (all highest in Italy and lowest in Barbados).

## Apparent national cultural effects

A small number of factors appeared to relate to national cultures. For example, staff in Barbados were in general most likely to engage in spontaneous staff-led musical interactions. This occurred even though levels of formal management support for staff to develop creative practice per se were lowest in Barbados (highest in Sweden, equally low in England and Italy). This finding was thought by staff to be due to the island's strong culture of singing and the continued affiliation with intergenerational, faith-related singing. This influence also appeared to draw in staff from overseas, who generally reported more comfort in singing in settings in Barbados than in the other countries. Staff from Sweden, where national community and choir singing was reported as most prevalent, tended to more strongly advocate musician-led sing-a-long events in their place of work, to which they would collectively contribute. Compared with other staff, staff from the Philippines and South Africa, who reported the highest levels of school-based musical training (singing/learning an instrument), tended to more strongly advocate live, high-quality music performances in care settings.

While the limitations of this small study render the findings non-generalizable, they nonetheless provide a view of the factors that help to shape current perceptions and behaviours. While reporting the positive value of music in supporting their own wellbeing and that of the people for whom they care, staff can find themselves at the heart of tensions around the role of music in the workplace, particularly in more clinically oriented settings. The findings indicate that more substantial and robustly designed research is needed to investigate the wider role of arts-grounded creativity in the training and practice of care-givers (e.g. Särkämö et al. 2014), particularly in view of the growing demand for a creative, flourishing, and sustainable workforce (Fig. 29.3).

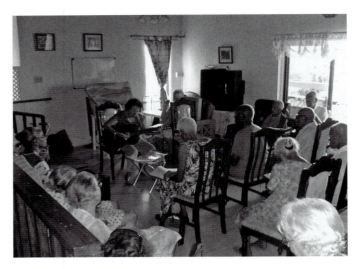

**Fig. 29.3** Ocean View Nursing Services, Christ Church, Barbados: music session with visiting musician.
Reproduced by kind permission of Trish Vella-Burrows. Copyright © 2015 Trish Vella-Burrows.

## Concluding comments

This chapter has explored the potential for participatory arts to help promote a good life and personal and social wellbeing in older age groups. It has shown that global concern about managing the future growth of older populations is spurring evidence-based policy. The case studies indicate that the provision of accessible participatory arts in older age has the potential to challenge notions of inevitable decline, target the health needs of people living with long-term conditions that threaten health and wellbeing, and support the needs of an increasingly important care-giving workforce. Ongoing research is needed to better understand the impact of creating participatory arts opportunities to affect social and cultural capital, to reconnect older people with their communities, and to engender the personal resilience with which older people may positively manage the challenges associated with old age. Some useful resources are listed in Box 29.1.

---

**Box 29.1**  Resources

**Campaigns for older people's health and wellbeing**

◆ Contact the elderly. A lifeline of friendship (End Loneliness campaign): <http://www.contact-the-elderly.org.uk/>

◆ Engage with Age. HOPE: hubs for older people's engagement (Northern Ireland): <http://engagewithage.org.uk/hope/>

◆ My Home Life (a UK-wide initiative that promotes quality of life and delivers positive change in care homes for older people): <http://myhomelife.org.uk/>

**Arts, health, and wellbeing research and campaign agencies**

◆ Sidney De Haan Research centre for Arts and Health, Canterbury Christ Church University: <http://www.canterbury.ac.uk/research/centres/sdhr/>

◆ Arts for Health, Manchester Metropolitan University: <http://www.artsforhealth.org>

◆ The Centre for Clinical and Health Services Research, University of the West of England: <http://www1.uwe.ac.uk/hls/research/clinicalandhealthresearch.aspx>

◆ Winchester Centre for Research into the Arts as Wellbeing, University of Winchester: <http://www.artshealthandwellbeing.org.uk/directory/university-winchester-research-centre-arts-wellbeing>

◆ National Alliance for Arts, Health and Wellbeing: <http://www.artshealthandwellbeing.org.uk>

## References

ACNI (Arts Council of Northern Ireland) (2013). *Evaluation of the Arts and Older People Programme. Final Report.* Available at: <http://www.artscouncil-ni.org/images/uploads/publications-documents/aopp_final_oct13.pdf>

Administration on Aging (2012). A profile of older Americans: 2012. Available at: <http://www.aoa.gov/aging_statistics/profile/2012/3.aspx>

Age NI (2012). *Age NI's Response to the Service Framework for Older People.* Belfast: Age NI.

Age of Creativity (2012) Age and Creativity Project. Available at: <http://www.ageofcreativity.co.uk/items/199>

Aked, J., Marks, N., Cordon, C., and Thompson, S. (2008). *Five Ways to Wellbeing.* London: New Economics Foundation.

Beaumont, J. (2011). *Measuring National Wellbeing: Discussion Paper on Domains and Measures.* London: Office of National Statistics.

Bishop, C. (2012). *Artificial Hells: Participatory Art and the Politics of Spectatorship.* London: Verso.

Bormans, L. (2011). *The World Book of Happiness.* Ontario: Firefly Books.

Bowers, H., Clark, A., Crosby, G. et al. (2009). *Older People's Vision for Long-term Care.* London: Joseph Rowntree Foundation.

Bungay, H. and Clift, S. (2010). Arts on prescription: a review of practice in the UK. *Perspectives in Public Health*, **130**, 277–281.

Campbell, J. (2010). *The Commissioner for Older People Bill.* Belfast: Northern Ireland Assembly Research and Library Services.

Clift, S. (2012). Creative arts as a public health resource: moving from practice-based research to evidence-based practice *Perspectives in Public Health*, 2012, **132**, 120–127.

Clift, S., Camic, P.M., Chapman, B., et al. (2009). The state of arts and health in England. *Arts & Health: An International Journal for Research, Policy and Practice.* **1**, 6–35.

Cohen, G. (2000). *The Creative Age: Awakening Human Potential in the Second half of Life.* New York: Harper Collins.

Cohen, G. (2006). *The Mature Mind: The positive Power of the Aging Brain.* New York: Basic Books.

Cohen, G. (2009). New theories and research findings on the positive influence of music and art on health with ageing. *Arts and Health*, **1**, 48–62.

Cohen, G., Perlstein, S., Chapline, J., et al. (2006). The impact of professionally conducted cultural programs on the physical health, mental health, and social functioning of older adults. *The Gerontologist*, **46**, 726–734.

Cuddy, A.J.C. and Fiske, S.T. (2002). Doddery but dear: content and function in stereotyping of older people. In T.D. Nelson (ed.), *Ageism: Stereotyping and Prejudice Against Older Persons*, pp. 3–26. Cambridge, MA: MIT Press.

Csikszentmihalyi, M. (1999). implications of a systems perspective for the study of creativity. In: R. Sternberg (ed.), *Handbook of Human Creativity*, pp. 313–338. New York: Cambridge University Press.

Cutler, D. (2009). *Ageing Artfully: Older People and Professional Participatory Arts in the UK.* London: Baring Foundation.

Department of Health (2007). *A Prospectus for Arts and Health.* London: Department of Health.

Dissanayake, E. (1992). *Homo Aestheticus: Where Art Comes From and Why.* Seattle: University of Washington Press.

EHRC (Equality and Human Rights Commission) (2011). *Close to Home: An Inquiry into Older People and Human Rights in Home Care.* London: Equality and Human Rights Commission.

Flood, M. and Phillips, K. (2007). Creativity in older adults: a plethora of possibilities. *Issues in Mental Health Nursing*, **28**, 389–411.

Greaves, C. and Farbus, L. (2006). Effects of creative and social activity on the health and wellbeing of socially isolated older people: outcomes from a multi-method observational study. *Journal of the Royal Society for the Promotion of Health*, **126**, 134–142.

Hackney, M. and Earhart, G. (2010). Effects of dance on gait and balance in Parkinson's disease: a comparison of partnered and non-partnered dance. *Neurorehabilitation and Neural Repair*, **24**, 384–392.

Hasselkus, B. (2011) *Meaning of Everyday Occupation.* Thorofare, NJ: Slack Incorporated.

HelpAge India (2013). Eldercare. Online at www.helpageindia.org/our-work/eldercare.html (accessed 20 September 2013).

Houston, S. and McGill, A. (2011). A mixed method study into ballet for people living with Parkinson's. *Arts and Heath*, **5**, 103–119.

Hrishikesh Centre of Contemporary Dance (2011a). Dance for Parkinson's Disease [video]. *YouTube* (uploaded 28 December 2011). Available at: <https://www.youtube.com/watch?v=bpohne_-bkq>.

Hrishikesh Centre of Contemporary Dance (2011b). 'Dance for Parkinson's Disease—Hrishikesh [video]. *YouTube* (uploaded 25 January 2011). Available at: <https://www.youtube.com/watch?v=_0ksmrhhu9m>

Hughes, M., Waite, L., Hawkley, L., and Cacioppo, J. (2004). A short scale for measuring loneliness in large surveys: results from two population-based studies. *Research on Aging*, **26**, 655–672.

Index Mundi (undated). Country facts. Available at: <http://www.index-mundi.com> (accessed 28 September 2013).

International Statistical Institute (2013). Developing countries. Available at: <http://www.isi-web.org/component/content/article/5-root/root/81-developing> (accessed 26 September 2013).

Kramer, A., Colcombe, S., Bherer, L., Dong, W., and Greenough, W. (2004). Environmental influences on cognitive and brain plasticity during aging. *Journal of Gerontology: Medical Science*, **59A**, 940–957.

NICE (National Institue for Health and Care Excellence) (2013). Mental wellbeing of older people in care homes. *NICE Quality Standard [QS50].* Available at: <http://www.nice.org.uk/guidance/qs50> (accessed 04 January 2013).

NISRA (Northern Ireland Statistics and Research Agency) (2013). *Population and Migration Estimates Northern Ireland 2012—Statistical Report.* Belfast: Northern Ireland Statistics and Research Agency.

NCCDPHP (National Center for Chronic Disease Prevention and Health Promotion) (2013). *The State of Healthy Ageing in America in 2013.* Atlanta, GA: Centers for Disease Control and Prevention, US Dept of Health and Human Service. Available at: <http://www.cdc.gov/aging/pdf/state-aging-health-in-america-2013.pdf> (accessed 02 June 2013).

National Endowment for the Arts (2009). *2008 Survey of Public Participation in the Arts.* Washington, DC: National Endowment for the Arts.

NIA, NIH, and WHO (National Institute of Aging, National Institutes of Health and World Health Organisation) (2011). *Global Health and Aging.* Available at: <http://www.who.int/ageing/publications/global_health/en/> (accessed 20 September 2013).

OFMDFM (2005). *Ageing in an Inclusive Society.* Belfast: Office of the First Minister and Deputy First Minister

Organ, K. (2013). *After You are Two: Exemplary Practice in Participatory Arts with Older People.* London: The Baring Foundation.

Owen, T., Mayer, J., Cornell, M., et al. (2012). *My Home Life: Promoting Quality of Life in Care Homes.* London: Joseph Rowntree Foundation.

Population Reference Bureau (2011). India's aging population. *Today's Research on Aging: Program and Policy Implications*, issue 25. Available at: <http://www.prb.org/pdf12/todaysresearchaging25.pdf> (accessed 02 June 2013).

Prescott-Allen, R. (2001). *The Wellbeing of Nations.* Washington, DC: Island Press.

Prince, M., Prina, M., Guerchet, M., and Alzheimer's Disease International (2013). *World Alzheimer Report 2013: Journey of Caring. An Analysis of Long-Term Care for Dementia.* London: Alzheimer's Disease International.

Public Health Agency (2012). *Director of Public Health Annual Report—2012.* Belfast: Health and Social Care Public Health Agency.

Quince, C. (2013) *Low Expectations: Attitudes on Choice, Care And Community for People with Dementia in Care Homes.* London: Alzheimer's Society.

Ryff, C. and Singer, B. (1998) The contours of positive human health. *Psychological Inquiry*, **9**, 1–28.

Särkämö, T., Tervaniemi, M., Laitinen, S., et al. (2014). Cognitive, emotional, and social benefits of regular musical activities in early dementia: randomized controlled study. *The Gerontologist*, **54**, 634–650.

Seedhouse, D. (1997). *Health Promotion: Philosophy, Prejudice and Practice.* Chichester: Wiley.

Seligman, M.E.P. (2011). *Flourish: A Visionary New Understanding of Happiness and Wellbeing.* London: Simon and Schuster.

Seltzer, K. and Bentley, T. (1999). *The Creative Age: Knowledge and Skills for the New Economy.* London: Demos.

Stickley, T. and Duncan, K. (2007). Art in mind: implementation of a community arts initiative to promote mental health. *Journal of Public Mental Health*, **6**, 24–33.

Sullivan, P. (2009). Gene D. Cohen, 65: psychiatrist broke ground in geriatrics. *Washington Post*, 11 November 2009. Available at: <http://www.washingtonpost.com/wp-dyn/content/article/2009/11/10/ar2009111018634.html>

Sung, H., Lee, W., Chang, S., and Smith, G. (2011). Exploring nursing staff's attitudes and use of music for older people with dementia in long term-care facilities. *Journal of Clinical Nursing*, **20**, 1776–1783.

Swindells, R., Lawthorn, R., Rowley, K., et al. (2013). Eudaimonic wellbeing and community arts participation. *Perspectives in Public Health*, **133**, 60–65.

UN (2002). *World Population Ageing 1950–2050.* New York: Department of Economic and Social Affairs Population Division, United Nations. Available at: <http://www.un.org/esa/population/publications/world-ageing19502050/pdf/preface_web.pdf>

UNDP (United Nations Development Programme) (2013). The rise of the South. Human progress in a diverse world. *Human Development Report 2013.* New York: United Nations Development Programme. Available at: <http://hdr.undp.org/en/2013-report>

Wali, A., Severson, R. and Longoni, M. (2002). *Informal Arts: Finding Cohesion, Capacity and Other Cultural Benefits in Unexpected Places.* Chicago, IL: Chicago Center for Arts Policy.

Vella-Burrows, T. (2011). Care staff perspectives of the role of music in the care of people living with dementia. PhD Thesis, Department of Music and Performing Arts, Canterbury Christ Church University.

White, M. (2009). *Arts Development in Community Health: A Social Tonic.* London: Radcliffe Publishing Ltd.

WHO (1946). Preamble to the Constitution of the World Health Organization as adopted by the International Health Conference, New York, 19–22 June, 1946; signed on 22 July 1946 by the representatives of 61 States (*Official Records of the World Health Organization*, no. 2, p. 100) and entered into force on 7 April 1948.

WHO (1986). *The Ottawa Charter for Health Promotion.* Geneva: World Health Organization.

WHO (2001). *International Classification of Functioning, Disability and Health.* Geneva: World Health Organisation.

WHO (2002). *Active Ageing: A Policy Framework.* Geneva: World Health Organization.

Wimo, A., Winblad, B., and Jonsson, L. (2010). The worldwide societal costs of dementia: estimates for 2009. *Alzheimer's and Dementia*, **6**, 98–103.

Winkler-Wagner, R. (2010). Cultural capital; promises and pitfalls in educational research. *Ashe Higher Education Report*, **36**(1), 1–144.

Yosso, T. (2005). Whose culture has capital? A critical race theory discussion of community cultural wealth. *Race Ethnicity and Education*, **8**, 69–91.

# CHAPTER 30

# Case study: engaging older people in creative thinking—the Active Energy project

Loraine Leeson

## Geezer power

I first met the members of the Geezers Club in 2007 through an art commission from SPACE Studios London, initiated in response to a research programme at Queen Mary University of London on the democratization of technology. The arts have always been a useful tool in helping communities instigate change by bringing their ideas into the public domain in an engaging and accessible way, and this commission followed several decades of my art practice doing just this. While educational or therapeutic outcomes had never been a central purpose of my work, these nevertheless often play a key part in its process.

The Geezers Club was set up in 2006 following research (Davidson 2006) on older people's attendance at clubs and classes in the London Borough of Tower Hamlets. Tower Hamlets is one of the poorest boroughs in the United Kingdom, and isolation for older people is a particular issue due to the lack of resources available to help residents have an active social life. In particular the research identified how few older men were taking part in group activities and that widowers often lacked the social infrastructure through which lone women alleviate loneliness, concluding that men are more likely to need activities addressed specifically to their needs and interests. The Geezers Club at AgeUK in Bow was founded to reduce the isolation of retired men over 50 by encouraging them out of their homes and back into the community. Members gain access to social activities, participate in outings, and receive talks by outside professionals, mainly on health-related topics. However, they are also keen to do more. Following my first visit, one member commented that they were always being talked to about their disintegrating bodies and how much they welcomed the opportunity to exercise their minds and develop their ideas. The group also placed immense value on the fact that the activity was not just for its own sake or to pass the time.

I have found an important aspect of the creative work I conduct with communities to be its functional outcome, achieved through each participant contributing his or her skills and expertise to a meaningful task, and bringing in outside expertise as required. To this I bring my own experience in visual media, creative facilitation, and knowledge of how to take on board the ideas of others. These may commence as individual contributions, but are combined through the project's structure to become part of a shared outcome, as in VOLCO, a planet in cyberspace created entirely out of the vivid imaginations of children. Over a period of 10 years a thousand young people between the ages of 7 and 13 interacted online with others of different cultures and life experiences to build a new virtual world based on cooperation and collective imagination. Another project drew on the local knowledge of 400 London teenagers, who created *The Young Person's Guide to East London* (<http://www.ypg2el.co.uk/>), subsequently used by thousands of visitors to the London 2012 Olympics. Similarly, the lifelong experiences of older people in the Active Energy project (http://www.active-energy-london.org/) have begun to inform new developments in technology with an altruism fuelled by the desire to leave a mark and a legacy for future generations. This is, after all, what most of us wish to do, but it can become forgotten in work with older people, whose experience too often becomes trivialized.

I have to admit that I too approached the group with limited expectations. My brief from SPACE was to create work over 6 weeks to be shown in their Not Quite Yet exhibition. Unused to such a short development period, I was tempted to imagine suggestions for gadgets and devices that would make life easier or more interesting for Geezers Club members. Nevertheless I adhered to the process of framing a proposition that would allow their ideas to emerge. My question 'What technology would you like to see developed that you feel would support your life, or that of your community?' was initially met with a few responses that supported my preconceptions. However, one member of the group posed a question in return: 'When electricity prices prevent older people from heating their homes, and the River Thames is just down the road, why are we not using it to power our city?' We debated the historical use of water wheels, one of which had been in use on London Bridge centuries earlier, and questioned the demise of the tidal power research that most remembered hitting the headlines in the 1980s before its support was withdrawn by the Thatcher government. By the end of our first session all 14 members of the group were fired up with the topic and wanted to take part in the project. While knowing nothing about the subject, my role was to enable the group to develop their idea, and I resolved to take them as far with this as I could.

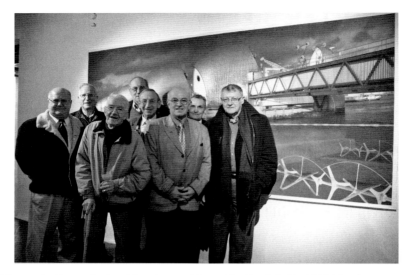

**Fig. 30.1** Visualization of tidal turbines on the Thames Barrier with project participants: The Not Quite Yet, SPACE, London, 25 January–29 February 2008. Reproduced by kind permission of Loraine Leeson. Copyright © 2015 Loraine Leeson.

A conversation with the director of the Sustainability Research Institute at the nearby University of East London revealed tidal power to be his pet project. Under his guidance the group organized minibus outings to look at locally sited wind turbines that would most easily adapt for underwater use and a visit to the Thames Barrier proved this to be a suitable ready-made barrage for potential turbine installation. From visual materials gathered in our research I was able to create a large-scale photomontage of how turbines might function in this location. The group's new knowledge coupled with their understanding of its potential benefits for the lives of local people made them highly effective advocates of the sustainability argument. To capture this, projected video interviews with its members accompanied the photovisualization in the exhibition, the enormous scale of the projections that towered over the viewer lending a weight of authority to the views of the speakers portrayed. The impact of this installation on gallery visitors was further reflected in its significant local press coverage. In the eyes of the media the senior years of the project's participants clearly added to the public interest. Despite little experience of public speaking, eight members of the group presented the project to great acclaim at the On the Margins of Technology symposium accompanying the exhibition (Fig. 30.1).

It could not stop there. After the exhibition we found funding to equip the Geezers Club with a laptop and other equipment that would allow its members to learn the skills to research online and share findings. Engineering expertise presented itself in the form of Toby Borland, a highly creative mechanical engineer who ran a prototyping laboratory at the University of East London, and Professor Stephen Dodds, renowned for his development of the control system for the European Space Commission. Both gave freely of their time and knowledge out of interest in the project. The SPACE arts organization, which had worked alongside Queen Mary University of London to offer the original arts commission, rejoined the project for similar reasons, raising funds to support intergenerational work with a local school and continue the project. This gave the Geezers an opportunity to further share their accumulated wisdom through mentoring teenage boys in workshops that introduced them to the concept of renewable energy—a touching scenario in which isolated men were able to support underachieving boys in their own community. The workshops culminated in the creation of a wind turbine for the roof of the AgeUK centre. As it spun, the turbine generated the energy to spell out in light the words 'Geezer power' (Fig. 30.2).

In tandem with the school workshops, the Geezers had been developing their own ideas for tidal turbines. As working class men with backgrounds in manual trades they held between them a range of practical skills. One had been a steam turbine engineer, another a mechanic, and it seemed that most knew how to strip down and reassemble a motorcycle. The group spontaneously came up with proposals for improvements to existing turbine designs, as well as some new ideas. With engineer Toby Borland's

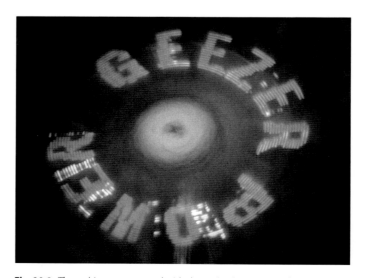

**Fig. 30.2** The turbine programmed with the project's message, February 2010. Reproduced by kind permission of Loraine Leeson. Copyright © 2015 Loraine Leeson.

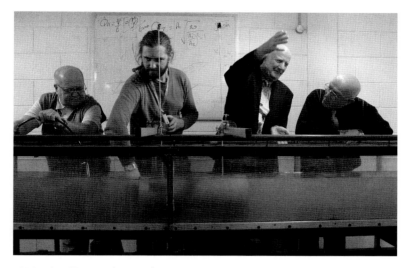

**Fig. 30.3** Testing turbine efficiency at University of East London, March 2010.
Reproduced by kind permission of Loraine Leeson. Copyright © 2015 Loraine Leeson.

help these were further developed at the university prototyping laboratory and tested in a specialist water tank where the energy output of each could be measured (Fig. 30.3).

In the meantime social scientist Professor Ann Light, who had led the original democratizing technology research, became interested in how the project had emerged as an initiative in its own right, and rejoined the expanding, though informal, project team. In 2011 she invited the group to the Participants United workshop at the University of Central Lancashire, where the group was studied as a model of good practice in how innovation can be successfully developed in a participatory setting. Here the Active Energy group presented the project for the second time as part of a growing multidisciplinary team, and have since contributed to other academic research.

In 2012 I was invited to participate in a residency and exhibition at the Mattress Factory Museum of installation in the United States and saw this as an opportunity to both enrich the project and test its methods. I put the question asked of the Geezers in London to a group from Northside Seniors in Pittsburgh, and showed them the work of their UK counterparts. Amid much excitement we were able to connect the two groups through Skype to share their experiences. Northside Seniors' choice of topic was Alzheimer's research. They felt concerned that not only was there still no cure for this disease, but also that lack of accessible information undermined their own generation's experience of warning signs and symptoms, preventing friends and family from adequately supporting sufferers. We found professional expertise on this topic at the Alzheimer's Disease Research Centre, University of Pittsburgh, where researchers welcomed the narrative of personal experiences supplied by participants that was able to give a human face to their work. Members of the seniors' group were similarly delighted that their concerns should be valued in this way. Together we put together an installation with large-scale video interviews of Northside Seniors, placing these alongside those undertaken with the Geezers from the first exhibition. Each was further accompanied by the factual information that supported the case they were making. The effect of the large room

filled with monumental 'talking heads' describing key contemporary issues, was a reminder of the seniority of the elders in the community and the value of their experience to society. Outside the exhibition room a video booth was available for visitors to add their experiences to those being expressed in the installation, and contribute to the research at the Alzheimer's Centre. An education programme also provided opportunities for young people to visit the gallery with members of the seniors' group available as experts to answer questions on ageing (Fig. 30.4).

In October 2013 the Geezers tested a turbine on a Thames barge opposite the Houses of Parliament, piloting what we was believed to be the first small-scale turbine for slow-moving tidal rivers. Its low-cost manufacture offers additional potential for use in developing countries. However, the Geezers will not cease their work until they see renewable energy powering their own East London community (Fig. 30.5).

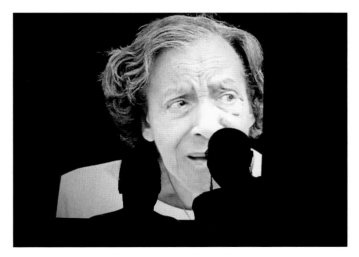

**Fig. 30.4** Active Energy, Pittsburgh, at the Mattress Factory, Pittsburgh, United States, September 2012–May 2013. A six-projector video installation.
Reproduced by kind permission of Loraine Leeson. Copyright © 2015 Loraine Leeson.

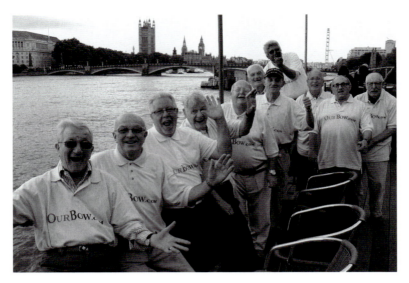

**Fig. 30.5**  Celebrating the testing of the Geezers' tidal turbine on the River Thames, 15 October 2013.
Reproduced by kind permission of Loraine Leeson. Copyright © 2015 Loraine Leeson.

## Conclusions

The significance of the Active Energy project in terms of the wellbeing of its participants lies in the motivation experienced by those involved. As an artist I worked alongside the people in these groups rather than delivering a service to them, supporting the choice of issues that they considered to be important. The project worked from the premise that the accumulated life experience of older people is of value to the wider society and its implicit task was to find creative ways to uncover what each had to offer. The Centre for Health Promotion at University of Toronto (2012) defines quality of life as: 'The degree to which a person enjoys the important possibilities of his or her life'. I see it as the business of the arts if not to create meaning per se, then to pull together meanings from lived experience, and in participatory arts this means facilitating

the realization of these possibilities. Art is also particularly effective in re-presenting these ideas within the public domain in a way that is able to engage others, promote dialogue, confer social value, and elicit feedback and respect for those who have shared their ideas. Energy levels certainly remained high for participants in both Active Energy groups, while in the longer-term engagement at the Geezers Club it was reported how some members suffering from depression had only come out of their shells through this project. Although the participatory approach described here may use less traditional forms than workshops offered through museum and gallery partnerships, such as the 'object handling' described by Camic and Chatterjee (2013, p. 67), its ability to place at its centre the needs and concerns of those involved gives it a distinct and effective role to play in stimulating older people's active creativity and contributing to their quality of life and wellbeing.

## References

Camic, P., and Chatterjee, H. (2013). Museums and art galleries as partners for public health interventions. *Perspectives in Public Health*, **133**, 66–71.

Centre for Health Promotion, University of Toronto (2012). The quality of life model. Available at: <http://sites.utoronto.ca/qol/qol_model.htm> (accessed 9 November 2013).

Davidson, K. (2006). Investigation into the social and emotional wellbeing of lone older men. In: *Working with Older Men—Improving Age Concern's Services* [Report of a Research into Practices Seminar, 26 September 2006, hosted by Age Concern Tameside], pp. 5–11. Available at: <https://www.menshealthforum.org.uk/sites/default/files/pdf/ageconcernoldermenseminar.pdf>

# CHAPTER 31

# Group singing as a public health resource

Stephen Clift, Grenville Hancox, Ian Morrison,
Matthew Shipton, Sonia Page,
Ann Skingley, and Trish Vella-Burrows

## The value of group singing for wellbeing and health

This chapter considers the developing evidence base for the idea that regular group singing can have important benefits for personal and social wellbeing, but more importantly for mental and physical health. It draws in the main on the findings from a progressive programme of work undertaken by the Sidney De Haan Research Centre for Arts and Health at Canterbury Christ Church University since 2005. The team within the centre, led by Stephen Clift and Grenville Hancox, has undertaken a series of innovative research studies which have demonstrated, we believe convincingly, that group singing can have an important role in tackling some growing public health challenges associated with increased life expectancy, namely a rise in the prevalence of long-term health conditions and growing costs of health and social care. These are challenges affecting not only the United Kingdom but other countries throughout the world whatever their levels of economic development and health and social care infrastructures.

The concern of the De Haan Centre has not simply been to test the idea that regular group singing can have benefits for health and wellbeing in the management and treatment of long-term health conditions. We have also pursued the idea that singing can be an activity, if supported on a sufficiently large-scale, that can make a significant cost-effective contribution at a public health level. Since the De Haan Centre began its work, the United Kingdom has seen a remarkable growth of interest in community singing and its personal, social, and wellbeing benefits, stimulated in particular by the work of Gareth Malone through his BBC TV series promoting choral singing in a wide variety of community and institutional settings. His work has had an enduring legacy, not least the network of Military Wives choirs (http://www.militarywiveschoirs.org), which at the time of writing numbered 58 groups across the United Kingdom with nine in Germany and five outside Europe. A number of other successful initiatives provide striking models of the potential for mobilizing the power of singing for wellbeing in the field of health and social care to achieve population-level impacts. Examples

include, Young Voices (http://www.youngvoices.co.uk), which works with primary schools bringing together children from all over the country to participate in large-scale singing events. Equally impressive is the growing phenomenon of the Rock Choir organization (http://www.rockchoir.com), which runs singing groups all over the United Kingdom and organizes regular mass-singing events. Currently, Rock Choir has over 16,000 members and groups meet in over 240 UK towns. The websites for Military Wives, Young Voices, and Rock Choir show the scale of these ventures and the huge number of people involved in their events. Testimonials from participants, together with film material, clearly reveal the powerful impact that joining together in singing with others can have.

Since 2000 there has also been a growth of scientific interest in singing, wellbeing, and health. When Clift and Hancox (2001) conducted their first small-scale, qualitative surveys on the perceived benefits of choral singing they were able to find only four previously published studies which reported very limited data on the possible health benefits of group singing. Ten years later, when Clift et al. (2010) undertook a systematic and critical review of the research on group singing and health, they found no fewer than 48 studies reported in 51 published papers. Additional reviews by Gick (2010), Wan (2010), and Clark and Harding (2012) identify further studies particularly with a focus on the use of group and individual singing in therapeutic settings. At the time of writing a simple Google Scholar search revealed yet more studies published between 2012 and 2014, with the Clift and Hancox (2001) study cited by no fewer than 158 publications. The field is thus a growing one, and the increasing body of evidence lends support to the value of group singing for wellbeing and health. Nevertheless, all of the reviews point to the need for further more robust research designs with larger controlled studies conducted over longer time periods using validated measures of wellbeing and health outcomes. A recent Cochrane Review on singing and bronchiectasis in adults and children is instructive in this respect: the review turned out to be empty, as no controlled trials were found on this topic following a very extensive search of the scientific literature (Irons et al. 2010).

Reference to two recent studies on singing which address some of the biological dimensions of group singing will help to provide contrast to the work pursued by the De Haan Centre. Vickhoff et al. (2013) have recently shown that when people sing together in groups their individual heart rhythms become synchronized, especially when the structure of the song leads to a coordinated pattern of breathing among the singers. The authors show that the heart rate decelerates during the out-breath and that this is experienced as soothing and may account for the stress-relieving effects that people often report when singing. In a further recent study, Kreutz (2014) reports that group singing leads to a higher level of the hormone oxytocin, often called the 'bonding hormone' as it is released in women during labour, childbirth, and breast feeding, and is associated with feelings of emotional closeness and love. The suggestion is that this hormone may play a part in the positive feelings of belonging people can report when they sing together in a group.

Both of these studies undoubtedly have relevance for the notion that group singing can have health and wellbeing benefits, as they identify some of the physiological mechanisms brought into play when people sing and make music together. However, both studies involved only small groups of young healthy participants singing for short periods of time, and neither provides direct evidence that singing can have sufficient measurable benefits for people experiencing challenges to their mental or physical health to be of interest to health and social care services. This point is reinforced by the fact that the findings from the Vickhoff et al. (2013) study are described on the NHS Choices website but their relevance to the treatment of heart disease is dismissed with a headline 'No proof that singing is good for the heart' and the comment that:

> '. . . these findings should be viewed in the light of that fact that only 11 teenagers were involved in the analysis, and none of the teenagers were followed up over time. This means that we can't say whether singing in a choir leads to better health.'
>
> NHS Choices (2013)

## The work of the De Haan Centre on singing, wellbeing, and health

The De Haan Centre is now (2015) in its eleventh year of a systematic programme of research on singing and health. Our continuing research mission is to build a robust and objective body of evidence on the ways in which, and the extent to which, regular engagement in group singing can be beneficial for wellbeing and health. Several substantial empirical projects have been undertaken to date to explore the wellbeing and health benefits of group singing with a variety of participating groups:

- a cross-national survey of singers in established choral societies and choirs in Australia, England, and Germany
- an evaluation of a network of singing groups for older people including many affected by memory problems
- a randomized controlled trial of the value of weekly group singing for people aged 60 and over living independently in the community
- an evaluation of a network of singing groups for people with enduring mental health issues, and

- a feasibility study to explore the value of group of singing for people with chronic respiratory illness.

As our work has progressed we have been increasingly focused on the contribution that singing can make to the wellbeing of people with long-term health conditions.

## A cross-national survey of choral singing, wellbeing, and health

The cross-national survey involved over a thousand members of choirs in Australia, England, and Germany (Clift et al. 2008, 2009, 2010a; Clift and Hancox, 2010). The principal aims were to build on an earlier study by Clift and Hancox (2001) to document definitively the perceived benefits of singing among choristers, and to describe the demographic and health profile of singers in established community singing groups. The survey included three open questions about singing and health and a specially constructed set of 24 statements on a range of potential effects and benefits associated with singing. It also made use of the WHOQOL-BREF, which measures four domains of quality of life, to place findings on perceptions of choral singing in the context of a conceptually strong and empirically grounded model of health and wellbeing.

A majority of choral singers were well-educated (over half had experienced higher education, and around a quarter further education). Many choir members were in retirement, with an average age of 58 across the three countries, and there were between two and three times as many women as men. Choristers had been singing on average for 25 years, and had been loyal members of their present choir for an average of 6 years. Generally speaking, self-assessed health was high in each of the three national samples, but a significant minority of respondents reported less than satisfactory health. Long-term health problems were reported by approximately half of all participants. Not surprisingly, such problems were more common among the older members of choirs. In order to construct a summary scale or scales to assess the benefits of choral singing the 24 items in the singing questionnaire were subject to factor analysis. A strong first component with substantial loadings from 12 items emerged (e.g. improved mood, enhanced quality of life, greater happiness, stress reduction, and emotional wellbeing) and these were used to create a single, highly reliable measure of the perceived effects of singing on wellbeing. Women scored more highly on this scale, confirming the finding of Clift and Hancox (2001) that women report stronger wellbeing effects from singing than men.

Answers given to the open questions about singing and health produced many rich accounts of the benefits choral singers believe they gained from singing. Here are some examples in which singers highlight the role of singing in promoting feelings of happiness and the more general effects they believe this has on their physical health (Clift et al. 2009):

> Having a good 'quality of life' and feeling at ease psychologically and socially helps me maintain a good mental state of health (at times in my life I have felt anxious/despair etc.). This, for me, is inextricably linked with my physical health, i.e. feeling happy helps my physical health.

> I believe I have a better immunity because I am happier than if I didn't sing . . . and I believe that if you're happier then you're healthier.

I am never happier than when I am singing this can only have a positive effect on my health and wellbeing.

'Because of the emotional experience of singing and the feeling of wellbeing it engenders, a positive attitude to life follows, which must have a positive effect on physical health.'

As these testimonies illustrate, the singers' accounts also expressed a range of intuitive hypotheses employed to explain how singing can be beneficial. From a careful analysis of such qualitative feedback, six mechanisms were identified which help to account for how singing can have an impact on health and wellbeing: positive affect, focused concentration, deep controlled breathing, social support, cognitive stimulation, and regular commitment. Each of these mechanisms serves to counter factors and processes that are potentially detrimental to wellbeing and health (Clift and Hancox 2010).

## Qualitative evaluation of singing groups for older people: Silver Song Clubs

From the outset, the Sidney De Haan Research Centre has sought to help promote and evaluate community singing projects, and helped to establish a charitable organization called Sing For Your Life which has created a network of Silver Song Clubs for older people (http://www.singforyourlife.org.uk).

At an early stage in the work of Sing For Your Life, researchers at the Sidney De Haan Research Centre undertook a 'formative evaluation' based on six Silver Song Clubs formed in the early stages of the project (Skingley and Bungay 2010). Given the rapid expansion of the network of song clubs following this initial study, the evaluation was followed up with a larger-scale survey of club participants (Bungay et al. 2010).

The initial formative evaluation sought to identify the key characteristics and processes of a Silver Song Club and to gain the views of participants, facilitators, volunteers, and centre managers regarding the health and social benefits of attending the clubs. Semi-structured interviews were conducted with 17 participants from three of the clubs. Participants valued the opportunity to sing with others and they liked the organization of the clubs, including the ways in which different facilitators presented the materials and choice of songs. Approximately three-quarters of those interviewed had quite extensive previous musical experience either as members of choirs or singing groups or playing musical instruments. The following themes were identified as potential benefits for the participants of attending Silver Song Clubs: enjoyment, promotion of wellbeing and mental health, social interaction, physical improvement, and cognitive stimulation.

On the basis of the formative evaluation, participants in all the clubs (32 in the south-east of England at the time) were surveyed to gather information on the age, gender, and living circumstances of participants, and to assess whether the views of those interviewed in the qualitative phase were held more widely (Bungay et al. 2010). A total of 369 members of 26 clubs completed the questionnaire. Ages ranged from 60 to 99, with an average age of 79 years. Most were female (77%) and living in their own homes (88%) as opposed to in nursing or residential care. More than half lived on their own (52%), and a third received some external support (33%). In general, large majorities of the participants enjoyed the clubs, looked forward to them, and felt that singing helped to make them feel better in themselves. Interestingly, however, previous experience of music and singing was an important factor in this respect. Most people with lower previous musical experience enjoyed the clubs (86%), and looked forward to them (82%), but to a lesser extent than those with higher previous experience (98 and 96%, respectively).

## A community randomized controlled trial of community singing for older people

On the basis of the qualitative evaluations of Silver Song Clubs, the De Haan Centre worked in partnership with Sing for Your Life and researchers at the University of Kent's Centre for Health Services Research to conduct a randomized control trial on group singing for older people (Clift et al. 2012; Skingley et al. 2014), with funding from the UK National Institute for Health Research.

The study took place in five locations across east Kent in south-east of England, and was open to people over the age of 60 living independently who were not currently members of a singing group or choir. A variety of means were employed to advertise the study (e.g. through newspaper advertising and door-to-door leafleting) and 265 people were enrolled in study who were willing to be randomized into either a weekly singing group running for 3 months or a usual activities control condition. Participants had an average age of 67.3 years and 84% were female. In terms of average age and sex composition, the sample was similar to that investigated in the cross-national study.

Participants completed a number of standardized health questionnaires before the start of the project, then at the end of the 3-month singing intervention, and then again after a further 3 months when no singing took place. The principal outcome measure for the study was the York SF-12, a short questionnaire which measures self-assessed mental and physical health. The Hospital Anxiety and Depression Scale (HADS) was also used to measure anxiety and depression There was consistent attendance at the singing groups and 80% of participants completed questionnaires on all three occasions.

The findings from the study showed clearly that regular singing resulted in a significant increase in mental wellbeing as measured by the York SF-12 immediately after the end of the intervention compared with the usual activity control. In addition, the improvement in mental wellbeing was maintained over a further 3 months, during which no singing took place (see Fig. 31.1). There were also significant reductions in depression and anxiety scores on the HADS at 3 months, although the benefits for depression and anxiety were not sustained on follow-up.

Attention was also given to the feedback provided by participants on the questionnaires completed, and this also clearly revealed that a wide range of benefits were experienced. Those in the singing group wrote positively about:

◆ enjoyment and pleasure
◆ impact on the quality of their singing
◆ impact on mental health and wellbeing
◆ social benefits through socializing and forming friendships
◆ improvements in breathing
◆ the quality of the facilitation of the groups and the repertoire, and
◆ their hopes for the continuation of the groups after the project.

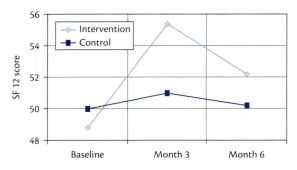

**Fig. 31.1** Silver Song Club randomized controlled trial: York SF-12 mental wellbeing component scores for participants in the intervention and control arms (differences between the groups are significant at 3 and 6 months). Reproduced with permission from Clift, S., Skingley, A., Coulton, S. and Rodriguez, J. *A controlled evaluation of the health benefits of a participative community singing programme for older people (Silver Song Clubs)*, The Sidney De Haan Research Centre for Arts and Health, Canterbury Christchurch University, Folkestone, UK. Copyright © 2012 The Sidney De Haan Research Centre for Arts and Health.

The following examples of comments given by participants express some of these themes:

'Many times on the morning of the project I haven't felt like coming, but always I came and felt so much better afterwards. Group singing lifts the spirits.'

'I started my participation in this project just after I retired from work and feeling a little anxious about future life. This project has been instrumental in showing me there is life after work.'

'The singing has, I feel, boosted my confidence as I tend to be rather shy. I am hoping I may be able to join a singing group/church choir in the near future.'

'Introspection is the curse of old age—this project reduces such self-awareness and actually offers the realization that there is more living to be done.'

As noted, this project recruited a cross-section of older people living independently in the community. Although many participants disclosed some existing health challenges, on average the

level of assessed mental wellbeing at the outset was close to the population norm and means on the anxiety and depression scales of the HADS were below the clinical threshold on this instrument. In further work of the De Haan Centre we have explored the potential value of singing for people who are experiencing mental and physical health challenges.

### The east Kent singing for mental health project

In 2009, the De Haan Centre established a network of seven singing groups for people with enduring mental health issues (the East Kent 'Singing for Health' Network Project) (Clift and Morrison 2011) in towns across east Kent. Over the course of 10 months, the choirs grew in size and involved over 100 mental health service users together with friends, family, and health professionals providing support. The choirs came together to form a large chorus for a public performance in February 2010 and then to mark the culmination of the project in June 2010 (see Fig. 31.2). A short film about the project based on the final performance has been produced, including interviews with members of the choirs (<https://www.youtube.com/watch?v=ITDAi9lWhyw>).

The project was evaluated qualitatively on the basis of observation and interviews, and more systematically employing the Clinical Outcomes in Routine Evaluation (CORE) questionnaire, an instrument widely used in clinical practice within the UK National Health Service (NHS). The questionnaire gives a total score measuring mental distress, but also four subscores measuring 'wellbeing', 'problems', levels of daily 'functioning', and 'risk' to self and others (with lower scores being positive; for details of this instrument see Gray and Mellor-Clark, 2007). For a sample of 42 choir members completing the CORE questionnaire at baseline then 8 month later, there was a statistically significant reduction in the total mental distress score, together with improvements in three of the four subscales (see Table 31.1).

These measurable changes were strongly supported by written feedback given by members of the choirs experiencing challenges of social anxiety, depression and other mental health issues:

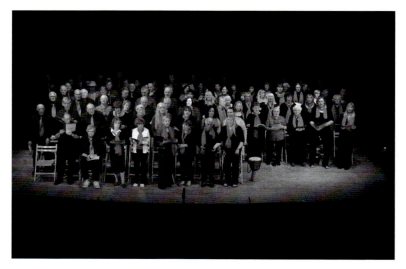

**Fig. 31.2** Singing for mental health: choirs in the network performing at the end of the project at the Granville Theatre, Ramsgate, UK, June 2010. Reproduced by kind permission of The Sidney De Haan Research Centre. Copyright © 2015 The Sidney De Haan Research Centre.

**Table 31.1** Singing for mental health: means (standard deviations) on the CORE questionnaire at baseline and the end of the project

|  | n | Baseline | End of project | P-values |
|---|---|---|---|---|
| Total score | 42 | 9.43 (6.58) | 6.85 (5.26) | 0.001 |
| Wellbeing | 42 | 1.33 (0.88) | 0.96 (0.74) | 0.003 |
| Problems | 42 | 1.11 (0.87) | 0.80 (0.65) | 0.005 |
| Functioning | 42 | 1.03 (0.71) | 0.74 (0.61) | 0.003 |
| Risk | 42 | 0.19 (0.45) | 0.15 (0.26) | n.s. |

n.s., not significant.

Higher scores represent greater mental distress. Risk scores are very low as few members of the group reported self-harming behaviour or conflicts with others.

'I have bipolar disorder. When I am depressed, singing in the group and coming together with other people lifts my mood and gives me something positive and productive to focus on. When I am manic, singing is something I can channel my extra energy into and express my enthusiasm for life through. The choir provides structure and purpose in an otherwise sometimes empty life. The group reminds me that there are many people with difficulties of one kind or another. We can understand each other's problems and support one another.'

'It helps me to structure my week, to have something to keep going for. I enjoy meeting all types of people. It has been very good to meet new people who have experiences similar to my own. If I feel I might have a panic attack, I know how to breathe properly which helps. I would have very little reason to leave the house if I wasn't doing choirs.'

'Singing helps as I can become withdrawn with depression, so it helps me express myself. It is nice to be able to express myself through singing. I can be quite self-conscious at times and it is nice to be able to do something in unison. I find my mood is lifted and find myself singing when alone. To be part of a group has helped my self-consciousness.'

## Singing for people with chronic obstructive pulmonary disease (COPD)

The most recent study completed by the De Haan Centre has explored the role that regular group singing may have in improving the wellbeing of people with chronic obstructive pulmonary disease or COPD (Morrison et al. 2013; Skingley et al. 2013). COPD primarily includes bronchitis and emphysema which involve damage to different regions of the lungs (most commonly due to smoking) and lead to difficulties with breathing. COPD worldwide is a major cause of ill-health and death, and in the United Kingdom alone it is estimated that approximately 3 million people are affected by this condition.

A number of small-scale studies, including three clinical trials, have shown that people with COPD find that singing is enjoyable and beneficial in terms of subjective wellbeing and health and helps with their breathing. However, little or no improvement has been found for standard lung function measures and assessments of physical activity (e.g. distance walked before feeling breathless) (Bonilha et al. 2009; Lord et al. 2010, 2012; Goodridge 2013). Possible reasons for the lack of improvement in lung function are that the length and intensity of the singing activities were insufficient to produce positive changes. All of the studies also took place in clinical settings, and in the Goodridge et al. (2013) study, singing was introduced as an adjunct to a more extensive pulmonary rehabilitation programme.

In planning a further study, therefore, a different community singing model was followed, similar to that adopted in our previous studies. A network of six small choirs was established for over 100 people with COPD (with supporters/carers welcome) meeting weekly over the course of 10 months. On three occasions during the project, groups were brought together for larger choral workshops and performances. As no other community-based study has been conducted before over this length of time, the project was designed as a feasibility study rather than a randomized controlled trial (see Fig. 31.3 for a photo of one of the groups involved in the project).

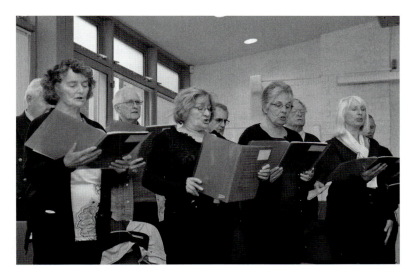

**Fig. 31.3** Singing for COPD: the Folkestone group which acted as a pilot for the feasibility study.

**Table 31.2** Singing for COPD: means (standard deviations) for measures of lung function and the SGRQ at baseline and the end of the project

| Measure | n | Baseline | End of project | P-value |
|---|---|---|---|---|
| $FEV_1$ | 66 | 1.29 (0.49) | 1.32 (0.51) | 0.094 |
| $FEV_1$% predicted | 67 | 54.34 (20.45) | 56.28 (21.98) | 0.006 |
| FVC | 64 | 2.43 (0.75) | 2.54 (0.75) | 0.027 |
| FVC% predicted | 65 | 81.72 (22.60) | 85.35 (21.70) | 0.034 |
| SGRQ total | 71 | 48.71 (16.95) | 45.42 (16.96) | 0.024 |
| SGRQ symptoms | 71 | 59.16 (23.49) | 56.04 (22.05) | 0.143 |
| SGRQ activities | 71 | 65.46 (22.41) | 63.33 (22.14) | 0.204 |
| SGRQ impact | 70 | 35.65 (17.56) | 32.21 (15.90) | 0.042 |

SGRQ, St George's Respiratory Questionnaire; FEV, forced expiratory volume; FVC, forced vital capacity.

Participants were assessed using standard spirometry before the start of the intervention and then at the conclusion of the project. Two key measures were taken: 'forced expiratory volume' or $FEV_1$ (the amount of air in litres that can be forcefully expelled from the lungs in one second) and 'forced vital capacity' or FVC (the amount of air that can be expelled in total when breathing out for a long as possible). These values naturally decline with age for everyone, so in addition to the raw scores, adjusted percentage scores relative to normative values were also calculated. In addition, participants completed a series of questionnaires, including the St George's Respiratory Questionnaire (SGRQ) with the total score as the principal outcome measure. This has been used internationally as a condition-specific measure of health status.

From a feasibility point of the view, the study proved to be highly successful. A sample of 106 participants with COPD was successfully recruited. They varied in the severity of their COPD, with 15% mild, 45% moderate, 30% severe, and 10% very severe. The mean age of the people in the sample was 69.5 (SD 7.64) years; a third were male.

Table 31.2 presents the results observed for the lung function measures and the SGRQ total and subscale scores. All the lung function measures increased, and all but $FEV_1$ to a statistically significant degree. These results are particularly striking as a decline in these values over this period of time would normally be expected. A significant improvement was also found on the SGRQ total score, with this improvement accounted for by the change in the reported impact of breathing problems on daily living.

Qualitative feedback from the participants provided further strong support for the perceived value of weekly singing in helping to improve breathing:

'Standing to sing helps posture, you think 'upright' automatically as this gives maximum output from your lungs. The relaxation exercises do just that, and learning to breathe bringing the muscles of the abdomen into play, as well as controlled exhalation, has helped me enormously.'

'This is the first winter I have not had to call an ambulance or be on several lots of antibiotics and have taken only maintenance doses of steroids. This maybe a coincidence or it may be better because of the breathing help we have received.'

'I believe that the project is teaching me how to understand my breathing and how to control it. This is very useful; it stops me hyperventilating when my breathing is under pressure, i.e. climbing a steep hill.'

'Helped mentally and physically. Somewhere to go with like-minded people. Have not for the first time in 5 years been admitted to hospital or casualty over the winter period. Opened up doors, i.e. joining the (BLF) Breathe Easy group.'

Personal testimonies on the benefits of singing are also featured in two of the three films produced about the project (<https://www.youtube.com/>, search for 'Sidney de Haan'). As the research was an uncontrolled feasibility study it is not possible to attribute the changes unequivocally to the intervention, but all the quantitative and qualitative evidence gathered points in that direction. It is worth mentioning that the cost to the NHS for one COPD hospital admission is estimated to be almost £2000 (NICE 2011). If this project had helped even one participant to avoid an emergency hospital admission, as described in the last the quotations, the cost saving involved would have been sufficient to run 20 weekly singing groups for 30 or more participants. Further research on community singing for COPD needs to include suitable control groups and also a detailed economic analysis of costs and benefits.

## Conclusions

The Sidney De Haan Research Centre is committed to researching the role of music and other participative arts activities in promoting the wellbeing and health of individuals and communities. It is pursuing this mission through a progressive and integrated research programme focused specifically on the value of group singing for wellbeing and health, and particularly for people with enduring chronic health conditions. We believe that our programme of research to date has shown conclusively that regular group singing can give rise to real benefits for the personal and social wellbeing of participants. We have also begun to show that regular singing can have measurable and clinically important benefits for people with existing mental and physical health challenges. As the population in the United Kingdom (and in countries throughout the world) continues to age and the burden of long-term health conditions continues to increase, new approaches will be needed in health and social care provision to meet these challenges. Group singing may well provide one cost-effective activity that can contribute to this growing public health challenge.

# References

Bonilha, A.G., Onofre, F., Vieira, L.M., Prado, M.Y., and Martinez, J.A. (2009). Effects of singing classes on pulmonary function and quality of life of COPD patients. *International Journal of COPD*, **4**, 1–8.

Bungay, H., Clift, S., and Skingley, A. (2010). The Silver Song Club project: a sense of wellbeing through participatory singing, *Journal of Applied Arts and Health*, **1**, 165–178.

Clark, I. and Harding, K. (2012). Psychosocial outcomes from active singing interventions for therapeutic purposes: a systematic review of the literature. *Nordic Journal of Music Therapy*, **21**, 80–98.

Clift, S. and Hancox, G. (2001). The perceived benefits of singing: findings from preliminary surveys with a university college choral society. *Journal of the Royal Society for the Promotion of Health*, **121**, 248–256.

Clift, S. and Hancox, G.(2010). The significance of choral singing for sustaining psychological wellbeing: findings from a survey of choristers in England, Australia and Germany, *Music Performance Research*, **3**, 79–96.

Clift, S. and Morrison, I. (2011). Group singing fosters mental health and wellbeing: findings from the east Kent 'singing for health' network project. *Mental Health and Social Inclusion*, **15**, 88–97.

Clift, S., Hancox, G., Staricoff, R., and Whitmore, C. (2008). *Singing and Health: A Systematic Mapping and Review of Non-clinical Research*. Canterbury: Canterbury Christ Church University.

Clift, S., Hancox, G., Morrison, I., Hess, B., Kreutz, G., and Stewart, D. (2009). What do singers say about the effects of choral singing on physical health? Findings from a survey of choristers in Australia, England and Germany. *European Society for the Cognitive Sciences of Music (ESCOM) Conference, Jyvaskyla, Finland, 12–16 August, 2009.* Available at: <https://jyx.jyu.fi/dspace/handle/123456789/20854>

Clift, S., Hancox, G., Morrison, I., Hess, B., Kreutz, G., and Stewart, D. (2010a). Choral singing and psychological wellbeing: quantitative and qualitative findings from English choirs in a cross-national survey. *Journal of Applied Arts and Health*, **1**, 19–34.

Clift, S., Nicols, J., Raisbeck, M., Whitmore, C., and Morrison, I. (2010b). Group singing, wellbeing and health: a systematic mapping of research evidence. *UNESCO e-Journal*, **2**, 1. Available at: <http://education.unimelb.edu.au/__data/assets/pdf_file/0007/1105927/clift-paper.pdf> (accessed 15 February 2014).

Clift, S., Skingley, A., Coulton, S., and Rodriguez, J. (2012). *A Controlled Evaluation of the Health Benefits of a Participative Community Singing Programme for Older People (Silver Song Clubs)*. Canterbury: Sidney De Haan Research Centre for Arts and Health. Available from: <http://www.canterbury.ac.uk/research-and-consultancy/research-centres/sidney-de-haan-research-centre/documents/community-singing-programme-for-older-people.pdf> (accessed 15 February 2014).

Irons, J.Y., Kenny, D.T., and Chang, A.B. (2010). Singing for children and adults with bronchiectasis. *Cochrane Database of Systematic Reviews*, (2): CD007729.

Gick, M. (2010) Singing, health and well being: a health psychologist's view. *Psychomusicology: Music, Mind and Brain*, **21**, 1–32.

Goodridge, D., Nicol, J., Horvey, K.J., and Butcher, S. (2013). Therapeutic singing as an adjunct for pulmonary rehabilitation participants with COPD: outcomes of a feasibility study, *Music and Medicine*, **5**, 169–176.

Gray, P. and Mellor-Clark, J. (2007). *CORE: A Decade of Development*. Rugby: CORE IMS. Available at: <http://www.coreims.co.uk/core_occasional_papers.html> (accessed 15 February 2014).

Morrison, I., Clift, S., Page, S., et al. (2013) A UK feasibility study on the value of singing for people with chronic obstructive pulmonary disease (COPD). *UNESCO e-Journal*, **3**, 3. Available at: <http://education.unimelb.edu.au/__data/assets/pdf_file/0003/1067421/003_morrison_paper.pdf> (accessed 14 February 2014).

Kreutz, G. (2014) Does singing facilitate social bonding? *Music & Medicine*, **6**, 2, 51–60.

Lord V.M., Cave, P., Hume, V., et al. (2010). Singing teaching as a therapy for chronic respiratory disease—randomised controlled trial and qualitative evaluation. *BMC Pulmonary Medicine*, **10**, 41. Available at: <http://www.biomedcentral.com/1471-2466/10/41>

Lord, V.M., Hume, V.J., Kelly, J.L., et al. (2012). Singing classes for chronic obstructive pulmonary disease: a randomized controlled trial. *BMC Pulmonary Medicine*, **12**, 69. Available at: <http://www.biomedcentral.com/1471-2466/12/69>

NHS Choices (2013). No proof that singing in a choir is good for the heart. Available at: <http://www.nhs.uk/news/2013/07july/pages/no-proof-that-singing-in-a-choir-is-good-for-heart.aspx> (accessed 15 February 2014).

NICE (National Institute for Health and Clinical Excellence) (2011). *Chronic Obstructive Pulmonary Disease Costing Report: Implementing the NICE Guidance*. National Institute for Health and Clinical Excellence. Available from: http://www.nice.org.uk/nicemedia/live/13029/53292/53292.pdf (accessed 15 February 2014).

Skingley, A. and Bungay, H. (2010). The Silver Song Club Project: singing to promote the health of older people. *British Journal of Community Nursing*, **15**, 135–140.

Skingley, A., Page, S., Clift, S., et al. (2013). 'Singing for breathing': Participants' perceptions of a group singing programme for people with COPD. *Arts & Health: An International Journal for Research, Policy and Practice*, **6**, 69–74.

Skingley, A., Bungay, H., Clift, S., and Warden, J. (2014). Experiences of being a control group: lessons from a UK-based randomized controlled trial of group singing as a health promotion initiative for older people. *Health Promotion International*, **29**, 751–758.

Vickhoff, B., Malmgren, H., Åström, R., et al. (2013). Music structure determines heart rate variability of singers. *Frontiers in Psychology*, **4**, art 334.

Wan, D.Y., Rüber, T., Hohmann, A., and Schlaug, G. (2010). The therapeutic effects of singing in neurological disorders. *Music Perception*, **27**, 287–295.

# CHAPTER 32

# Intergenerational music-making: a vehicle for active ageing for children and older people

Maria Varvarigou, Susan Hallam, Andrea Creech, and Hilary McQueen

## The benefits of intergenerational music-making

A strong corpus of research highlights the positive and long-lasting impact of intergenerational activities on active ageing, cultural exchange, and reciprocal learning (Newman et al. 1997; Newman and Hatton-Yeo 2008; St John 2009; Creech et al. 2014a). In this chapter 'active ageing' is defined as 'a comprehensive strategy to maximize participation and wellbeing as older people age' (Walker 2013, p. 86). Walker argues that active ageing should operate at all stages of the life course and at individual (lifestyle), organizational (management), and societal (policy) levels.

The main purpose of intergenerational practice is to bring together different generations to 'collaborate on purposeful activities, while supporting and nurturing each other in meaningful ways' (Herrmann et al. 2006, p. 124). These interactions amongst different generations provide 'the kind of purposeful existence that is important to human development' (Newman et al. 1997, p. 19). Intergenerational programmes in music have reported a wealth of benefits for children and older adults alike. Music-making and listening to music are valued, enjoyable activities across the life span with numerous implications for social and personal development (Hallam 2001), identity negotiation (Macdonald et al. 2002; Lally 2009), physical development, health and wellbeing (Ashley 2002; Clift, et al. 2010; Varvarigou et al. 2012), and cognitive development and learning (Hallam 2005; Cohen 2009). Active music-making in groups, in particular, has been found to facilitate learning and teaching experiences and at the same time to confront and manage 'conflict and situations of living together' (Cunha and Lorenzino 2012, p. 74). Active music-making also supports the development of cognitive skills related to purposeful listening, concentration, attention, and sharing of ideas, which lead to expressions of creativity (Hickson and Housley 1997).

One significant contribution of intergenerational music programmes is the integration of diverse populations and people of differing abilities in activities that enhance the creation of interpersonal attachments and promote social involvement and engagement (Darrow et al. 2001; Cusicanqui and Salmon 2005; Springate et al. 2008; de Vries, 2012). In addition, through active musical interactions participants in intergenerational activities develop a sense of mutual concern, caring, and respect for each other's abilities and interests (Darrow et al. 2001; Conway and Hodgman 2008; St John 2009, 2012). For example, Conway and Hodgman (2008) examined the experiences of college students and older people in an intergenerational choral project in the United States and found that working towards a collaborative choral performance heightened the experience of all involved, enabled a better understanding of others, and led to enhanced musical and social connections and a greater respect for each other.

Benefits specifically experienced by older adults have been linked to improved health and wellbeing, including a reduced sense of isolation as the older adults often go out to meet other people, interact with them, and 'make friends' (Dallman and Power 1996), and a renewed sense of worth and productivity through passing on knowledge, skills, and life experience to younger generations (Frego 1995; Rubinstein 2002; West 2003; Garber 2004; Springate et al. 2008). This phenomenon, where older people impart values, culture, and life skills to members of the succeeding generation in their endeavour to improve the world, offer service to others, and 'contribute something worthwhile to the betterment of society' (Herrmann, et al. 2006, p. 135), is known as 'generativity'. Erikson (1963, p. 267) advocated that 'the concept of generativity is meant to include such popular synonyms as productivity and creativity, which, however, cannot replace it'. In the absence of generativity the individual may feel a 'pervading sense of stagnation and personal impoverishment' (Erikson 1963, p. 267).

Benefits reported by younger participants are related to the dissolution of negative stereotypes and the creation of interpersonal attachments and relationships that boost their self-esteem (Herrmann et al. 2006; Springate et al. 2008; Meshel and McGlynn 2010). Frego (1995) recognized that through intergenerational contact children or young people dispel negative images of ageing, with older people often being presented by the media as 'being over the hill, out of date, out of touch, frail, sick and in need of services and support' (Kerschner and Pegues 1998, p. 2; Alcock et al. 2011). Similarly, older adults observe young people in creative and productive activities and develop positive attitudes about them (Darrow et al. 2001; Dabback 2005; de Vries, 2012). For instance, Darrow et al. (2001) explored the attitudes of teens and older adults, who acted as an audience, towards an intergenerational choral performance by teens and older adults. They reported that teens talked about older people's 'quality music performance' and had the opportunity to 'appreciate active ageing, by recognising that personal independence and musicianship can continue throughout one's life' (Darrow et al. 2001, p. 48).

Active ageing through lifelong learning and development of skills for both young and old has been the focus of several music studies, with the latest research in neuroscience supporting the significance of learning in later life (Cohen 2009; Mehrotra 2011; Schneider 2011; Koelsch and Stegemann 2012) and the power of music in facilitating physical interactions, communication, and active learning.

There is no single definition for describing intergenerational practice around the world. In the United Kingdom this term is used to refer to 'purposeful activities, which are beneficial to both young people (normally 25 or under) and older people (usually aged over 50)' (Hatton-Yeo 2006, p. 12). Nevertheless, groups of older people can in themselves be intergenerational, often covering several decades (Frego 1995; O'Neill and Heydon 2013). There is also an intergenerational dynamic when groups leaders and facilitators representative of the 'middle generation' (i.e. 25–50 years old) work alongside older people in creative activities (Springate et al. 2008). In this chapter we explore the benefits and challenges of active music-making with children under the age of 16 and adults aged over 50 (New Dynamics of Ageing 2009; Schuller and Watson 2009) in intergenerational musical activities. Examples of three different types of programmes where (1) older adults provide service to children or young people, (2) children or young people assist older adults, and (3) cooperative programmes where different generations collaborate in musical activities as equal partners serving others (Newman et al. 1997) illustrate how music could facilitate intergenerational expression, communication, understanding and model active ageing.

## Case study 1: older adults provide service to children or young people

When older adults share their time, skills, and experiences with children and young people they become a valuable resource to the school, teacher, parent, student, and community (Newman et al. 1997). De Vries (2012) explored intergenerational active music-making through the interactions of three senior Australians with children. Through sharing music as a common interest, the older adults became the children's friends, advocates, and motivators. The first was 67-year-old Irene, who started receiving piano lessons again after a gap of 60 years, who played the piano together with her granddaughter, Chelsea (11 years old). In Irene's words, playing the piano with her granddaughter fostered a special connection between them, 'a way of communicating, of being together' (de Vries 2012, p. 343). The second was 75-year-old Margaret, who volunteered as a piano accompanist for a rural primary school choir and taught the violin to one of the children in the choir, 8-year-old Kylie. Margate saw great musical potential in Kylie. Kylie's family, however, could not afford to purchase a musical instrument for her or offer her music lessons. Margaret brought her half-sized violin from home to the school and started teaching Kylie the violin free of charge. The third was 72-year-old Bruce, who played keyboard, piano, and guitar in his 1950s style rock and roll band. His friend's son, 15-year-old Josh, played the saxophone but wanted to give it up, so his father asked Bruce if Josh could 'sit in the band' as a way of motivating him to keep playing. Bruce not only welcomed Josh to the band but, as time went by, also encouraged him to have a greater say in the choice of repertoire of the band, recognizing that young people and older adults alike have a need to be heard and for independence (Frego 1995). De Vries' study illustrated the significance of reciprocity of learning between generations and the great sense, amongst the older people, of being valued and respected by the children and others connected to the children (e.g. the school principal). The older adults in the study acknowledged that the children had taught them how to use technology (iPod, Finale Notepad, and the ProTools software program), had motivated them to engage with music, and had also helped them to become familiar with the modern repertoire. What is more, there was a recognition amongst the older adults that their contribution to the children's musical learning had been significant. Irene expanded Chelsea's piano repertoire by introducing duets that they could play together, Kylie would not have had the opportunity to learn to play the violin if Margaret had not volunteered to teach her for no charge, and Bruce supported Josh's development of technique on the saxophone through regular rehearsals and performances with the band. Combined with the feeling of making a lasting contribution to the children's learning and social development, this study also advocated for intergenerational music-making by promoting the development of older adults as teachers/mentors or fellow musicians (Markus and Nurius 1986; Creech et al. 2014b) who not only taught and guided the younger generation, fulfilling their desire for generativity, but also modelled active ageing and the 'vitality that is possible to later life' (Rubinstein 2002, p. 38).

## Case study 2: children and young people assist older adults

The Hand-in-Hand outreach programme in Canberra, Australia (Garber 2004) facilitated active music-making of primary school children with older adults in residential homes and with other disadvantaged members of the community. The philosophy of the programme was rooted in the altruistic use of music, and the core aim was 'not to make music for others but with others, with specific intent to benefit all those involved' (Garber 2004, p. 2). Susan West, the founder of the programme, explained that encouraging altruism through music is a 'life affirming, therapeutic activity' (West 2003, p. 1) founded on five principles:

> '(i) involvement with music is naturally human; (ii) making music is of more value for the individual than consuming music; (iii) making music in order to have a beneficial effect on another is more valuable than simply making music for oneself alone; (iv) making music with another in order to engage the other in music making is more beneficial for both giver and receiver, and (v) making music so as to encourage the receiver to, in turn, make music to have a beneficial effect on another is more beneficial for both and society as a whole.'
>
> West (2003)

The programme involved groups of young children visiting nursing homes and singing songs from the Tin Pan Alley era with the residents. Garber underlined that although singing was the key activity, children and older people sang together without intending to produce a performance or just a 'sing-a-long'. Instead the focus was on using singing as a tool for a therapeutic communication between the children and the older people. In essence, the programme encouraged altruistic behaviour in children through the use of music; children and teachers were making music together for the benefit of others. Percussion instruments were initially used but were later found to prevent close contact during singing, so the children were encouraged to physically interact with the older adults instead. For example, once the singing started, the children would 'take hold of the residents' hands, look into their eyes and sing with great gusto and confidence' (Garber 2004, p. 147).

The impact of this intergenerational programme on the participants, especially with reference to improving their health and wellbeing, was noteworthy: (1) children expressed a great sense of enjoyment, enthusiasm, and interest in learning about music; (2) at-risk or disabled children 'displayed a heightened sense of maturity' resulting in behavioural and attitudinal improvement towards learning at school; (3) the children displayed no signs of stage fright or performance anxiety during and outside the sessions; and (4) the older adults demonstrated increased social and emotional wellbeing and raised self-esteem through opportunities to share life experiences and make a contribution to the children through their responses. With reference to the increased emotional and social wellbeing of the older adults, West reported that victims of stroke, people with depression, and residents with various forms of dementia were observed to sing and talk with the children and share spoken memories triggered from the songs. Furthermore, wheelchair-bound and ambulatory residents were observed to dance (children and 'dancing wheelchairs') as well as sing with the children. Box 32.1 shows some responses from the participants in the Hand-in-Hand programme. The responses illustrate children's strong sense of purpose in 'making people happy' driven by their innate desire to have a place and role in society and to make a contribution (Frego 1995; Newman et al. 1997; Springate et al. 2008). The teachers' responses emphasized the children's maturity and immediacy in their musical interactions with the older adults, and they referred extensively to the positive impact of the interactive experience on social

***

**Box 32.1** Hand-in-Hand: quotes from the participants

**Children**

I like visiting them once a month because making people feel happy makes me happy.

I enjoy making people happy, but sometimes they won't let go of your hand or they smell funny. It's good when they sing along or better when they get up and dance.

I like it because they are always happy and it's me making them happy. We get to know the people there and make them happy.

**Teachers**

Often teachers are surprised by particular children who are right into it. The experience is humanizing. So often children are just sitting in front of a computer and passive. In this situation they are giving out, giving out some energy.

My kids really surprised me. They went right forward toward the residents; they didn't stay in a group. They were confident on their own and approached some of the frailest and most unapproachable residents. One child in the class had cerebral palsy and was legally blind. He went right up close to the resident and really sang out. Another child was developmentally delayed and particularly neglected but he gravitated toward the Ainslie [school name] kids. He was comfortable and felt safe with them, more so than with the residents. Another child I taught used to really look forward to going to the nursing home and seeing one particular resident who would tell him stories.

However it is not just the singing. It is not a performance. It is the eye contact, the holding hands and sometimes getting them to dance or just (if they are too sick to sing) a reaction like humming, tapping with a foot or fingers. You can feel that in their way they participate and enjoy the music making.

Source: data from Garber, S.J. (2004). The Hand-in-Hand community music program: a case study. PhD Dissertation, Australian National University, Canberra. Copyright © 2004 S.J. Garber.

***

relationships, which often created feelings of belonging, enjoyment, and appreciation. This highlights that, given the opportunity to experience social affirmation, being accepted, and valued (Creech et al. 2013), children can make a significant contribution to enhancing the wellbeing of older adults.

## Case study 3: cooperative programmes—children and older adults as equal partners

The Music for Life project (Hallam et al. 2012b) was funded by the New Dynamics of Ageing Strand of the UK Research Councils to: (1) explore the way in which participating in creative music-making activities could enhance the lives of older people, (2) consider the extent to which this may impact on social, emotional, and cognitive wellbeing, and (3) consider the specific process through which this occurs. One part of the project comprised an intergenerational music programme for older adults who were residents in two sheltered housing establishments ($n = 11$) and children ($n = 35$) from two East London primary schools. Sheltered housing accommodation is accommodation

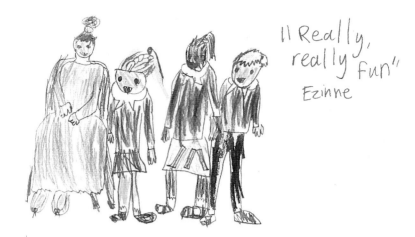

**Fig. 32.1** 'Really, really fun'—the positive impact of intergenerational musical interactions on older people (the figure on the left) and children as drawn by one of the participating pupils.

provided specifically for older people. Such schemes usually have the services of a warden or scheme manager, though increasingly this person lives off site, or the service is provided as 'floating support', with periodic visits from a member of staff. The programme lasted for 2 months and culminated in a concert at the Pitt Theatre, Barbican Centre, London (for a detailed description of the intergenerational project, please refer to Varvarigou et al. 2011).

Between October 2009 and January 2010, the older adults engaged in weekly creative music sessions, which included singing, song writing, and experimentation with untuned percussion instruments. Three music facilitators who all had great experience in working with young people in the community led the sessions. From March until May 2010 the music facilitators visited each of the two participating children's groups for an hour in order to teach the children the songs that they rehearsed with the older adults, how to play untuned percussion instruments, and how to use body percussion to accompany singing. After the school rehearsal the children joined the older adults for an additional hour in a collaborative music session. The findings from this music programme emphasize the positive impact that intergenerational interactions can have on modelling active ageing and on supporting children's and older adults' sense of purpose, control/autonomy, and social affirmation, i.e. the human need for affection and behavioural confirmation, that lead to enhanced cognitive, physical, social, and emotional wellbeing (Fig. 32.1).

First, through engagement in intergenerational activities the older adults had opportunities to fulfil their desire for generativity and regain a possibly neglected sense of worth as members of society who can make a lasting contribution (Frego 1995; Boulton-Lewis et al 2006; Boulton-Lewis 2010; Mehrotra 2011). Allowing the older adults to share experiences and their favourite musical repertoire with the children facilitated this. Learning new musical repertoire and skills in playing untuned percussion instruments gave the older adults a reason for regularly attending the sessions. Moreover, the older people played a central role in

a musical performance for their families, community members, and for the younger people. The performance itself gave the older adults the opportunity to contribute to making a rich experience for the younger people, and to contribute to a most moving performance for the audience (Darrow et al. 1994, 2001; Cusicanqui and Salmon 2005; Conway and Hodgman 2008 ). Opportunities for creative music-making were also offered, which resulted in one of the older adults writing a song and in the children creating body percussion and instrumental improvisation to accompany this song at the Barbican Centre performance (Varvarigou et al. 2013). Because of their beauty and productivity, art programmes have a reason for continued participation that fosters sustained involvement (Cohen et al. 2006; Chapman 2013).

Secondly, intergenerational music-making encouraged a sense of control in the interactions of the participants. For example, the children were invited to choose the actions to accompany each musical phrase of 'El Café', a traditional song from Argentina taught by the music facilitators. This process helped everyone to remember the lyrics. Likewise, the older adults were encouraged to devise an instrumental accompaniment for the song using untuned percussion and to show it to the children, who then joined in with their maracas. The more physically able older adults engaged in all musical activities including action games, action songs, and body percussion to accompany singing, which had a positive impact on their sense of physical and cognitive wellbeing. Those who were more physically frail joined in the singing and derived enjoyment from observing children's vitality and enthusiasm. The older adults emphasized that the experience of working with the children was rejuvenating as it 'made them feel younger' and they were happy to chat with the children and answer their questions. Learning and development in music was also evident throughout the course of the programme. The older adults were challenged to develop their concentration and memory in learning and remembering new songs (Fig. 32.2).

Thirdly, musical interactions promoted the development of social relationships, supporting social affirmation and emotional wellbeing; the children found the older adults funny, kind, and

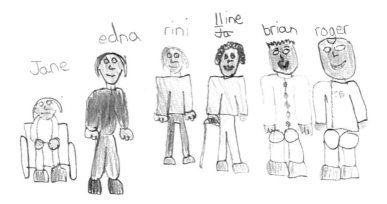

**Fig. 32.2** A drawing depicting older people's happiness (smiling faces) after the children's visit to the sheltered housing accommodation.

---

**Box 32.2** The Music for Life project: quotes from the participants

### Children

The best thing about singing and playing music with older people was seeing the old people happy.

I liked singing to the seniors and playing the instruments.

When we were at [sheltered housing building] these were some of the most fun days of my life with A., G. [the older adults] and the rest of the crew.

I liked one thing about older people; that they really helped us and they played music and instruments very well.

### Older adults

Music makes you feel younger.

I enjoyed the company of the children . . . [they] were wonderful; the way they sing.

Well, it [music-making] helps me. It makes me young. Without music . . . , I wouldn't be here [Barbican Centre] . . . Instead of sitting, watching TV, doing nothing. Look, we are here, we meet people, meet you, meet lovely people . . . For a start, we miss the band. We feel empty without them. It was fantastic; very good idea. I would be happy to be with the group . . . and I feel so young to be honest with you. And I am happy.

As soon as we warmed up and we started singing, I had this lovely feeling of heart being in harmony. I mean it was hard work. It was a big commitment. It ran for about six months but it was worth every minute of it really. And a big thank you to everyone . . . I am interested in how you can get kids to read music as painlessly as possible because you have so many things to remember . . . I have been attending the courses run by J and L [the facilitators] and their colleagues for about six months now and I really enjoyed them very much indeed because at school I had a lot of bad experiences in music.

### Teachers

And it was such an interesting environment, and being on the stage and working with the other school and then obviously working with the older people and them being centre stage. And finding out about S.'s [one of the older adults] song—he'd actually written that himself. It just felt that they were part of something really special.

The whole participation, the whole collaboration with the singing and also playing instruments and just the whole interaction I think. That was probably the highlight for them. Going there [sheltered housing], singing with them, singing to them and then with them and the instruments and everything.

### Music facilitators

One of the key things that stayed with me from this project has been this kind of real opening up of personalities and confidence in using music.

Each group completely changes the dynamic of the other group.

I think for the older participants the benefits were to get the sense of energy from the children, for musical support, you know, the children really could help to hold that altogether.

Source: data from Varvarigou, M., Creech, A., Hallam, S., and McQueen, H. (2011). Bringing different generations together in music-making—an intergenerational music project in East London. *International Journal of Community Music*, **4**, 207–220. Copyright © 2011 The Authors.

loving and they enjoyed making music with them. The teachers emphasized that the children bonded with the older adults and developed respect for them. Although the children were 'a bit worried at first', after the first visit they 'were looking forward to going back again and again'. Both the children and the older adults were excited about giving a performance in front of an audience, and they also felt a great sense of achievement in working hard together in order to produce a successful performance for their friends and relatives. Box 32.2 shows some responses from the children, the older adults, the facilitators, and the school teachers on the impact of this intergenerational music programme on supporting wellbeing and promoting active ageing.

## The challenges of intergenerational music-making and ways forward

We have illustrated that intergenerational music projects can have a lasting impact on the cognitive, physical, social, and emotional wellbeing of the participants and can encourage and sustain lifelong learning and active ageing. There are, however, challenges for the participants and the facilitators related to planning and realizing intergenerational practice. Facilitators report challenges related to the management of mixed-ability groups and creating a sense of inclusion for all involved (Cusicanqui and Salmon 2005), finding appropriate repertoire (Conway and Hodgman 2008; de Vries 2012), gaining the respect of the older adults, setting an appropriate pace for the sessions, and using appropriate language (Hallam et al. 2012a). The children report challenges related to stereotypes about older adults being physically frail, 'needy and sad' (Frego 1995, p. 17).

Children and older adults, however, have reciprocal and shared needs which are 'related to the placement and role of these generations within the life continuum', and which 'reflect treatment of the young and the old by the larger society' (Newman et al. 1997, p. 18); both older adults and children need to feel secure, accepted, valued, and to have a place and role in society (St John 2009). These shared needs are reflected in the model of subjective wellbeing proposed by the Music for Life project (Creech et al. 2013) which suggests that promoting a sense of purpose, control/autonomy, and social affirmation (i.e. positive social relationships, competence, and a sense of recognized accomplishment) through intergenerational music-making could support active ageing and wellbeing.

Some of the challenges in maximizing the potential benefits to be derived from intergenerational practice related to the particular training needs of facilitators who work with older people. Whilst the facilitators of the Music for Life project were highly skilled and experienced in their work with young people, this project revealed some particular pedagogical issues relating to effective practice when working with older people. Myers (1995, p. 12) recognized that 'the thrust of teaching and research in music education has historically been directed towards school-age population', therefore, there is a pressing need for music facilitators who lead intergenerational activities to be well aware of the relationship between active ageing and engagement

in music-making amongst older people with particular reference to social, emotional, physical, and cognitive wellbeing. Organizing musical activities that provide a variety of options and take account of different interests, abilities, experiences, and needs (Mehrotra 2011) could create a sense of inclusion during intergenerational music-making and create a sense of control and feeling of empowerment for the participants who can then choose the intensity of their interactions (Garber 2004; Darrow and Belgrave 2013). In addition, in order for intergenerational musical activities to be inclusive, music facilitators should take account of frailty, not ignore it (Walker 2013). Musical activities need to consider the physical or other limitations of older adults or children (Darrow and Belgrave 2013) and run at a pace that allows older adults to interact with the children with vibrancy and enthusiasm while the young people experience the physical and emotional care and support offered by the older adults. Some practical suggestions from Chapman (2013) and St John (2009) include: settling the children or young people when they arrive through fun warm-up exercises which are often quite physical to shake off any jitters; ensure that all the activities provide an opportunity for interaction and/or team work across the generations, for example, when singing in parts, make sure that each part (team) includes both generations; use songs with actions which require people to look at/gesture to each other/touch hands; encourage teams of older and younger people to come up with creative ideas together; encourage eye contact and verbal communication; try to communicate to schoolchildren that they are not in school so different rules apply, for instance, encourage them to make noise, be physical, move around, and chat with the older adults; and acknowledging efforts with genuine praise in a voice appropriate for each population dignifies responses with authenticity (St John 2009, p. 744).

Facilitators should draw on the wealth of knowledge and experience that the participants bring to the music session, 'honour multiple interpretations of the presented task' (St John 2009, p. 743) and support the older adults' sense of generativity allowing them to model active ageing. Facilitators should also allow the children to have their voices heard and to show their care or physical and emotional support to older adults (West 2003; Garber 2004; Cusicanqui and Salmon 2005). Supporting generativity and the need for contributions from all participants makes the musical interactions purposeful and helps the facilitators to gain the respect from both older adults and children. Finally, music, through its general appeal, can serve as a vehicle to bring about understanding between the generations, encouraging the development of relationships and friendships, and respect for one another and for each person's unique contribution to the musical activities, which leads to strengthening the sense of being accepted and valued for both older adults and children.

## Summary

By describing three case studies, this chapter has provided evidence that intergenerational music-making can offer numerous benefits to both children and older people. These benefits are related to enhanced physical, cognitive, social, and emotional wellbeing as well as lifelong learning. Through intergenerational active music-making older people have the opportunity to recover a sense of worth (that is often diminished) by making a valuable contribution to a child's experience of shared music-making and by positively influencing children's perceptions of active ageing while enhancing their own learning and growth. Likewise, children or young people have the opportunity to share their vitality, enthusiasm, and energy with older adults, facilitating the dissolution of stereotypes and both generations' sense of purpose in participation and a sense of control and autonomy over the choice of repertoire and quality of interactions. Finally, intergenerational musical interactions could promote social affirmation, through a sense of belonging and an appreciation of the contribution that both older adults and children can make to joint music-making. Intergenerational practice is an ideal platform for modelling active ageing and lifelong learning, serving as a vehicle to bring about exchange of ideas between the generations.

## References

Alcock, C.L., Camic, P.M., Barker, C., Haridi, C., and Raven, R. (2011). Intergenerational practice in the community: a focused ethnographic evaluation. *Journal of Community and Applied Social Psychology*, **21**, 419–432.

Ashley, M. (2002). Singing, gender and health: perspectives from boys singing in a church choir. *Health Education*, **102**, 180–186.

Boulton-Lewis, G. (2010). Education and learning for the elderly: why, how, what. *Educational Gerontology*, **36**, 213–228.

Boulton-Lewis, G., Buys, L., and Lovie-Kitchin, J. (2006). Learning and active aging. *Educational Gerontology*, **32**, 271–282.

Chapman, F. (2013). Musical Connections and Intergenerational Practice. York: City of York Council.

Clift, S., Hancox, G., Morrison, I., Hess, B., Kreutz, G., and Stewart, D. (2010). Choral Singing and psychological wellbeing: quantitative and qualitative findings from English choirs in a cross-national survey. *Journal of Applied Arts and Health*, **1**, 19–34.

Cohen, G.D. (2009). New theories and research findings on the positive influence of music and the art on health with ageing. *Arts & Health: An International Journal for Research, Policy and Practice*, **1**, 48–62.

Cohen, G.D., Perlstein, S., Chapline, J., Kelly, J., Firth, K.M., and Simmens, S. (2006). The impact of professionally conducted cultural programmes on the physical health, mental health and social functioning of older adults. *The Gerontologist*, **46**, 726–734.

Conway, C. and Hodgman, T. (2008). College and community choir member experiences in a collaborative intergenerational performance project. *Journal of Research in Music Education*, **56**, 220–237.

Creech, A., Hallam, S., Varvarigou, M., McQueen, H., and Gaunt, H. (2013). Active music making: a route to enhanced subjective wellbeing among older people. *Perspectives in Public Health*, **133**, 36–43.

Creech, A., Hallam, S., Varvarigou, M., and McQueen, H. (2014a). *Active ageing with music: Supporting wellbeing in the Third and Fourth Ages*. London: Institute of Education, University of London.

Creech, A., Hallam, S., Varvarigou, M., Gaunt, H., McQueen, H., and Pincas, A. (2014b). The role of musical possible selves in supporting subjective wellbeing in later life. *Music Education Research*, **16**, 32–49.

Cunha, R. and Lorenzino, L. (2012). The secondary aspects of collective music-making. *Research Studies in Music Education*, **34**, 73–88.

Cusicanqui, M. and Salmon, R. (2005). Seniors, small fry, and song: a group work libretto of an intergenerational singing group. *Journal of Gerontological Social Work*, **44**, 189–210.

Dabback, W. (2005). Examining the gap between theory and emerging practices in the instrumental music education of older adults. *International Journal of Community Music*, **B**(1), 1–16.

Dallman, M.E. and Power, S. (1996). Kids and elders. *Forever Friends*, No. 27.

Darrow, A.A. and Belgrave, M. (2013). Students with disabilities in intergenerational programmes. *General Music Today*, **26**, 27–29.

Darrow, A. A., Johnson, C.M., and Ollenberger, T. (1994). The effect of participation in an intergenerational choir on teens' and older persons' cross age attitudes. *Journal of Music Therapy*, **31**, 119–134.

Darrow, A.A., Johnson, C.M., Ollenberger, T., and Miller, M.A. (2001). The effect of an intergenerational choir performance on audience members' attitudinal statements towards teens and older persons. *International Journal of Music Education*, **38**, 43–50.

Erikson, E. (1963). *Childhood and Society*. New York: W.W. Norton.

Frego, D. (1995). Utilising the Generations with Music programmes. *Music Educators Journal*, **81**, 17–19, 55.

Garber, S.J. (2004). The Hand-in-Hand community music program: a case study. PhD Dissertation, Australian National University, Canberra.

Hallam, S. (2001). *The Power of Music: the Strength of Music's Influence on our Lives*. A study commissioned by the Performing Right Society. London: Performing Right Society.

Hallam, S. (2005). *Enhancing Motivation and Learning Throughout the Lifespan*. London: Institute of Education, University of London.

Hallam, S., Creech, A., Varvarigou, M., and McQueen, H. (2012a). The characteristics of older people who engage in community music making, their reasons for participation and the barriers that they face. *Journal of Adult and Continuing Education*, **18**, 21–43.

Hallam, S., Creech, A., Varvarigou, M., and McQueen, H. (2012b). Perceived benefits of active engagement with making music in community settings. *International Journal of Community Music*, **5**, 155–174.

Hatton-Yeo, A. (2006). *Intergenerational Programmes: An Introduction and Examples of Practice*. Stoke-on-Trent: Beth Johnson Foundation.

Herrmann, S., Sipsas-Herrmann, A., Stafford, M., and Herrmann, N. (2006). Benefits and risks of intergenerational program participation by senior citizens. *Educational Gerontology*, **31**, 123–138.

Hickson, J. and Housley, W. (1997). Creativity in later life. *Educational Gerontology*, **23**, 539–547.

Kerschner, H. and Pegues, J.M. (1998). Productive aging: a quality of life agenda. *Journal of the American Dietetic Association*, **98**, 1445–1448.

Koelsch, S. and Stegemann, T. (2012). The brain and positive biological effects in healthy and clinical populations. In: R. Macdonald, G. Kreutz, and L. Mitchell (eds), *Music, Health, and Wellbeing*, pp. 436–456. New York: Oxford University Press.

Lally, E. (2009). The power to heal us with a smile and a song: senior wellbeing, music-based participatory arts and the value of qualitative evidence. *Journal of Arts and Communities*, **1**, 25–44.

Macdonald, R., Miell, D., and Hargreaves, D. (eds) (2002). *Musical Identities*. Oxford: Oxford University Press.

Markus, H. and Nurius, P. (1986). Possible selves. *American Psychologist*, **41**, 954–969.

Mehrotra, C. (2011). In defence of offering educational programs for older adults. *Educational Gerontology*, **29**, 645–655.

Meshel, D. and McGlynn, R. (2010). Intergenerational contact, attitudes, and stereotypes of adolescents and older people. *Educational Gerontology*, **30**, 457–479.

Myers, D. (1995). Lifelong learning: an emerging research agenda for music education. *Research Studies in Music Education*, **4**(June), 21–27.

New Dynamics of Ageing (2009). NDA programme specification. Available at: <http://www.newdynamics.group.shef.ac.uk/music-for-life.html>

Newman, S. and Hatton-Yeo, A. (2008). Intergenerational learning and the contribution of older people. *Ageing Horizons*, **8**, 31–39.

Newman, S., Ward, C., Smith, T., Wilson, J., and McCrea, J. (1997). *Intergenerational Programmes—Part, Present and Future*. Washington, DC: Taylor and Francis.

O'Neill, S. and Heydon, R. (2013). Elders connecting to young people through singing: evidence of generativity and wellbeing among older adults in an intergenerational program. Paper presented at the Advancing Interdisciplinary Research in Singing 5th Annual Meeting. Abstract available at: <http://www.airsplace.ca/5th_annual_meeting_abstracts#eldersconnecting>

Rubinstein, R.L. (2002). The third age. In: R.S. Weiss and S.A. Bass (eds), *Challenges of the Third Age: Meaning and Purposes in Later Life*, pp. 29–40. New York: Oxford University Press.

Schneider, K. (2011). The significance of learning for aging. *Educational Gerontology*, **29**, 809–823.

Schuller, T. and Watson, D. (2009) *Learning Through Life: Inquiry into the Future for Lifelong Learning*. Leicester: NIACE.

Springate, I., Atkinson, M., and Martin, K. (2008). *Intergenerational Practice—a Review of the Literature*. LGA Research Report F/SR262. Slough: NFER.

St John, P.A. (2009). Growing up and growing old: communities in counterpoint. *Early Child Development and Care*, **179**, 733–746.

St John, P.A. (2012). Unforgettable: musical memories with infants and seniors. Paper presented at the International Society of Music Education World Conference, Thessaloniki, Greece, 15–20 July 2012.

Varvarigou, M., Creech, A., Hallam, S., and McQueen, H. (2011). Bringing different generations together in music-making—an intergenerational music project in East London. *International Journal of Community Music*, **4**, 207–220.

Varvarigou, M., Creech, A., Hallam, S., and McQueen, H. (2012). Benefits experienced by older people in group music-making activities. *Journal of Applied Arts and Health*, **3**, 183–198.

Varvarigou, M., Hallam, S., Creech, A., and McQueen, H. (2013). Different ways of experiencing music-making in later life: Creative music sessions for older learners in East London. *Research Studies in Music Education*, **35**, 103–118.

de Vries, P. (2012). Intergenerational music making: a phenomenological study of three older Australians making music with children. *Journal of Research in Music Education*, **59**, 339–356.

Walker, A. (2013). Commentary: the emergence and application of active aging in Europe. *Journal of Aging and Social Policy*, **21**, 75–93.

West, S. (2003). Mining Tin Pan Alley: the songs of Tin Pan Alley as a social, musical and educational resource in the development of music making based on a community-focused social/altruistic philosophy. *Youth Studies Australia*, **22**, 25–31.

# PART 4

# Creative arts and public health in different settings

33 **The arts therapies: approaches, goals, and integration in arts and health** *271*
Amy Bucciarelli

34 **Museums and art galleries as settings for public health interventions** *281*
Helen J. Chatterjee

35 **Case study: creativity in criminal justice settings—the work of the Koestler Trust** *291*
Tim Robertson

36 **Quality of place and wellbeing** *299*
Bryan Lawson and Rosie Parnell

37 **Creative arts in health professional education and practice: a case study reflection and evaluation of a complex intervention to deliver the Culture and Care Programme at the Florence Nightingale School of Nursing and Midwifery, King's College London** *309*
Ian Noonan, Anne Marie Rafferty, and John Browne

38 **Case study: singing in hospitals—bridging therapy and everyday life** *317*
Gunter Kreutz, Stephen Clift, and Wolfgang Bossinger

39 **Case study: the value of group drumming for women in sex work in Mumbai, India** *325*
Varun Ramnarayan Venkit, Anand Sharad Godse, and Amruta Anand Godse

# CHAPTER 33

# The arts therapies: approaches, goals, and integration in arts and health

Amy Bucciarelli

## Introduction

The science of healthcare is most effective when it is combined with empathetic communication, a humanistic approach, and comprehensive medical interventions that address the physical, spiritual, and emotional wellbeing of a whole person (Robichaud 2003; Serwint 2013). This chapter discusses the arts therapies as an important component of arts and health. The professional roles, settings, and training of arts therapists are defined; the philosophies that underlie how the arts therapies work are outlined; and the five foundational principles that guide arts therapies practices are highlighted. Finally, how the arts therapies can work in partnership with arts in medicine is described. A case example is used to illustrate how collaboration between fields leads to strong care in arts and health.

## Defining the arts therapies

The arts therapies are a group of counselling disciplines that combine the fields of fine arts and psychology (Malchiodi 2005; Brett and McHarg 2011). Art therapy, dance/movement therapy, drama therapy, music therapy, and poetry therapy are mental health professions that use their discipline-specific art form as a therapeutic tool (ADMP 2003; BAAT 2011; BADTH 2011; BAMT 2012; AMTA 2013; NAPT 2013). Professionals with formal training and credentials for multiple arts therapies disciplines are called expressive therapists (IETA 2012). Sometimes 'expressive therapies' or 'creative arts therapies' are used as umbrella terms to describe collective disciplines, associations, or tracks within degree programmes (NCCATA 2013). For the purposes of this chapter, the field of professions is referred to as the 'arts therapies'. The professions are identified by their training-specific name: art therapy, dance/movement therapy, drama therapy, music therapy, or poetry therapy.

The arts therapies are a separate field from arts in medicine. Arts in medicine employs professional artists who *do not* pursue psychotherapeutic goals and are purely focused on promoting wellbeing in healthcare settings (Graham-Pole 2007). Collaboration between arts in medicine and the arts therapies will be discussed later in this chapter.

The arts therapies are closely related to psychology, counselling, and social work in addressing both psychological and physical wellbeing in healthcare settings (Malchiodi 2003a; AMHA 2013; APA 2013; NASW 2013). These fields employ similar theoretical models of human development, behaviour, social systems, multicultural issues, psychopathology, and assessment. A defining goal of these fields, including the arts therapies, is to provide clients with non-judgmental counselling that encourages changes in thoughts or behaviours to increase emotional and physical health (ADMP 2003; Malchiodi 2003a; BAAT 2011; BADTH 2011; BAMT 2012; APA 2013; AMHA 2013; NAPT 2013; NASW 2013).

The arts therapies stand apart from traditional forms of therapy because they combine non-verbal communication, creativity, and multisensory experiences into recovery tools. Instead of simply talking about thoughts and feelings, arts therapists guide people to express themselves through visual art, dance, movement, drama, music, or poetry (Levy 1988; Bruscia 1998; Rubin 1999; Mazza 2003; Malchiodi 2005; Langley 2006; Serlin 2007).

## How the arts therapies work

The arts are known to facilitate creative expression (Dissanayake 2000; Malchiodi 2005; Graham-Pole 2007). People instinctively use the arts to acknowledge emotions, feel understood, and discover deeper meaning (Jung 1933). Furthermore, when people encounter adversity they are often motivated to seek creative solutions through curiosity, imagination, and flexible thinking (Torrance 1993) which can lead to increased resilience against negative emotions (Maslow 1968; Torrance 1993). Different levels of creative expression, from kinaesthetic and sensory to cognitive and symbolic, can aid progress toward wholeness through the arts (Lusebrink 1990). Arts therapists use the benefits of creativity to enhance self-understanding and healing for their clients.

Arts therapists also utilize the multisensory nature of the arts to assist therapeutic processing and physiological restoration. Information from the external world enters the body through senses like sight, sound, touch, and smell. Then, the brain hierarchically processes behaviours, emotions, thoughts, and memories related to the experience of the senses (Perry, 2009; Moore et al. 2009; Rosen and Levenson 2009). Verbal therapies employ language to process this complex information. However, psychological conditions, disease, neglect, and trauma all affect healthy neuroprocessing, which can limit the use of purely verbal therapies (Gantt and Tinnin 2009; Perry 2009; Chatterjee 2010). If the body and brain are not optimally functioning, initiating change through high-level cognition is difficult.

The arts simultaneously engage multiple brain processes (Malchiodi 2003b; Gantt and Tinnin 2009; Chanda and Levintin 2013). Music can moderate autonomic nervous system functions like heart rate and muscle tension while stimulating a positive neurochemical release to give an uplifted mood (Chanda and Levintin 2013); visual art allows a victim of trauma or brain degeneration to retrieve memory images from non-verbal sections of the brain and communicate them in a comprehensible way (Gantt and Tinnin 2009; van Buren et al. 2013); and dance studies show that the cortical regions that perceive body movements are different from those that execute body movements, resulting in brain plasticity that could affect divergent thinking and problem-solving (Cross and Ticini 2012). Observing the ways that the arts influence the brain and body brings understanding to the powerful whole-person work of the arts therapies.

When creative expression is delivered in a therapeutic setting, a three-pronged dialogue blossoms between the client, artwork, and therapist (Lusebrink 1990; Brett et al. 2011). Arts therapists are skilled at offering experiences approachable to people with a range of artistic abilities and knowledge (Payne 1993). An arts therapist guides the client to choose materials and interventions that will enable a successful creative experience (Lusebrink 1990). The process of art-making informs the participant and the therapist about cognitive, emotional, or physical distress which can unlock conscious and unconscious meaning, opening the door for authentic self-expression. Focus is not on the aesthetic composition or value of the art piece (Malchiodi 2003a), and the therapist does not judge or impose interpretation on the work. The outcome is tangible, like lyrics to a song or a theatrical skit, and builds a bridge from psychological content to verbal processing and holistic healing. The client leads the session path and the arts therapist shepherds the work so it can be communicated in a meaningful and safe way. Acting in a counselling role, arts therapists have the responsibility to nurture the therapeutic relationship by understanding transference, boundaries, and issues of self-care (Bruscia 1988; Levy 1988; Rubin 1999; Mazza 2003).

Each arts therapies discipline has inherent similarities and characteristic differences (Knill et al. 2004). An art therapy session might be silent. A turn inward arouses visual images that evoke personal reflection. A dance/movement therapy session might shift a participant's awareness outward, experiencing relationships through rhythm as they synchronize movement to a beat. Clients may prefer one form of the arts therapies over another. Different disciplines are more or less suited to particular therapeutic settings and treatment goals. The ultimate objective of all arts therapies is to promote mental, social, physical, and spiritual health (ADMP 2003; BAAT 2011; BADTH 2011; BAMT 2012; NAPT 2013).

## Settings for the arts therapies

The arts therapies can be incorporated into any setting where psychotherapy is suggested as a treatment (Malchiodi 2003a).

They are particularly indicated for people who have challenges communicating, problems navigating their environment, or difficulty making sense of the world around them (Payne 1993). Arts therapies can benefit people of all ages and cultural backgrounds. Sessions are administered to individuals, couples, families, or groups depending on the setting and goals of therapy.

Arts therapists work with clients in private practice or institutions including medical hospitals, schools, adult day homes, addiction recovery centres, eating disorder treatment centres, prisons, military settings, physical rehabilitation, and psychiatric hospitals. Emerging areas of arts therapy service include international outreach, risk prevention, and community health initiatives (Camic 2008; Stuckey and Nobel 2010; Levin and Levin 2011). In all these settings caregivers can also benefit from the arts therapies to decrease burnout and stress-related illnesses (Koff-Chapin 2013).

## Training in the arts therapies

Practice as a psychologist or counsellor requires intensive training about the complexities of human thought and behaviour. Similarly, it takes years of study and discipline to master the studio arts. Arts therapists have a specialized training that combines preparation in the arts and counselling psychology (Rubin 1999). In order to practice professionally, most of the arts therapies disciplines require corresponding accredited master's degrees in addition to registration, board certification or licensure (ADMP 2003; BAAT 2011; BADTH 2011; BAMT 2012; NAPT 2013). In the United States, music therapists are currently educated to bachelor level or higher (AMTA 2013). The American Music Therapy Association (AMTA) is discussing transition to require master's level entry into the field which would align the educational requirements of music therapists with the other arts therapies (AMTA 2014). Each arts therapies discipline has its own governing associations and accreditation boards throughout the world. These organizations establish educational standards, codes of ethics, and professional expectations (ADMP 2003; BAAT 2011; BADTH 2011; BAMT 2012; IETA 2012; NAPT 2013).

In parts of the world where the arts therapies are new or undeveloped, responsible professionals obtain accredited training. Some traditional psychologists and counsellors use art in therapy, but before doing so they are encouraged to seek training from endorsed arts therapies instructional programmes (see ADMP 2003; BAAT 2011; BADTH 2011; BAMT 2012; NAPT 2013). These professionals are mindful that arts therapists have extensive knowledge about how arts materials, processes, and outcomes can affect the safe delivery of therapy.

The arts therapies are growing in recognition as evidence-based treatments (Dileo and Bradt 2009). In order to continue the development of these fields, students and professionals are encouraged to contribute to educational development, programme evaluation, policy reform, and research efforts that continue to expand the reach of health outcomes and employment opportunities for arts therapists.

## Foundational principles of the arts therapies

A range of health goals and outcomes are available when people participate in the arts therapies. Transformative capabilities are only limited by available resources and the openness of a client. Most arts therapies interventions develop from the core principles that art can be inherently therapeutic, art can be used to assess symptoms, behaviours, and developmental levels, art can provide emotional safety and containment, art can activate progress towards goals, and art can be used as a form of communication.

## Art is inherently therapeutic

Internal ideas, beliefs, and energies are released though artistic expression (Knill et al. 2004; Malchiodi 2005). The art process *itself* can be therapeutic. Csikszentmihalyi (1997) noticed increased focus, motivation, and self-awareness through the 'flow' of creative activities. Intentional art-making is grounding. It mirrors other evidence-based techniques, such as mindfulness-based stress reduction (MBSR), which prompts body awareness and a focused, non-judgemental mind (Gard et al. 2012). The arts therapies offer a goal-directed diversion from physical and emotional pain (Malchiodi 2005). Art-making also bolsters the goals of other therapies. In music therapy, a child with speech difficulties is guided to play a recorder for the purpose of strengthening the coordination of his or her mouth muscles (Young 2011). Simultaneously, the child meets speech therapy goals and gains a feeling of accomplishment, which can reinforce positive mood and self-image, as the result of playing an instrument.

## Art assesses

Arts therapists are knowledgeable about developmental milestones expressed through the arts. Children first scribble, then draw circles before squares (Lowenfeld and Brittain 1987). Eventually, they add shapes and lines together that represent objects. By knowing how humans progress as they age, arts therapists can notice when development is inhibited.

Arts therapists know how to assess emotional, behavioural, and physical states (Feder and Feder 1998). Each arts therapies discipline has methods for identifying psychopathology, such as anxiety, depression, or cognitive degeneration, through the specific art form. The tone in a piece of writing or the line-quality in a drawing offers important diagnostic information when it is considered within the clinical picture. Formal and informal arts therapies assessments advise the healthcare team in quick and economical ways about treatment recommendations (Payne 1993; Feder and Feder 1998; Betts 2006). The arts create archives, like a song or phrase of movement, that document change over time and help navigate the course of therapy.

## Art is safe and containing

Art, music, dance, drama, and creative writing are familiar leisure activities. When arts modalities are available in therapy they remain approachable even when treatment seems foreign or overwhelming (Lusebrink 1990). Drama therapists direct war veterans to act out untold stories of combat through mime, gesture, and tone (Johnson 2010). The whole-body approach opens a dialogue about traumatic experiences that is less threatening than talking about difficult memories. At the same time, the structure of the activity and guidance by the therapist offer safety for processing sensitive issues. In another example, a child squirts paint from medical syringes onto a canvas to release aggressive energies in a productive way. The experience makes hospitalization seem less threatening and provides a fun, empowering experience.

Particular diagnoses result in a loss of control. Dance can help 'organize movements, calm dystonia, and improve gait and balance' in patients with Parkinson's disease (ADTA undated, p. 1). Similarly, a hyperactive child can feel more focused and controlled with structured art materials, like colouring pencils (Lusebrink 1990). Arts therapists understand how materials, sound, movement, and composition influence behaviour and the psyche. For example, movement can elicit body-based responses that trigger memories of trauma; or finger painting can cause regression from well-organized behaviours to a less controlled child-like state.

## Art activates

The arts therapies mobilize participants to be active in treatment (Rubin 1999; Malchiodi 2005). Jumping, strumming, reciting, and transcribing alleviate helplessness and instil control. Activity is physiologically beneficial and it grounds personal awareness to stimulate psychological growth (Csikszentmihalyi 1997). A poetry therapist asks a bed-ridden adult to recite a poem—the poem's imagery evokes a personal story that is energizing despite the patient's immobility (Integrative Medicine Committee 2004).

Arts processes, tasks, and outcomes become a metaphor for life skills outside the dance studio or art room. Children naturally explore their world and learn how to interact with it through engagement with the arts (Rubin 1999). Clients of all ages rehearse problem solving, conflict resolution, and positive coping through the arts therapies. For example, a drum circle teaches assertiveness, responsiveness, and risk-taking through rhythms (Snow and D'Amico 2010). These skills are translated to relationships outside the therapy room.

## Art communicates

Arts are a fundamental form of communication (Dissanayake 2000; Chandara and Levitin 2013). Humans learn to move, draw, and respond to music before communicating through speech (Lowenfeld and Brittain 1987; Bruscia 1998). People who have developmental or cognitive learning deficits benefit from communication delivered through the arts. For instance, a child with autism can learn about social cues through dance (Levy 1988).

In a more complex way, arts therapists understand that non-verbal language originates from inner perceptions, thoughts, or emotions (Knill et al. 2004). Difficult or undiscovered experiences, like sexual abuse or grief, may surface through art (Payne 1993; Malchiodi 2005; Serlin 2007). Arts therapists help clients reflect, respond, and interpret personal meaning from the art while providing a sense of safety through their therapeutic approach and intentional choice of arts methods (Malchiodi 2005). They use the art as an objective tool to verbally process psychological content, gain insights, or promote catharsis.

A teenager who demonstrates defiant behaviour can make a lyrical rap to express frustrations about an unsupportive home life and distaste for rules. The rap is a constructive release of emotions. The arts therapist can use the themes communicated in the rap to help the teenager gain insights and increase psychosocial development. The rap is a tangible product that can be revisited and used throughout the course of therapy. If the teenager shares the rap with others, it becomes a vehicle for an audience to experience empathy and understanding.

## Arts and health

Arts-based services are ideal for healthcare settings. They are preventative, non-invasive, cost-effective, and accessible with few to no side effects (Malchiodi 2005; Sonke 2011; Chandara and Levintin 2013). They can even be *fun*! Arts and health is a broad term describing a group of fields that contribute to the practice of, education about, and research into arts-based services that are integrated into hospitals and public health settings. Some of the fields comprising arts and health include medicine, health administration, community health, arts therapies, and arts in medicine or arts in healthcare (Dileo and Bradt 2009; Camic 2011; Tesch and Hansen 2013).

### Differentiating the arts therapies from arts in medicine

Within arts and health two fields are commonly discussed: arts in medicine and the arts therapies. In the United States, arts in medicine developed primarily in medical hospitals (Sonke et al. 2009) and the arts therapies evolved in psychiatric, medical, and educational settings (Levy 1988; Bruscia 1998; Mazza 2003; Vick 2003; Malchiodi 2005; Langley 2006; Serlin 2007;). Their origins directly influenced the approach and scope of practice for each field. Clear differences distinguish artists in residence from arts therapists in healthcare settings (Dileo and Bradt 2009; Broderick 2011).

#### Arts in medicine

Arts in medicine integrates the arts into the environment and provides creative activities as a way to humanize the healthcare experience and enhance personal wellbeing (Sonke-Henderson and Brandman 2007; Lee 2013). Artists employed in arts in medicine are commonly called artists in residence (Graham-Pole 2007). Artists in residence demonstrate excellent proficiency in specific art forms such as visual art, dance, music, theatre, or writing (Sonke et al. 2009). Within art forms, an artist in residence may have specialized techniques, styles, instruments, or media that they tailor to their healthcare work.

Artists in residence work alongside the healthcare team, but they are not considered clinicians and, therefore, work independently of patients' diagnoses and treatments (Sonke 2011; Lee 2013). The artist's relationship with participants shifts between that of mentor, facilitator, and fellow-artist (Brett and McHarg 2011). Artists in residence work with people who are motivated to participate in the arts (Lee 2013). Artwork begins on a conceptual level and the process is led by the patient. Artwork is kept private or is publicly exhibited. As such, artists in residence may view the work with an aesthetic lens and influence the creative process or product (Brett and McHarg 2011). A skilled artist in residence has knowledge about the healthcare environment, a high level of artistic expertise, and clearly understands the scope of practice (Sonke et al. 2009).

Arts in medicine programmes are typically supported by trained volunteers who work under the supervision of artists in residence (Sonke et al. 2009). Volunteer support lengthens the reach of cost-effective arts programming and provides hands-on education for developing arts and health professionals.

#### The arts therapies in healthcare settings

Arts therapists are allied health professionals: members of an interdisciplinary team of clinicians including physicians, nurses, social workers, psychologists, psychiatrists, case managers, physical therapists, occupational therapists, recreation therapists, and child life specialists, among others (Lee 2013). Arts therapists use arts-based interventions to assist physical and psychological healing. In hospital or clinic settings, arts therapists are referred to work with specific concerns that affect medical outcomes such as anxiety, compliance, or palliative issues (Goodill 2005; Malchiodi 2013). Arts therapists have access to confidential patient files including information on states of health and psychosocial–spiritual histories (Brett and McHarg 2011). They support medical treatment plans (Councill 2003; Malchiodi 2013), and therefore communication with clinicians through medical record notes and team meetings is essential for care delivery (Brett and McHarg 2011).

Art therapy comforts a child adjusting to a new diagnosis by having familiar materials, like crayons, available during unfamiliar hospital experiences. Analysing song lyrics helps a patient talk about his or her fears of death and dying. A dance therapist and a physical therapist collaborate on rehabilitation goals. A patient paints an image to show clinicians what the pain feels like. A poem written for nurses and physicians assists the transition from a long hospitalization to home life. Patient stories captured through a theatrical performance make meaning out of illness and offer an opportunity for personal reflection and psychological development. The arts therapies build communication and rapport, enabling the patient to actively participate in treatment and assisting the healthcare team to effectively deliver care (Goodwill 2005; Malchiodi 2013).

Figure 33.1 offers a visual example that illustrates the professional distinctions between artists in residence and arts therapists. Both patients were asked to create a 'winter scene'. The image on the left was made in a workshop with an artist in residence. During the process, the artist in residence suggested choices for the scene like 'a carrot nose' and 'a yellow sun'. The goal was to deliver a fun experience and a product the child was proud of. The image on the right replicates a drawing made in an art therapy session with a patient on dialysis. The art therapist fostered a safe space for expression, but did not direct the process. Even on a basic examination, some elements of the picture seem unusual. One colour, red, is used for almost all the picture, which makes the 'melting' snowman look like it was 'shot or bleeding'. The sun is darkened, the tree has an odd-looking branch, and the overall quality seems disorganized compared with the image on the left. An art therapist would use this drawing to explore themes of emotional or physical distress with the patient.

### Arts therapies and arts in medicine collaborations

Increasingly, artists in residence and arts therapists are working together in healthcare (Graham-Pole 2007). Both fields recognize that the arts give physiological benefit, normalize the healthcare environment, create empowerment, produce positive feelings, facilitate meaning through expression, build cultural awareness, engage people in community, and offer tools for practitioner self-care (Malchiodi 2003c; Sonke-Henderson and Brandman 2007; Brett and McHarg 2011). Arts in medicine and the arts therapies are accessible for individuals, groups, families, and communities. To the untrained eye, the work of arts therapists and artists in residence appears very similar.

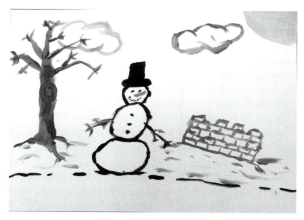 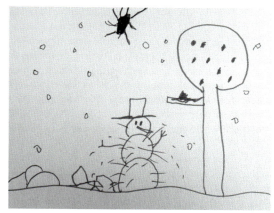

**Fig. 33.1** An example to illustrate the professional distinctions between an artist in residence and an art therapist (see text for explanation).
Reproduced by kind permission of Amy Bucciarelli. Copyright © 2015 Amy Bucciarelli.

Every arts therapist is an artist (Brett and McHarg 2011). A foundation in studio arts is a pre-requisite to enter arts therapies degree programmes. Conversely, every artist has experienced how the arts transform thoughts, emotions, and behaviours. Mutual understanding and collaboration between the two professions equals fruitful arts and health practices (Brett and McHarg 2001; Sonke et al. 2009).

An arts therapies department without artists in residence lacks critical arts support. Artists in residence extend their creative reach to every person in the healthcare picture: from facilities workers, to patients, to administrators (Sonke-Henderson and Brandman 2007). Clinical settings transformed into theatrical performance stages or public art galleries establish a visible culture of arts for everyone to enjoy. Although there is therapeutic benefit to these initiatives; facilitating, promoting, and advocating for the arts takes arts therapists away from focusing on rehabilitation goals.

Concurrently, arts in medicine programmes without arts therapists are limited in their scope of service. Medical health does not discriminate between developmental disorders, behavioural challenges, and psychological diagnoses. Arts therapists have the skills and techniques to work with clients who experience difficulty, are resistant to treatment, and have physical challenges that prevent benefit from other services. Table 33.1 displays a guide for artists in residence and healthcare clinicians to recognize appropriate arts therapies referrals. The behaviours listed could be symptoms that indicate mental health issues. For example, someone who has difficulty sleeping counter-indicated to medical issues could be depressed.

The arts therapies are uniquely positioned to open up communication and understanding between medical communities and arts in medicine practices. Arts therapists speak the clinical discourse *and* the language of the arts. Arts therapists become translators, of sorts: they have the clinical terms to describe arts-based care to medical staff. Similarly, arts therapists know a patient's medical status. They can help steer artists in residence to care for a patient with complex health issues in the most supportive way.

Patients have ebbs and flows in their psychotherapeutic and physical needs during treatment, particularly during long-term hospitalization. Artists in residence can utilize arts therapists as a

**Table 33.1** Indicators for arts therapies referrals

| Behavioural indicators for arts therapies *or* other psychosocial referrals | Arts-based indicators for arts therapies referrals |
| --- | --- |
| • Talks about being down or sad | • Makes art, music, writing, or is moving frequently |
| • Overly quiet: only responds with nods or shrugs | • Content of arts expression is odd or chaotic |
| • Stays in bed despite medical indications that ambulation is appropriate | • Arts expression has a heaviness or intensity to it |
| • Lights off and blinds closed frequently | • Art outcome seems 'flooded': patient completes it extremely quickly, or fills it with emotional charge |
| • Apathetic: lack of emotions/behaviours | • Not naturally engaging in the arts despite it being developmentally appropriate for communication (i.e. 3–6 years old) |
| • Angry frequently or inexplicably | |
| • Engages in play that has themes of excessive violence, dismemberment, monsters, symbols of death or other scary things (for older patients, obsession with any of these things) | • Telling stories through metaphors and symbols in the arts |
| | • Themes of weapons, monsters, death, or scary things repeated in the art |
| • Talks about dying or wanting to disappear | • Behaviours with arts materials or arts processes are not appropriate |
| • Difficulty sleeping or nightmares | • Treatment team cannot find medical basis for physical complaints or pain (arts-based assessment could help) |
| • Major change in behaviour | |
| • Fearful when family members leave the room | |
| • Acts much younger than developmental age | |
| • Anxious | |
| • Excessive energy | |
| • Poor attention | |
| • Hyper-vigilance | |
| • Confusion | |
| • Psychosis | |
| • Addictions | |
| • Non-compliant with medical recommendations | |

resource when arts-based indicators suggest a patient is in need of a higher-level of care (see Table 33.1). When a patient has low therapeutic needs, artists in residence can promote general wellbeing through the arts as an adjunct to therapy. Artists in residence and arts therapists can join together on sophisticated legacy projects like doll-making or personal memoirs. Artists have expertise about specialized arts tools and techniques that can amplify an art therapist's work. In partnership, the arts therapist is holding the therapeutic space while the artist in residence is expanding creative capacity.

Distributing arts care between professionals is a successful method for delivering cost-effective care. When a patient has a positive relationship with one arts professional the groundwork for openness and trust is established. Meaningful work with the next arts professional is unlocked quickly and easily. Communication and collaboration lowers the burden on individual caregivers and develops a network when difficult outcomes like death happen, as they inevitably do.

Artists in residence and arts therapists can learn from each other. Artists in residence practice their art professionally outside the healthcare environment. Their art strengthens their hospital practice and promotes self-care (Brett and McHarg 2011). Analogously, the arts therapies model educational programmes, professional ethics, standards of practice, and practitioner–patient boundaries for arts in medicine (Moss and O'Neil 2009).

## A reflective case example

Khandice was a 20-year-old admitted to the hospital for treatment of osteosarcoma, discovered while she was playing basketball. An ambitious young woman, she had a passion for school and hopes of becoming a music producer. I was referred to visit her as the art therapist on a paediatric palliative care team. The team served all cancer patients at the recommendation of the American Academy of Pediatrics (2012).

I met Khandice a week into her 10-month treatment. She told me she loved to sing and do theatre, but it had been a long time since she had made art. In our first session, Khandice was intensely focused on the technical aspects of drawing a baby elephant. After spending a significant time on it, she dismissed the drawing because it was 'frustrating' her. She couldn't verbalize why there was a tear streaming down the baby elephant's trunk—just that 'it was cute and belonged there'. A girl moving into womanhood was admitted to the paediatric haematology–oncology unit with her mother by her side. Her drawing seemed symbolic of grief for her diagnosis and the vulnerability this independent young adult was experiencing with her hospitalization.

I quickly learned that Khandice needed complex, sophisticated art interventions to be satisfied in therapy. This seemed like her attempt to assert maturity in a hospital unit geared toward children. Her adult freedom was taken away. Art seemed like her avenue to maintain it. Together, we explored thoughts, feelings, and general catharsis through mask-making, mixed-media collages, drawings, and large-scale paintings.

During treatment, Khandice had some of the most severe reactions to chemotherapy I've ever seen. However, no matter the pain or how incapacitated she appeared she insisted on art therapy. Khandice self-proclaimed that it helped her manage her pain and take her mind away from the side effects of chemotherapy. There were days when art-making would energize her for hours. Other days, it would lull her to sleep. She used our sessions as a vehicle for what she needed in that moment. I, as the art therapist, followed her directions down that road. The treatment team was aware of our therapeutic relationship and looked to me to assess how she was coping.

As Khandice became stabilized in her treatment—she made it through surgery and her side effects were better managed—she began to vocalize goals: like learning how to play the ukulele and writing a personal memoir. It seemed appropriate to introduce her to my arts in medicine colleagues.

Because Khandice and I had good rapport, she easily trusted anyone bringing arts and health services. Introductions into her room were easy and the artists in residence could instantly engage in meaningful work. Hand in hand with the artists, I supervised therapy goals while they involved her in arts in medicine activities. Our collaborations allowed Khandice to have almost daily arts care while still spreading resources among many other patients.

One of our musicians in residence familiarized her with chords on the ukulele. They developed a musical composition together. The following day, the musician told me they had a melody but needed lyrics. In my next session with Khandice, I did an art therapy intervention that used collage to create a visual poem. She fashioned together personally meaningful strings of words. The poem seemed to carry themes about family relationships, loss, perseverance, and hope. When the musician in residence returned, he helped her blend the poem into a musical composition. His expertise conducted the technical tweaking it needed. Later that week I listened to Khandice play and sing her beautiful song. We continued using themes from the song in our next art therapy piece.

Under the physician's approval, an artist in residence taught her mindfulness techniques and movements, similar to the martial arts, to help supplement physical therapy goals. Another musician played her music to help her through a painful procedure. One of the most powerful collaborations was when a writer helped her transcribe her 'memoirs'.

I was seamlessly able to pass the baton to him to interview Khandice about her life story. What evolved was a series of stunning poems that documented her journey through cancer treatment. The writer in residence had a particular ability to unfold genuine creativity and form it with sensitivity into the work; and I was able to sit with Khandice to process, mourn, laugh, and celebrate the words as they flowed from the page. When she finished reading the first draft, she looked up to me as a tear rolled down her cheek. This time, Khandice had words for the tear: she said, 'I've come so far'.

## Conclusion

Arts and health has much to offer healthcare. The arts therapies are a vital part of addressing the emotional and physical needs of people in health settings. Integration with medical staff, other therapy services, and arts in medicine enable the arts therapies to help address the needs of the whole person. In particular, a partnership between arts therapists and artists in residence constructs a culture of rich arts care.

Khandice benefited from comprehensive healthcare. She used the arts to navigate through one of the most difficult life experiences.

Art therapy helped her address her emotions as they were authentically communicated. The supportive relationship between her art therapist and artists in residence amplified her creative capabilities resulting in increased expression, self-esteem and power.

**My Super Powers**

Chemo is my power reserve.
It's my special power.
I can use it
but the more I use it
the more it makes me sick.
Love: it's something
I can pull from people
and it restores me.

Khandice Long (written with Dylan Klempner)

Khandice verbalized desire to give back to arts and health in the way it had given to her. As a result, she gave permission for her story to be shared. Let us use Khandice as our inspiration to pull professional strengths from each other and walk hand-in-hand as we restore health through the informative, compassionate, and collaborative power of the arts.

## References

ADMP (Association for Dance Movement Psychotherapy UK) (2003). What is dance movement psychotherapy? Available at: <http://www.admt.org.uk/dance-movement-psychotherapy/what-is-dance-movement-psychotherapy/> (accessed 25 September 2013).

ADTA (American Dance Therapy Association) (undated). Dance/movement therapy and Parkinson's disease. Available at: <http://www.adta.org/resources/documents/info-sheet-dmt-parkinsons-with-resource-bib.pdf> (accessed 27 September 2013).

American Academy of Pediatrics (2012). What is palliative care? Available at: <http://www2.aap.org/sections/palliative/> (accessed 30 September 2013).

AMTA (American Music Therapy Association) (2013). Education and clinical training information. Available at: <http://www.musictherapy.org/about/requirements/> (accessed 26 September 2013).

AMTA (American Music Therapy Association) (2014). Fall MLE progress report. Available at: <http://www.musictherapy.org/assets/1/7/2014_Fall_MLE_Progress_Report.pdf> (accessed 23 March 2014).

APA (American Psychological Association) (2013). About APA. Available at: <http://www.apa.org/about/index.aspx> (accessed 29 September 2013).

BAAT (British Association of Art Therapists) (2011). What is art therapy? Available at: <http://www.baat.org/about-art-therapy> (accessed 25 September 2013).

BADTH (British Association of Drama Therapists) (2011). Welcome. Available at: <http://badth.org.uk> (accessed 25 September 2013).

BAMT (British Association for Music Therapy) (2012). What is music therapy? Available at: <http://www.bamt.org/music-therapy.html> (accessed 25 September 2013).

Betts, D.J. (2006). Art therapy assessments and rating instruments: do they measure up? *The Arts in Psychotherapy: An International Journal*, **33**, 422–434.

Brett, M., Kuczaj E., and McHard, J. (2011). Working on the edge. *Journal of the Irish Association of Creative Arts Therapists*. Available at: <http://www.mariebrett.ie/files/working-on-the-edge.pdf> (accessed 26 September 2013).

Broderick, S. (2011). Arts practices in unreasonable doubt? Reflections on understandings of arts practices in healthcare contexts. *Arts & Health: An International Journal for Research, Policy and Practice*, **3**, 95–109.

Bruscia, K.E. (1998). *Defining Music Therapy*, 2nd edn. Gilsum, NH: Barcelona Publishers.

Csikszentmihalyi, M. (1997). *Finding Flow: The Psychology of Engagement With Everyday Life*. New York: Basic Books.

Camic, P.M. (2008). Playing in the mud: health psychology, the arts, and creative approaches to health. *Journal of Health Psychology*, **13**, 287–298.

Chatterjee, A. (2010). Neuroaesthetics: a coming of age story. *Neuroscience*, **12**, 53–62.

Chanda, M.L. and Levitin, D.J. (2013). The neurochemistry of music. *Trends in Cognitive Sciences*, **17**, 179–193.

Councill, T. (2003). Medical art therapy with children. In: C. A. Malchiodi (ed.), *Handbook of Art Therapy*, pp. 207–219. New York: Guilford Press.

Cross, E.S and Ticini, L.F. (2012). Neuroaesthetics and beyond: new horizons in applying the science of the brain to art of dance. *Phenomenology and the Cognitive Sciences*, **11**, 5–16.

Dileo, C. and Bradt J. (2009). On creating discipline, profession, and evidence in the field of arts and healthcare. *Arts & Health: An International Journal for Research, Policy and Practice*, **1**, 168–182.

Dissanayake, E. (2000). *Art and Intimacy: How the Arts Began*. Seattle, WA: University of Washington Press.

Feder, B. and Feder, E. (1998). *The Art and Science of Evaluation in the Arts Therapies: How do we Know What's Working?* Springfield, IL: Charles C. Thomas.

Gantt, L. and Tinnin, L.W. (2009). Support for neurobiological view of trauma with implications for art therapy. *The Arts in Psychotherapy*, **36**, 148–153.

Gard, T., Holzel, B.K., Sack, A.T., et al. (2012). Pain attenuation through mindfulness is associated with decreased cognitive control and increased sensory processing in the brain. *Cerebral Cortex*, **22**, 2692–2702.

Goodill, S.W. (2005). *An Introduction to Medical Dance/Movement Therapy: Health care in motion*. London: Jessica Kingsley.

Graham-Pole, J. (2007). Applications of art to health. In: I.A. Serlin (ed.), *Whole Person Healthcare: The Arts in Health*, Vol. 3, pp. 1–21. Westport, CT: Praeger Perspectives.

IEATA (International Expressive Arts Therapy Association) (2012). Registered expressive arts therapist. Available at: <http://www.ieata.org/reat.html> (accessed 26 September 2013).

Integrative Medicine Committee (2004). Integrative medicine packet. National Association for Poetry Therapy. Available at: <http://www.poetrytherapy.org/pdf/integrativemedicinepacket.pdf> (accessed 27 September 2013).

Johnson, D.R. (2010). Performing absence: the limits of testimony in the recover of the combat veteran. In: E. Leveton (ed.), *Healing Collective Trauma Using Sociodrama and Drama Therapy*, pp. 56–80. New York: Springer.

Jung, C.G. (1933). *Modern Man in Search of a Soul* (transl. W.S. Dell and C.F. Baynes). San Diego: Harcourt, Inc.

Knill, P.J. Barba, H.N., and Fuchs, M.N. (2004). *Minstrels of Soul: Intermodal Expressive Therapy*, 2nd edn. Toronto: EGS Press.

Koff-Chapin, D. (2013). Beyond the patient: art and creativity for staff, management, executives, and organizational change. In: C.A. Malchiodi (ed.), *Art Therapy and Healthcare*, pp. 316–332. New York: Guilford Press.

Langley, D. (2006). *An Introduction to Dramatherapy*. London: Sage.

Lee, J. (2013). How do you distinguish an arts therapist from an artist in residence? Available at: <http://artsinmedicine.ufhealth.org/about/faq/> (accessed on 30 September 2013).

Levin, E.G. and Levin, S.K. (eds). (2011). *Art in Action: Expressive arts therapy and Social Change*. London: Jessica Kingsley.

Levy, F.J. (1988). *Dance Movement Therapy: A Healing Art*. Reston, VA: American Alliance for Health, Physical Education, Recreation, and Dance.

Lowenfeld, V. and Brittain, W.L. (1987). *Creative and Mental Growth*, 8th edn. New York: Macmillan.

Lusebrink, V.B. (1990). *Imagery and Visual Expression in Therapy*. New York: Plenum Press.

Malchiodi, C.A. (2003a). The art and science of art therapy. In: C.A. Malchiodi (ed.), *Handbook of Art Therapy*, pp. 1–3. New York: Guilford Press.

Malchiodi, C.A. (2003b). Art therapy and the brain. In: C.A. Malchiodi (ed.), *Handbook of Art Therapy*, pp. 16–24. New York: Guilford Press.

Malchiodi, C.A. (2003c). Art therapy with medical support groups. In: C.S. Malchiodi (ed.), *Handbook of Art Therapy*, pp. 352–361. New York: Guilford Press.

Malchiodi, C.A. (2005). Expressive therapies: history, theory, and practice. In: C.A. Malchiodi (ed.), *Expressive Therapies*. pp. 1–15. New York: The Guilford Press.

Malchiodi, C.A. (2013). Introduction to art therapy in health care settings. In: C.S. Malchiodi (ed.), *Art Therapy and Healthcare*, pp. 1–11. New York: Guildford Press.

Maslow, A.H. (1976). Creativity in self-actualizing people. In: A. Rothenberg and C.R. Hausman (eds), *The Creativity Question*, pp. 86–92. Durham, NC: Duke University Press.

Mazza, N. (2003). *Poetry Therapy: Theory and Practice*. New York: Brunner-Routledge.

Miller, S.Z. and Schmidt, J. (1999). The habit of humanism: a framework for making humanistic care a reflexive clinical skill. *Academic Medicine*, **74**, 800–803.

Moore, D.W., Bhadelia, R.A., Billings, R.L., et al. (2009). Hemispheric connectivity and the visual-spatial divergent-thinking component of creativity. *Brain and Cognition*, **70**, 267–272.

Moss, H. and O'Neil, D. (2009). What training do artists need to work in healthcare settings? *Medical Humanities*, **35**, 101–105.

NAPT (National Association for Poetry Therapy) (2013). Where and how is poetry therapy used? Available at: <http://www.poetrytherapy.org/> (accessed 25 September 2013).

NASW (National Association of Social Workers (2013). Practice. Available at: <http://www.naswdc.org/practice/default.asp> (accessed 29 September 20130.

NCCATA (National Coalition of Creative Arts Therapies Association) (2013). About NCCATA. Available at: <http://www.nccata.org/#!aboutnccata/czsv> (accessed 28 September 2013).

Payne, H. (ed.) (1993). *Handbook of Inquiry in the Arts Therapies: One River Many Currents*. London: Jessica Kingsley.

Perry, B.D. (2009). Examining child maltreatment through a neurodevelopmental lens: clinical applications of the neurosequential model of therapeutics. *Journal of Loss and Trauma*, **14**, 240–255.

Robichaud, A.L. (2003). Healing and feeling: the clinical ontology of emotion. *Bioethics*, **17**, 59–68.

Rosen, H.J. and Levenson, R.W. (2009). The emotional brain: combining insights from patients and basic science. *Neurocase*, **15**, 173–181.

Rubin, J.A. (1999). *Art Therapy: An Introduction*. Philadelphia, PA: Brunner/Mazel.

Serlin, I.A. (2007). Theories and practices of art therapies: whole person integrative approaches to healthcare. In: I.A. Serlin (ed.), *Whole Person Health Care: The Arts in Health*, Vol 3, pp.107–119. Westport, CT: Praeger Perspectives.

Serwint, J. (2013). *Humanism in Pediatric End of Life Issues* [Pediatric Grand Rounds Presentation, 9 August]. Gainesville, FL: University of Florida.

Sonke J. (2011). Music and the arts in healthcare: a perspective from the United States. *Music and Arts in Action*, **3**, 5–14.

Sonke, J., Rollins, R., Brandman, R., and Graham-Pole, J. (2009). The state of the arts in healthcare in the United States. *Arts & Health: An International Journal for Research, Policy and Practice*, **1**, 107–135.

Sonke-Henderson, J. and Brandman, R. (2007). The hospital artist in residence programs: narratives of healing. In: I.A. Serlin (ed.), *Whole Person Healthcare: The Arts in Health*, Vol. 3, pp. 67–86. Westport, CT: Praeger Perspectives.

Snow, S. and D'Amico, M. (2010). The drum circle project: a qualitative study with at-risk youth in a school setting. *Canadian Journal of Music Therapy*, **16**, 12–39.

Stuckey, H.L. and Nobel, J. (2010). The connection between art, healing, and public health: a review of current literature. *American Journal of Public Health*, **100**, 254–263.

Tesch, L. and Hansen, E.C. (2013). Evaluating effectiveness of arts and health programmes in primary health care. *Arts & Health: An International Journal for Research, Policy and* Practice, **5**, 19–38.

Torrance, E.P. (1993). Understanding creativity: where to start? *Psychological Inquiry*, **4**, 232–234.

Van Buren, B., Bromberger, B., Miller, B., Potts, D., and Chatterjee, A. (2013). Changes in painting styles of two artists with Alzheimer's disease. *Psychology of Aesthetics, Creativity, and the Arts*, **7**, 89–94.

Vick, R.M. (2003). A brief history of art therapy. In: C.A. Malchiodi (ed.), *Handbook of Art Therapy*, pp. 5–15. New York: Guilford Press.

Young, H.E. (2011). Music therapy for speech disorders and speech rehabilitation [video]. Available at: <http://www.youtube.com/watch?v=_06vjUQvMF4> (accessed 27 September 2013).

# CHAPTER 34

# Museums and art galleries as settings for public health interventions

Helen J. Chatterjee

## Introduction to museums and galleries in public health

> Museums and galleries have always served a number of purposes other than the evident one of enabling visitors to appreciate their collections of art and artefacts. They are a site for social interaction and for acquiring and conveying an air of cultural authority. They may provide a cool place on a hot day or a quiet retreat.
>
> Classen (2007, p.897)

Over the past decade or so the notion that museums (here the term is used to include art galleries) can help to bring about social change has gained considerable support. Several authors have discussed the social role of museums (Sandell 2002; Classen 2005; Silverman 2010) and there are numerous examples of museum programmes which seek to address social inclusion, including working with young offenders, the unemployed and those on low incomes, older adults, and disadvantaged minorities (Brown et al. 2009). Lois Silverman (2002) was one of the first authors to suggest that museums could expand their social role to recognize their therapeutic potential. In more recent work, Silverman has gone on to propose that museums contribute to the pursuit of health in five major ways: promoting relaxation; providing immediate intervention by bringing about beneficial change in physiology, emotions, or both; encouraging introspection which can be beneficial for mental health; fostering health education; advocating public health and enhancing healthcare environments (Silverman 2010, p. 43). To date, however, robust evidence to substantiate these outcomes has been hard to come by, despite a wealth of anecdotal evidence supporting the role of museums in health and wellbeing.

The impact of museums on health and wellbeing is explored extensively in Chatterjee and Noble's recent book *Museums, Health and Wellbeing* (2013). The book brings together a large body of research and practice-led examples which help to define a new museum movement called 'museums in health' (Chatterjee and Noble 2013, p. 2). Chatterjee and Noble advocate that museums in health is grounded in the wider field of arts and health, and there is considerable cross-over between the types of activities and programmes offered by both the museums sector and the arts sector in relation to improving health and wellbeing. Many museums now offer an array of programmes, events, resources, and activities targeting a range of audiences (Chatterjee and Noble 2013, pp. 54–55):

◆ public health education

◆ mental health services/users

◆ older adults and reminiscence

◆ children and hospital schools; including services for children with learning difficulties/autism spectrum disorders/physical health problems

◆ health professionals/carers training

◆ others, including rehabilitation and intergenerational health projects.

Some of the best known examples of museums in health might equally be termed 'arts in health'. In the United Kingdom, Dulwich Picture Gallery's Good Times programme offers creative workshops, art appreciation talks, and gallery tours for older adults, targeting socially isolated members of the local community. The gallery's prescription for art service is run in association with local GPs and nurses with special responsibilities for older adults encourage patients to attend creative workshops in the gallery. Qualitative research undertaken by the Oxford Institute of Ageing at Oxford University used post-session questionnaires, diaries and personal testaments, interviews with participants, and observations from creative workshops to evaluate the impact of the Good Times programme. The research found that the programme enhances the lives of local people, helps combat social isolation, and enhances the efficacy of conventional medical treatment (Harper and Hamblin 2010). In the United States, the New York Museum of Modern Art's Meet Me project provides guided tours for small groups of people with dementia plus their family members and carers. Research undertaken by New York University used a psychosocial framework, including a variety of scales, to assess participants' responses to the sessions. The research found improved interaction and happiness for adults with dementia after viewing and discussing artworks, and improved relationships with carers (Rosenberg et al. 2009).

## Museums in health: examples from the field

Chatterjee and Noble (2013) outline a range of examples of museums in health work from the United Kingdom and internationally, some highlights of which are discussed in this section (for further details and examples see Chatterjee and Noble 2013, Chapter 4). Under the banner of public health education, museums are using their collections and spaces to address a variety of public health issues. Through temporary and permanent exhibitions, displays, and road shows, issues such as mental health, obesity, and ageing are being tackled by museums. Chatterjee and Noble (2013) propose that museums are ideally placed to use their spaces to tackle challenging and potentially contentious issues, as unlike many public sector institutions their agendas are traditionally geared towards inclusivity, engagement, and education.

Some of the best known examples of public health education in museums come from medical and science museums, exemplified by the 2013 'Mind Maps: Stories from Psychology' exhibition at London's Science Museum which was curated in collaboration with the British Psychological Society. The exhibition focused on the treatment and assessment of psychological disorders over the past 250 years, demonstrated using objects from the museum's medical collections plus artworks and archive images. In another UK example, the Wellcome Collection in London offers a public exhibitions programme about various aspects of health and disease which attracts hundreds of thousands of visitors per year. Several other medical museums, such as the Thackray Medical Museum in Leeds, United Kingdom and the Medical Museion, Copenhagen, Denmark, also use their collections as a vehicle to explore public health challenges such as obesity, as well as exploring medical history. The Medical Museion is part of the University of Copenhagen's Faculty of Health and Medical Sciences; as with many university medical museums, in addition to training healthcare professionals it seeks to raise public awareness about the importance of medical science and technology, in the past, present, and future, through public exhibitions, events, and an interactive website. In other European examples, European Union culture funding has been used to build networks of medical museums, such as the Connecting the European Mind project which funded a network of psychiatric museums including Museum Dr Guislain (Belgium), the Wellcome Collection (United Kingdom), Museum Ovartaci (Denmark), and MuSeele (Germany), focused on sharing and exchanging knowledge, exhibitions, and collections.

The Museu da Vida (The Museum of Life) in Brazil uses its space to provide information and educational opportunities in science, health, and technology in a creative and entertaining way, through permanent exhibits, interactive activities, theatre, and videos. The Museu da Vida serves both as a place to contemplate health-related information and somewhere to tackle current health challenges within the community. The museum's initiative Travelling Science: Life and Health for Everyone is based inside a large truck that moves from city to city, taking with it an interactive exhibition, handling collections, games, workshops, interactive equipment, videos, story-tellers, and talks about health. The truck operates in the south-west region of Brazil where many smaller towns in the region do not house museums, galleries, or other public institutions that can address local health needs, so the Museu da Vida fulfils this role in an interactive and kinaesthetic way, using a community arts and health model.

The majority of work in museums targeting mental health service users is focused around creative and participatory arts practice. A good example is the Lightbox in Woking (United Kingdom) which has been running community programmes since 2007. The Arteffact project in North Wales involved four museums (Bodelwyddan Castle, Llandudno Museum, Gwynedd Museum and Gallery Bangor, and Oriel Ynys Môn in Anglesey) and used art workshops in the museums to improve the mental health and wellbeing of people who had a history of mental health problems or who were experiencing an episode of stress. Similar programmes offered by National Museums Liverpool, Bolton Museum, the Harris Museum in Preston, Leicestershire Open Museum, Colchester and Ipswich Museums Service, and the Tate Modern in London have also targeted users of mental health services and in several examples the museums work closely with healthcare providers. Colchester and Ipswich Museums Service went a step further and used project funding to employ a mental health project officer, who had a background in psychotherapy, in an innovative 2-year project to develop new programmes geared towards users of mental health services. As with many museum programmes the service was reliant on external funding, and when the funding came to an end the post was sadly disestablished. This innovative project and use of funding, however, shows that through collaboration with health and social care providers museums have the ability to offer novel public health interventions.

Older adults and older adults with dementia also constitute a significant area of provision for museums and art galleries. Much activity in this area is focused around reminiscence work, whereby both museums and art galleries use their collections as a vehicle for exploring memories, sharing stories, and to provide opportunities for museum object handling and for viewing and discussing visual art. Well-known examples such as London's Dulwich Picture Gallery and New York's Museum of Modern Art have already been mentioned, but many other museums and art galleries have services directed at older adults including: in the United Kingdom the British Museum, the Tate Modern, the Beamish Museum, Tullie House Museum and Art Gallery, the Museum of Liverpool; in the United States Amon Carter Museum of American Art; and in Australia the Tasmanian Museum and Art Gallery, Macquarie University Art Gallery, Hurstville City Museum and Gallery, and Museum Victoria.

Children and schools form a large part of the educational programming for many museums and art galleries, yet despite this there are relatively few examples of health and wellbeing programmes targeting young people. Provision in this area has largely been focused around children with special needs, including autistic spectrum disorders. In the United States, the Please Touch Museum's therapeutic membership scheme was designed for organizations that serve children with disabilities. Therapists pay to join the scheme which provides access to a range of therapeutic resources for children receiving physical therapy, occupational therapy, early intervention, and special instruction. In another US example, Boston's Museum of Fine Art runs an Artful Healing programme which offers art-making activities for children, young adults, and their families, in hospitals and healthcare centres in the Boston area.

Finally, there are a host of programmes run in the United Kingdom and elsewhere focused around general health and wellbeing and targeting a variety of users. Glasgow's Open Museum, for example, has worked with asylum seekers and refugees, users of day care, those on low incomes, and users of mental health services, through a variety of community-based, museum-led interventions. All the projects use museum objects, often in association with group activities such as workshops. In another example, the House of Memories project at the National Museums Liverpool (NML) is a training programme for carers, social workers, and family members supporting people with dementia. The project has attracted nationwide interest and is mentioned in the British prime minister's Challenge on Dementia report (DH 2013, p. 8).

## Measuring impact: evaluating success

Many museums and art galleries have undertaken, or commissioned, their own evaluations regarding the impact of their work on their target audiences, and there is now a considerable body of evaluative evidence demonstrating how museums contribute to health and wellbeing (Wood 2008; Davenport and Corner 2011; Renaissance North West 2011; Balshaw et al. 2012; Bodley 2012; NML 2012). Chatterjee and Noble have reviewed and summarized the various studies and evaluations to list the many positive outcomes that museums in health can bring about (Chatterjee and Noble 2013, p. 115):

◆ positive social experiences, leading to reduced social isolation

◆ opportunities for learning and acquiring news skills

◆ calming experiences, leading to decreased anxiety

◆ increased positive emotions, such as optimism, hope, and enjoyment

◆ increased self-esteem and sense of identity

◆ increased inspiration and opportunities for meaning making

◆ positive distraction from clinical environments, including hospitals and care homes

◆ increased communication between families, carers and health professionals.

While the weight of museum-led evaluation is compelling, the most persuasive evidence of the impact of museums in health comes from the sector's collaboration with academics. In the following examples, discussed in detail in Chatterjee and Noble (2013), mixed-methods or quasi-experimental approaches have often been used to obtain a deeper understanding of the impact of activities on participants' health and wellbeing. This is an advantage because the research tends to use methods which have been tested for repeatability and reliability, adding weight to the findings, such that the outcomes can be more effectively tied to real changes in participants' health and wellbeing. Examples include:

◆ London's Dulwich Picture Gallery with Canterbury Christ Church University in the United Kingdom (Eeckelaar et al. 2012; Camic et al. 2014) and the Oxford Institute of Ageing, Oxford University (Harper and Hamblin 2010)

◆ Woking's Lightbox with Brunel University, London (Bryant et al. 2011)

◆ Tyne and Wear Museums (with the Institute for Ageing and Health, Newcastle University)

◆ Manchester Museums, Manchester's Whitworth Art Gallery, Manchester Art Gallery, Carlisle's Tullie House and Art Gallery, Bolton Library and Museum Service, and Preston's Harris Museum as part of the Who Cares? programme, with the Psychosocial Research Unit at the University of Central Lancashire (Froggett et al. 2011),

◆ Colchester and Ipswich Museum Service, with SE-SURG (South Essex Service User Research Group) and Anglia Ruskin University,

◆ the Heritage2Health project (coordinated through the Faculty of Health and Social Care Sciences, St George's University of London),

◆ New York's Museum of Modern Art with New York University (Rosenberg et al. 2009),

◆ the National Gallery of Australia with New South Wales Aged Care Evaluation Unit and Australian National University (MacPherson et al. 2009)

◆ UCL (University College London) Museums' 'Heritage in Hospitals' project (coordinated through UCL Museums and Public Engagement and the School of Life and Medical Sciences (Chatterjee et al. 2009; Ander et al. 2011; Thomson et al. 2011; Lanceley et al. 2012; Ander et al. 2012a,b; Thomson et al. 2012a,b).

Froggett et al. (2011), for example, used a qualitative psychosocial framework in their evaluation of the Who Cares? museums, health, and wellbeing programme which involved six museums in the north-west of England. The aim of the research was to investigate the effect of access to museum activities on health and wellbeing across disadvantaged groups in each museum. Froggett et al.'s approach focused on the meaning and uses of objects and artworks by individuals, the relationships between participants and museum staff and partners, and the implications of the programmes for cultural inclusion. The study used self-evaluation questionnaires, video, semi-structured and narrative style interviews, in-depth observation of groups, and creative outputs such as artworks. Results showed that practice which specifically targets small group work with museum objects promotes a sense of cultural inclusion and also that 'interaction with museum collections in favourable conditions offers people the opportunity to find new cultural forms in which to express their experience. Personal experience can then be communicated to others' (Froggett et al. 2011, p. 72). Froggett et al. go on to propose that this is a distinctive contribution that museums can make to wellbeing which draws on the nature of their collections and their symbolic cultural significance, and the personal symbolic significance the collections hold for individuals (Froggett et al. 2011, p. 72).

Other studies have also drawn upon the unique potential of multisensory interaction with museum objects as a vehicle for improving aspects of health and wellbeing. The Heritage in Hospitals project run by UCL took handling collections from UCL Museums and partner museums (the British Museum, Reading Museum, Oxford University Museums) into hospitals and care homes in London, Reading, and Oxford. The project involved over 300 hospital patients and care home residents, and employed a mixed-methods framework to assess the impact of a 30- to 40-minute museum object handling session on participants. Psychological and subjective wellbeing measures before and after the session were used alongside qualitative methods based on grounded theory (Thomson et al. 2011, 2012a,b; Ander et al. 2012a). Quantitative measures showed that there were significant increases in participant's wellness and happiness scores (Thomson et al. 2011, 2012a,b). Qualitative analysis revealed that 'once patient participants were engaged, museum objects provided unique and idiosyncratic routes to stimulation and distraction. The data showed that patients used the heritage objects combined with tailored and easy social interaction, sensory stimulus and learning opportunities to tap into concerns about identity, emotions, energy levels and motivation' (Ander et al. 2012a, pp. 8–12). As well as scholarly outputs this research resulted in a guide to using museum collections in hospitals and other healthcare settings (Ander et al. 2012b).

In follow-up work, Thomson and Chatterjee developed the Museum Wellbeing Measure and Toolkit containing various approaches for assessing the impact of museum activities on psychological wellbeing (Thomson and Chatterjee 2013, 2014) (see Figs 34.1 and 34.2). Staff (*n* = 58) from 32 specialist UK museums and galleries and their audiences (*n* = 207; including groups of mixed adults, older adults with dementia, and younger adults) were involved in the development of measures. Various prototypes of existing and adapted measures of psychological wellbeing were tested with participants, including a shortened version of the Positive Affect–Negative Affect Scale (PANAS) (Watson et al. 1988) and visual analogue scales (VAS) to measure wellness and happiness (EurolQol 1990). The final toolkit contains Generic Wellbeing Questionnaires (a short six-item version and a longer 12-item version) and Generic Wellbeing Umbrellas, which are based on words derived from the PANAS and use a rating scale from 1 to 5.

There are other examples of museum evaluations which have employed quantitative health measures, with the Warwick–Edinburgh Mental Wellbeing Scale (WEMWBS

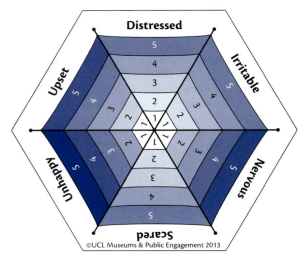

**Fig. 34.2** Thomson and Chatterjee's (2013) UCL Museum Wellbeing Measure: the generic negative wellbeing umbrella.
Reproduced with permission from University College London. Copyright © 2015 University College London, UK.

2006) being a popular choice. The Arteffact project carried out in museums in North Wales used the WEMWBS to assess the mental wellbeing of participants at the start and end of the project, and the Museum of Hartlepool used the shortened version of the scale (SWEMWBS 2007) in their evaluation of an intergenerational dance project.

In support of the mixed-methods approach, the Centre for Wellbeing at the New Economics Foundation published a guide to measuring wellbeing to help practitioners measure wellbeing outcomes (NEF 2012). The guide recommends using three sets of wellbeing questions: the Short Warwick–Edinburgh Mental Wellbeing Scale (SWEMWBS 2007), the Office for National Statistics subjective wellbeing questions, and a question on social trust, which they suggest is a key factor for wellbeing.

There are many arts in health studies which have explored the impact of arts participation within museums and art galleries, discussed in this volume and elsewhere (Staricoff 2004, 2007; Clift et al. 2009; White 2009; Chatterjee and Noble 2013). Some recent informative examples have focused on people with dementia (PWD). In MacPherson et al.'s (2009) study, PWD visited the National Gallery of Australia once a week for 6 weeks to discuss artworks. Levels of engagement were studied through direct observation and focus group sampling using a qualitative approach. Results revealed that participants showed increased levels of engagement, and this was particularly apparent for those individuals who were generally withdrawn or behaviourally disturbed in their usual environments. In a mixed-methods study using a pre-test and post-test design, Eeckelaar et al. (2012) showed that viewing and making art by PWD in an art gallery had an impact on episodic memory and verbal fluency. In a similar follow-up study, Camic et al. (2014) focused on comparing PWD participating in art activities in a traditional and a modern art gallery. The study demonstrated no significant difference in quantitative measures in either setting, but found a non-significant trend towards reduced carer burden and positive

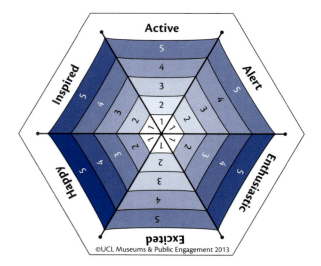

**Fig. 34.1** Thomson and Chatterjee's (2013) UCL Museum Wellbeing Measure: the generic positive wellbeing umbrella.
Reproduced with permission from University College London. Copyright © 2015 University College London, UK.

benefits for wellbeing, including self-reports of greater social inclusion, enhanced cognitive capacities, and quality of life at both gallery sites. Although these studies have tended to involve relatively small numbers of participants (fewer than 20), they exemplify the value of undertaking focused research in museums and art galleries in order to better understand the impact of such encounters on health and wellbeing.

## Understanding museums in health

The aforementioned evaluation and research regarding museums in health has provided a more nuanced view of how and why museum encounters bring about improvements in health and wellbeing. In particular, it is the unique cultural perspective afforded by museums and their collections which appears to be the key to improvements in health and wellbeing. As the custodians of cultural heritage, museums can provide a window into what it means to be human, providing opportunities for meaning-making, self-reflection, and a chance to explore identity. Whilst many museums explicitly encourage this through exhibitions and public programming, it is encounters with the collections housed in museums which appear to help explain why museum visits may elicit changes in health and wellbeing. But why it is that physical interaction with museum collections is so significant?

> 'The moon rock is an actual piece of the moon retrieved by the Apollo 17 mission. There is nothing particularly appealing about the rock; it is a rather standard piece of volcanic basalt some 4 million years old. Yet, unlike many other old rocks, this one comes displayed in an altar-like structure, set in glass, and is complete with a full-time guard and an ultrasensitive monitoring device (or so the guards are wont to say). There is a sign above it which reads, 'You may touch it with care'. *Everyone touches it.*'
>
> Meltzer (1981, p.121)

This excerpt from Meltzer (1981) describes a piece of moon rock that went on display in the National Air and Space Museum in Washington, DC. Although the moon rock is apparently not any more physically or aesthetically interesting than an ordinary piece of basalt, the intrinsic and material properties of the moon rock and those ascribed to it by placing it on display in a museum render the object culturally important. It is this process of 'added value' that appears to tie into people's views and perspectives of interacting with museum collections. Cultural value is ascribed to objects by connecting and presenting relevant, often intrinsic, information about the objects. In doing so, museums afford an opportunity to learn, reflect, and contemplate the materiality of the world around us.

Froggett et al. (2011) argued that when individuals interact with museums and their collections, the object's properties (including its intrinsic, physical, and material properties) trigger memories, projections, sensory, emotional, and cognitive associations. This could be because museum objects function as symbols of various factors which may affect, or be important to, our lives such as identity, relationships, nature, society, and religion, as advocated by Pearce (1995). Pearce proposes that museum experiences can lead to a process of symbolization due to the symbolic significance of the object. The psychosocial evidence suggests that objects function as a 'mental representation of possible relationships among things, events, and relationships' and further that 'Humans bring their own knowledge, experiences and values to objects and make meaning' (Baumeister 1991, p. 15). Several authors have discussed the role of material objects in meaning-making (e.g. Rowe 2002) and others have argued that it is the multisensory experience which elicits ideas and meaning (Gregory and Whitcomb 2007; Dudley 2010). Further, Vygotsky (2002) suggested that objects play a role in the development of self-awareness through multisensory interaction.

The symbolic, meaning-making, properties of objects could account for their intrinsic therapeutic potential. Camic et al. (2011) showed that the use of found objects (referred to as material objects that are found or discovered, are not usually purchased, hold no intrinsic financial value, and have personal significance) in psychotherapy helped to enhance engagement, increase curiosity, reduce difficult feelings, evoke memories, and provide a sense of agency through increased physical activity and environmental action. Several authors have suggested that museum objects trigger memories, ideas, and emotions in ways that other information-bearing materials do not (Kavanagh 2000; Phillips 2008; Lanceley et al. 2012; Chatterjee and Noble 2013).

Given the symbolic and cultural significance of museum objects, their value in psychotherapy offers a fascinating area of future research. Lanceley et al. (2012) explored the therapeutic potential in cancer care of handling museum objects. The study was grounded in Kleinian theory, conceived by the psychoanalyist Melanie Klein (1997). Klein used various objects (animal figures, small cars, pencils, and paper) as a means to provide a vocabulary to facilitate expression of the thoughts and feelings of children. The objects were used to explore the child's conscious and unconscious phantasies during therapy. Klein proposed that the inner phantasy world (where the word 'phantasy' is used to distinguish unconscious phantasy from conscious 'fantasy') is as important as the external world because it shapes our view of the internal world. Lanceley et al. (2012) proposed that the use of museum objects in clinical practice may draw on the same principles, given that museum objects carry symbolic meaning for individuals if feelings are projected onto them. They went on to propose that the object can act as a repository or container for different and difficult states of mind, and set out to test this with female cancer patients.

The Lanceley et al. (2012) study recruited ten women: five who had recently had surgery for a gynaecological cancer and knew their diagnosis, and five who had a significant family history of ovarian cancer and were attending the clinic for screening. Qualitative methods were used to elicit and describe patients' responses during a museum object handling session using a mix of natural and human-made objects from UCL Museums, including Egyptian artefacts, fossils, and artworks. The sessions were conducted and audio-taped by gynaecological cancer nurse specialists who were subsequently interviewed by the study researcher and invited to reflect on the session. Field notes were made immediately following these interviews and analysed alongside transcripts of the nurse–patient sessions to highlight contextual issues that might have a bearing on the interpretive analysis (Knowles 2008). The constant comparative method was used to identify themes (Glaser and Strauss 1967) and psychodynamic interpretation was based on Kleinian theory. The following themes resulted from the analysis: survival, fear of cancer, powerlessness, reproductive capacity, and (female) family history. The study revealed the patients' symbolic use of the objects and how the women transferred their thoughts and feelings onto the objects. The following excerpts from session transcripts demonstrate how patients described the symbolic role of the object:

'This one (an object) I picked because I see it as a weapon . . . I have felt extremely angry and this makes me feel very powerful. I could use it to attack, to damage, to deface, you know, all of that stuff. This could be, as it were, the symbol of all the bad stuff. It intrinsically isn't bad but it's symbolic of bad and I like the way it is a cross section. I suppose in many ways this represents my potential cancer from the outside. None of us know what's going on inside, the little horror is growing away.'

> Lanceley et al. (2012, p. 817)

'The attraction (of the object) was somebody who is powerful, has survived, holds a rattle, 'don't mess with me', you know, that um and I want to be like that, I want to say leave me alone or I will smash you across the head, swing my handbag at you (Laughs). She [a small Egyptian bronze cat figurine] gives me that sense of possibility of strength, but it's a private thing.'

> Lanceley et al. (2012, p. 815)

'. . . So this (the object) is giving me perhaps a little sense of the ability to strike back.'

> Lanceley et al. (2012, p. 817)

'N: Can you tell me why you have chosen this object [small Egyptian bronze cat figurine]?
S: Yeah. Well it is maternal isn't it? It has a maternal appearance with the basket and everything. Also though it's small it has survived and it's old. It has existed for many generations.
N: What does it feel like to handle the object?
S: It is smooth and for its size heavy and compact
N: Mmm
S: It feels nice. It is comforting to hold her.
N: Comforting. I see and so do you feel in need of comfort? Is that something you feel now?
S: Well we all do don't we.
N: Mmm
S: It will be the anniversary of my mother's death in two days time.
N: Oh is it?
S: Mmm Oh . . . I think it's a powerful figure. I like the little kittens she's carrying but what . . .
N: Well that's interesting because this figure used to be carried by women wishing to have children.
S: Oh I want kids in the future . . . I don't want it (the object) to affect me in a bad way.
N: Do you think it has the power to do that?
S: Yes, probably. But I like it because it's strong and will endure. I mean it won't break easily will it? (Laughs) Can I keep it?
N: Well it must go back in the box I'm afraid but er I wonder what you will substitute for its comfort in the next day or so?
S: (Laughs) Alcohol! No only joking! (Laughs)'

> Lanceley et al. 2012, p. 814; N, nurse; S, patient)

In these examples, and others explored in the study, it is apparent that the museum objects are acting as a vehicle which enabled the participants to explore issues of fear, loss of the healthy self, fertility, and death. In this sense they are transitional objects (Winnicott 1992) which elicit a sense of power, comfort, and support.

One issue that is frequently raised by studies such as this is the facilitator effect. In other words is it the object or the facilitator which elicits the perceived outcomes? This is raised by a participant in the Lanceley et al. study who queried 'I don't know whether it's that (the object) or just talking to you that's relaxing' (Lanceley et al. 2012, p. 818). Results from this study and others (see Chatterjee et al. 2009; Thomson et al. 2011, 2012a,b; Ander et al. 2012a), however, suggest that it is the nature and depth of the conversations elicited by museum objects which is significant. As demonstrated in the extracts, the symbolic power and properties of the objects are cited as the conduit for exploring emotions, facilitating discussion, and expressing opinions.

The object effect was tested in UCL's Heritage in Hospitals project, whereby hospital patients and care home residents took part in facilitated sessions handling museum objects. In the experimental condition participants were encouraged to discuss and handle the objects, but in the control condition a subset of participants were not allowed to see or touch the real objects and instead images of the objects were used. The study employed a mixed-methods approach involving the PANAS (Watson et al. 1988) and two VAS to measure wellness and happiness (EurolQol 1990), alongside qualitative approaches. Quantitative measures and scales were completed before (pre-test) and after (post-test) a 40-minute session facilitated by researchers. In a cohort of 100 hospital patients from a variety of wards (oncology, acute and elderly, surgical admissions), 70 were recruited to the experimental condition and 21 for the control condition. The results showed statistically significant differences between the experimental and control conditions for PANAS and VAS wellness and happiness scores. In the experimental condition there was a significant increase in PANAS and VAS scores in pre- and post-test results. In the control condition there was less change or a negative difference in pre- and post-test results. This indicates that participants' perceptions of their positive emotions, wellness, and happiness were significantly better when they were allowed to touch the real museum objects as opposed to simply viewing pictures of them (Thomson et al. 2012).

Whilst it would be possible experimentally to test the facilitator effect there is a question of the feasibility and purpose of such a test. In scenarios such as museum object handling sessions or participatory art viewing sessions the facilitators play a key role in encouraging engagement; this is often necessary both for the optimal running of sessions and also for the safety of the participants and museum collections alike. Given that museum encounters are intrinsically social and often interactive experiences, the fact that a facilitator may play a role in contributing to improved health or wellbeing need not be seen as problematic but part of the overall 'therapeutic' approach. Notwithstanding these challenges, a more robust approach to analysing the impact of museum encounters on health and wellbeing will be beneficial for both the museums and health/social cares sectors and their associated audiences.

## Conclusions

There is now a range of evidence which suggests that museum and art gallery encounters can help with a range of health issues, enhance wellbeing, and build social capital and resilience. These organizations have the potential to address a wide spectrum of health, wellbeing, and social needs, including: healthy ageing; health education; reduction of stress; social isolation; pain intensity (possibly linked to reduced drug consumption); enhanced mental health (possibly linked to reduced reliance on mental health services); increased mobility; cognitive stimulation; and sociality and employability (Chatterjee and Noble 2013, p. 123). However, although there is good evidence in support of some of these outcomes, others such as increased mobility and reduction in pain intensity have not been tested.

Museums in health is a new field of study, although in practice many museums and art galleries have been running programmes targeting the specific health and wellbeing needs of their audiences for some years. In order to fully understand the range of benefits resulting from museum encounters, however, further work is needed to demonstrate the specific psychological, physical, and physiological benefits that these interactions bring about. Notwithstanding the need for further evidence, it is extremely timely to consider a new public health role for museums and galleries, as has been proposed by Chatterjee et al. (2009), Camic and Chatterjee (2013), and Chatterjee and Noble (2013). The future is likely to be characterized by increasing pressure on health and social services. For example, many western populations are living longer but are experiencing more age-related diseases such as dementia and lifestyle-related health problems such as obesity and diabetes. The museums sector is well placed to tackle many aspects of health and wellbeing as there is considerable evidence to suggest that museums are effective agents of social change. Museums have a strong track record of delivering social and learning outcomes, and extending these services and programmes to meet the public health needs of their audiences is easily within reach.

## References

Ander, E.E., Thomson, L.J., Lanceley, A., Menon, U., Noble, G., and Chatterjee, H.J. (2011). Generic wellbeing outcomes: towards a conceptual framework for wellbeing outcomes in museums. *Museum Management and Curatorship*, 26, 237–259.

Ander, E., Thomson, L., Lanceley, A., Menon, U., Noble, G., and Chatterjee, H.J. (2012a). Heritage, health and wellbeing: assessing the impact of a heritage focused intervention on health and wellbeing. *International Journal of Heritage Studies*, 19, 229–242.

Ander, E., Thomson, L.J., Noble, G., Menon, U., Lanceley, A., and Chatterjee, H.J. (2012b). *Heritage in Health: A Guide to Using Museum Collections in Hospitals and Other Healthcare Settings*. London: UCL. Available at: <http://www.ucl.ac.uk/museums/museums-old/research/touch/publications/heritage-in-health> (accessed 22 October 20130.

Balshaw, M., Daniel, J., Mount, P.W., and Regan, D. (2012). *How Museums and Galleries Can Enhance Health and Wellbeing*. Available at: <http://www.healthandculture.org.uk/about/> (accessed 22 October 2013).

Baumeister, R.F. (1991). *Meanings in Life*. New York: Guilford Press.

Bodley, A. (2012) *History to Health: Research into Changing Health Agendas for the UK Medical Collections Group*. Available at: <http://www.thackraymedicalmuseum.co.uk/ThackrayMuseum/media/Attachments/historytohealth.pdf> (accessed 22 October 2013).

Brown, C., Wood, E., and Salgado, G. (eds). (2009). *Inspiring Action: Museums and Social Change*. Edinburgh: MuseumsEtc.

Bryant, W., Wilson, L., and Lawson, J. (2011) *Ways of Seeing Evaluation*. London: Brunel University. Available at: http://www.brunel.ac.uk/__data/assets/pdf_file/0010/256069/ways-of-seeing-evaluation-2.pdf (accessed 12 March 2015).

Camic, P.M. and Chatterjee, H.J. (2013). Museums and art galleries as partners in public health interventions. *Perspectives in Public Health*, 133, 66–73.

Camic, P.M., Brooker, J., and Neal, A. (2011). Found objects in clinical practice: preliminary evidence. *The Arts in Psychotherapy*, 38, 151–159.

Camic, P.M., Tischler, V., and Pearman, C. (2014). Viewing and making art together: an eight-week gallery-based intervention for people with dementia and their caregivers. *Aging and Mental Health*, 18, 161–168.

Chatterjee, H.J. and Noble, G. (2013). *Museums, Health and Wellbeing*. Farnham: Ashgate Publishing.

Chatterjee, H.J., Vreeland, S., and Noble, G.(2009). Museopathy: exploring the healing potential of handling museum objects. *Museum and Society*, 7, 164–177.

Classen, C. (2005). *The Book of Touch*. Oxford: Berg.

Classen, C. (2007). Museum manners: the sensory life of the early museum. *Journal of Social History*, 40, 895–914.

Clift, S., Camic, P.M., Chapman, B., et al. (2009). The state of arts and health in England. *Arts & Health: An International Journal of Research, Policy and Practice*, 1, 6–35.

Davenport, B. and Corner, L. (2011). *Review of Policy and Research Evidence relating to the Ageing, Health and Vitality Project*. Newcastle University. Available at: <http://objecthandling.files.wordpress.com/2012/05/policy-research-review-for-ahv1.pdf> (accessed 18 October 2013).

DH (Department of Health) (2013) *The Prime Minister's Challenge on Dementia. Delivering Major Improvements in Dementia Care and Research by 2015: A Report on Progress*. Available at: <https://www.gov.uk/government/publications/the-prime-ministers-challenge-on-dementia-annual-report-of-progress> (accessed 12 March 2015).

Dudley, S.H. (2010). Museum materialities: objects, sense and feeling. In: S.H. Dudley (ed.), *Museum Materialities: Objects, Engagements, Interpretations*, pp. 1–17. London: Routledge.

Eeckelaar, C., Camic, P.M., and Springham, N. (2012). Art galleries, episodic memory and verbal fluency in dementia: an exploratory study. *Psychology of Aesthetics, Creativity and the Arts*, 6, 262–272.

EuroQol Group (1990). EuroQol: a new facility for the measurement of health-related quality of life. *Health Policy*, 16, 199–208.

Froggett, L., Farrier, A., and Poursanidou, K. (2011). *Who Cares? Museums Health and Wellbeing: a study of the Renaissance North West Programme*. University of Central Lancashire, Preston. Available at: <http://clok.uclan.ac.uk/3362/> (accessed on 12 March 2015).

Glaser, B.G. and Strauss, A.L. (1967). *The Discovery of Grounded Theory: Strategies for Qualitative Research*. Chicago: Aldine.

Gregory, K. and Whitcomb, A. (2007). Beyond nostalgia: the role of affect in generating historical understanding at heritage sites. In: S.J. Knell, S. MacLeod, and S.E.R. Watson (eds), *Museum Revolutions: How Museums Change and are Changed*, pp. 263–275. New York: Routledge.

Harper, S. and Hamblin, K. (2010).*This is Living. Good Times: Art for Older People at Dulwich Picture Gallery*. Available at: <http://www.ageing.ox.ac.uk/system/files/This%20Is%20Living-Good%20Times%20Art%20for%20Older%20People-1.pdf> (accessed 22 October 2013).

Kavanagh, G. (2000). *Dream Spaces: Memory and the Museum*. London: Leicester University Press.

Klein, M. (1997). *The Psychoanalysis of Children*. New York: Vintage Books [first published 1932].

Knowles, J.G. and Cole, A.L. (2008). *Handbook of the Arts in Qualitative Social Science Research: Perspectives, Methodologies, Examples and Issues*. Los Angeles: Sage.

Lanceley, A., Noble, G., Johnson, M., Balogun, N., Chatterjee, H.J., and Menon, U. (2012). Investigating the therapeutic potential of a heritage-object focused intervention: a qualitative study. *Journal of Health Psychology*, 17, 809–820.

MacPherson, S., Bird, M., Anderson, K., Davis, Y., and Blair, A. (2009). An art gallery access programme for people with dementia: 'You do it for the moment'. *Ageing and Mental Health*, 13, 744–752.

Meltzer, D.J. (1981). Ideology and material culture. In: R.A. Gould and M.B. Schiffer (eds), *Modern Material Culture: The Archaeology of Us*, p. 121. New York: Academic Press.

NML (National Museums Liverpool) (2012). *House of Memories. An Evaluation of National Museums Liverpool: Dementia Training Programme*. Available at: <http://www.liverpoolmuseums.org.uk/learning/documents/house-of-memories-evaluation-report.pdf> (accessed 18 October 2013).

Pearce, S.M. (1995). *On Collecting: An Investigation into Collecting in the European Tradition*. London: Routledge.

Phillips, L. (2008) Reminiscence: Recent Work at the British Museum. In: H. J. Chatterjee (ed.), *Touch in Museums: Policy and Practice in Object Handling*, pp. 199-204. Oxford: Berg.Rosenberg, F., Parsa, A., Humble, L., and McGee, C. (2009). *Meet Me: Making Art Accessible to People With Dementia*. New York: Museum of Modern Art.

Rowe, S. (2002). The role of objects in active, distributed meaning-making. In: S.G. Paris (ed.), *Perspectives on Object-Centred Learning in Museums*, pp. 19–35. Mahwah, NJ: Lawrence Erlbaum Associates.

Sandell, R. (2002). *Museums, Society, Inequality*. London: Routledge.

SWEMWBS (Short Warwick–Edinburgh Mental Wellbeing Scale) (2007) NHS Health Scotland, University of Warwick and University of Edinburgh. Available at: http://www.healthscotland.com/uploads/documents/14092-swemwbssept2007.pdf (accessed 18 October 2013).

Silverman, L.H. (2002). The therapeutic potential of museums as pathways to inclusion. In: R. Sandell (ed.), *Museums, Society, Inequality*, pp. 69–83. London: Routledge.

Silverman, L.H. (2010). *The Social Work of Museums*. London: Routledge.

Staricoff, R.L. (2004). Arts in health: a review of the medical literature. *Arts Council England Research Report* no. 36.

Staricoff, R.L. (2007). *A Prospectus for Arts and Health*. London: Arts Council England. Available at: <http://www.artscouncil.org.uk/publication_archive/a-prospectus-for-arts-and-health> (accessed 16 January 2014).

Thomson, L. and Chatterjee, H.J. (2013). *The UCL Museum Wellbeing Measures Toolkit*. Available at: <http://www.ucl.ac.uk/museums/research/touch/ucl-museum-wellbeing-measures-toolkit.pdf> (accessed 18 October 2013).

Thomson, L. and Chatterjee, H. J. (2014) Assessing wellbeing outcomes for arts and heritage activities: Development of a Museum Wellbeing Measures Toolkit. *Journal of Applied Arts & Health,* **5,** 29–50. doi: 10.1386/jaah.5.1.29_1

Thomson, L., Ander, E., Menon, U., Lanceley, A., and Chatterjee, H.J. (2011). Evaluating the therapeutic effects of museum object handling with hospital patients: a review and initial trial of wellbeing measures. *Journal of Applied Arts and Health,* **2,** 37–56.

Thomson, L., Ander, E., Lanceley, A., Menon, U., Noble, G., and Chatterjee, H.J. (2012a). Enhancing cancer patient wellbeing with a non-pharmacological, heritage-focused intervention. *Journal of Pain and Symptom Management,* **44,** 731–740.

Thomson, L., Ander, E., Lanceley, A., Menon, U., Noble, G., and Chatterjee, H.J. (2012b). Quantitative evidence for wellbeing benefits from a heritage-in-health intervention with hospital patients. *International Journal of Art Therapy,* **17,** 63–79.

Vygotsky, L. (2002). Play and its role in the mental development of the child [originally published in 1933]. *Psychology and Marxism Internet Archive*. Available at: <https://www.marxists.org/archive/vygotsky/works/1933/play.htm>

Warwick Edinburgh Mental Wellbeing Scale (WEMWBS) (2006). The Warwick Edinburgh Mental Wellbeing Scale. NHS Health Scotland, University of Warwick, and University of Edinburgh. Available at: <http://www.healthscotland.com/documents/1467.aspx> (accessed 8 October 2013).

Watson, D., Clark, L., and Tellegen, A. (1988). Development and validation of brief measures of positive and negative affect: the PANAS scales. *Journal of Personality and Social Psychology,* **54,** 1063–1070.

White, M. (2009). *Arts Development in Community Health: A Social Tonic.* Radcliffe Publishing: Oxford.

Winnicott, D.W. (1992). Transitional objects and transitional phenomena [first published 1951]. In: *Through Paediatrics to Psychoanalysis: Collected Papers,* pp. 229–242. London: Brunner-Routledge.

Wood, C. (2008). *Museums of the Mind: Mental Health, Emotional Wellbeing, and Museums.* Bude: Culture Unlimited.

# CHAPTER 35

# Case study: creativity in criminal justice settings—the work of the Koestler Trust

## Tim Robertson

## Context and outline

Prisoners have always produced art. On the walls of the Tower of London there are highly accomplished carvings by sixteenth-century prisoners—names, dates, family emblems, sacred symbols, and ardent declarations of faith or regret (Thurley 1996). Plainly, these Tudor inmates needed a pastime, and—especially when awaiting execution for their religion or politics—graffiti offered a precious outlet for an assertion of allegiance and passion that might reach a sympathetic audience. The survival of the carvings indicates both that the work was tolerated or even supported by the Tower authorities and that the captives ultimately achieved their artistic goals.

In twenty-first-century prisons, inmates still take up the arts as a pastime, an expression of identity within an institution that removes liberty, and a communication to others of feeling, viewpoint or hope. Of course, though, criminal justice is now directed at offending against property or person, not political or religious dissent. Modern prisons are tasked not just with the containment and punishment of criminals, but also with their rehabilitation—that is, with individual and public health, in the sense of long-term wellbeing for offenders and the community. The National Offender Management Service (NOMS)—the UK government agency that has managed prisons and probation in England and Wales since 2004—states its purpose as:

> '... to protect the public and reduce reoffending by delivering the punishment and orders of the courts and supporting rehabilitation by helping offenders to reform their lives.'
>
> NOMS (2013)

Finding the right balance of punishment and rehabilitation is a perennial debate in penal practice. It is largely through the rehabilitation agenda that organized arts activities have found a place in the service provision of prisons and probation. This extends even to national policy. In England and Wales, the government commissions, co-funds, and meets regularly with the National Alliance for Arts in Criminal Justice (<https://www. artsincriminaljustice.org.uk>), a coalition of arts companies that work with offenders, which aims to promote good practice and makes a case for the work. In Scotland, the government has also coordinated and funded a strategy for arts and justice. At an operational level, however, there are wide variations in the size and reach of the arts activities, and in the degrees of credibility and support they win from local justice agencies. Moreover, the punishment agenda—especially when oversimplified in the media and political rhetoric—poses an ongoing threat of stereotyping the arts as too 'soft' or enjoyable to be appropriate for criminals (Fig. 35.1).

This chapter summarizes the types of arts taking place in the British criminal justice system, identifies three theories offering a rationale for this activity, and considers the kinds of evidence that can demonstrate its impact. Each of these areas is also related to the work of the Koestler Trust, a prison arts charity that has for over 50 years made Britain the only country in the world with a nationwide arts awards scheme to motivate creative achievements by offenders, and a national programme of exhibitions to showcase those achievements to the public.

## How arts are created in criminal justice settings

Prisoners and other offenders create the arts through four channels: education, therapy, arts projects and independent creativity.

### Education

All prisons have education departments, funded by government and delivered through contracts with colleges or private companies. The curriculum is focused on literacy, numeracy and vocational skills, but most departments also offer some arts courses—which can include painting and drawing, music, creative writing and graphic design. Prisoners are allocated to courses depending on an assessment of need and the availability of places. Less than a third of prisoners are in education at any one time (House of Commons 2005, p. 54). All the courses

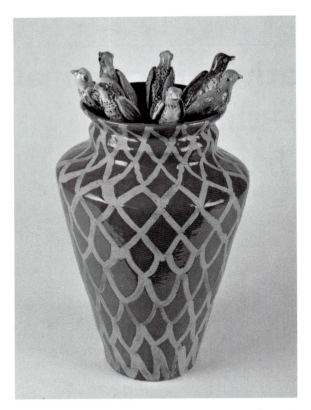

**Fig. 35.1** 'Birds of a Feather' by a prisoner at HM Prison Pentonville, London. Koestler Commended Award for Pottery, 2012 (glazed ceramic 40 × 22 × 22 cm). Reproduced by kind permission of The Koestler Trust. Copyright © 2015 The Koestler Trust.

lead to qualifications, generally at a basic level. Some prisoners progress to higher education, for example by obtaining grants for Open University courses. Most submissions to the Koestler Awards come through prison education departments (Koestler Trust 2013).

### Therapy

Many prisons have special units for prisoners with learning difficulties or emotional needs. Usually provided through the National Health Service, these often include arts-based occupational therapy. Some prisons also offer drama therapy or art therapy to address offending behaviour. The focus is on psychological benefits for the participants rather than on a finished artistic product, but some of the resulting artworks are entered for the Koestler Awards.

### Arts projects

Many arts activities with offenders are projects of arts charities. These range from major national companies, like the National Gallery (<http://www.nationalgallery.org.uk/learning/outreach-projects/inside-art>) or the Hallé Orchestra (<http://www.halle.co.uk/young-offenders.aspx>), which run the projects as part of their education or outreach programmes, to small

organizations, sometimes with one or two staff, which specialize in engaging offenders through specific art forms. Most are one-off or short-term projects, involving a group of offenders for a week or two, culminating in a performance or publication; some are longer partnerships, such as residencies for writers or artists over months or years. Prisons occasionally commission arts projects; more often the arts charity devises the project, raises funds from philanthropic sources, then approaches a prison to provide the venue, the support staff, and a financial contribution. Arts charities and freelancers make up most of the 600+ members of the National Alliance for Arts in Criminal Justice.

### Independent creativity

Today's equivalent of the Tower of London graffiti is the creative writing, drawing, painting and composing that prisoners pursue on their own initiative. Most prisoners have done nothing artistic since school. Some discover a talent that gives them currency: they make drawings from photographs of the family or pets of other inmates, or write love poems or children's stories in return for cigarettes and other goods. Some practice traditional prison crafts like matchstick modelling, soap carving, or bread sculpting (Meadows 2010) (Fig. 35.2).

Hundreds of these works are entered for the Koestler Awards, often directly from the prison wing, using an entry form published in *Inside Time*, the national newspaper for prisoners. With evidence emerging that, because of staffing cuts, prisoners are spending longer periods in their cells (Prison Reform Trust 2013), the need for in-cell creativity looks set to increase. Some arts charities—notably Fine Cell Work (<http://www.finecellwork.co.uk/>) and the Burnbake Trust (<http://www.burnbaketrust.co.uk/>)—address this need by providing training and materials.

## Theoretical models

Arts in criminal justice stem from a variety of beliefs and goals that can be summarized in three broad theoretical models. Each model helps explain current activity and offers a rationale for future development.

### The model of individual change

Offenders are, by definition, people who need to change. Society needs them to stop harming more victims, and most offenders themselves want to improve their lives. Here the role of arts is to benefit individual offenders, a change which will in turn benefit others. Within prisons, the arts can be valuable simply by keeping inmates occupied and calm, averting harm to staff and other prisoners, arguably by making resistance innocuous (Cheliotis 2012). But in policy statements and for most criminal justice professionals—as well as many arts organizations—the overriding aim of any provision for offenders is to reduce reoffending. Almost half of prisoners released from custody in England and Wales in 2010 reoffended within a year, and the failure to reduce this rate over the last decade has made fresh solutions a political priority (Ministry of Justice 2013).

Recognizing the difficulty of pinpointing a direct causal relationship between intervention and rehabilitation, NOMS policy

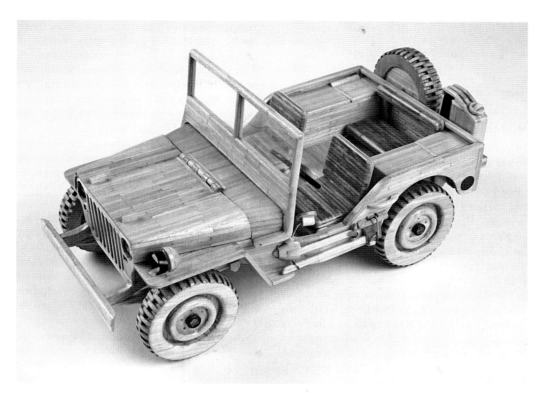

**Fig. 35.2** '1942 Willys Jeep' by a prisoner at HM Prison Isle of Wight. Koestler Platinum Award for Matchstick Modelling, 2013 (matchsticks and mixed media 7 × 8 × 15.5 cm). Reproduced by kind permission of The Koestler Trust. Copyright © 2015 The Koestler Trust.

includes commissioning services targeted at 'intermediate outcomes' which can *contribute* to reduced offending (NOMS 2012). These include improved attitudes and thinking, closer family relationships, withdrawal from substance misuse, and housing and employment on release. Some arts activities are designed specially to address these factors. For example, graphic design courses equip offenders for specific employment; Geese Theatre Company (<http://www.geese.co.uk/>) uses masks and role-plays to teach insight into offending behaviour; and Safe Ground (<http://www.safeground.org.uk/>)uses drama to enhance prisoners' family relationships. Other arts projects—like poetry or music workshops—are not specifically applied to functional outcomes, but still aim to enhance intellectual and interpersonal abilities, which offenders can then use to improve their relationships and access practical services.

The process through which offenders move out of crime is the subject of the recent criminological discourse of 'desistance theory' (McNeill et al. 2012). This identifies a personal journey followed by most offenders in which the frequency and severity of their offending decline as they grow older, until they desist from crime altogether. The process may meander, but the outcome is profound—the offender's identity is transformed to that of non-offender. Indicators of desistance include shifting from a self-narrative of failure to one of potential, from passivity to a sense of agency, from self-doubt to an appropriate level of self-esteem. Desistance theorists are often wary of translating their observations into a blueprint for services, but they have specifically cited the arts as reinforcing and potentially speeding up desistance (Anderson et al. 2011).

The breadth and depth of the impact of the arts on individual offenders is perhaps best conceptualized through four realms of human wellbeing: physical, intellectual, emotional, and spiritual (or body, mind, heart, and soul). Most interventions with offenders operate on one or two of these areas, for example job-based training on intellectual skills, psychology on cognitive and emotional development, chaplaincy on spiritual growth. The arts are unique in engaging and nurturing all four fields as the following examples indicate:

- Physical: sight for visual arts; hearing for music; dexterity for ceramics or needlecraft; agility for dance or drama; capturing sensuality in writing.

- Intellectual: literacy for writing; numeracy for measurements in visual arts or rhythms in music, poetry, and dance; observing and interpreting the realities to be represented; studying and implementing forms, traditions, and techniques; constructing viewpoint, narrative, and shape.

- Emotional: finding a perspective on feelings in order to express them; empathizing with others' feelings, for example to create a portrait or character; communicating passion to the audience, reader, listener, or viewer.

- Spiritual: discovering and conveying a sense of meaning or purpose, often connected to an innermost self or to an external sphere of hope and power, and founded on a profound conviction of truth.

Certainly many offenders themselves identify the arts as transformational as the writer, artist and curator Eve McDougall has:

'I have been involved with the Koestler Trust in different ways over the years and find it a great platform for changing lives through art. I am an ex-prisoner, and art changed my life: it taught me how to structure my life—beginning, middle and end. Every piece I create is a new adventure.'

From an interview with the author (January 2014)

## The model of social change

Rehabilitation requires change not just by offenders but also by society. Prisoners may become model citizens, but can resettle on the outside only if they are accepted and ideally supported back into family, community, employment and other social opportunities. Many ex-prisoners find social attitudes the biggest barrier to resettlement. There is evidence of prejudice from some employers (Working Links 2010), and public misconceptions are widespread: 66% of people in England and Wales believe crime is increasing, when it is in fact falling and is now at its lowest level since 1981 (Prison Reform Trust 2013, p. 76). Sociologists have long identified media representation as fuelling fears about offending (Kidd-Hewitt and Osborne 1995), and press coverage has had a severe impact on some arts projects, including cancellation of a Comedy School course in a prison in 2008, following claims in the *Sun*, a British tabloid newspaper, that participants included an al-Qaida terrorist, and in 2009 removal of a Koestler Award-winning sculpture from display in the Royal Festival Hall in London after *The Times* reported that the artist was a high-profile murderer. In 2011, a *Sunday Express* report on a Koestler exhibition in

Liverpool typified the stereotypes used by the press, describing the exhibition as a sick display of art by killers, funded by tax-payers. It also alleged that a small ceramic exhibit entitled 'Man in Black' was a bust of Moors murderer Ian Brady, whom the article labelled as a monster (Faulkner and Evans 2011). Responding in a BBC interview, the Koestler Trust pointed out that the ceramic was in fact of the singer Johnny Cash, whose albums include *The Man in Black*.

Art submissions are accepted by the Trust only when accompanied by signed authorization from the artist and an appropriate member of staff: the Trust does not ask about entrants' offending, nor disclose their identities.

Arts charities are rarely campaigning organizations, and the arts are inherently open to varied interpretations by audiences, but clearly part of the rationale for bringing prison arts to the public is to challenge the branding of all offenders as 'monsters'. The Koestler Trust states this aim in neutral terms—'to promote public awareness and understanding of arts by offenders' (see Fig. 35.3)—but visitors to Koestler exhibitions repeatedly comment that the displays help them to see offenders as human beings:

'I didn't think art was something offenders should do, or would even want to do. The exhibition makes you realise they are just people. You see them painted in a different light—quite literally!'

Visitor to Koestler UK exhibition 2012

Most interventions with offenders need to happen in confidential settings, but a distinctive feature of many arts projects is an artistic output that can communicate more widely. Public

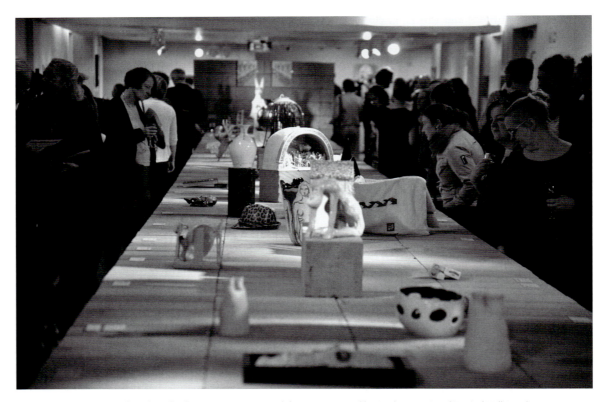

**Fig. 35.3**  Koestler 2012 UK exhibition of arts by offenders, secure patients and detainees, curated by Sarah Lucas, Royal Festival Hall, London.
Reproduced by kind permission of The Koestler Trust. Copyright © 2015 The Koestler Trust.

showcasing is integral to the practice of many offender arts charities—with publications like *Not Shut Up* magazine (<http://www.notshutup.org/>), theatre performances by Clean Break (<http://www.cleanbreak.org.uk/>), Pimlico Opera (<http://www.grangeparkopera.co.uk/2014/01/pimlico-opera-in-prison/>)and Synergy Theatre (<http://www.synergytheatreproject.co.uk/>), and gigs by Music in Prisons (<http://www.musicinprisons.org.uk/>) and Changing Tunes (<http://www.changingtunes.org.uk/>). In conveying the talents and humanity of offenders, these platforms may help prevent reoffending by making society more open to rehabilitation.

## The human rights model

There are two dangers in justifying the arts on the basis of individual or social change. One is that creativity is necessarily open and unpredictable: it cannot guarantee outcomes that are calming or civilizing; on the contrary, much art is troubling and disruptive. The second danger is of creating a patronizing distinction between arts for the affluent classes—who may pursue creativity as a profession or a leisure activity—and arts for poor or marginalized people—which are justified by the evidence that it does them good.

A human rights model avoids these pitfalls by not seeking to bring about specific change at all. Under this model, arts are justified in prison because they are justified everywhere, as enshrined in Article 27 of the Universal Declaration of Human Rights:

> 'Everyone has the right freely to participate in the cultural life of the community [and] to enjoy the arts.'
> Reproduced from the Universal Declaration of Human Rights, by the United Nations. Copyright © 1948 United Nations. Reprinted with the permission of the United Nations.

This is central to the ethos of London's Southbank Centre, an internationally respected arts venue that has significantly raised the profile of offender art by hosting the annual UK Koestler Exhibition since 2008. As its artistic director Jude Kelly says:

> 'Everyone has an imagination. Everybody is expressive. Everybody, therefore, can enjoy other people's expressiveness. Art should be for everyone—it's a human right.'
>
> Kelly (2012)

This is the impulse behind most prisoners' participation in the arts: they have no particular outcome in mind—they simply pursue their enjoyment. As one Koestler Award-winner puts it: 'For me, art rises above all else. I will continue to paint because it brings me joy.' A punishment agenda would question the appropriateness of enjoyment in prison; a rehabilitation agenda would argue that enjoyment enables offenders to discover their pro-social potential; but many prisoner-artists are aspiring simply to create the best possible art.

## Research evidence

The National Alliance for Arts in Criminal Justice maintains an on-line Evidence Library of relevant research reports at <http://www.artsevidence.org.uk/>. The focus is on individual change, and the Alliance has itself commissioned two reports that epitomize two main methodologies: a quantitative study of reoffending, and a qualitative study of desistance. In the quantitative research, Johnson et al. (2011) made a statistical analysis of data from three offender arts programmes and measured significant reductions in the expected rates of reoffending. For the qualitative research, Bilby et al. (2013) interacted with offenders during four arts projects, and identified numerous personal signs that the projects were reinforcing desistance.

However, a recent NOMS review of 134 studies assessed only 16 to be 'good-quality research', concluding that 'no solid evidence was found that arts projects are able to have a direct impact on reoffending' (Burrowes et al. 2013). Meanwhile desistance theorists argue that reoffending rates are themselves misleading: an offender not caught between particular dates may remain prone to continue offending, while a repeat offender may be undergoing profound positive change, with offending growing less severe. Desistance can be ascertained only by nuanced, contextualized appraisal of individuals.

This mixed picture of evidence for individual change at least offers an array of information for practitioners. In terms of social change, almost no research is available, although a survey of visitors to a Koestler exhibition has found an impact on attitudes (Exley 2014). Equally scarce is research by arts academics into the aesthetic quality or cultural value of arts by offenders—though there is some artistic critical analysis in Meadows (2010) and Cheliotis (2012). Yet the experience of the Koestler Trust is that arts evidence—offenders' paintings, poems and performances themselves—can be the most instructive evidence of all.

## Artistic judgement and the Koestler Trust

The Koestler Trust's work can be summarized as a springboard for offenders, artists and audiences to reach new levels of artistic judgement. The Trust's half-century history makes its awards uniquely prestigious as a motivator of creative achievement by offenders, generating over 8000 entries a year in 60 art forms from over 300 establishments across the United Kingdom. It also has a high profile with the public, with over 50,000 visitors to Koestler exhibitions in 2013 in Cardiff, Gateshead, Glasgow and London.

When encouraging offenders to submit artworks, and inviting arts professionals to judge for the awards and curate the exhibitions (including distinguished artists like Jeremy Deller, Sarah Lucas, and Grayson Perry, and writers like Wendy Cope, Douglas Dunn, and Will Self), the Trust deliberately sets no criteria for their judgements. In the Koestler mentoring programme, artist-volunteers are trained to provide one-to-one mentoring to ex-offenders; they are given strict boundaries to minimize personal risk but allowed complete discretion about the creative content of the mentoring sessions. Viewing a Koestler exhibition, visitors cannot fall back on the reputation or market value of the artists: told no more than the artist's first name and prison, they have to judge for themselves. The Koestler ethos is that this freedom from imposed expectations and formulaic targets—coupled with strong recognition of beauty and excellence—generates a transformative encounter for all involved.

Two Koestler Award-winning works—a painting and a poem—will serve as evidence for this transformation. They also

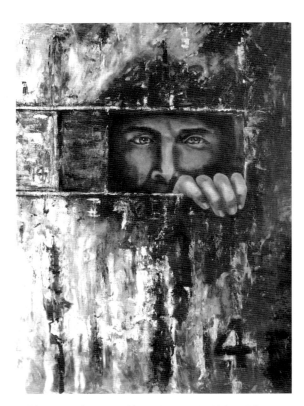

**Fig. 35.4** 'The Lost and Forgotten' by a prisoner at HM Prison Whatton, Nottinghamshire. Koestler Awards 2011 (acrylic on canvas 79 × 58.5 cm)
Reproduced by kind permission of The Koestler Trust. Copyright © 2015 The Koestler Trust.

exemplify two recurring motifs of prisoner art: entrapment and escape. The painting (see Fig. 39.4), by an adult male prisoner from HM Prison Whatton in Nottinghamshire, was exhibited at the 2011 Koestler UK exhibition at Southbank Centre. A technically accomplished representation of a prisoner's eyes looking out from the small communication window in a cell door it makes a blunt, perhaps political point about the harshness of imprisonment, underlined by its title 'The Lost and Forgotten'. The Prison Service deserves credit for allowing such freedom of expression, and the piece is characteristic of inmate art in contrasting the individual—the human face—with the system—the metal door that almost obliterates him by filling most of the picture's area.

But the painter has made two artistic decisions that both reinforce and transgress this contrast. First, the prisoner strives to breach the divide to the viewer outside the cell—with his fingers through the window and with the intensity of his stare—simultaneously defiant and defeated. Secondly, while the prisoner is painted in photorealistic style—details sharp, colours smooth and strong—the door is impressionistic—in light colours and rough textures. On one hand, this makes the prisoner more substantial than the door: the prison might melt away like a dream. On the other hand, what the door makes vivid is the artist—his painterly energy palpable in the brushstrokes. Instead of limiting him to metallic grey, the door unleashes his variety and dynamism: it is imaginatively opened. By applying his creativity to the prison itself, the offender-artist transfigures it into a field of possibility.

This paradox of captivity releasing opportunity was also experienced by Arthur Koestler (1905–83), the writer-philosopher who founded the Koestler Awards in 1962, who had been a political prisoner in the Spanish Civil War and Second World War. He wrote that his 'periods of confinement in prisons and concentration camps . . . each turned into a spiritual blessing', because—though he would have preferred a self-imposed retreat—the solitude expanded his consciousness at moments into an 'oceanic experience' (Koestler 1952, p. 130). In 2013, the Koestler Gold Award for Poetry went to an inmate of HMP Stafford who uses a similar marine image:

### Back To the Sea

Show me the sea, the shining sea
and let me breathe it in
bit by salty bit.
I'll close my arms around the waves
and wash my soul in it.

Reproduced by kind permission of the Koestler
Trust and the author

The rapturous evocation of a place of spiritual renewal (that will 'wash my soul') is clinched by the poem's physicality—especially the taste of the salt and the sound of 'bit' and 'it'. This confident escape seems the antithesis of the locked door in 'The Lost and Forgotten'. But ultimately the poem is suffused with the same poignancy of looking out from prison. In both works frustration generates the urgency of aspiration. This is the drama that grips and moves visitors to Koestler exhibitions: every exhibit is a cry to reconnect with the outside, thwarted but hopeful. And the dialectic of ambition and setback is fundamental to the way offenders build new lives through the arts—by reaching through instead of sidestepping, by realizing a selfhood in balance with, even springing from, life's barriers and contradictions.

If a crime is an act of poor judgement—misguided, dishonest or cruel—then everybody needs criminals to learn to judge, and to be judged, with integrity and humanity. There is no better training-ground for this than the arts. The arts set goals that can be attained only through originality, accuracy and empathy. There are no shortcuts: artistic decisions have to be genuinely owned. Creativity is uniquely transformative because the only ultimate judgement in art is truthfulness, in all its human complexity.

## References

Anderson, K., Colvin, S., McNeill, F., et al. (2011). *Inspiring Change: Final Project Report of the Evaluation Team*. Available at: <http://www.art-sevidence.org.uk/evaluations/inspiring-change-final-project-report-evaluation-t/> (accessed January 2014).

Arts Alliance (2015). *Annual Review 2014/15*. Available at: <https://www.artsincriminaljustice.org.uk/national-alliance-arts-criminal-justice-annual-review-2014-15-0> (accessed March 2015).

Bilby, C., Caulfield, L., and Ridley, L. (2013). *Re-imagining Futures: Exploring Arts Interventions and the Process of Desistance*. London: Clinks. Available at: <http://www.artsalliance.org.uk/re-imagining-futures-exploring-arts-interventions-and-process-desistance> (accessed January 2014).

Burrowes, N., Disley, E., Liddle, M., et al. (2013). Intermediate Outcomes of Arts Projects: A Rapid Evidence Assessment. Available at: <https://www.gov.uk/government/uploads/system/uploads/attachment_data/file/254450/intermediate-outcomes-of-arts-projects.pdf> (accessed January 2014).

Cheliotis, L. (2012). *The Arts of Imprisonment: Control, Resistance and Empowerment*. Edinburgh: Ashgate.

Exley, E. (2014). Unpublished survey of visitors to UK Koestler Exhibition 2013 for criminology dissertation at Cardiff University.

Faulkner, A. and Evans, N. (2011). Fury at Ian Brady 'artwork'. *The Sunday Express*, 13 March 2011. Available at: <http://www.express.co.uk/news/uk/234188/fury-at-ian-brady-artwork>

House of Commons Education and Skills Committee (2005). *Prison Education: Seventh Report of Session 2004–05*. Available at: <http://www.publications.parliament.uk/pa/cm200405/cmselect/cmeduski/114/114i.pdf> (accessed January 2014).

Johnson, H., Keen, S., and Pritchard, D. (2011). *Unlocking Value: The Economic Benefit of the Arts in Criminal Justice*. London: New Philanthropy Capital. Available at: <http://www.thinknpc.org/publications/unlocking-value/> (accessed January 2014).

Kelly, J. (2012). What i See. Meet the ambassadors: Jude Kelly [interview]. Available at: <http://whatiseeproject.com/news/meet-the-ambassadors-jude-kelly> (accessed January 2014).

Kidd-Hewitt, D. and Osborne, R. (1995). *Crime and the Media: The Post-Modern Spectacle*. London: Pluto Press.

Koestler, A. (1952). *Arrow in the Blue* [reprinted 2005]. London: Vintage.

Koestler Trust (2013). Koestler Awards 2013 entrants statistics. Available at: <http://www.koestlertrust.org.uk/pdfs/entrants_graphs2013.pdf> (accessed January 2014).

McNeill, F., Farrall, S., Lightowler, C., and Maruna, S. (2012). How and why people stop offending: discovering desistance. *IRISS Insights*, no. 15. Available at: <http://www.iriss.org.uk/sites/default/files/iriss-insight-15.pdf> (accessed January 2014).

Meadows, M. (2010). *Insider Art*. London: A&C Black.

Ministry of Justice (2013). *Transforming Rehabilitation: A Strategy for Reform*. London: The Stationery Office.

NOMS (2012). *NOMS Commissioning Intentions for 2013–14*. Available at: <http://www.justice.gov.uk/about/noms/commissioning> (accessed January 2014).

NOMS (2013). *National Offender Management Service Business Plan 2013–14*. London: Ministry of Justice. Available at: <http://www.justice.gov.uk/downloads/publications/corporate-reports/noms/2013/noms-business-plan-2013-2014.pdf> (accessed January 2014).

Prison Reform Trust (2013). *Bromley Briefings Prison Fact File. Autumn 2013*. Available at: <http://www.prisonreformtrust.org.uk/portals/0/documents/factfile%20autumn%202013.pdf> (accessed January 2014).

Thurley, S. (1996). *The Tower of London: Official Guide*. London: Historic Royal Palaces.

Working Links (2010). *Pre-judged: Tagged for Life. A Research Report into Employer Attitudes to Ex-Offenders*. Available at: <http://www.workinglinks.co.uk/all_about_us/our_research/tagged_for_life.aspx> (accessed January 2014).

# CHAPTER 36

# Quality of place and wellbeing

Bryan Lawson and Rosie Parnell

## Introduction to quality of place and wellbeing

In this chapter we deal with the setting, rather than the art that might reside in or take place in that setting. It is the art of the architecture itself that is our concern here. We focus on healthcare and educational settings since those are the settings for which we have most data, but we shall also argue that there are good reasons for being optimistic about the extent to which it may prove possible to generalize from these data.

In its constitution the World Health Organization defines 'health' as 'a state of complete physical, mental, and social wellbeing not merely the absence of disease . . .' It is therefore argued that health must include measures of wellbeing and quality of life beyond purely medical ones.

There are now several well-regarded and frequently referenced measures of quality of life that are regularly published by established authorities. Some focus on economic and political stability, along with climate and other factors. Two in particular, from *The Economist* and Mercer, operate at the national and city level. There tends to be quite a high correlation between these two indices, with cities such as Melbourne and Vancouver often showing very high scores; both indices include attempts to record the quality of architecture. By contrast the WHO quality of life indices can be used at the personal level. The WHO indices include several factors such as physical and mental health, personal independence, and socialization. However, they still include an environmental factor that embraces architecture.

The idea that the natural and designed environments contribute to our quality of life and wellbeing is therefore hardly new or strange, but the extent to which this is true and the detailed factors that are chiefly responsible have not featured highly in political policy-making or economic expenditure. Good architecture, in particular, is often viewed as an expensive luxury rather than a basic element responsible for our productivity and wellbeing.

In 2003 the UK Construction Research and Innovation Strategy (nCRISP) published its report on the social and economic value of construction (Pearce 2003). It claimed that 'Good design contributes to physical and mental health, to a sense of identity and wellbeing, to good social relationships, reduced crime, and higher productivity. Bad design and dilapidated capital stock has the opposite effect' (Pearce 2003, p. 50). It talked about good design as offering 'significant but as yet, largely unquantified benefits in terms of human wellbeing' (Pearce 2003, p. 59).

In fact, many of these benefits are increasingly well quantified, and we shall argue that we could be more assertive about the extent to which our designed environment contributes, through quality of place, to our sense of wellbeing. We shall also argue that, if we work with the evidence that is already available, then there are benefits to both the occupants and users of these environments as well as wider economic benefits that may be quite significant.

At Sheffield University, work has been taking place on healthcare environments for nearly 20 years and on educational environments for about 10 years. We do not necessarily think that these two settings are somehow more important than others, but they do offer relatively good research opportunities. In both settings (particularly hospitals and schools) large numbers of people, patients, or students pass through in relatively short periods of time and their progress is well documented on a number of measures.

With regard to healthcare settings, the team at Sheffield University was asked by an agency of the British government to survey all the work in this field and produce a structured database of research relevant to the ways in which our designed environment, specifically but not exclusively architecture, could contribute to the wellbeing of patients as well as staff. Initially we found around 500 references, this quickly rose to over 1000 and it is now well over 2000, though not all have yet been reviewed and analysed into a formal database.

In educational settings many different aspects of schools have been examined through a range of mainly small-scale studies. There have been a number of significant reviews of this research (Weinstein 1979; McGuffey 1982; Earthman and Lemasters 1996; Higgins et al. 2005) citing over 400 separate references. More recently, Peter Lippman, an architect and researcher working in a US context, published a book drawing on various disciplines including environmental psychology and education, as well as research in different kinds of settings such as offices, in order to build an evidence-based framework for school design (Lippman 2010).

This body of research on healthcare and educational settings varies in the extent to which it is rigorous. Some is merely anecdotal while other work is based on action research in the settings themselves. There is work that surveys, in various ways, the preferences and satisfaction of users, and there is work that correlates aspects of the setting with objective measured outcomes. Some work is highly controlled, but a considerable amount is field based and we are increasingly seeing longitudinal studies and studies where aspects of settings are parametrically varied. There are of course considerable ethical problems involved in direct experimentation on such vulnerable subjects as patients and students, so even in these settings not all the work that we might like to carry out for scientific reasons is actually possible.

Among the measures used and shown to relate in some way to the hospital setting are patient satisfaction, quality of life, treatment times, levels of medication, displayed aggression, sleep patterns, and compliance with treatment regimes. In the school context comparable measures include student attainment, levels of attention, mood, and motivation, levels of aggressive or disruptive behaviour, teacher and student self-esteem, and physical health and wellbeing—from discomfort to major ailments (Higgins et al. 2005, p. 11).

Research of this kind involving very young children requires a more creative approach to give them opportunities to express their feelings. Similarly some people in care, particularly in mental health settings, also demand more sophisticated research methods. However, overall, if asked in the right way, people can express satisfaction or otherwise with a setting and how important it is to them. This kind of work suggests strongly that the environmental setting makes a significant contribution to what someone regards as their quality of life. We shall return to the research itself later, but before doing so we want to review its significance in terms of the extent to which these settings can be more efficient and effective, and the scale of the resulting economic consequences.

Lawson and others conducted a longitudinal study in two hospitals, one in general medicine and one in mental health (Lawson and Wells-Thorpe 2002). The first part of the study was conducted in wards that had existed for some time and the second after these wards had either been significantly redesigned or completely rebuilt. In both cases, however, the pattern of patient referral and treatment remained very substantially the same and the staff were generally the same with only normal turnover. Patients were invited to express their views about a series of factors, and a whole host of normally gathered data about health outcomes were studied. Some of the data are very dramatic. In the new wards in the general hospital patients were released significantly earlier, with non-operative acute patient treatment times reduced by 21%. They also took dramatically less Class A analgesic medication. The average number of days when Class A drugs were given was reduced by 22% and the average dose reduced by 47%. In the new mental health hospital the average length of stay was reduced by 14% and the number of patients classed as making good progress increased significantly. The need to place patients in a secure restrained environment dropped by a remarkable 70%, and levels of patient aggression and abuse were also significantly reduced.

It is also interesting to note that in this study patients assessed their overall treatment and the performance of the staff caring for them as significantly better in the newly designed settings. It was clear that they felt their life overall in these new settings was of a higher quality.

We turn now to a survey done by Lawson and Phiri (2003) of all the research available into the impact of the design of the setting on health outcomes. Lawson and Phiri suggested that, taken together, all the operational savings that could reasonably be expected from an evidence-based design approach might be in the region of 20% annually compared with most British National Health Service hospitals. They also showed that the cost of running a hospital typically exceeds the cost of building as early as the second year of operation. A theoretical study called Fable Hospital, using data from the United States and building on the work of Roger Ulrich, suggested that an additional capital cost of only about 5% might be needed in order to achieve these very significant annual savings (Berry et al. 2004).

Taken together, then, this new evidence-based approach has the potential simultaneously to improve the quality of patient experience and health outcomes while also saving time and costs. So we now have a great deal of data on hospitals. What can we learn from it generically?

## Research findings on healthcare and educational settings

Lawson and Phiri undertook a large-scale content analysis of all this research and managed to structure the findings under only a few headings—each leading to recommendations for designers (Lawson 2007). We will now summarize them briefly as they structure much of the subsequent discussion and also form the basis of some design tools.

1. *Privacy, company, and dignity.* Design to give people privacy, company, dignity. Design to enable them to be alone and to be with others when they wish to. Enable them to control their levels of privacy. There is considerable evidence that neglecting these factors can lead to significant levels of stress and unhappiness.

2. *Views.* Design to give occupants and visitors views out of buildings. The evidence about such things is not just a woolly expression of niceness. It has been demonstrated that hospital patients who have views outside actually recover more quickly. Not just views; even daylight is actually good for us. Desirable views are not always those that architects assume. Patients waiting at a clinic where they may be concerned about some test results might benefit most from a calming view. On the other hand patients in more long-term care may prefer views that are interesting and stimulating rather than beautiful but relatively static scenes.

3. *Nature and outdoors.* Design to give building occupants contact with nature. Ideally and in the right climate this may be a matter of physical access. Views of nature are known to be therapeutic. Internal planting and even pictures can help significantly where gaining access to the outdoors is not possible or sensible. Even pictures of nature have some effect.

4. *Comfort and control.* Give all building occupants environmental comfort and, most importantly, control over that comfort. This most obviously involves heat and light. However, it also includes sound. It is absurd that many new hospitals are notoriously noisy places. Some of Roger Ulrich's research has shown that patients in a cardiac unit had their heart rates significantly reduced by decreasing background sound levels (Blomkvist et al. 2005). Giving immobilized patients bed head controls of lights, blinds, and curtains and doors is really very cheap to do and remarkably effective in reducing stress levels.

5. *Legibility of place.* Create places that have spatial legibility. Make places that people understand and can find their way around in. We navigate using our own mental map of the world. Places

that are confusing prevent us from building that map and add to stress levels. Design so that there is some hierarchy of space, so that public and private places are clearly demarcated, so that entrances and ways out are obvious, so that different parts of buildings have different qualities.

6. *Interior appearance.* This is much more subjective, but, in general, places that people will spend time in should feel homely, light, and airy, with a variety of colours and textures. Design them to look clean, tidy, and cared for. Use art to provide stimulation or distraction. This may be paintings, sculpture, and even the nature of the spaces themselves. However, it can also be performance. The Chelsea and Westminster Hospital in London has famously shown and measured the value of this (Staricoff et al. 2001). The effects of composed and performed art are discussed further in other chapters of this book.

7. *Facilities*/8. *Staff.* These headings include the provision of facilities that are specific to the functioning of the particular healthcare building in question. An example would be the provision of overnight stay facilities for relatives of long-term patients. The staff provisions also tend to be specific to the conditions under which the staff work in such buildings.

The first five of these points reflect a very high proportion of the research findings that could account for all the benefits to patients and economic savings already discussed. We could certainly phrase the first five of these points without any reference to healthcare and hospitals, and we have largely done so here. These factors are hardly concerned with the specific functionality of hospitals, rather they are more about the making of good places in general and about the ability of good places to improve our overall quality of life. The final points about facilities and staff provisions certainly relate much more specifically to the nature and purpose of healthcare buildings.

So a provisional conclusion here is that although the research upon which all this is based is exclusively about buildings for healthcare, the bulk of the data indicate the importance of generally good place-making rather than issues specific to the highly specialized nature of hospitals and other healthcare facilities.

Rokhshid Ghaziani provided evidence for this conclusion when she constructed a framework for the school design process based on the existing research evidence and the reflections of children (Ghaziani 2012). The process included analysis of three previous UK studies which had elicited children's opinions about and aspirations for their school environments: 'The school I'd like' (Birkett 2001a,b; Burke and Grosvenor 2003), *Joinedupdesignforschools* (Sorrell and Sorrell 2005), and the Sorrell Foundation's Young Design Programme (see <http://www.thesorrellfoundation.com/young_design_programme.php>). Six categories of concern to the students emerged from the data (Ghaziani 2008, p. 232), revealing significant overlaps with the points discerned in the hospitals context:

1. Indoor spaces (interior): the interior of school buildings and how they look.
2. Comfort and control: the comfort levels of pupils and teaching staff in school buildings and the extent to which these can be controlled.
3. Activity spaces: specific design features required for different activities.

4. Nature and outdoors: the extent to which pupils have contact with the natural world, whether they can see and access nature both indoors and outdoors.
5. Facilities: those facilities that are important for pupils.
6. Exterior: the exterior of school buildings and their appearance.

With the exception of a general section on views, this list maps very closely onto our healthcare-derived list of factor, indicating that these data do seem to have generic value. This also aligns with our more common-sense everyday implicit knowledge about good places. Think for instance about how you choose a seat in a restaurant: most people prefer a seat with a protected back affording some privacy and yet with a good view. Hotel rooms with the best views attract higher rates. The great Dutch architect Herman Hertzberger taught us, among many things, about the delight that old people take in watching life going on (Hertzberger 1991). Whereas a patient in a short-stay clinic or at the dentist may benefit from a calming view, longer-term residents are more likely to prefer an interesting one.

Ever since Kevin Lynch's seminal work (Lynch 1960) we have appreciated the value of creating cities that are legible and understandable, and such ideas are clearly applicable to large-scale building complexes such as shopping malls, airports, hospitals, university campuses, and many others.

Is it possible, then, that our five or six major headings begin to give us a picture of the key aspects of the design of settings in general that most help to continue to improve our sense of wellbeing and quality of life? If we are right about this then of course we would also expect to see a change of emphasis and priority in different settings. Our analysis of the research has shown this even within healthcare—for example in mental health, or for older people and children, or even the difference between short- and long-stay patients. Similarly, general best practice today would suggest that privacy and dignity are more important for adults, and single-room accommodation is a target in general hospitals and a norm in mental hospitals. However, children's hospitals still tend to be provided with space that enables children to have company rather than privacy.

We might also expect to see different pathologies resulting from settings not designed to comply with research. For example, in poorly designed hospitals patients might take more medication, be more aggressive and less cooperative in complying with treatment regimes, and take longer to recover. In schools we might expect to see teachers and students with low self-esteem, lacking motivation and engagement, reflected in higher than usual rates of absenteeism and lower levels of attainment.

Of course there are many settings in which it is difficult to identify objective performance criteria. In the domestic setting there are so many activities and a high proportion of them may have little or no recognizable purpose against which success could be measured. However, research by Judith Torrington at Sheffield University on residential care homes for older people has succeeded in building a series of measures which add up to an index of quality of life in this context (Torrington et al. 2004). Using this index, it has been possible to look at the aspects of building design that correlate either positively or negatively with residents' quality of life. Torrington's studies found positive associations with the extent to which the buildings offered choice and control of the environment. This includes such factors as free access to outdoor spaces, choice between a shower or a bath, and control over bedroom heating—linking strongly to points 3 (nature and outdoors) and 4 (comfort and control) in our list for the healthcare context. Further positive associations were found with the extent to which buildings offered support for frailty, which inevitably becomes more important for older people. Next a positive association was also found with the extent to which buildings supported their residents cognitively. This includes such things as way-finding and the extent to which different parts of the building are recognizable—linking clearly to the healthcare study point 5 (legibility of place). Finally a positive association was found with factors referred to in the study as 'community'. These included the siting of the building and its links to the wider community in terms of transport, nearby facilities, and spaces that allowed for family and friends to visit and gather. We can see links here with the healthcare study point 1 (privacy, company, and dignity).

Disturbingly, two separate studies showed negative associations between quality of life and health and safety factors (Parker et al. 2004; Torrington et al. 2004). This latter point perhaps needs more open debate as we have come to allow the health and safety factors in design to become value-free. That is, health and safety are regulated for, and must be satisfied, whatever the negative consequences of complying might be. It may be that, in environmental terms, wellbeing involves some small degree of risk. In older people this might be the danger of falling while taking a walk in a garden. If we are not careful gardens might even be designed out altogether on the grounds of health and safety, but not of wellbeing! In particular those buildings created for and on behalf of people who themselves may not have a loud voice, such as hospitals, schools, and care homes, might easily become over-institutionalized without this as an explicit intention, and as a result the wellbeing of their occupants might diminish.

## Current design practice

Next we examine how design practice is keeping up with and exploiting all this scientific evidence. Although we are arguing here that our findings may have generic value, in order to investigate this fairly we shall first examine current design practice in healthcare and educational settings. There is no question that in recent years some outstanding pieces of architecture have been created for the category of hospital buildings, but they are surprisingly small in number. Most architects familiar with the data we have presented here would almost certainly cite a similar fairly short list of buildings they admire that have been designed around these principles. However, the generality of practice is rather more disappointing.

A recent study based on our analysis of the evidence base for healthcare environments was published by CABE (the Commission for Architecture and the Built Environment, which merged with the Design Council in 2011), the UK government architectural watchdog. The study showed very disappointing results achieved in a major expansion of primary-care design. In fact the report suggested that the weakest features of some 20 primary-care centres were actually in the very aspects of their design where the research evidence was at its strongest. Only 32% of buildings were rated as 'good' and 6% as 'excellent' in relation to a factor that covered the 'overall experience of a building and gives an impression of the standard of service delivery' (CABE 2008).

A post-occupancy evaluation of 18 buildings for treating patients affected by cancer showed similarly poor results overall in relation to the evidence base, and no improvement in the quality of design over a 4-year period. Recent reviews of newly constructed schools are generally no more encouraging. In a leaked government-commissioned report evaluating 25 schools in England, peer review by design, education, information and communication technology (ICT), and sustainability specialists resulted in only nine of the schools (36%) being rated as 'very good' over all, with the remaining 16 schools (64%) assessed as 'pass', i.e. acceptable (Hayman 2012). Factors often highlighted as being unsuccessful included the school grounds, environmental performance in use (particularly over-heating in summer), and sound insulation (Partnerships_for_Schools 2011).

In fact four of the points identified in our healthcare analysis were used by one of the authors as principles of design for a major urban redevelopment strategy of over 100 hectares at Grangegorman in the centre of Dublin, Ireland working with the Santa Monica-based architects Moore Rubell and Yudell (Lawson 2014). This scheme included a complete university campus, healthcare facilities, commercial, residential, and cultural buildings, as well as a large park and sports ground. The floor plates of the healthcare buildings were specifically shallow in plan in order to ensure that whatever detailed design was developed subsequently would have a high likelihood of giving occupants views out over the extensive landscaping. An axis was developed that provided increasing levels of privacy and dignity moving towards the mental health facilities. The overall layout was devised so that new routes had a strong sense of direction and gave views along them of significant existing and largely historic Dublin landmarks. The scheme subsequently won awards from the World Architecture Festival, the Chicago Athenaeum, and the American Institute of Architects (AIA). So there is no reason to believe that designing on the basis of scientific evidence cannot lead to creative and internationally admired design. So what is going wrong? Why is practice generally not making use of this overall evidence base about how to design for quality of life?

## Problems of implementation in design practice

There are probably several major obstacles to overcome here. The primary difficulty is to do with the nature of design education as opposed to scientific education, and the modes of thinking and problem-solving used in these two very disparate general fields. Most designers are not well educated in terms of research methods in general. They probably lack the skills needed to read and critically evaluate work involving the measurement of human performance, feelings, perceptions, and attitudes and the consequent use of descriptive and inferential statistics. Expecting an architect to read a thousand pieces of such research before designing a hospital is clearly unrealistic. One of the consequences of this is that much of the empirical research that evidence-based design must rely on is not conducted by designers. Designers then are neither setting the research agenda nor significantly contributing to the acquisition of such knowledge. They are thus not usually seen by governments and sophisticated clients as being at the forefront of the field.

These problems could be seen to exist at what we might call the policy level. However, there is the much more fundamental question of how design knowledge and scientific knowledge can be combined. Nigel Cross famously asked if there was indeed a 'designerly way of knowing', and there is probably now a consensus in the design research field about this (Cross 1982). Designers generally lack an overarching theory of their field. As a general rule there is little or no theory that helps a designer get from problem to solution in the way we would find in engineering for example. There are no theories or formulae to learn. Actually, designers' knowledge is very heavily biased towards an understanding and appreciation of solutions. The designer tackles ill-defined problems, learning more about them largely through a process of proposing solutions. This process involves what has been termed 'constructive' thinking (Cross 1982, p. 225) and prioritizes synthesis as opposed to analysis.

This inevitably leads us on to the vexed question of how problems and solutions map onto each other in design. Scientific evidence tends to be parametric and atomistic. It is the very nature of such research that much of it works at a highly specific level. For example, we are now well aware of the benefits not just of views and contact with nature but also of the presence of daylight and even sunlight. One study even suggested that patients in rooms facing east might do better than patients in rooms facing west (Beauchemin and Hays 1996). Light is also the topic of a large proportion of the studies into the relationship between school buildings and learning (Higgins et al. 2005, p. 9). However, it has also been found that the recommendations resulting from such studies on different isolated factors can be in direct conflict with each other when compared. One straightforward example of this is found in the recommendation to prioritize daylight in classrooms alongside the parallel recommendation to avoid glare. Similarly, recommendations for improved air quality, through mechanical ventilation or air-conditioning for example, can be in direct conflict with the recommendation to reduce background noise (Higgins et al. 2005, p. 9).

This closer look at the nature of the evidence base therefore reveals several tricky problems. First, that in order to make sense of, and critically evaluate, such evidence we need some theories. These are likely not to be known or understood by designers since they will probably be from the realms of psychology, sociology, biology, or any number of other related fields, but certainly not from design. So architects and other environmental designers are unlikely to be able to read and make critical evaluative sense of the research, and indeed may well not even hear about it.

This is compounded by a second problem. Knowledge of this kind from environment–behaviour studies is not some detailed knowledge coming from a theory of structural mechanics or some evidence about the kinds of materials and systems that might contribute to sustainability. This is evidence about the performance of the designed object as part of a human system such as a hospital, a school, a law court, and so on. Thus it lies firmly in the domain of what have been called 'radical constraints' (Lawson 2006). These are matters to do with the very central purpose and reason for the designed object rather than the technicality of making and maintaining it. In other words, the 'why' is central and the 'what' peripheral. Such ideas cannot be brought into play late in the design process when detailing the construction, structure, and services of buildings. We are talking here about the very things that are likely to give form and organization to the design. We have come to call such matters primary generators (Darke 1978). They permeate the whole design and thus need to be very well understood. The scientific knowledge then needs to be embedded

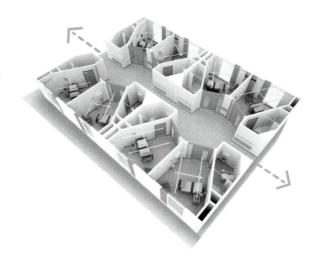

**Fig. 36.1** Southmead Hospital, Bristol, UK: a design for hospital wards that made integrated use of all the available research evidence.
Image reproduced by kind permission of BDP, Carillion plc and the North Bristol NHS Trust.
Copyright © 2015 BDP, Carillion plc and the North Bristol NHS Trust.

in these primary generators and hence positioned right at the very heart of the design process.

Thirdly, design, if it is to be successful, cannot address the evidence base in the atomized way in which it is often presented. Instead, a designerly synthesis of factors is required and in a specific context. The challenge before us then lies in finding a way to express such scientific knowledge in a 'designerly way of knowing'. In the context of this book it is perhaps important to make the distinction here between art and design. While these two are often understandably confused, in this case the distinction is a vital one. Designed elements of buildings have many roles to play. In this sense problems and solutions in design do not easily or directly map onto each other. Rather each designed element may address many aspects of the problem. A window in a hospital room, for example, not only lets in light and possibly fresh air, but also offers a view out while affecting privacy and dignity too. Each of these factors can be separately researched, but the architect must integrate the solution across all of them. What is even more problematic here is that the window also has to solve other technical and legislative problems that lie beyond our research findings altogether. Thus a window cannot simply be adjusted in the design to accommodate one piece of atomistic research without potentially impacting widely across other factors (Fig. 36.1).

## Possible ways forward

So what can be done to tackle these apparently intractable obstacles and make better use of our hard-earned empirical evidence in professional design practice? First we must put conscious effort into surveying, structuring, and summarizing the available research in a form that can be used in design. Lawson and Phiri have shown several ways in which this can be done. For healthcare, two computer-based tools called ASPECT and IDEAs were created towards this end. ASPECT is an evaluative tool that allows designers and their clients to ask simple questions about a design or an existing building, and from this produces a profile set of scores that indicate how well the design complies with the

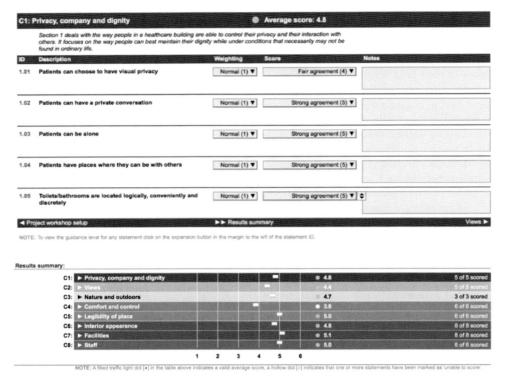

**Fig. 36.2** ASPECT: a tool for assessing the extent to which hospital designs comply with the research evidence.
Reproduced by kind permission of Bryan Lawson. Copyright © 2015 Bryan Lawson.

research findings under each heading. Inevitably this also then points the way to areas that could be improved. The points in our earlier list are part of ASPECT (Lawson 2007) (Fig. 36.2).

IDEAs works almost the other way round. It shows images of designs that are particularly strong in addressing particular features of the research. It shows the range of design features that can be brought into play to create the desired effects. It acts as a sort of interactive design resource enabling designers and clients to discuss issues and get ideas about the design they want to create (Fig. 36.3).

A similar resource, IMAGINE, developed by the Bureau—Design + Research (BDR) at Sheffield University presents existing school designs, analysing them thematically to highlight principles of good practice (Chiles 2013). Commentaries, photographs, and architectural drawings situate these principles in their various geographical, social, cultural, and political contexts, allowing designers, other specialists, and their clients and users to learn from applied examples. These tools are probably far from perfect and could be improved. But it is really only possible to begin to create them or work on them if you have an understanding both of the scientific research and of the nature and process of designing (Fig. 36.4).

Another way forward is to educate designers in some of the sciences that generate this knowledge so they can work as specialists in larger design teams. One barrier to this is the persistent refusal of the architectural profession to allow for specialism. Our degree courses, and the way the professional bodies regulate and recognize them, tend towards requiring us all to be general practitioners capable of designing anything and running our own practice. The role models put in front of students tend to be signature architects, and normative architectural culture is such that anyone with a technical or scientific specialism is seen as a lesser being. Alternatively, architectural education might seek to equip students with the critical and analytical skills and the practical knowledge that they require to gather the existing evidence base, integrating this into the everyday dialogue of the design studio.

We should perhaps end with a caveat. While promoting this approach we must also guard against the tyranny of scientific authority. Environment–behaviour studies research is beginning to be understood by large-scale professional clients. This is certainly happening in hospital design. There is a danger that successful evidence-based designs become authoritative in the eyes of major clients who then instruct their architects to replicate them. In a major review of school construction in England commissioned by the British government (James 2011) it was indeed recommended that 'New buildings should be based on a clear set of standardized drawings and specifications that will incorporate the latest thinking on educational requirements and the bulk of regulatory needs.' (James 2011, p. 6). While the government did not go so far as to introduce standardized designs, it did create the so-called 'baseline designs for schools'—a number of sets of drawings created for the purpose of either being applied directly or as the basis for discussions with planning authorities during the design development phase of government-sponsored school building. Whether or not these particular designs leave space for designers to synthesize, envision, and innovate is open to debate. However, this is exactly what is needed: a form of evidence-based design that nevertheless allows for creative innovation.

To illustrate this in practice we would cite the highly innovative Evelina London Children's Hospital (Lawson 2010). Way

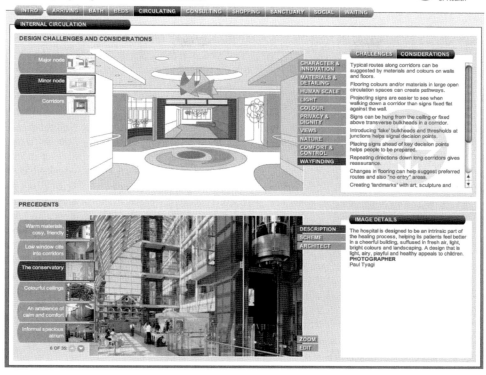

**Fig. 36.3** IDEAS: a tool for assisting designers to use the research evidence during briefing and design.
Reproduced by kind permission of Bryan Lawson. Copyright © 2015 Bryan Lawson.

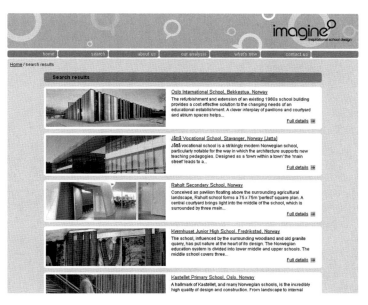

**Fig. 36.4** IMAGINE: marketing material for the school design resource.
Reproduced by kind permission of Bureau—Design + Research, University of Sheffield; Education Funding Agency; Balfour Beatty Investments. Copyright © 2015 Bureau—Design + Research, University of Sheffield; Education Funding Agency; Balfour Beatty Investments.

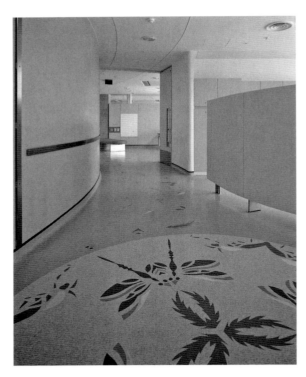

**Fig. 36.5** The flooring pattern at Evelina London Children's Hospital.
Reproduced by kind permission of Paul Tyagi. Copyright © 2015 Paul Tyagi.

finding in large hospitals is always an issue and there are many well-documented techniques involving maps, signage, and even lines along the floor. The Evelina architects commissioned an artist to create mosaics of animals in the flooring. These mosaics present the complete animal once you reach a major circulation node, but as you penetrate deeper into the building the animal fragments. So under your bed you may have just the wing of a butterfly. To get out of the ward and towards the entrance the task is to assemble the whole butterfly. The animals are also themed to various types of habitat such as ocean or forest on different floors. In this particular case, art clearly meets architectural design and the result is a delight as well as a sound evidence-based solution (Fig. 36.5).

The Evelina hospital, then, offers an example of what we should all be aiming for, a creative evidence-based approach to design. A great deal of evidence is now in place and although we have concentrated here on healthcare and educational settings, our analysis is that much of the evidence and its emergent themes are remarkably generic. The key issues we have identified are designing for community, privacy, and dignity, creating views, promoting contact with nature, creating comfortable environments over which people have control, and making understandable places. Of course we would like to see more evidence gathered, but translating the existing evidence into designerly knowledge that allows for creative innovation remains one of the greatest challenges. The evidence we have strongly suggests this will pay dividends not only in terms of quality of life but also economically in many settings.

# References

Beauchemin, K.M. and Hays, P. (1996). Sunny hospital rooms expedite recovery from severe and refractory depressions. *Journal of Affective Disorders*, **40**, 49–51.

Berry, L.L., Parker, D., Coile, R.C., Hamilton, D. K., O'Neill D.D., and Sadler, B.L. (2004). The business case for better buildings. *Frontiers of Health Service Management*, **21**, 1–24.

Birkett, D. (2001a). The school we'd like. *Guardian*. Available at: <http://www.guardian.co.uk/guardianeducation/story/0,3605,501372,00.html> (accessed 24 November 2013).

Birkett, D. (2001b). Future perfect. *Guardian*. Available at: <http://education.guardian.co.uk/schools/story/0,5500,501387,00.html> (accessed 24 November 2013).

Blomkvist, V., Eriksen, C.A., Theorell, T., Ulrich, R., and Rasmanis, G. (2005). Acoustics and psychosocial environment in intensive coronary care. *Occupational and Environmental Medicine*, **62**, e1.

Burke, C. and Grosvenor, I. (2003). *The School I'd Like: Children and Young People's Reflections on an Education for the 21st Century*. London: Routledge Falmer.

CABE (2008). *LIFT Survey Report*. London: Commission for Architecture and the Built Environment.

Chiles, P. (2013) Not brave enough: building schools for the future—the process versus the product. In: A. Neely and M. O'Kane Boal (eds), *Building our Children's Future*, pp. 48–61. Belfast: PLACE..

Cross, N. (1982). Designerly ways of knowing. *Design Studies*, **3**, 221–227.

Darke, J. (1978). The primary generator and the design process. In: W.E. Rogers and W.H. Ittleson (eds), *New Directions in Environmental Design Research: Proceedings of EDRA 9*, pp. 325–337. Washington: Environmental Design Research Association.

Earthman, G.I. and Lemasters, L. (1996). Review of research on the relationship between school buildings, student achievement, and student behavior. *Council of Educational Facility Planners, International Annual Meeting Tarpon Springs, Florida, October 8, 1996*. Available at: <http://www.eric.ed.gov/pdfs/ed416666.pdf> (accessed 2 November 2013).

Ghaziani, R. (2008). Children's voices: raised issues for school design. *CoDesign*, **4**, 225–236.

Ghaziani, R. (2012). An emerging framework for school design based on children's voices. *Children, Youth and Environments*, **22**, 125–144.

Hayman, A. (2012). Exclusive: third of previous government's new schools 'very good'. *Building.co.uk*. Available at: <http://www.building.co.uk/exclusive-third-of-previous-governments-new-schools-very-good/5035562.article> (accessed 2 November 2013).

Hertzberger, H. (1991). *Lessons for Students in Architecture*. Rotterdam: Uitgeverij.

Higgins, S., Hall, E., Wall, K., Woolner, P., and McCaughey, C. (2005). *The Impact of School Environments*. London: The Design Council.

James, S. (2011). *Review of Education Capital*. Available at: <https://www.education.gov.uk/consultations/downloadabledocs/james%20reviewpdf.pdf>

Lawson, B.R. (2006). *How Designers Think*. Oxford: Architectural Press.

Lawson, B.R. (2007). Design indicators. In: D. Stark (ed.), *UK Healthcare Design Review*, pp. 88–95. Glasgow: Keppie Design.

Lawson, B.R. (2010). Healing architecture. *Society for Arts in Healthcare Journal*, **2**, 95–108.

Lawson, B.R. (2014). *The Healthcare Campus at Grangegorman. The Grangegorman Master Plan in Dublin—An Urban Quarter with an Open Future*. Kinsale: J.M. O'Connor.

Lawson, B.R. and Phiri, M. (2003). *The Architectural Healthcare Environment and its Effects on Patient Health Outcomes*. London: The Stationery Office.

Lawson, B.R. and Wells-Thorpe, J. (2002). The effect of the hospital environment on the patient experience and health outcomes. *Journal of Healthcare Design and Development*, **March**, 27–32.

Lippman, P. (2010). *Evidence-Based Design of Elementary and Secondary Schools*. Hoboken, NJ: Wiley.

Lynch, K. (1960). *The Image of the City*. Cambridge, MA: MIT Press.

McGuffey, C.W. (1982). Facilities. In: H.J. Wahlberg (ed.), *Improving Educational Standards and Productivity*, pp. 237–288. Berkeley, CA: McCutchan Publishing.

Parker, C., Barnes, S., McKee, K., Torrington, J., and Tregenza, P. (2004). Quality of life and building design in residential and nursing homes for older people. *Ageing and Society*, **24**, 941–962.

Partnerships_for_Schools (2011). Post-occupancy evaluation of schools 2010–2011. A leaked report published by Building. *Building.co.uk*. Available at: <http://www.building.co.uk> (accessed 26 July 2013).

Pearce, D. (2003). *The Social and Economic Value of Construction: The Construction Industry's Contribution to Sustainable Development*. London: nCRISP.

Sorrell, J. and Sorrell, F. (2005). *Joinedupdesignforschools*. London: Merrell.

Staricoff, R.L., Duncan, J., Wright, M., Loppert, S., and Scott, J. (2001). A study of the effects of the visual and performing arts in healthcare. *Hospital Development*, **32**, 25–28.

Torrington, J., Barnes, S., McKee, K., Morgan, K., and Tregenza, P. (2004). The influence of building design on the quality of life. *Architectural Science Review*, **47**, 193–197.

Weinstein, C.S. (1979). The physical environment of the school: a review of the research. *Review of Educational Research*, **49**, 577–610.

# CHAPTER 37

# Creative arts in health professional education and practice: a case study reflection and evaluation of a complex intervention to deliver the Culture and Care programme at the Florence Nightingale School of Nursing and Midwifery, King's College London

Ian Noonan, Anne Marie Rafferty, and John Browne

## Introduction to creative arts in health professional education and practice

In 2012, Jane Cummings, Chief Nursing Officer for England, launched her *Compassion in Practice* strategy for nursing and midwifery which has become known for the headline six Cs: care, compassion, competence, communication, courage, and commitment (DH 2012). This chapter proposes that engagement with the creative arts in nursing and midwifery education offers one route to explore, expand, and enhance students' non-normative ethics and values that underpin the sustained delivery of person-centred compassionate care and will demonstrate how students have applied creative arts learning to meet these core domains.

In starting the debate about whether compassion can be taught, Pence (1983) emphasized the importance of *imagination* and *imaginative thinking* and cited the George Bernard Shaw quip 'Do *not* do unto others what you would have done to you: their tastes might be different.' In order to achieve what Pence described as self-transposal, to feel compassionately someone else's pain and suffering, requires not just a moral interest in social justice, but a virtue achieved through 'an intimacy . . . built on related moral

qualities between listener and sufferer of trust, honesty, and the time and willingness to listen' (Pence 1983, p. 189). Beauchamp and Childress (2001) expand on the importance of compassion in their description of the non-normative virtues that underpin healthcare practice: compassion, discernment, trustworthiness, integrity, and conscientiousness. Using creative arts in health education provides an opportunity for students to engage with narrative and hermeneutic analysis that helps them to understand patients' lived experiences of their illnesses and receiving care, and to explore their own virtues and values so that a professional intimacy can be achieved while also developing their imaginations and imaginative thinking.

This chapter will explore a further six Cs—culture and care, complex intervention, collaboration, composer in residence, choir, and creativity—at the Florence Nightingale School of Nursing and Midwifery, King's College London. The model of a complex intervention will explore how a multifaceted approach helped embed culture and care in both individual modules of learning and as a philosophy throughout the school. Collaboration was key to the success of the project and generated novel ideas and further projects. The reflections of John Browne, composer in residence in the school, on the creative processes and outcomes from his residency, and participants' evaluations of The Nightingale Choir and the nursing and humanities module will be used to demonstrate how students link their experiences to care, compassion, competence, communication, courage, and commitment.

## Culture and Care

Culture and Care is a programme of activities placing creativity at the heart of the educational experience, releasing talent and energy from staff and students. Health professions in the United Kingdom are highly regulated and the curriculum notoriously congested. Culture and Care explores ways in which we can create a sense of space to enable staff to move from the 'crowded' to the 'creative' curriculum. This involves opening up an imaginative space in which staff and students can explore their emotional responses to care and the role that creativity might play in their practice, drawing on a diverse range of arts based performance and experiential tools.

The programme aims to:

◆ enable staff and students to explore their practice from a cultural perspective and enhance their communication skills and

◆ celebrate and reflect diverse identities and varied experiences, strengthening a sense of community.

Nursing and midwifery require many different skills and capabilities: the sensory, social, and emotional as well as the intellectual. All need to work in harmony, playing like finely tuned instruments. A growing body of scientific evidence demonstrates that arts and culture programmes can play a central role in preparing healthcare professionals for the challenges that will face them throughout their working lives. Such programmes can bring specific and measurable benefits to both staff and patients (Lelchuck-Staricoff 2004; Scott et al. 2013).

To celebrate the 150th anniversary of the school we commissioned the renowned portrait photographer Eileen Perrier to set up a studio and take portrait photographs of staff and students to build a sense of community. The portraits were intended as a talking point and reflective resource for staff, students, and friends of the school to visualize the diversity and strength of our community. We also commissioned Laura Potter, a jewellery maker, to fashion a series of ceremonial neck-pieces derived from objects, material culture, and exhibits in the Florence Nightingale Museum. We organized a collaborative workshop with the Imperial War Museum 'Screening the Nurse', unearthing early nursing films in the museum's collection which had never been screened before. Drawing upon the musical talents of the school we convened a choir and wrote a proposal to the Performing Arts Society and Arts Council England to secure funding to engage a composer in residence.

The Culture and Care programme also included the Handle with Care event funded by and staged at the Wellcome Collection—this was an all-building spectacular designed to demonstrate the use of all the senses in the scientific practice of nursing. We offered tastings of Crimean cooking in full regalia and costume; historical nursing films including biopics and silent films accompanied by pianist Stephen Horn; evening talks on the representation of nurses were given at the National Portrait Gallery by Professor Ludmilla Jordanova; a symposium Navigating Nightingale

examined the life of Florence Nightingale from celebrity to statistician, epidemiologist, public health reformer, and theological and religious beliefs; exploring Nightingale's links with literary London; an edited book, *Notes on Nightingale* (Nelson and Rafferty 2010); and the launch of a interactive walking tour app also called Navigating Nightingale.

## Complex interventions

The introduction of arts interventions into organizations with therapeutic intent is akin to a complex intervention. Complex interventions in health care, whether therapeutic or preventative, contain a number of separate interacting elements which seem essential to the proper functioning of the intervention, although the 'active ingredient' of the intervention that is effective is difficult to specify (MRC 2008). Complexity may have several different levels: target population, intervention, behaviours, and outcomes. If we were to consider a randomized controlled trial of a drug versus a placebo as being at the simplest end of the spectrum, then we might see a comparison of a stroke unit with traditional care as being at the most complex end of the spectrum. The greater the difficulty in defining the active ingredients of an intervention and how they relate to each other, the greater the likelihood that it is a complex intervention.

There are key phases in the evaluative framework developed for a complex intervention. These are laid out in the most recent Medical Research Council (MRC) guidance from development through feasibility testing and piloting to implementation and evaluation (MRC 2008). Even if we can specify precisely what such an arts intervention might be, for example to introduce singing into the care of patients with dementia as a means of stimulating musical memory, it may be that carers are also interacting with patients in a deeper and more intense way: supporting their relatives and teaching them to sing and communicate with each other; stimulating physical movement and using the song as a trigger for reminiscence; and building a sense of shared experience and community. Each of these elements may be an important contribution to the effectiveness of a singing intervention. If we now hypothetically consider evaluating a singing intervention, the song is but one potentially complex contribution to a larger and more complex combination of diverse inputs. Interventions can be delivered at different levels: individual through to professional, organizational, and population. The Culture and Care programme functioned as a series of feasibility, testing, and pilot activities implementing a range of creative arts which can be evaluated in terms of the outcomes, participant evaluation, and collaborations created as a result.

## Collaboration

King's College is situated in the heart of London and on the doorstep of many national and international arts organizations. Without question the collaborations both within the college and with external agencies contributed to the success and momentum of the integration of creative arts in the pre-registration programmes. Many arts organizations have educational leads who were keen to engage new audiences and visitors. 'Internal' collaborators included existing partnerships with National Health Service (NHS) Trusts and independent placement providers within King's

Health Partners, an academic health sciences centre. Two brief case study examples illustrate the synergy that emerged from these collaborations.

With seed-funding from London Centre for Arts and Cultural Exchange (LCACE) a project led by the Guildhall School of Music and Drama explored the interprofessional learning of musicians, actors, music therapists, nurses, and doctors through 3 days of 'live-labs' improvising in mixed genres and media around the themes of engagement, listening, and touch. Three strong themes emerged: a sense of individual learning and relating this to the participants' own practice; learning specifically about communication; and a theme of seeing this work as the start of an exciting process and trying to answer the question—where next? (Gaunt et al. 2009).

'Where next?' was answered in a 2-day workshop with Elinor Tolfree who helped devise a performance of her hemiplegic migraine using improvisation with actors, musicians, nurses, and a dancer for a performance at a public engagement event at the Wellcome Trust. *Elinor's Migraine* was performed to a capacity audience as part of the Handle with Care public engagement event in September 2010. Elinor reflected ' . . . never before have I felt so listened too . . . the musicians and actors found it easier to hear and acknowledge my story without trying to modify, quantify, or make it better. There was something about the urgency to act amongst the health professionals that it, at times, felt like they had come to their conclusions without hearing the end of my story.'

## Composer in residence

John Browne was appointed as composer in residence in the school for 2 years in a project jointly funded by the Performing Rights Society for Music Foundation and Arts Council England. John has offered the following reflections on his experience of the residency:

'The standout feature for me was the rich thematic context: caregiving; suffering; death; birth; human connection; joy; pain; and love. What a gift for a composer!'

'The practical context, however, was trickier: a university with five campuses; the NHS; students working in various hospitals; a many-tentacled beast. There were other obstacles too like the oppressive architecture of the school, bureaucracy, institutional drag, engaging an exhausted, overloaded staff. But against all this I had solid support and encouragement and pretty much *carte blanche* to conceive ideas that would bring music and care together.'

'So, what to do? How could I create music that involved and engaged this community, that would be meaningful, suitably ambitious, affecting, rigorous in quality, and authentically enhance the training and practice of the students and staff?'

'I set about absorbing the values, issues, and perspectives of the school, its curriculum, and people. I found myself leading music exercises and teaching songs to the students at their induction day event. This gave me a very good idea of the community within which I had been placed—and it was very heartening. I discovered smart, empathetic young people with a willingness to be involved. I visited wards in the partner hospitals, attended nursing skills training, got involved in the Nightingale Choir and began to tease out ideas for the residency. The big and very obvious realization dawned on me: this was not an arts institution and so I needed to adapt.'

'I decided to focus in on music's capacity to help us process difficult emotions and experiences and to facilitate the forming of or deepening human connections.'

'I conceived a menu of ideas and tested their potential in terms of resources, spaces, and budgets and mounted a series of discrete events and projects that could all be components of a larger event: a community cantata at the Southbank Centre which I titled *A Nightingale Sang*.'

'Across the 2 years leading up to this event I ran creative music workshops for staff and students, composed choral works for Westminster Abbey Choir commemorating Florence Nightingale, for St Thomas' Hospital choir and the Nightingale Choir for BBC Radio 4 Sunday Worship, and another for the King's College Chapel Choir. I worked with students on a Songbook—a collection of songs to be used as a tool in children's nursing. I curated a Salon—an evening of music, poetry, art-making, and film and presented the first set of Hospital Ragas—instrumental pieces to be played at specific times of the day, week, or year in partner hospitals to affect mood.'

'*A Nightingale Sang* brought all this (and all the above choirs) together with a choir of mental health service users and staff from the Maudsley Hospital, King's College London Symphony Orchestra, and a nurse's gamelan group. At the core were a number of soloists who came from a key project of my residency entitled Songs of the Afflicted. I had wanted to create a piece that focused on mental health so I interviewed a number of mental health patients, staff, and students. They were encouraged to share their experience of mental health. Together we formed these into lyrics and musicalized them, the idea being to have very simple sung phrases accompanied by more complex, rich orchestral colours and textures with the accompaniment functioning as a sort of warm, empathetic blanket wrapped around the soloist.'

'I was of course concerned with the idea of excellence in the performance. With my soloists I didn't get the kind of excellence I got with the Rolls Royce choir of Westminster Abbey. Instead I got the excellence of authenticity, of communication, and of relevance.'

'In the end the most interesting point of connection that arose for me between music and health was the spiritual. That is spiritual in the broadest non-faith-aligned sense that created empathy as the central theme of *A Nightingale Sang*. The work functioned on many levels: as a reflection on the dynamics of care, an opportunity for human connection, a means of processing the complex emotions around the nature of suffering (mentally and physically), advocacy for the de-stigmatization of mental health, and to be a forum for a larger meditation on one of the key issues of the day for nursing—empathy.'

Browne (2010)

## Choir

With initial support from the King's Annual Fund, The Nightingale Choir was founded in 2007 in partnership with Mary King and Laka D of VoiceLab at Southbank Centre. The aim was to find a forum for students and staff to be creative together, have fun singing, and, importantly, sing at the launch of the Culture and Care programme. What was a fixed-term project quickly grew, and the choir, consisting of approximately 45 staff and students, meets weekly and sings at a variety of events. These have included being part of *A Nightingale Sang* by John Browne at the Queen Elizabeth Hall (Figs 37.1 and 37.2); being broadcast on BBC Radio 4; sharing the bill with the cast of *Mama Mia* for a Christmas celebration at the Evelina London Children's Hospital; and singing with the Mind and Soul Choir, King's College Jazz Band, and the Gospel Choir at Guy's Hospital.

One of the key dates in the choir's calendar is singing to welcome the new students on their first day—before any enrolment

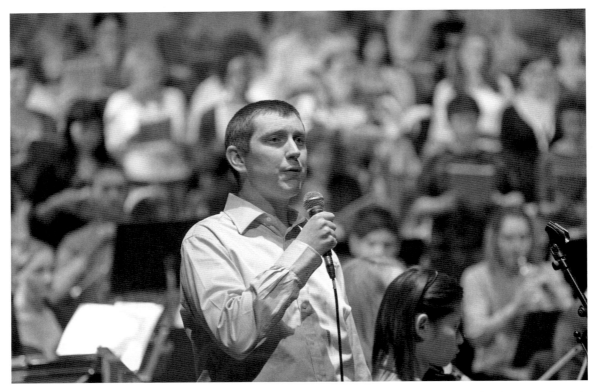

**Fig. 37.1** BSc mental health nursing student, Thomas Alexander, in *A Nightingale Sang* at the Queen Elizabeth Hall. His text, set by John Browne, focused on his experience working in an acute admissions ward.

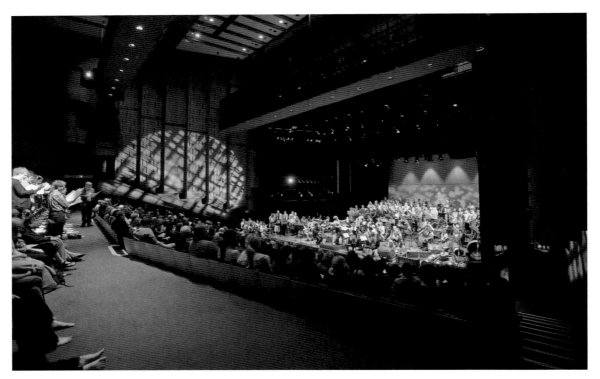

**Fig. 37.2** The Nightingale Choir on stage and King's College London Chapel Choir singing from the audience in *A Nightingale Sang* by John Browne.

**Table 37.1** Choir participant feedback illustrating the six generative mechanisms of psychological wellbeing

| Generative mechanism | Participant feedback |
| --- | --- |
| Positive affect | 'I took part in the workshops and thoroughly enjoyed it. I was a bit apprehensive at first but the coaches were so laid back and funny and that undoubtedly contributed to the relaxed atmosphere . . . It was excellent; up-beat and really fun to perform.' Student |
| Focused attention and cognitive stimulation | 'I found singing in the choir uplifting and energizing especially after a hard day at work. The sound we made was amazing (as was the response from our audience) and I taught with more energy and focus that day—I wish every day started with a song.' Academic staff |
| Focused attention and deep breathing | 'I had an amazing experience in the choir—first of all that it worked. At a time when work feels really pressured to take something else on seemed fool-hardy and yet after every rehearsal I felt exhausted and exhilarated all in one. At the end of a rehearsal I couldn't remember the stresses of strains of the day and even slept better. With each breath when we warm up it is as if I am letting go of something I have been holding all day. There seems to be something so liberating about singing.' Administrative staff |
| Social support | 'It was a great experience working with other members of the school staff and students in this collaborative venture. I really enjoyed meeting students in this forum and valued the expertise that they had in this area. It established relationships with students from a different perspective to the classroom and certainly developed a common ethos amongst those of us who took part and this seemed to me to be a desire to share our delight in having the opportunity to sing together and to sing for the school.' Academic staff |
| Regular commitment | I really looked forward to the workshops each week. It wasn't just a commitment to the choir but a reason to stop other tasks which can seem endless. The revision will still be there after the rehearsal!' Student |

begins, a lecture theatre of some 400 new and nervous first years are greeted by staff and students singing their hearts out. Members of the choir and audience were invited to submit free text feedback about this experience and a survey of their responses clearly captures the impact that singing, being sung to, and singing with, have for this group of students.

Although the function and experience of choir members is well documented (Clift et al. 2007; Clift and Hancox 2010), little research has investigated the impact on the audience. In terms of audience impact the core themes identified in the feedback included being made to feel welcome, feeling warm, and that the singing broke the ice or demystified the institution they

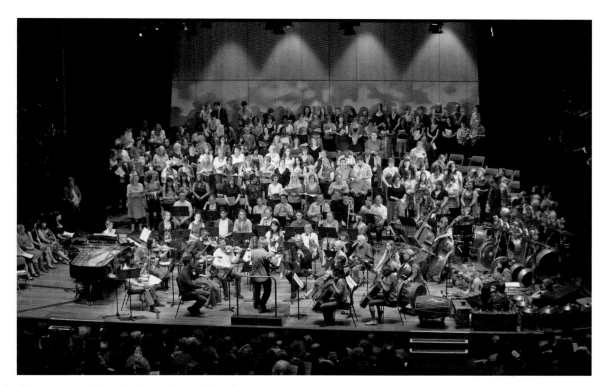

**Fig. 37.3** The full community choir and orchestra for *A Nightingale Sang*.
Reproduced by kind permission of King's College London. Copyright © 2012 King's College London, UK.

**Table 37.2** Student evaluation of the nursing and humanities module demonstrating learning related to the values expressed in the six Cs of *Compassion in Practice*

| Component | Student evaluations |
|---|---|
| Care | 'I think this module has helped me look at the care given to patients and will help me think of different methods of care to give to patients when in practice.'<br><br>'I'm more aware of the impact of noise; talking and laughing on the ward—this has increased my self-awareness.' |
| Compassion | 'I have been reminded of the value of thinking beyond my own point of view; I believe this will make me a more empathic practitioner.' |
| Competence | 'I have learned about analysing portraiture and it has helped me think in much more detail about what I observe in patients in my care.' |
| Communication | 'How to analyse, interpret, and explore—not just art, music, and literature, but experience. Ultimately, this module has helped me to understand the experiences of the people I work with, and to think, if I don't understand it at first, how else can I try?' |
| Courage | 'I have learnt that as an individual there is more I must question in practice: the how, the why, etc. as it is important to acknowledge how history has shaped our practice today.' |
| Commitment | 'Using art, music, and literature opens a whole new and creative way of interacting with patients and getting to know who they are and who I am.' |

were joining by representing the staff and students as 'human'. Students also reported feeling less nervous; feeling part of something; wanting to be part of the choir and that it was a beautiful experience:

'The choir was absolutely fabulous—delightful and a clever way to set the tone, break the ice, and have fun.'

'Feeling quite nervous I found the choir fantastic. They lifted the mood and made us feel relaxed. Brilliant!'

'I thought the introduction [first ever meeting] of our tutors singing was a lovely way to meet. It showed they were human too and all 'sang from the same hymn sheet.''

'Just to say that the choir was the first encounter I had with King's College London in any form other than the interview. I was sitting first thing in the morning, first day ever, on my own, the choir made me feel that this place . . . is very 'human' and not to be overwhelmed by the whole thing. It was the nicest way to welcome anyone that I can think of.'

Clift et al. (2007) identified six generative mechanisms that explained the impact on psychological wellbeing for choir participants: positive affect, focused attention, deep breathing, social support, cognitive stimulation, and regular commitment. Table 37.1 shows examples of participant feedback that replicate the findings in Clift et al. (2007).

The issue of commitment also featured in the comments of the audience who wanted to join the choir. Students undertake placements at different times of the year and often some distance from the main college campus. People expressed anxiety about joining but not being able to commit to all of the rehearsals, particularly when working shifts. For this reason an 'open' community choir model was adopted (Fig. 37.3), accepting and acknowledging that not all participants would be able to come to all rehearsals. This was supported by having music, text, and audio files of individual lines and all parts on a shared server site so people could practice and access the musical director's arrangements between rehearsals.

## Creativity

It is difficult to measure outcomes from the use of creative arts in health education, and as the aim is to broaden learners' vision and experience and enhance their values, the measurable outcomes may not be seen for years to come. However, it is possible for participants to evaluate their experience. These evaluations come from a module in nursing and humanities.

The module comprises a series of seminars and visits/events/workshops linking theory and practice explicitly through experiential learning theory, metaphor, hermeneutics, and narrative in order to enhance students' knowledge and understanding of the lived experience of illness and care and the socio-historical context of nursing.

Using a nominal group technique, participants were invited to evaluate the module. Table 37.2 shows how their experience and learning impacted on each of the six Cs of *Compassion in Practice* (DH 2012). This was revealed through an analysis of their free-text statements.

Overall, students seemed to be able to apply the learning to their practice at a more conceptual level than is typical in module evaluations:

'This module has helped me step away from the constraints of a scientific method/evidence-base, and spend time trying to understand illness and nursing as a lived experience. It has expanded my analytical skills and given me new frameworks with which to examine my own experiences, the experience of others, and evidence from nursing literature.'

'I have thoroughly enjoyed this module as it made me think of the service users' experience of mental health care, nursing role and my professional development in the widest context of the nursing theory, evidence, history and how thinking about, reflective activities and utilising various sources available to us such as music, arts and film can be of great utility not only towards trying to understand the sufferers' experience of mental illness and treatment but also in effectively engaging the service users.'

One fear of both lecturing colleagues and NHS Trust partners was that a creative arts-based module would be seen as a soft option or irrelevant to nursing practice. It is hoped that this chapter has demonstrated some of the ways in which a broad approach to using creative arts as an organization-wide strategy as well as within individual projects can prove, as one student put it, 'Nursing and humanities is a rigorous academic discipline not just 'fluffiness and interpretive dance'.'

## References

Beauchamp, T.L. and Childress, J.F. (2001) *Principles of Biomedical Ethics*, 5th edn. Oxford: Oxford University Press.

Browne, J. (2015). Composer in residence [website] <http://brownejohn.wordpress.com/>

Clift, S. and Hancox, G. (2010). The significance of choral singing for sustaining psychological wellbeing: findings from a survey of choristers in England, Australia and Germany *Music Performance Research*, **3**, 79–96.

Clift, S., Hancox, G., Morrison, I., Hess, B., Kreutz, G., and Stewart, D. (2007). Choral singing and psychological wellbeing: findings from English choirs in a cross-national survey using the WHOQOL-BREF. *International Symposium on Performance Science*, pp. 201–207. Available at: <http://www98.griffith.edu.au/dspace/bitstream/handle/10072/17825/48495_1?sequence=1>

DH (Department of Health) (2012). *Compassion in Practice: Nursing, Midwifery and Care Staff. Our Vision Our Strategy.* London: Department of Health. Available at: <http://www.england.nhs.uk/wp-content/uploads/2012/12/compassion-in-practice.pdf>

Gaunt, H., Noonan., I., and Ford, B. (2009). *Improvisation in Music, Drama and Nursing: An Exploratory Study of Inter-professional Learning.* London: Guildhall School of Music and Drama.

Lelchuck-Staricoff, R. (2004). *Arts in Health: A Review of the Medical Literature*. Research Report 36. London: Arts Council England. Available at: <http://www.artsandhealth.ie/wp-content/uploads/2011/08/ahreview-of-medical-literature1.pdf>

MRC (2008). *Developing and Evaluating Complex Interventions: New Guidance*. London: Medical Research Council. Available at: <http://www.mrc.ac.uk/documents/pdf/complex-interventions-guidance/>

Nelson, S. and Rafferty, A. (eds) (2010). *Notes On Nightingale: The Influence and Legacy of a Nursing Icon*. Ithaca, NY: Cornell University Press.

Pence, G.E. (1983). Can compassion be taught? *Journal of Medical Ethics*, **9**, 189–191.

Scott, S.D., Brett-MacLean, P., Archibald, M., and Hartling, L. (2013). Protocol for a systematic review of the use of narrative storytelling and visual-arts-based approaches as knowledge transition tools in healthcare. *Systematic Reviews Journal*, **2**, 19.

# CHAPTER 38

# Case study: singing in hospitals—bridging therapy and everyday life

Gunter Kreutz, Stephen Clift, and Wolfgang Bossinger

## History of singing in hospitals

Following a career as a music therapist with over 25 years of experience in the field of singing and mental health, the third author of the present chapter felt a need to explore the potential of an open singing group in the context of a psychiatric hospital. The key idea was to address potential singers inside and outside the hospital walls and reach out into the neighbouring communities to promote therapeutic singing. This inclination was particularly fuelled by Betty Bailey's and Jane Davidson's seminal studies (Bailey and Davidson 2005). These researchers observed significant improvement in quality of life in individual members of a choir consisting of homeless men in an urban environment in Canada. In response to their findings, an informal exploratory study was initiated in 2006 at the Christophsbad Göppingen psychiatric hospital in southern Germany. The main idea was that singing for everyone might provide an aid to develop social networks to overcome the isolation and stigma often experienced by people with mental health problems. The open singing group started with just four to six individuals who met once a month. The group expanded significantly after singing was offered weekly instead of monthly due to the higher motivation of the group members. In 2009, 60 to 90 people followed the invitation to join the open singing group every week. It comprised patients from the hospital, former patients, members of staff, visitors and friends of the patients, and people from the city and the neighbouring community. It turns out that this mix of people is typical for most of the singing groups associated with the network today. From its inauguration, the singing group received support from the hospital management through both its music therapy and cultural programme budgets. To date, it is free of charge to patients, former patients, staff, and visitors.

From early on, many singers reported strong and consistent positive effects of singing on their individual health and wellbeing. They found it so helpful that they suggested similar groups should be founded in every hospital. Two of the patients, in particular, a medical doctor and a business manager who were both suffering from clinical depression, suggested launching an association specifically devoted to singing in health institutions in order to underscore and disseminate its therapeutic value. Hence, the Singing Hospitals Association was founded by the third author in collaboration with former patients and colleagues in 2009, before it was acknowledged officially as a not-for-profit association a year later in 2010.

## Mission and dissemination

Singing Hospitals today is an international network to promote singing in health facilities under the patronage of Gerlinde Kretschmann, the wife of the Prime Minister of Baden–Württemberg. During the years before its official inauguration in 2010, singing groups had already become widespread throughout numerous health facilities. Up to date information can be retrieved from the official Singing Hospitals website <http://www.singende-krankenhaeuser.de> (in German).

The network's mission is to promote singing groups and individual singing across the health sector. Singing is believed to strengthen self-healing through the mobilization of individual resources that are still available to patients despite the presence of mental and physical illness (e.g. Clift 2012). These resources entail psychological processes such as positive emotions, optimism, as well as a belief in the possibility of recovery. More recent research on singing and mental health has confirmed the clinical benefits of regular group singing for people with a history of severe and enduring mental health challenges (Clift and Morrison 2011). Research on clinical effects using placebos underscores the psychological dimension in a wide range of medical treatments (Humphries 2004). Importantly, the network's mission also includes the dissemination of guidelines and ethical principles promoting a humanistic and holistic understanding of health and wellbeing in line with the well-known WHO definition of health. They ensure, as far as possible, the protection of dignity, self-image, and self-esteem and accommodation of the cultural and aesthetic needs for all individuals involved.

Singing leaders operate in diverse clinical settings including with hospitalized patients in psychiatry, in rehabilitation clinics and general hospitals, but also in medical centres and even in a funeral parlour. Singing groups associated with the network have been established in various states across Germany and in a number of countries outside Germany. The network comprises a range of activities at societal, political, and academic levels. Increasing memberships and continued inauguration of new singing groups reflect a growing general appreciation of cultural values in the context of recovery from ill-health as well as disease prevention and health promotion. Over 45 certified singing leaders are now active in hospital settings throughout Germany as well as in Austria and Switzerland.

Since May 2011 Singing Hospitals has organized annual meetings to disseminate practical experiences, research, and other developments in the field. The conferences also serve as platforms for informed discussions among practitioners, higher-level administrators, and researchers in the field. A list of previous and future meetings is posted on the network's website.

## Why singing in hospitals?

Singing in healthcare is based on the view that appropriate adjuvant therapies, in general, and therapeutic singing, in particular, are needed to enhance individual healing processes. Specifically, singing is thought to activate health resources in terms of psychological and physical wellbeing as well as increasing the quality of life for both patient and non-patient groups, providing opportunities for goal-oriented social interaction.

Locating singing groups within and outside hospital wards is advantageous for several reasons. First of all, it provides opportunity for singing across the entire population within and in the neighbourhood of health facilities. Secondly, there are usually no prerequisites for participation with respect to individual singing experience, age, sex, health status, or any differential variable. Thirdly, because singing activities occur on a regular basis and include people who are not patients, they provide opportunity for building social relationships and friendships. In sum these advantages may provide significant aid to bridge therapy and every-day life for individuals with poor health in the process of convalescence.

Singing group members, whether they are current patients, former patients, or non-patients, may benefit in a number of ways that resemble clinical outcomes (Kreutz et al. 2014). Ideally, singing activities may directly strengthen both individual and social resources to promote wellbeing and health, but they may also support non-verbal communication and pro-social behaviours within and between the various groups that work and live together in medical contexts.

## International collaboration and musical ambassadors

One of the goals of Singing Hospitals is to identify and recruit high-profile individuals around the world who are willing to collaborate and function as ambassadors for the network. Their main task, if agreed, is to represent Singing Hospitals and promote the idea of group singing in health settings. The current board of international ambassadors can be retrieved from the website which is continuously updated to include new members as well as exclude individuals who have left the board for various reasons. Some individuals have been specifically recruited as musical ambassadors, some of whom are well-known celebrities. In addition to representing Singing Hospitals they also contribute to extending the musical repertoire for specific target groups. Musical ambassadors currently include, for example the songwriters/performers

Reinhard Horn, Roland Kaiser, and Konstantin Wecker, and the classical musicians Samuel Youn, Cornelius Hauptmann, and Franz Josef Selig.

The international expansion of the Singing Hospitals network involves the foundation of singing groups in both German-speaking and non-German-speaking countries across Europe. Moreover, centres for training singing leaders for retirement homes and seniors have been established in Switzerland, while further expansion of training into Austria is under way.

## Quality control

Measures of quality control resemble those that are in use in other types of psychotherapeutic and psychophysiological interventions. They entail two main components, namely training and research. Both components are subject to continued development and mutual refinement. In particular, singing leaders graduating from the Singing Hospital Association's training programmes must comply with its ethical guidelines and principles. For example, they are trained to explore, respect, and accept the systems of beliefs and the convictions of their clients and refrain from superimposing their own beliefs and conceptions.

One milestone for the establishment of singing groups was the development of nationwide certified training programmes, such as the 'Singing leader in healthcare institutions and hospitals' comprising five 2-day modules as well as the more recent workshop 'Singing leader in retirement homes and for seniors' comprising four 2-day modules (inaugurated in February 2012).

As regards research, once evidence-based practice is established it will continuously provide feedback to improve training programmes and eventually refine underlying principles and guidelines. Singing leaders are also encouraged to continuously extend their training with respect to current issues, for example in consciousness research, transpersonal psychology, or religious studies.

## Certification of hospitals, health facilities, and retirement homes

On the basis of continued provision of singing by qualified singing leaders, health institutions may apply for a certification as 'Singing Hospital/Singing Health Institution' or 'Singing For Elderly People' at respective venues. It is assumed that certified Singing Hospitals and Singing Retirement Homes benefit from certification beyond the provision of singing itself. For example, singing may also mark a particularly positive and pro-social working environment, a friendly atmosphere, an appreciation of art and culture, as well as a holistic approach towards individuals' needs at physical, psychological, and spiritual levels of medical treatment and therapy.

Institutions complying with the certification guidelines are granted certification as 'Singing Hospital', a 'Singing Retirement Home', or a 'Singing Health Facility' and this enhances the public image of the given institution. For example, member institutions can print and use the logo of the Singing Hospitals Association for advertising purposes and benefit from their extensive media attention. They may also participate in research projects, and will receive a 10% discount on all charges for seminars and conferences for all their employees. In return, the

Singing Hospitals Association benefits from the certification of each institution, because each means a significant extension of the network and a multiplication of opportunities to promote its goals and ideals.

## Research

The second component serving quality control is scientific research, which is conducted under the leadership of members from the Singing Hospitals Association's scientific board. To investigate the effects and mechanisms involved in singing groups, practice-based approaches are of primarily used in the search for appropriate research strategies. The accumulation and dissemination of research is thus in the interest of a better understanding of the ways in which group singing may or may not meet the visionary goals of the movement. Moreover, research is also needed to identify good practices and to provide feedback to singing leaders as well as to patients in order to develop more objective ways of determining potential outcomes of singing interventions (Fig. 38.1).

## Research project: singing leaders

### Singing leaders

Singing leaders are key to the success of group singing, as are choir masters in amateur and professional choral societies. However, there are important differences between the role of singing leaders and choir masters. For example, for singing leaders there is a greater demand to acknowledge the physical and mental

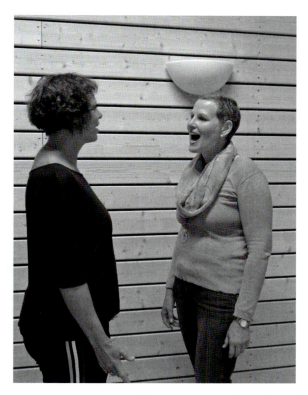

**Fig. 38.1** Resonance. Two patients of the singing group in the Paracelsus-Klinik Scheidegg, Germany.
Reproduced by kind permission of Elke Wünnenberg. Copyright © 2015 Elke Wünnenberg.

conditions of patient singers as well as their heterogeneous musical backgrounds. Therefore, numerous questions arise concerning the personal musical and professional backgrounds of singing leaders, their strategies for accommodating the diverse challenges of leading groups consisting of patients and non-patients, as well as their experiences in terms of perceived risks and benefits associated with group singing. To address these questions an interview study was conducted (Kreutz et al. 2014) involving 20 singing leaders (14 female; age range 19 to 58 years). Nine were trained music therapists, whereas a further nine had different therapeutic or medical backgrounds. Only two of the leaders, one male and one female, had no such background at all. Thirteen of those worked in psychiatric hospitals, while the remaining singing leaders had worked in diverse institutions including a general hospital, rehabilitation centres, general medical centres and a funeral home. Accordingly, their work addressed a wide range of patient and non-patient populations across these diverse settings.

Each singing leader was a trained musician. Experience of vocal training and voice coaching, including choral conducting, was of course widespread in this group. However, there was variation in the level of musical proficiency. In sum the therapeutic and musical backgrounds suggest the leaders were highly qualified in both domains. In addition, each singing leader graduated from one of the Singing Hospitals training centres.

### Singing groups

The singing groups were founded between 2003 and 2011. The size of each group varied from at least four to more than 70 participants. Most groups comprise 20 to 30 singers. Due to high fluctuation within the groups it is difficult to estimate the total number of individuals reached by those 20 singing leaders.

### Interviews

Singing leaders were initially briefed with an outline of the themes and questions to be asked during interviews and provided informed consent before the interviews were conducted. Transcriptions of the interviews were sent by email to each participant for corrections. Questions entailed general demographic information including education, with some emphasis on therapeutic and musical skills. The central questions first concerned their perceived role as singing leaders, their strategic approach and the design of group singing sessions, and the rationale for and nature of the vocal exercises and repertoire that were being sung. In the second part of the interview, the singing leaders were asked to reflect on their own experiences with the singers, the perceived risks and benefits, and, finally, the role of the Singing Hospitals network in the context of their work. The interviews were between approximately 20 and 45 minutes long.

### Content analysis

Following confirmation of the content of the interviews, the singing leaders' responses were transferred into a format which was readable by the software package MAXQDA®. This programme offers a number of tools for coding and analysing verbal data. The procedures for identifying themes and topics in these data followed the principles outlined by Mayring (1985, p. 191, Fig. 1). Importantly, content analysis requires several readings of the material and discussion of items in the event of conflicting interpretations. Two trained musicologists at the Carl von Ossietzky

University of Oldenburg were enrolled to read and discuss the materials in association with the second author.

## Results and discussion

The interviews provided an extremely rich set of responses. The scope of the data precludes a differentiated discussion within this chapter. The following examples thus highlight some of the themes and issues from the point of view of the singing leaders. As they are necessarily taken out of the context, some care was taken to include responses for which some convergence between at least a subgroup of interviewees emerged.

### Roles, concepts, and strategies

For many singing leaders their perceived role is intimately connected with the communication strategies they adopted in the group. One of these strategies is to provide motivation for inexperienced singers in order to overcome reservations:

> 'People who are assigned to the singing group are not necessarily keen to participate. The idea is, that it may be beneficial to try out something new and accept a degree of potential inconvenience at times . . . There are individuals who do not want to join in singing and just follow the physical movements. It rarely happens though, that people leave the room during a session'
>
> Anne (b. 1956, psychiatric hospital)

> 'Many patients, who assert that they cannot sing, realize how quickly they can change their mind. I am particularly impressed, when men, who claim not to be able to sing at all, all of a sudden start singing wholeheartedly.'
>
> Simon (b. 1958, psychiatric hospital)

> 'It is important to me to send the message to the participants, that singing is fun and that singing is an expression of joy of life and life itself. . . . It is good, when the sound is edgy . . . just as life can be rough, there can be roughness in music that may become resolved.'
>
> Petra (b. 1963, psychiatric hospital)

Taken together, the responses concerning roles and basic approaches suggest that singing leaders are well aware of the need to establish a confidential as well as a both cheerful and a respectful general setting before any musical goals may be addressed. Therefore, adjustment to individual needs and competences are essential rather than expecting adherence to preconceived programmes of singing activities.

With respect to the ways in which singing sessions are conducted, a temporal frame marking opening, middle, and closing phases was found important. Opening with welcoming rituals, for example, provides the opportunity to welcome new or returning members as well as help each individual to adjust to the group situation, which may in itself pose a challenge to some psychiatric patients. It is also common, particularly in smaller groups, to welcome group members personally by including their names in songs to facilitate bonding and to establish trust and confidence:

> 'During the initial phase . . . the focus is directed to the outside and inside. It is about feeling oneself within the present situation. This kind of self-exploration continues throughout the session.'
>
> Sandra (b. 1975, oncological rehabilitation centre)

Relaxation plays a major role during the initial phase. There is emphasis on physical arrival, breathing, and—sometimes—imaginative exercises, while lying comfortably on the floor. Singing leaders also mentioned that the voices of some patient group members may be harmed as a result of the medical treatments they are undergoing.

Subsequent phases often follow the dynamics that evolve from the initial phase. Therefore, the singing leaders adopt flexible strategies of planned components as well as seeking feedback from the group about the choice of repertoire and/or exercises to be performed. It is of note that therapeutic goals are rarely stated. Instead emphasis is given on enjoyment, fun, and positive feelings. Although the voice and various kinds of vocal repertoires are at the focus of the activity, a sense of humour and physical contact are frequently mentioned components of typical sessions:

> 'Laughing is quite essential because it takes out the sting from severe depression. Songs involving physical contact may also have a strongly relaxing effect.'
>
> Peter (b. 1960, psychiatric hospital)

### Benefits and risks

From the perspective of the singing leaders, the positive effects of singing by far outweigh more negative issues. There is consensus that psychological wellbeing, social contact and appreciation, building of trust and friendship, as well as psychosomatic changes are noted. In addition, there are occasionally reports of reductions of pharmaceutical medication in some participants in response to singing:

> 'Singing together and dancing is found easier than talking by many—there is a deep sense of connectedness and communality. Regular attendants often become friends. Meanwhile, some of them meet before the session in the cafeteria and socialize at other occasions. [ . . . ] Singing often has a strong anti-depressant effect. Many patients and other participants are beaming with happiness and joy.'
>
> Peter (b. 1960, psychiatric hospital)

> 'They [the singers] are more relaxed, happier, forget about pain and problems. People arrive with depressed moods. Their thoughts are caught up with negative episodes and pain. Their thinking is quite negative. . . . Singing may have positive effects, because it encourages people . . . and stimulating the body as a whole.'
>
> Anne (b. 1956, psychiatric hospital)

> 'One can see it in their faces that people are happier, more agile and vivid. It is still always surprising to me, when the depressed start to laugh.'
>
> Simon (b. 1958, psychiatric hospital)

Beyond such immediate effects, the reports also indicate that the positive effects carry on during the day following the singing session, sometimes even for several days until the next meeting. In sum, the singing leaders' observations indicate some clinical and non-clinical value in their work, and some role for the singing group in bridging therapy and every-day life.

However, most interviewees are well aware of the limits as well as of certain risks of their work. Three singing leaders stated that group singing did not entail any general or specific risk at all, while one interviewee did not respond to this question:

> 'Some are unable to tolerate the group situation.'
>
> Nina (b. 1974, psychiatric hospital)

> 'The condition of some individuals does not allow closeness to other people, or rather very little contact at all.'
>
> Lisa (b. 1963, psychiatric hospital)

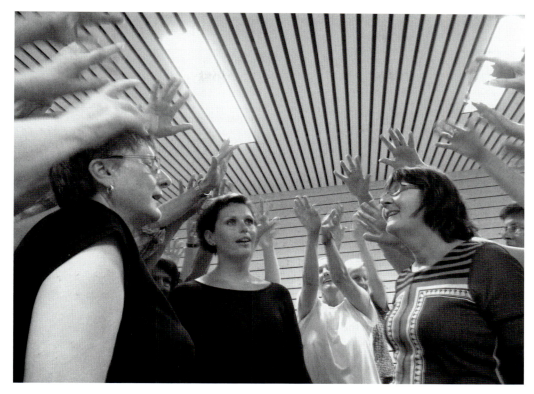

**Fig. 38.2** Protected, sheltered. Singing group in the Paracelsus-Klinik Scheidegg, Germany.
Reproduced by kind permission of Elke Wünnenberg. Copyright © 2015 Elke Wünnenberg.

Some singing leaders observe that at times it can be difficult to accommodate strong individual behaviours and emotions such as weeping or depression. They also find it difficult to attribute negative events, such as a sudden psychotic crisis, to the group singing, although some suspect that singing provides a strong stimulation that is not always easy to deal with. Some lyrics and songs can under certain circumstances be perceived as threatening. The discussion of risks seems important, because it highlights the conflict between, in principle, a non-therapeutic intervention on the one hand, and quasi-clinical or therapeutic outcomes on the other. Although psychotic episodes and withdrawals from singing groups are rare, the reports indicate a need for risk management strategies, which are already informally adapted by a number of singing leaders (Fig. 38.2).

## Research project: patients, former patients, and non-patients

This part of the research entailed both quantitative and qualitative responses from members of singing groups in various hospital settings. In addition to singing groups in hospitals, a further cohort of amateur choristers was included for comparison purposes. The general aim of this research was to see whether previously reported levels of perceived psychological benefits of singing were similar in both patient and non-patient groups. It was assumed that there was no systematic influence of previous choral experience on singing-related psychological wellbeing. A second goal was to examine some of the verbatim responses

about the benefits of singing from the point of view of the participating patients.

### Participants

A total of 725 choral singers comprising two large subgroups of Singing Hospitals ($n = 400$) and amateur choristers ($n = 325$) were included in the sample. Table 38.1 presents an overview of the various health institutions from which the former group was recruited. The remaining choristers were the German subsample of a previous cross-national study on amateur singing (Clift et al. 2010).

Closer inspection of the Singing Hospitals group revealed that about half of the sample consisted of current patients, the next largest group consisted of former patients (Table 38.2). The remainder of the sample included small numbers of staff or relatives of patients. However, the majority of the non-patient group did not

**Table 38.1** Distribution of participants across amateur choristers and Singing Hospitals groups ($n = 725$)

| Location | No. of participants |
|---|---|
| Freelance amateur choirs ($n = 7$) | 325 |
| Psychiatric hospitals ($n = 6$) | 219 |
| Oncological rehabilitation ($n = 2$) | 91 |
| General hospitals ($n = 2$) | 60 |
| Medical centres ($n = 2$) | 15 |
| Funeral home ($n = 1$) | 15 |

**Table 38.2** Distribution of participants within the Singing Hospitals cohort (*n* = 325)

| Participant groups | *n* |
|---|---|
| Patients | 205 |
| Former patients | 93 |
| Staff | 8 |
| Relatives | 7 |
| Status not disclosed | 66 |

disclose a direct relation to patients or the hospital. In other words, these individuals either refrained from indicating their status or should be considered as individuals who participated in the singing group for reasons that remain unexplored in the present study.

It is of interest that the gender distribution is strongly female biased among the amateur choristers (female 215, male 110, age range 18 to 81 years). The gender distribution in the Singing Hospitals cohort is even more pronounced in favour of females, whereas the age range is similar with respect to the largest sub-groups, namely patients and former patients (female 238; male 59, age range 19 to 89 years) with mean the age being between 49 and 53 years across the different cohorts.

## Questionnaires

The set of questionnaires administered to each participant asked for information on demographic and musical background. The most relevant inventories with respect to the present analysis were the 12-item questionnaire on singing and wellbeing (Clift et al. 2010) and the World Health Organization quality of life inventory in its shorter version (WHOQOL-BREF; Hawthorne et al. 2006).

## Results

### Singing experience

Naturally, all amateur choristers were experienced singers, most having sung regularly for a number of years (mean 25.9 years) in at least one choral society. By contrast, the majority of members of Singing Hospitals groups had little or no experience in singing (experienced singers *n* = 127; little or no experience in singing *n* = 168). Taken together, the average singing experience in that group was less than 6 months. Moreover, 22% of the Singing Hospitals singers reported having been told at least once in their life that they could not sing.

### Psychological effects

Table 38.3 summarizes the descriptive statistics with respect to self-reported psychological wellbeing related to singing. This analysis included only amateur singers, patients, and former patients. There is an overall high confirmation of positive effects across the various items. It is of note that on some scales former patients rated perceived benefits significantly higher than patients or amateurs. There was no effect of prior choral experience on these variables. Moreover, there was also lack of correlation between the amount of previous choral experience and perceived benefits, even when singers without such experience were excluded. In short, even singers with very little general singing experience reported the singing as highly rewarding.

**Table 38.3** Mean ratings (and standard deviations) of perceived psychological benefits related to group singing

| Item | Group | | |
|---|---|---|---|
| | Patients (*n* = 205) | Former patients (*n* = 93) | Amateur (*n* = 325) |
| Singing makes my mood positive | 4.30 (0.82) | 4.63 (0.57) | 4.31 (0.69) |
| Makes me feel a lot happier afterwards | 4.29 (0.82) | 4.49 (0.73) | 4.05 (0.76) |
| Relaxing and helps deal with stress | 4.24 (0.90) | 4.43 (0.78) | 4.09 (0.82) |
| Doesn't help general emotional wellbeing | 1.93 (1.11) | 1.60 (0.98) | 1.86 (0.91) |
| Promotes a positive attitude to life | 4.12 (0.87) | 4.29 (0.81) | 4.09 (0.78) |
| Helps make me a happier person | 3.91 (0.99) | 4.15 (0.92) | 4.01 (0.80) |
| Doesn't release negative feelings in my life | 2.49 (1.26) | 2.03 (1.21) | 2.38 (0.96) |
| Doesn't give me that 'high' | 2.07 (1.09) | 1.88 (1.17) | 2.05 (0.89) |
| Provides no deep significance compared with other things | 2.52 (1.18 | 1.91 (0.97) | 1.91 (0.97) |
| Improves wellbeing | 3.91 (1.01) | 4.29 (0.82) | 3.86 (0.88) |
| Releases negative feelings | 4.14 (0.87) | 4.34 (0.82) | 4.02 (0.75) |
| Positively affects quality of life | 4.16 (0.87) | 4.45 (0.75) | 4.35 (0.63) |

Values represent level of agreement on a scale from 1 (low agreement) to 5 (high agreement).

Table 38.4 presents the quality of life scores differentiated by the subscales physical health, mental health, social relationships, and environment. Perceived quality of life was significantly higher in amateurs compared with the patients and former patients in all four dimensions. It is of note that patients and former patients still had similar levels of quality of life. In particular, social relationships were not superior in the latter group. This could be a driving factor in the continued interest in singing, and a subject for future research.

**Table 38.4** Mean scores (and standard deviations) of perceived quality of life represented by the four dimensions of the WHOQOL-BREF

| Item | Group | | |
|---|---|---|---|
| | Patients (*n* = 205) | Former patients (*n* = 93) | Amateurs (*n* = 325) |
| Physical health | 13.07 (2.79) | 13.38 (2.99) | 16.88 (2.04) |
| Mental health | 12.60 (2.72) | 13.44 (2.75) | 15.64 (2.05) |
| Social relationships | 13.12 (3.54) | 12.99 (3.13) | 15.19 (2.99) |
| Environment | 14.64 (2.60) | 15.04 (2.29) | 16.58 (1.74) |

Values fall in a range from 4 (minimum) to 20 (maximum); higher values represent higher levels of perceived quality of life.

## Conclusions

To our knowledge, this is the first research project to have documented the views of singing leaders concerning their work with different patient groups in health institutions as well as the perceived effects of singing on psychological wellbeing in patient and non-patient choristers. Perhaps the most important finding is that both patients and non-patients benefit equally from group singing, irrespective of previous singing experience. Moreover, interviews with singing leaders reveal strategies which show similarities to and differences from amateur singing in non-patient choirs. It is of note that singing leaders in hospitals are challenged by both the heterogeneous musical backgrounds and health status of their singers.

It must be kept in mind that although group singing in hospitals is often termed therapeutic, the therapeutic effects may be considered primarily as outcomes rather than specific components of individual health interventions. This means that the focus of singing is clearly on the patients' resources, positive thoughts, and behaviours rather than deficits and specific considerations of medication. In this vein, psychophysiological mobilization, positive engagement in social processes, and psychological self-regulation are recurrent aspects in the singing activity that may be of direct value for health. Some of these effects are even reflected at the level of endocrine functions, including the release of the social binding hormone oxytocin (Grape et al. 2003).

Limitations of singing in hospitals emerge with respect to cases in which individual psychiatric patients have difficulty in coping with the group situation. Although such cases are rare, they suggest that supervision and continued reflection to identify best practices and strategies are crucial to the further development of group singing in health institutions. Reports from singing leaders suggest that the network as such must be considered as a relevant resource for their own work, providing a platform for further education and the exchange of concepts, ideas, and experiences. The professional and administrative network comprising the Singing Hospitals initiative also provides a means for gaining professional acknowledgment, which appears appropriate in light of the highly positive responses from patients, former patients, and other individuals who love to sing in groups.

## References

Bailey, B.A. and Davidson, J.W. (2005). Effects of group singing and performance for marginalized and middle-class singers. *Psychology of Music*, **33**, 269–303.

Clift. S. (2012). Singing, wellbeing and health. In: R. MacDonald, G. Kreutz, and L. Mitchell (eds), *Music, Health, and Wellbeing*, pp. 113–124. Oxford: Oxford University Press.

Clift, S. and Morrison, I. (2011). Group singing fosters mental health and wellbeing: findings from the east Kent 'Singing for Health' network project. *Mental Health and Social Inclusion*, **15**, 88–97.

Clift, S., Hancox, G., Morrison, I., Hess, B., Kreutz, G., and Stewart, D. (2010). Choral singing and psychological wellbeing: quantitative and qualitative findings from English choirs in a cross-national survey. *Journal of Applied Arts and Health*, **1**, 19–34.

Grape, C., Sandgren, M., Hansson, L.O., Ericson, M., and Theorell, T. (2003). Does singing promote wellbeing?: an empirical study of professional and amateur singers during a singing lesson. *Integrative Physiological and Behavioral Science*, **38**, 65–74.

Hawthorne, G., Herrman, H., and Murphy, B. (2006). Interpreting the WHOQOL-Bref: preliminary population norms and effect sizes. *Social Indicators Research*, **77**, 37–59.

Humphries, N. (2004). The placebo effect. In: R. Gregory (ed.), *The Oxford Companion to the Mind*, pp. 45–51. Oxford: Oxford University Press.

Kreutz, G., Bossinger, W., Böhm, K., and Clift, S. (2014). Singen im Krankenhaus aus Sicht von Singleitern: Eine qualitative Untersuchung. [Singing in hospital wards from the perspective of singing leaders: a qualitative study]. *Musiktherapeutische Umschau*, **35**, 5–15.

Mayring, P. (1985). Qualitative Inhaltsanalyse. In: G. Jüttemann (ed.), *Qualitative Forschung in der Psychologie*, pp. 187–211. Weinheim: Beltz.

# CHAPTER 39

# Case study: the value of group drumming for women in sex work in Mumbai, India

Varun Ramnarayan Venkit, Anand Sharad Godse, and Amruta Anand Godse

## Introduction to group drumming in rehabilitation

The present case study is a description of a practice-focused report based on a special group drumming project undertaken by Taal Inc. Training and Research, an arts-based training organization based in Pune in association with FLOW: Social Sciences Research for Health and Wellbeing, India. The project was conducted with two groups of girls and women in sex work living in a rehabilitation home in Mumbai. This chapter highlights the background of sex work in India, the process of group-drumming exercises, the reaction of the participants, and, most importantly, the potential of arts interventions with such a group. Additional data for the chapter were collected through in-depth interviews with various organizations working mainly in the state of Maharashtra, central India.

'In my happiness and sadness, I play drums', said one of the participants on the last day of a nine-session group drumming intervention at a government rehabilitation home for young women in sex work in Mumbai. She was one of many to report an opportunity to freely express her feelings (Fig. 39.1).

## Sex work in India

Prostitution is one of the oldest professions known in India and, largely, the world (Milman 1980; Chatterjee 1992). The *Devdasis* (temple girls/Geishas) were accepted and played a central role in the religious and cultural life of India from the tenth century; however, there is a big difference between the *Devdasis* in historical times and the *Jogins* (women in sex work) of today (Pande 2008). There has been a great deal of change over the years, and today in India the main reasons for entry into this profession are poverty, caste, and ritualized prostitution (Sahni et al. 2008). Broadly, there exist two kinds of institution that work for women in prostitution: those that work to organize women in sex work to reduce sexually transmitted infections among them, for example the Durbar Mahila Samanway Committee and Veshya AIDS

Mukabla Parishad, Sangli (VAMPS), and those non-governmental organizations (NGOs) that work to rehabilitate and 'prevent' prostitution (Gangoli 2008). Social stigma, violence, substance use, trauma, and various issues associated with these women have been a major concern for psychologists, sociologists, anthropologists, social workers, and rehabilitation workers in India (Venkit et al. 2013). Hence women's movements have arisen to address issues such as dignity of labour, non-stigmatization, spreading awareness of sex work as sexual exploitation, and sex work as an occupational choice. To add to this there has been conflation of trafficking with prostitution which makes the entire scenario rather complex (Sahni et al. 2008).

There are many institutions (government and private) working towards the organization and prevention of prostitution and rehabilitation of women in prostitution all over the country. Prerana, a Mumbai-based anti-trafficking agency, works to end second-generation prostitution and to protect women and children from the threats of human trafficking by defending their rights and dignity, providing a safe environment, supporting their education and health, and leading major advocacy efforts. It offers educational support, institutional placement, night care centres, and post-rescue operations (Prerana 2013).

Neehar is located in Pune, and its main goal is the upbringing, care for, and rehabilitation of children of prostitutes. Fulwa (meaning a 'bunch of flowers') is an educational project in the red light district for the children of sex workers and is a supportive partner to Neehar offering day care centre services, *Balwadi* (kindergartens), non-formal education, remedial education, and a literacy class for the women (Vaanchit Vikas 2013). Similar to these are institutes like Snehalaya (Mumbai and Pune), Swadhar (Mumbai and Pune), Eklavya (Pune), Jagruti (Bengaluru), and Sanlaap (Kolkata) that work with women and children to help them become independent in spirit, thought, and action, and have full control over their lives rather than be victims.

Vanchit Vikas and Mukta operate two dispensaries and counselling centres in Maharashtra offering healthcare and education to women in prostitution to control the spread of HIV and

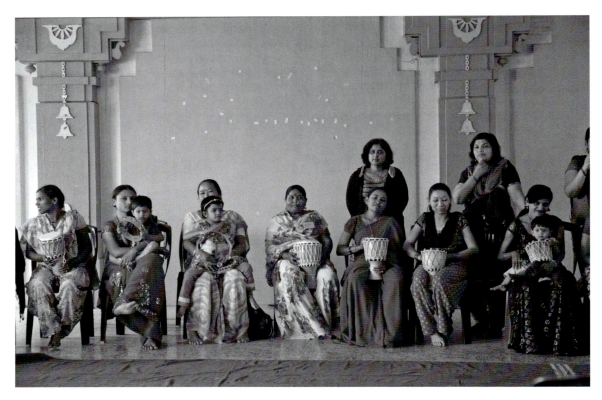

**Fig. 39.1** 'One, two, ready, drum!' Volunteers and women in sex work during a group drumming session for a women's group in Pune, India.
Reproduced by kind permission of Saheli HIV/AIDS Karyakarta Sangh. Copyright © 2015 Saheli HIV/AIDS Karyakarta Sangh.

offer free or subsidized medication. They aim to increase access for these women to affordable medical care in the city, expand the range of services to include preventive and curative services, improve the quality of services to prevent sexually transmitted infections, and increase awareness about and utilization of these services (Vaanchit Vikas 2013).

### Prevalence of art in the life of women in prostitution: then and now

Having a strong knowledge of traditional dance forms, the temple girls were employed as singers, dancers, and musicians to offer certain services to the deities. They played a central role in the religious and cultural life of India from the tenth century onwards (Pande 2008). The performing arts were always highlighted as an integral part of a *Devdasis*' life (Chawla 2002). In India today the place of the performing arts seems to have receded due to the advent of issues such as violence, social stigma, and trafficking, but nevertheless the arts, especially singing and dancing, are major areas of talent or interest for women in prostitution. Most of the girls we have worked with in drumming workshops know the latest Bollywood songs and dance steps, which are typically love songs with steps which have a noticeable sexual connotation (Venkit et al. 2013). Hence using drumming as a therapeutic intervention or a tool for expression seemed to be a natural progression for them. As the sessions progressed and mutual trust grew stronger, the participants would volunteer to sing songs from their culture, expressing a strong connection to their homes and heritage with a bittersweet reminiscence.

### Arts interventions with women in prostitution

Apart from the aforementioned drumming project, Hrishikesh (founder of the Hrishikesh Centre for Contemporary Dance) has started the Love in Dark Times project where he works with children of women in sex work, alcoholics, parents with HIV, and single parents, in partnership with a school in Pune (Pawar 2010). During one of our interviews the theatre activist Sushma Deshpande, who worked with VAMPS, explained:

> Theatre exercises, predominantly role play gave them [women in sex work] a way to look at their own selves objectively. Performing on stage boosted the participants' confidence. Never before had they interacted with communities with such energy. It accelerated the process of overcoming stigma associated with their profession. The stage became a platform to express themselves leaving behind all their inhibitions.

### Group drumming as therapy for women in sex work: delivery and evaluation methods

Taal Inc. Training and Research, an arts-based training organization based in Pune, undertook a special project pioneering the use of group drumming for women in prostitution as a therapeutic tool. The aim of this work was to explore the potential of group drumming as group therapy for women in sex work following a programme of residential rehabilitation in two homes in Mumbai, India. The objectives of the study were to monitor changes in the groups, during and after drumming sessions, with regard to the behavioural parameters of relaxation/stress reduction, confidence/ motivation, attention/concentration, and group cohesiveness.

Group drumming interventions were conducted at two homes. Home A housed adults (over 18 years of age) and Home B housed girls (under 18 years of age). Both homes are residential institutions where the inhabitants live once they have been rescued. The probation period in Home A is 21 days. Homes A and B focus on rehabilitation, reintegration, occupational therapy and education, recreation, and healing, respectively.

The initial session (session zero) was a rapport-building session where the team of facilitators and observers got to know the participants and vice versa. Sessions were held once a week. During the following session we started the drumming programme while pre-programme interviews were conducted with the participants who were most likely to be present throughout the nine-session programme. Given the 21-day probation period, there was a good deal of uncertainty with respect to the regularity of attendance of the participants in Home A. In addition to this, the authors did not have access to any standardized checklists or tests to assess behaviour during these sessions and hence constructed these tools from scratch.

To collect data through the sessions an observation checklist was devised to record the behaviour of participants while drumming. The checklist was built by enlisting behaviour indicators that represented the parameters being researched. For example 'listens actively during session' would represent the 'attention/ concentration' parameter and 'interrupts session' or 'helps fellow participant' would represent the 'group cohesiveness' parameter. Forty such indicators were listed and all the observers were briefed to avoid unnecessary bias. There were three trained observers per session who were each assigned a maximum of eight to ten participants to observe (based on the roll numbers provided in the first session). Each time a behaviour indicator was observed, a tally mark would be entered. A total of five tally marks would decide if the participant showed the behaviour significantly and be assigned a value of 'one' otherwise 'zero' in the data sheet. A coefficient at the group level for each indicator of the variables being studied was derived by calculating the ratio of the number of participants exhibiting the behaviour to the total number of participants. The proportion was presented on a scale of zero to one. This served as our strongest tool and showed results with the least social desirability, unlike the 'drum circle after-effects checklist'. This 44-item questionnaire was rated on a five-point scale and data were collected pre- and post-programme. The questionnaire was in English but had been translated into Hindi and administered to the group, only for it to be realized that the participants were not adept at, fluent, or comfortable with such questionnaires due to their levels of literacy and inclination and hence gave us inconsistent, non-representative results.

To simplify data collection by retaining authenticity another brief questionnaire (form 'B') was constructed to assess the participants' eating and sleeping habits on the day of the sessions. This was administered in a group and served its purpose well.

At the end of the drumming intervention, post-programme interviews were conducted with as many as possible of those participants who were present for the pre-programme interviews and also those participants who wanted to voluntarily share their experience after the drumming programme. The questions were aimed at increasing our understanding of the overall experience,

confidence about drumming, interest, motivation, self-awareness, group cohesiveness, other remarks/stories, and the participant's opinion about changes within themselves after the drumming programme.

The facilitator, co-facilitator, and observers maintained a diary for each session recording their impressions and observations. These diaries consisted of a detailed report of the activities in each session, any special observations or occurrences, and their reflections.

Finally, feedback was collected from the staff members of the rehabilitation homes and the social workers who were in contact with the participants at both homes on a regular basis. These respondents reported any significant change that they observed in the participants during the days of the sessions and also during the rest of the week.

## Reflections on the drumming therapy sessions

Drumming is accessible, expressive, and communicative (Stevens and Burt 1997), and considering the musical inclinations of our participants we started off on a confident note. Hence, during our first interaction with the participants they made their best effort as would be the case when any outsider came to visit the home. This was session zero, our rapport-building session, and our opportunity to break the ice, especially since our facilitator was male there was a noticeable 'giggly' phase that we had to work through.

The instruments used were medium to small sized djembes, tambourines, shakers, and wood-blocks. Since the homes did not possess chairs for all the participants and they were more comfortable sitting on the ground the technique for playing the djembe had to be modified to suit that sitting posture. The first session was spent in understanding this new drum and truly getting a feel for the activity and the atmosphere. The sheer novelty of the activity and curiosity of the participants saw the session through successfully.

By the second session the participants realized that we were not just one-off visitors and started challenging, trusting, opening up, and even taking more liberties during the sessions. On the one hand, the level of stress and lack of engagement amongst the group was very high; consequently a group rhythm, which would usually be set up in a matter of minutes, could take more than four sessions to become confidently established. On the other hand some participants genuinely took to the djembe with great fondness and reported feeling light and calm after drumming. It was after a rhythmic catharsis exercise that the group would be led into a guided visualization of a picture that was a source of 'happiness' in their lives. The aim of this was to remind them of their ability to experience this very basic emotion. Almost all participants reported 'seeing' an image of their families of whom they are very fond, but since they were separated from them they felt sadness at that moment. This marked the start of their therapeutic journey using the drums.

Even though each session did not begin from where the previous one left off in terms of participants' responses, their persistence or will to learn did not diminish, and hence therapeutic progress was not deterred. In the third session we decided to address the presence of subgroups within these homes by emphasizing the existing interdependence when playing a group rhythm. One of the participants said that 'Sharing happiness with everybody, even one's enemies is good', which goes to show that many were pleasantly surprised to be able to create a rhythm with peers in the group with whom they would otherwise not mingle. We also reinforced the visualization of happiness to strengthen that quality amongst the participants by creating a conscious 'mental peg' or 'anchor of happiness'. We realized that not all the stress they faced was due to their occupation but in fact to their current circumstances.

The attention span of the participants could be limited at times, and to address this some interesting rhythm games were devised. The fourth session was dedicated to introducing activities involving drumming, singing, verbalizing rhythms, and introspection that were rapidly rotated to keep them occupied.

By the fifth session the drumming activity was familiar to them and there was a well-evolved group rhythm. The concept of being in a 'bridge space' seemed to throw some light on why this took so long. From a daily reality where one's freedom is questionable, to being rescued and put into a rehabilitation home, decreases the women's perceived independence. Generally speaking the facilities provided by these homes do not address the psychological need for expressing feelings. 'I would like to introduce drumming in my Mahila Sangh [women's group] back home', said one of the participants who found that group drumming helped her to gain a sense of self-empowerment. Another interesting point arose with Home B. Due to the age of the participants we had issues with cohesiveness and mutual respect. After in-depth interviews with the care-givers we realized that these girls would be reprimanded on a continuous basis and only seldom were they allowed free expression. The drumming sessions supported that internal movement towards acceptance and personal freedom.

The sixth session was our therapeutic turning point. We divided the group into two smaller groups to ensure more one-on-one attention and engagement. A group size of 10 to 15 is optimum for such therapeutic interventions. This gave room for more questions and hence clarifications. We introduced 'resource accessing', a group cohesiveness exercise devised by one of the authors (Venkit) based on a series of anchors where each participant reinforces an inherently positive quality. Thereafter each participant identifies a negative or counter-productive quality followed by a 'remedy' quality. The remedy qualities identified are usually a majority of the positive qualities identified earlier by some of the other participants. During the development stages of group drumming the participants showed interdependence and underwent a process wherein each participant acted as a source to help sustain the rhythm when one participant faltered. It is this invisible transaction that is generalized when the remedy quality replaces the negative quality that is invariably present within the group. This is an exercise to rekindle the inherent interdependence of participants in a group.

As we drew closer to our penultimate session we thought it best to equip the participants with motivation to apply the behavioural qualities shown during these drumming sessions in their everyday lives. Participants were encouraged to play the role of a facilitator and experience the process of controlling a group. Even though most were shy to start off with, all participants came forward and led the group to a 'start' or a 'stop' at the very least. 'My fears and inhibitions that I felt during the first sessions have all disappeared now', said one of the participants on being asked how she felt after drumming for seven sessions. By this last session, the

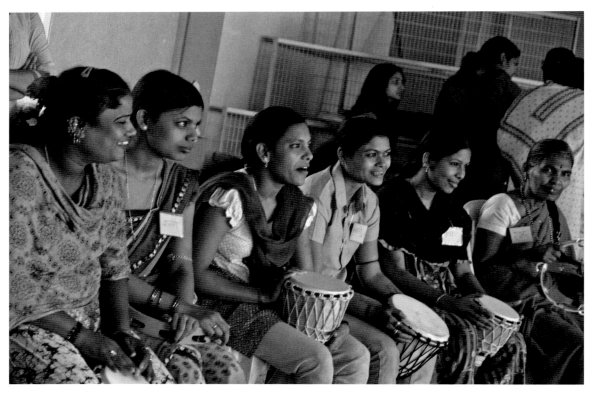

**Fig. 39.2** 'More smiles per beat.' Volunteers and women in sex work during a group drumming session for a women's group in Pune, India.
Reproduced by kind permission of Saheli HIV/AIDS Karyakarta Sangh. Copyright © 2015 Saheli HIV/AIDS Karyakarta Sangh.

group was able to rely on themselves for the group rhythm and less on the facilitator. The group progression resembled the 11 group therapy principles of universality, instillation of hope, recollection of primary family group, altruism, catharsis, group cohesiveness, giving information, freedom to experiment, socialization skills, interpersonal learning, and existential factors.

It was reported that interventions at the rehabilitation homes usually do not extend beyond a 5-week threshold due to a lack of funding, interest of the participants, and disinclination of the institutions to see the programmes through. The group drumming intervention created a lot of opportunity for the participants to take an active interest in their present circumstances and, hence, their futures.

## Conclusion

'On the first day we were only listening to others but on the last day we were playing and listening to others', said one of the participants and sums up the value of group drumming for this population.

The group drumming intervention using various participatory musical elements was well received by the participants and led to positive changes as reported by the participants and observed by the group of facilitators. Such an activity helped at both the individual and group levels by creating a platform for expression and exchange during the process of rehabilitating the women engaging in sex work. The intervention was an effective medium and seemed to address the women's latent psychological needs. This could be used as a starting point for beginning a one-on-one counselling relationship to focus on the women's mental health, which seems to be neglected in the current scenario in India. Social stigma, violence, substance use, trauma, and various other issues associated with this population have been a major concern for psychologists, sociologists, anthropologists, social workers, and rehabilitation workers. It is suggested that drumming has potential as a group therapy, using drumming as a metaphor and incorporating the principles of group therapy. Further research and practice using this intervention with other groups with special needs will have applications in rehabilitation programmes on a general level. There exist a large number of NGOs working for the physical, social, and economical betterment of women in sex work. Their psychological condition however, needs more attention. More such arts-based group interventions such as dance movement therapy, fine art therapy, and music therapy could be introduced along with their existing social rehabilitation methods to ensure holistic healing (Fig. 39.2).

## Acknowledgements

For this chapter we would like to thank our team Miss Kohinoor Darda, Miss Mrinmayi Kulkarni, Mr Swatcchanda Kher, Miss Rajeshwari Baxi, Mr Kaustubh Tambhale, Miss Nupur Moudgill, and all at team Taal Inc. We would also like to thank Dr Mrs Rohini Sahni for her expertise and support and Saheli—Sex Workers Collective for their cooperation.

## References

Chatterjee, R. (1992). *The Queens' Daughters: Prostitutes as an Outcast Group in Colonial India*. Bergen: Chr. Michelsen Institute, Department of Social Science and Development.

Chawla, A. (2002). *Devdasis: Sinners or Sinned Against*. New Delhi: Samarth Bharat.

Gangoli, G. (2008). Immortality, hurt or choice: Indian feminists and prostitution. In: R. Sahni, K.V. Shankar, and H. Apte (eds), *Prostitution and Beyond: An Analysis of Sex Work in India*, pp. 21–22. New Delhi: Sage Publishers.

Milman, B. (1980). New rules for the oldest profession: should we change our prostitution laws? *Harvard Women's Law Journal*, **3**, 1.

Pande, R. (2008). Ritualized prostitution: Devdasis to Jogins—a few case studies. In: R. Sahni, K.V. Shankar, and H. Apte (eds), *Prostitution and Beyond: An Analysis of Sex Work in India*, pp. 101–102. New Delhi: Sage Publishers.

Pawar, H. (2010). Hrishikesh Centre of Contemporary Dance. Available at: <http://www.hrishikeshpawar.com/project.php?page=project> (accessed September 2013).

Prerana (2013). Website. Available at: <http://www.preranaantitrafficking.org/> (accessed 27 September 2013).

Sahni, R., Shankar, K.V., and Apte, H. (eds) (2008). *Prostitution and Beyond: An Analysis of Sex Work in India*, 1st edn. New Delhi: Sage Publishers.

Stevens, C.K. and Burt, J.W. (1997). Drum circles: theory and application in the mental health treatment continuum. *Continuum*, **4**, 175–184.

Vaanchit Vikas (2013). Website. Available at: <http://vanchitvikas.org/> (accessed 20 September 2013).

Venkit, V.R., Godse, A.A., and Godse, A.S. (2013). Exploring the potentials of group drumming as a group therapy for young female commercial sex workers in Mumbai, India. *Arts & Health: An International Journal for Research, Policy And Practice*, **5**, 132–141.

# Index

*46664* campaign, South Africa 8

**A**
abreaction 15
Abreu, José Antonio 193, 196
Access Arts Queensland 136
access to healthcare
　Australian Aboriginal and Torres Strait
　　Islander population 148, 149
　community-based arts for health 106–7
Acorn Foundation, Mumbai, India 154
acquired immune deficiency syndrome *see*
　HIV/AIDS
Action for Autism (India) 154
action research and participatory action
　research, comparison between 78
Active Energy project, London, England 245–8
activity spaces, design for 301
Adams, D. 49
adolescents *see* children and young people
adverse effects of cultural activities 56, 59
Aesop 7
Africa, arts in healthcare 123
Afternow project 22–4
age factors
　cognitive effects of music training 68, 69
　public health and cultural experiences
　　cultural consumption 56, 57
　　life span perspective 60
　singing 252, 253
　　chronic obstructive pulmonary disease 256
　　in hospitals 322
　　Silver Song Clubs 253
　*see also* children and young people; older age
ageing of population
　China 164
　interest in arts and health, growth of 8
　USA 113
　*see also* older age
AIDS *see* HIV/AIDS
AIDS Support Organization Drama
　Group, Mulago Hospital, Kampala,
　Uganda 125–6
Aiken, N.E. 55
Airis project, Västra Götaland, Sweden 176
air quality considerations in design 303
alcohol use 182
Aleksandersen, Åge 175
alexithymia 65–6
al Sayah, F. 79
Amber Creative Club, India 158
American Music Therapy Association
　(AMTA) 272
American Red Cross 117

Americans for the Arts 51, 117
Amin, Idi 124
Amon Carter Museum of American Art,
　Texas, USA 282
amygdala 65
Anantharaman, Ganesh 154
Ancient Egypt 14
Ancient Greece 14–15
Ander, E.E. 284
Animating Democracy 51–2
Annable-Coop, Carly 228, 229, 230
anonymity 85, 88
Antonovsky, A. 213
anxiety
　China 164
　cultural consumption in general
　　population 58
　India 153, 154
　psychophysiology 70
　　art psychotherapy 70
　　neurobiology 65
　singing
　　older age 253, 254
　　Singing for Health Project, east Kent,
　　　England 254, 255
　social determinants 30
　trends 21
Apollo 14
*Applied Arts and Health* 3
architecture and wellbeing 299–306
　current design practice 302
　problems of implementation in design
　　practice 302–3
　research findings 300–2
　ways forward 303–6
Aristotle 3, 13, 14–15
Armstrong, J. 12
art
　Barefoot Artists 107
　community health and education 42–7
　criminal justice settings 189, 296
　cultural consumption in general
　　population 57
　ethical issues 83, 85, 86
　evolutionary perspective 55
　health promotion 176
　hospitals 113, 119, 135–6
　India 158
　Kids Company 219–24
　life span perspective 60–1
　low-birth-weight and prematurity 108
　murals
　　Barefoot Artists 107
　　psychosis 85, 86

　US prisoners 189
　Norway 176
　older age
　　Active Energy project, London,
　　　England 245–8
　　Arts and Older People Programme,
　　　Northern Ireland 238–9
　　Norway 176
　sexual assault victims 106–7
　social inclusion 107
　socially engaged 51
　therapies *see* arts therapies
　*as* therapy vs art *in* therapy 13
　Uganda 123, 124
　　HIV/AIDS 126
　　Karamoja in the Eyes of her Children 125
　USA
　　hospital collections 119
　　hospital displays 113
　　military-based programmes 117
　*see also* fine arts
Arteffact project, Wales 282, 284
Artes y Salud en Immokalee, Florida,
　USA 107
art galleries 281–7
　examples 282–3
　impact measurement 283–5
　understanding galleries in health 285–6
artists in residence 274, 275–6
　Australia 136
Art of Good Health and Wellbeing
　conference 138–9
ArtPlace America 52
art psychotherapy in rehabilitation 70
*Arts & Health* 3, 42
Arts Access Australia 137, 138
Arts and Health Alliance (formerly Society for
　the Arts in Healthcare) 3, 4, 8
Arts and Health Australia (AHA) 4
Arts and Health Foundation, Australia 138
*Arts and Medicine* 137
Arts and Older People Programme (AOPP),
　Northern Ireland 238–9
arts-based health research (ABHR) 83–9
　benefits 83–4
　challenges 84
　ethical issues 84–9
arts-based qualitative research
　methods 78–9
Arts Becomes Therapy (ABT, India) 154, 158
ArtScape Toronto 52
ArtsCare 239
　Northern Ireland 106
　Oregon, USA 116

Arts Council England (ACE)
  Be Creative Be Well 95–7
  *A Prospectus for Arts and Health* 11
  *The Value of Arts and Culture to People and
    Society* 11
Arts Council Northern Ireland (ACNI) 238
ArtsHealth Centre for Research and Practice,
  University of Newcastle, Australia 139
Arts Health Institute (AHI, Australia) 139
Arts Health Network Canada (AHNC) 4
Arts in Health, Flinders Medical Centre,
  Adelaide, Australia 136
Arts in Healthcare Certification Commission
  (AHCC) 118
Arts in Healthcare for Rural Communities,
  Florida, USA 109, 116
Arts in Healthcare Research Database (USA) 114
arts in medicine 274
Arts in Motion (India) 156
Artsite Scheme, Tasmania, Australia 135
Arts on Fire (Australia) 137
Arts SA 139
arts therapies 271–7
  arts and health 274–6
  Australia 136
  criminal justice settings 292
  defined 271
  foundational principles 272–3
  how they work 271–2
  India 152
  referrals indicators 275
  settings 272
  training 272
Art Talks project, Pune India 207
Asclepius 14
Ashforth, A. 131
Asociación Ak'Tenamit, Guatemala City,
  Guatemala 109
ASPECT 303–4
Assam Autism Centre (India) 154, 158
Atlantic Philanthropies 238
audience misinterpretation 86
Audience of One, Mumbai, India 154
audience vulnerability 87
auditory cortex 69
Austin, E.W. 108
Australia
  Arts and Health Australia 4
  arts and health in 135–40
    arts and humanities 136–7
    art therapy 136
    community-based arts 137
    evaluation 137–8
    first national steps 137
    government policy 139–40
    healthcare design 135
    healthcare services 135–6
    national consolidation 138–9
  community cultural development 53
    Cultural Development Network 51
  community health and education, arts in 41, 45
  Gomeroi Gaayanggal, Tamworth, New
    South Wales 108
  indigenous people *see* Australian Aboriginal
    and Torres Strait Islander people
  intergenerational music-making 260–1
  museums and art galleries 282, 283
  National Arts and Health Framework
    (NAHF) 135, 136, 138, 139–40
  public health 119

life span perspective 61
  singing 252
Australia Council 137, 139
  *Art and Wellbeing* 138
  Community Arts Committee (CAC) 137
  *Strategy Options in Arts and Health* 139
Australian Aboriginal and Torres Strait
  Islander people 145–9
  community singing project 146–9
  Gomeroi Gaayanggal, Tamworth, New
    South Wales 108
  mental illness and chronic disease
    prevention needs 145
Australian Centre for Arts and Health
  (ACAH) 138–9
Australian Health and Hospitals
  Association 138
Australian Institute for Patient and Family
  Centred Care (AIPFCC) 139
Australian Institute of Medical and Biological
  Illustrators (AIMBI) 136
*Australian Medical Observer* 137
Australian Network for Arts and Health
  (ANAH) 137, 138
Austria, singing in hospitals 318
authorship 87, 88
Autism Care (India) 154
autism spectrum disorders
  dance therapy 273
  India 156
    music therapy 154
  museums and art galleries 282
Avenida Brasil, Rio de Janeiro, Brazil 179–85
  Crescer e Viver 184–5
  Grupo Cultural AfroReggae 181–4

**B**
Bacharach, D.W. 67
Baganda people, Uganda 123–4
Bagisu people, Uganda 123
Bailey, Betty 317
Balsara, Zubin 154
Bangert, M. 69
Barbados, dementia 240–2
Barefoot Artists 107
Barry, Gerald 35
Barthes, R. 77
Bartlett, D. 214
Barton, Kelvin 37
Barz, Gregory 125
Batmanghelidjh, Camila 220
Bauer, Ida 15
Baumann, M. 12
Baumgartner, T. 70
Beah, Ishmael 203
Beamish Museum, England 282
Beauchamp, T.L. 309
Beck, R.J. 214
Be Creative Be Well 95–7
Belgium, museums 282
Belliveau, G. 84
Bentley, T. 237
Benzon, W. 55
bereavement 14
Bergen University, Norway 173
Berglund, A. 131
Bermann, Gregorio 5
Bernardi, L. 214
Bernays, Jacob 15

Berry, Drew 137
Beveridge, William 19
Bharata, *Natya Shastra* 155
Bhupatkar, Maithily 237, 238
Bible 14
bibliotherapy 16
Big Noise, Scotland 196
Bihar School of Yoga, Munger, India 157
Bilby, C. 295
bipolar disorder 255
Bipolar UK 230
Bittman, B.B. 174
Blackstone, Mary 84
Blair, Tony 39
Bloom, T. 13
Boal, Augusto 78, 187, 188
Bock, Thomas 136
Bodbole 158
Bodelwyddan Castle, Wales 282
body painting 123
Bojner Horwitz, E. 69
Bolton Library and Museum Service,
  England 283
Bolton Museum, England 282
Bonde, L.O. 194, 197
bonfire night parade, Rye, East
  Sussex, UK 52
books 56
Booth, E. 194
Booth, T. 201
Borland, Toby 246
Bossinger, Wolfgang 317
Boston University, Prison Education
  Program 187
Botton, Alain de 12
Bourriaud, Nicolas 88
Boydell, K.M. 85, 89
Bradbury, Helen 106
Brady, Ian 294
Braun, A. 115
Braun, V. 75
BRAVO Youth Orchestras 194, 195, 196
Brazil
  Avenida Brasil, Rio de Janeiro 179–85
    Crescer e Viver 184–5
    Grupo Cultural AfroReggae 181–4
  Gruppo Cultural AfroReggae, Rio de
    Janeiro 8
  museums 282
Brett Lee Foundation 158
BrightHearts App 136
British Museum, London, England 282, 283
Broca's area 69
bronchiectasis 251
Brooklyn Parkinson Group (BPG) 104
Browne, John 309–10, 311, 312
BUDEA, Buwolomera Village, Uganda 125
Budhan Theatre (India) 156
Burkhardt, J. 227
Burnbake Trust 292
burnout 173–4
Butabika Hospital, Kampala,
  Uganda 124, 125
Butcher, S.H. 14
Butler-Kisber, L. 87
Buys, N. 146
Bwakeddampulira AIDS Patients Educational
  Team, Masindi, Uganda 125
Bygren, L.O. 57, 60, 211
Byrne, Ellie 75

**C**

Cadbury Brown, H.T. 36
Cameron, Drew 117
Camic, P.M. 248, 284, 285, 287
Campbell, Don 12–13
Campo, Rafael 13–14
Canada
  Arts Health Network Canada 4
  ethical issues in arts-based health
    research 84
  public health 119
  singing, by homeless men 317
Canada Public Health Agency 204
Canadian Hospice Palliative Care
  Association 116
cancer
  arts therapies 276–7
  museums 285–6
  public health and cultural experiences 57
capabilities approach 30
Carabine, J. 76
caregivers
  arts therapies 272
  dementia 281–2, 284
  Tanpopo-no-ye, Nara City, Japan 107
Cash, Johnny 294
Casson, Hugh 36
catharsis
  group drumming, female sex workers in
    India 327
  history of art and healing 13, 14–16
ccd.net 137
Centre for Culture, Health, and Care,
  Levanger, Norway 172
Centre for Health Promotion, University of
  Toronto 248
cerebellum 69
Chabukswar, Anand 156
Chadwick, Edwin 19
Changing Tunes 295
Chapman, F. 264
Chatterjee, H.J. 248, 281, 282, 283, 284, 287
Cheliotis, L. 295
Chelsea and Westminster Hospital, London,
  England 301
chemotherapy 154
Chikte, Vidya 152
children and young people
  abused 219–24
  applied theatre, risky moments in 85, 88
  Artes y Salud en Immokalee, Florida,
    USA 107
  arts therapies 219–24, 273, 274
  Brazil
    Crescer e Viver 184–5
    Grupo Cultural AfroReggae 182–3
    mortality 180
  community health and education, arts in 42–7
  dance 227–32
  education in creativity and wellbeing
    promotion 201–8
    barriers to healthy development 203–8
    healthy child development 202–3
    right to healthy development with
      wellbeing 203
  emotional competence 66–7
  health literacy 109
  India 154
  Kids Company, England 219–24
  museums and art galleries 282

music 215
  cognitive effects of music training 69
  India 154
  intergenerational music-making 259–65
Norway 175
public health and cultural
  experiences 58–9
quality of place and wellbeing 300
singing 214–15
  Young Voices 251
Sistema programmes 193–7
social competence 66
social determinants of health
  intergenerational equity 29–30
  social capital and participation 31
  stress 30
Sweden 174–5
Uganda 125
  HIV/AIDS 126
USA 115
vintage photographs, perceptions of 113
Children's Trust Fund 42
Childress, J.F. 309
China
  creative arts and public health 163–9
    cultural participation in general
      population 164
    engagement with creative arts 163–4
    health benefits of creative arts 166–8
    implications of creative arts
      engagement 168
    research study 166–8
    traditional cultural activities 164–6
  older age 235
Chisholm, Brock 5
choice anxiety theory 21
choirs see singing
Christophsbad Göppingen psychiatric
  hospital, Germany 317
chronic diseases
  Australian Aboriginal and Torres Strait
    Islander people 145, 148, 149
  China 163, 164, 166, 167, 168, 169
  see also specific diseases
chronic obstructive pulmonary disease
  (COPD) 255–6
cinemas
  cultural consumption in general
    population 56
  Culture Palette in Healthcare Centres,
    Stockholm, Sweden 173 173
  life span perspective 59
Cintra, Marily 135, 138
circumcision 123
circus performance 184–5
Clark, I. 251
Clarke, V. 75
Classen, C. 281
Clean Break 295
Clift, Stephen
  evaluation of research 16
  evidence 55, 138
  research questions 95
  role of arts in health promotion 8
  singing 251, 252, 314
climate change 21, 22
Clinical Outcomes in Routine Evaluation
  (CORE) questionnaire 254, 255
cognitive decline 32
  see also dementia

cognitive development, and music
  training 58, 68–9
cognitive reserve 215
Cohen, Gene 61, 115, 239–40
Colchester and Ipswich Museums Service,
  England 282, 283
Cole, A.L. 79
Collaborative Environments for Creative
  Arts Research (CeCAR), University of
  Newcastle, Australia 139
Combat Paper Project, USA 117
Comedy School 294
comfort, design for 300, 301, 302
Commission for Architecture and the Built
  Environment (CABE) 302
Commission on the Social Determinants of
  Health (CSDH) 27
Commonwealth Games, Manchester 41
communication
  arts therapies 273
  children and young people 203
    Speech Bubbles programme 204–5
community
  concept 103
  defined 49
community arts 78
community-based arts for health
  promising practices 103–9
    access to healthcare 106–7
    health literacy 107–9
    wellness 104–5
  Well London programme 95–100
community cultural development
  (CCD) 49–53
  international initiatives 50–1
  local communities 52–3
  national programmes 51–2
community health and education, arts in 41–7
  emergence 41
  future 47
  international dimensions 44–5
  lessons learned 47
  Roots and Wings project 42–4
  Tilery lanterns project 45–7
company, design for 300, 301, 302
compassion 309
composers in residence 309–10, 311
Conaghan, Angeline 205, 206
Concerts Norway 172
conferences on arts and health 3, 5, 7
  Australia 138
confidentiality 83, 85
Connecting the European Mind project 282
consent see informed consent
constructive thinking (designers) 303
constructivism 74, 75
consumerism 22
control
  design for 300, 301, 302
  social determinants of health 30, 32
Convention on the Rights of the Child
  (CRC) 202, 203
Conway, C. 259
Cope, Wendy 295
Corbin, J. 75
coronary heart disease 165
corpus callosum 69
cortisol 66, 69–70
Costa-Giomi, E. 58
Cox, S.M. 87

Craemer, R. 138
Creating Social Capital (Australia) 137
Creative Ageing Centre, Brisbane,
        Australia 139
Creative Australia 139
Creative Cities Network (UNESCO) 50–1
Creative Europe 51
Creative Expression Centre for Arts Therapy
        (CECAT), Perth, Australia 136
Creative Nation (Australia) 137
Creative Partnerships 43
Creative Partnerships Australia 138
Creative People and Places 97
creative placemaking 52
creativity, definition of 201, 236–7
Creativity and Aging Study, USA 240
credentialling, USA 118
Crescer e Viver, Rio de Janeiro, Brazil 184–5
criminal justice settings 291–6
        Animating Democracy 51–2
        artistic judgement and the Koestler
                Trust 295–6
        how arts are created in 291–2
        research evidence 295
        theoretical models 292–5
        USA 187–90
Critical Appraisal Skills Programme
        (CASP) 80
Cross, Nigel 303
Crummett, A. 78
Cruz, Oswaldo 179, 184, 185
Csikszentmihalyi, M. 202, 236–7, 273
Cuesta 195
cultural capital 235
Cultural Development Network (CDN),
        Australia 51
Cultural Ministers Council (CMC,
        Australia) 138
Cultural Walking Stick, Norway 172
culture, definition of 49–50, 202
Culture for Life (Norway) 172
Culture, Health and Wellbeing Conference 7
Culture Palette in Healthcare Centres,
        Stockholm, Sweden 173–4
Cummings, Jane 309
Cunha, R. 259
Cunningham Dax, Eric 136
curiosity
        art 113
        children's 42, 44
Cuypers, K. 211

D
DADAA 45
dance
        adverse effects 56
        children and young people 227–32
                Usinga World Centre for Dance and
                        Music, Bagamoyo, Tanzania 206
        China 165, 166–8
        Culture Palette in Healthcare Centres,
                Stockholm, Sweden 174
        Dancing Well: The Soldier Project 117
        emotional competence 67
        evolutionary perspective 55
        health literacy 107
        health professional education and
                practice 311
        India 151–3, 154–6, 158
                female sex workers, Mumbai 326

intergenerational 120, 261
older age
        Dance for PD, Pune, India 237–8
        Hip Op-eration Hip Hop Crew, New
                Zealand 105
        Parkinson's disease 104–5, 114, 237–8
        psychophysiology 68, 69–70
        representing mental healthcare
                pathways 85, 86
        Sweden 175
        therapy 272, 273
        Uganda 123, 124
                HIV/AIDS 125
        value of 215
Dance All (India) 156
Dance for PD 114
        India 155, 156, 237–8
        USA 104–5
Dance for Young People project, Sweden 175
Dance United 227–32
Dancing Well: The Soldier Project 117
Darpana Academy of Performing Arts,
        Gujarat, India 8
Darrow, A.A. 260
data analysis, qualitative research 75–7
data collection, qualitative research
        74–5, 79
Date, Suchitra 152
Davar, Shiamak 156
Davidson, Jane 317
Dax Centre, Melbourne, Australia 136
Day, Lucienne 36
Day, Robin 36
Daykin, Norma 75, 77
D'Cruz, Natasha 152
debt 30
De Haan Centre, Canterbury Christ Church
        University, England 251, 252–6
de Leeuw, S. 119
Deller, Jeremy 295
De Manzano, Ö. 68
dementia
        art 176
        dance 215
        drumming 174
        museums and art galleries 281–2,
                283, 284–5
        music 211, 240–2
                Norway 172
        Northside Seniors, Pittsburgh,
                USA 247
        social determinants of health 32
        TimeSlips, Wisconsin, USA 105
demographics
        ageing see also ageing of population
        global 235, 236
Denmark, museums 282
depression
        art psychotherapy 70
        Australia
                Aboriginal and Torres Strait Island
                        population 148, 149
                evaluation 138
        children and young people 175
        cultural consumption in general
                population 58
        India 153, 154
        Iroquois 'condolence ritual' 14
        life course approach 29, 59
        psychophysiology 67, 70

resilience 163
singing
        in hospitals 317, 320, 321
        older age 253, 254
        Singing for Health Project, east Kent,
                England 254, 255
        social determinants 30
                older age 32
                social contact 31
        'Time Being 2' project, Isle of Wight,
                England 12
        trends 21
DeSalvo, Louise 16
Deshpande, Sushma 152, 326
desistance theory 293, 295
development
        child 202–8
        definition 50
Dharap, Sujata 158
Dharavi Rocks, India 154
diet and food 22–3, 184
dignity, design for 300, 301, 302, 303
Diodorus Siculus 14
disability-free life expectancy
        (DFLE) 57
        health inequalities 28, 29
discourse analysis (DA) 75
        case study 75–7
        Foucauldian 76–7
Dissanayake, Ellen 55, 66, 103
Dodds, Stephen 246
Doll, Sir Richard 20
Doshi, Anubha 152
Doyle, D. 138
drama
        children and young people
                Speech Bubbles programme,
                        England 205
                Usinga World Centre for Dance and
                        Music, Bagamoyo, Tanzania 207
        criminal justice settings 292, 293
        female sex workers, India 326
        foundational principles of drama
                therapy 273
        health professional education and
                practice 311
        India 151, 156
        Uganda 123, 124
                HIV/AIDS 125
        see also theatre
drawing see art
drug use 182–3
drumming
        dementia 17
        India 153, 154
                Art Talks project, Pune 207
                children and young people 207
                female sex workers, Mumbai 325–9
        transferable skills 273
        We beat drums project, Skåne,
                Sweden 174–5
Dulwich Picture Gallery, England 281,
        282, 283
Duncan, K. 12
Dunn, Douglas 295
Durbar Mahila Samanway Committee,
        India 325
Durham University, Centre for Medical
        Humanities (CMH) 42, 44, 45, 46
dysphonia severity index (DSI) 214

**E**

Earhart, G.M. 104
economic issues *see* financial issues
Editions in Craft 132
education
    attainment, level of
        appeal of cultural activities 173
        cultural involvement 59, 60
        singers 252
        social determinants of health 30
    criminal justice settings 291–2
    health *see* health literacy
    of health professionals 309–14
    lifelong learning *see* lifelong learning
    maternal 30
    *see also* community health and education,
        arts in; schools
Eeckelaar, C. 284
Egypt, Ancient 14
Eklavya, Pune, India 325
elderly people *see* older age
El Sistema *see* Sistema programmes
Emerson, R.W. 44
emotional balance 60
emotional competence 65–7
emotional exhaustion 59
emotional intelligence 203
employment *see* working age
empowerment
    arts therapies 273
    Crescer e Viver, Rio de Janeiro,
        Brazil 184–5
    empowering song approach 189
    social determinants of health 30, 32
End to Loneliness campaign, UK 236
energy use 21
Engage with Age (EWA), Northern Ireland 238
England
    Active Energy project, London 245–8
    children and young people
        Haringey Nursery Schools Consortium
            Lullaby Project 205–6
        Kids Company 219–24
        Speech Bubbles programme 204–5
    community cultural development 49
    criminal justice settings 291, 292, 294, 295
    health inequalities 27, 28, 31
    health professional education and
        practice 309–14
    intergenerational music-making 261–4
    museums and art galleries 281, 282,
        283–4, 285–6
    National Alliance for Arts, Health and
        Wellbeing 4
    older age
        dementia 240–1
        wellness-focused services 236
    public health and cultural experiences 61
    quality of place and wellbeing 302, 303, 304
    singing 251, 252, 253
        Silver Song Clubs 252
        Singing for Health Project, east
            Kent 254–5
    Sistema programmes 195, 196
    Southbank Centre London 35–9
    Time Being 2 project, Isle of Wight 12
    Well London programme 95–100
Erikson, E. 259
ethical issues 83–9
    artworks by people with mental illness 136

challenges and solutions 85–8
community health and education, arts
    in 44, 45
dance 230–1
food 22–3
health education, USA 118
in practice 84, 88
procedural ethics 84, 88
public health 23
qualitative research 74, 75, 79–80
quality of place and wellbeing 300
singing in hospitals 318
ethics committees 83, 84, 89
    challenges and solutions 85, 87
    procedural ethics 84
    qualitative research 79–80
European Action Plan 51
European Capitals of Culture 52
European Commission 104
European Review of Social Determinants of
    Health 29, 32
European Union 282
evaluation of arts for health interventions 16
    Australia 137–8
    evidence question 12
    qualitative research 73, 74
    role 6–7
Evelina London Children's Hospital,
    England 304–6
Every Child Matters strategy (UK) 42
evidence
    hierarchy of 6, 16, 55
    question of 12
evidence-based medicine 116
evolutionary perspective on cultural
    experiences 55
expressive therapists 271
exterior design of schools 301

**F**

facilities, design for 301
family planning 108
*favelas*, Rio de Janeiro, Brazil 179–85
Fearon, Pasco 219
Fernandez, Arthur 152
Festival of Britain 35–6, 37, 38, 39
festivals 41, 49, 50
    Southbank Centre London 35–9
fêtes, village 52–3
fibrinogen 68
fibromyalgia 69–70
films *see* cinemas
financial issues
    Australia 135, 138, 140
        art therapy 136
    China, public health in 163
    chronic obstructive pulmonary
        disease 256
    community health and education,
        arts in 44
    European Capitals of Culture 52
    evidence question 12, 16
    health inequalities 27
    Sistema programmes 195–6
    Tanzania, Usinga World Centre for Dance
        and Music 206
    USA
        arts in healthcare settings 114
        USA 240
fine arts *see* art

Fine Cell Work 292
Finland
    cultural consumption in general
        population 57
    life span perspective 59
Finnegan, Lesley 43
Flinders Medical Centre, Adelaide,
    Australia 136, 139
Flood, Bill 49–50
Florence Nightingale School of Nursing and
    Midwifery, King's College London,
    England 309–14
flow 202, 273
    psychophysiology 68
    singing 215
FLOW: Social Sciences Research for Health
    and Well-being, India 325
focus groups 74–5
folk art, India
    dance 155
    drama 156
folk dance, China 165
food and diet 22–3, 184
Foucauldian discourse analysis (FDA) 76–7
found poetry 85, 86–7
Franklin, Benjamin 104
Fraser, K.D. 79
Freedom in Creation (FIC), Uganda 125
Frego, D. 260
Freud, Sigmund 15
Friends of Ruwenzori, Kabarole District,
    Uganda 125
Froggett, L. 283, 285
From War to Home project, USA 117
Fulwa, Pune, India 325
functional magnetic resonance imaging
    (fMRI) 115

**G**

Gabrielsson, A. 67
galleries *see* art galleries
Garber, S.J. 261
Gardner, H. 9
Gaser, C. 69
Gaztambide-Fernandez, R. 187
Geese Theatre Company 293
Geezers Club, London, England 245–6
gender factors
    HIV/AIDS, South Africa 129, 130
    public health and cultural experiences
        cultural consumption 56, 57, 58
        life span perspective 60
    singing 252, 253
        chronic obstructive pulmonary
            disease 256
        in hospitals 322
        Silver Song Clubs 253
    *see also* men; women
generativity 259, 264
Germany
    museums 282
    public health and cultural
        experiences 61
    singing 252
        in hospitals 317–23
        Military Wives choirs 251
Ghaziani, Rokhshid 301
Gick, M. 251
Gillam, L. 84
Gilroy, A. 13

Global Alliance for Arts and Health (GAAH)
    Arts in Healthcare Certification
        Commission 118
    *Bringing the Arts to Life* 115
    Conference 7
    public health 119
Gold, Christian 173
Goldbard, A. 49, 50
Goleman, D. 203
Gomeroi Gaayanggal, Tamworth, New South
    Wales, Australia 108
Goodridge, D. 255
Good Shepherd Support Action Centre,
    Kampala, Uganda 125
Gordon Healing Arts, Kampala, Uganda 125
Gough Whitlam, Edward 137
Govias, J. 194
Grangegorman, Dublin, Ireland 302
Grape, C. 214
Greece, Ancient 14–15
grey matter 68–9
grief 14
gross national income (GNI) 235
Grounded Ecotherapy 37
grounded theory 74, 75
Groussard, M. 69
Grupo Cultural AfroReggae, Rio de Janeiro,
    Brazil 8, 181–4, 185
Guatemala, Asociación Ak'Tenamit 109
Guildhall School of Music and Drama,
    London, England 311
Guillemin, M. 84
Gütay, W. 215
Gwynedd Museum and Gallery Bangor,
    Wales 282

H
Halle Orchestra 292
Hancox, Grenville 251, 252
Hand-in-Hand programme, Canberra,
    Australia 260–1
Harding, K. 251
Haringey Nursery Schools Consortium
    Lullaby Project, London,
    England 205–6
Harris Museum, Preston, England
    282, 283
Hasselkus, B. 236
Hathaway, Baxter 14
Hatton-Yeo, A. 260
Hauptmann, Cornelius 318
Hawkes, J. 49
health
    behaviour 147–8
    definitions 3–6, 104, 211, 236, 299, 317
    education *see* health education
    improvements 19–20
    Indian perspective 153
    inequalities 8
        children and young people 202
        community health and education,
            arts in 42
        urban vs rural communities 103, 116
        modernity 20–1
        *see also* social determinants of health
    literacy 107–9
    music(k)ing 194, 195, 197
    promotion 6, 104
        art 176
        Australia 137, 138

community health and education,
    arts in 46
    participatory arts 236
    social determinants of health 30
public *see* public health
Health 2020: 51
health and safety factors in design 302
Health Benefits Questionnaire 166
health education
    Grupo Cultural AfroReggae, Rio de Janeiro,
        Brazil 182, 183
    HIV/AIDS
        South Africa 130
        Uganda 125–6
        USA 118
HealthPlay (Australia) 139
health professional education and
    practice 309–14
Healthy People 2020 (USA) 113, 114, 119
heart disease/surgery 85, 87, 252
hedonic treadmill theory 21
Hendrix, Jimi 36
Heritage2Health project, England 283
Heritage in Hospitals project,
    England 283–4, 286
Heron, J. 78
Herrmann, S. 259
Hertzberger, Herman 301
hierarchy of evidence 6, 16, 55
Hildenfoso, Johayne 182–3
Hinduism 151
Hip Op-eration Hip Hop Crew, Waiheke
    Island, New Zealand 105
hippocampus 69
Hippocratic Oath 119
history of art and healing 13–16
HIV/AIDS
    Asociación Ak'Tenamit, Guatemala City,
        Guatemala 109
    awareness 8
    health education 108
    Names Project, California, USA 108
    palliative care, USA 115
    sex workers, India 325
    Siyazama Project, South Africa 129–32
    SPREAD programme, Rwanda 108
    Uganda 125–6
Hodgman, T. 259
Hodgson, Dorothy 36
Homer 14
homicide, Brazil 180, 181
Horn, Reinhard 318
Horn, Stephen 310
hospices 116
Hospital Anxiety and Depression Scale
    (HADS) 253, 254
Hospital Audiences Incorporated 137
hospitals
    architecture 299–301, 302, 303, 304–6
    art
        collections 119
        displays 113
    singing in 317–23
        benefits 318
        certification 318–19
        history 317
        international collaboration and musical
            ambassadors 318
        mission and dissemination 317–18
        quality control 318

research 319–22
    Uganda 124
housing 30
Houston, S. 104
Howarth, Alan 7–8
Hrishikesh 326
Huber, M. 5
Hubs for Older People's Engagement (HOPE),
    Northern Ireland 238
Hui, A. 78
human development index (HDI) 235
human immunodeficiency virus *see* HIV/AIDS
human rights model, criminal justice
    settings 295
Hurstville City Museum and Gallery,
    Wales 282
Hyde, K.L. 69
hyperactivity 273
hypertension 66
hypothalamic–pituitary–adrenocortical (HPA)
    axis 69–70
Hyyppä, M.T. 57

I
IDEAs 303, 304, 305
IMAGINE 304, 305
immunoglobulin 68
Imperial War Museum, London, England 310
India
    art in 151–3
    arts and health initiatives 151–9
        dance 154–6
        drama 156
        fine arts 158
        future 159
        music 153–4
        research and training 158–9
        yoga 156–8
    Art Talks project, Pune 207
    children and young people 107
    current health issues 153
    Darpana Academy of Performing Arts,
        Gujarat 8
    group drumming for female sex
        workers 325–9
    health perspective 153
    life expectancy 30
    older age 235
    Dance for PD, Pune 237–8
Indian Council for Mental Health 158
Indian School of Martial Arts 158
indigenous people
    art for public health 119
    Australia *see* Australian Aboriginal and
        Torres Strait Islander people
    Guatemala 109
Indigenous Risk Impact Score (IRIS) 146
individual change, model of 292–4
industrialization 19, 164
informed consent
    ethical issues 85, 86, 87, 88
    qualitative research 75, 79
Ingeberg, M.H. 176
Ings, R. 109
In Harmony England 195, 196
In Harmony Lambeth 37
Inside Me programme 44
Institute for Creative Health (ICH),
    Australia 138, 140
Institute of Health Equity 32

Institute of Psychiatry (IoP) 229–30, 231, 232
intellectual health and wellbeing, children 202
intelligence
    musical ability 67
    musical training 58, 215
interest in arts and health, growth of 3, 7–8
intergenerational equity 29–30, 32
intergenerational music-making 259–65
    benefits 259–60
    challenges 264
    cooperative programmes 261–4
    future 264
    older people assisting younger 260
    younger people assisting older 260–1
interior design 301
international conferences on arts and
        health 3, 5, 7
International Labour Organization 207
interviews 74–5
IQ see intelligence
Ireland, Republic of
    community health and education,
        arts in 41
    quality of place and wellbeing 302
Iroquois 'condolence ritual' 14
irritable bowel syndrome (IBS) 68
Islam 151
Italy, dementia 240–1
Iyengar, B.K.S. 157

J
Jagruti, Bengaluru, India 325
James, S. 304
James Irvine Foundation 50
Japan
    life expectancy 27
    Tanpopo-no-ye, Nara City 107
Jategaonkar, N. 85
Johnson, H. 295
Jolles, Frank 131
Jordanova, Ludmilla 310
journals
    ethical approval of research 80
    interest in arts and health, growth of 3
Judeo-Christian tradition 14

K
Kaiser, Roland 318
Kaivalyadham, Lonavala, India 157
Karamoja in the Eyes of her Children,
        Uganda 125
Kashyap, Tripura 155, 158
Kattenstroth, J.-C. 70
Katti, Shashank 154
Katz, G. 16
Keene, New York, USA 117
Kelly, Jude 36–7, 38, 295
Khare, Susan 152, 158
Kids Company 219–24
Kirklees Primary Care Trust, England 44
Kitojo Integrated Development Association,
        Kabarole District, Uganda 125
Klein, Melanie 285
Klempner, Dylan 277
Knaus, C.S. 108
Knell, J. 100
Knowles, J.G. 79
Koch, Robert 19
Koelsch, S. 214
Koestler, Arthur 296

Koestler Trust/Awards 37, 291, 292,
        294, 295–6
Konlaan, B.B. 57, 60
Krantz, G. 69
Kretschmann, Gerlinde 317
Kreutz, G. 214, 252
Krige, E. 132
Krishnamacharya 157
KROKUS project, Västernorrland County,
        Sweden 175
Krumhansl, C.L. 67
Kulkarni, Shekhar 154

L
Laban Movement Analysis 231
Lafrenière, D. 87
Lalit Kala Academi, India 158
Lanceley, A. 285–6
lanterns parades 45–7
Lapum, J. 87
Larundal Psychiatric Hospital, Melbourne,
        Australia 136
latent meaning 75
Laverack, G. 103
Lawrence, D.H. 6
Lawson, B.R. 300, 303
laxative pill consumption 60, 61
learning, science of 202
Leavy, P. 79
Leclerc-Madlala, Suzanne 130
Ledgard, Anna 88
Le Doux, Joseph 65
legacy 100
legibility of place, design for 300–1, 302
Leicestershire Open Museum, England 282
Leventhal, David 105
Lewis, A. 138
Lewis, Terence 156
Lewis-Williams, D. 55
Liamputtong, P. 79
libraries 56
life course approach
    arts in healthcare settings, USA 115
    cultural participation and health 58–61
    social determinants of health 29–30, 32
life expectancy
    health inequalities 27, 28, 29, 30
        social contact 31
    public health and cultural experiences 57
lifelong learning
    active ageing 260
    intergenerational music-making 265
    USA 115
Light, Ann 247
Lightbox, Woking, England 282, 283
light considerations in design 303
Limb, D. 115
Lindblad, F. 59
Linsell, Helen 228
Lippman, Peter 299
literacy
    health 107–9
    social determinant of health 44
Living House Project, Rio de Janeiro,
        Brazil 179
Llandudno Museum, Wales 282
Loca 44
London Bubble Theatre Company 204
London Centre for Arts and Cultural
        Exchange (LCACE), England 311

London Health Commission 11
London Transport, colourful condom
        campaign 49
Long, Khandice 276–7
Lorenzino, L. 259
Love in Dark Times project, Pune, India 326
low-birth-weight 108
Lucas, Sarah 295
Lynch, Kevin 301

M
McDonald, M. 107–8
McDougall, Eve 293–4
McGill, A. 104
McNiff, Shaun 13, 79
Macquarie University Art Gallery, Sydney,
        Australia 282
Madden, C. 13
Majno, M. 193, 196
Makerere University, Kampala, Uganda 124,
        125, 126
Mäki, J. 57
Malaysia, Teach for Malaysia
        programme 207–8
Malchiodi, C.A. 13
Malone, Gareth 251
managers, 60
Manchester Art Gallery, England 283
Manchester Museums, England 283
Mandela, Nelson 8, 129, 130
Marcus, M. 193, 194
Margaret Trowell School of Art,
        Uganda 124, 125
Mark Morris Dance Group (MMDG) 104,
        114, 237
Marmot, Sir Michael/Marmot Review 8,
        27, 30, 32
    community health and education, arts in 42
    healthy child development 202
Marsden, Sally 135, 137
Martinez, Juan 193
Matarasso, François 103, 119, 137
maternal education 30
MatrixInsights 12
Mattress Factory Museum, Pittsburgh, USA 247
Mayr, Franz 131
Meadows, M. 295
Medical Museion, Copenhagen, Denmark 282
Medical Research Council (MRC) 7
    health professional education and
        practice 310
    mixed-methods research programmes 73
    social interventions, evaluation of 7
Meethbhakre, Pankaj 152
Mehr, S.A. 58
Meltzer, D.J. 285
men
    Active Energy project, London,
        England 245–8
    see also gender factors
mental health problems
    Australian Aboriginal and Torres Strait
        Islander people 145
    dance 229–31
    India 153
        drama 156
    life course approach 29
    quality of place and wellbeing 300
    singing 254–5, 317–23
    see also specific problems

meta-analysis 6
Metamorphosis Group, Chattisgarh, India 158
MEWSIC 158
microethics 84
midwifery education and practice 309–14
Miles, Andrew 228
military-based programmes, USA 117–18
Military Wives choirs 251
Mills, D. 119
mindfulness 174, 273
mirror neurons 67
Mithen, S. 55
Mittal, Nikita 152
mixed-methods research 73–4
  case study 75–7
modernity
  benefits 22
  crisis in 21–2
  dis-eases of 20–1
  health improvements 19–20
money, exponential increase in 21–2
Moore Rubell and Yudell 302
Morrison, Herbert 35
Moss, H. 118
motor cortex 69
movies see cinemas
Mozart effect 12–13, 16
Mponda, John 206
Mthethwa, Bongani 131
Muirhood, A. 119
Mukta, India 325–6
Muktangan de-addiction rehabilitation centre,
    India 158
Mulago Hospital, Kampala,
    Uganda 124, 125–6
Mulligan, M. 51, 53
multiculturalism 113
multimodality, emotional education 66–7
multiple sclerosis 215
Mumbai Education Trust (MET), India 158
murder, Brazil 180, 181
Murphy, Natalie, Child Waiting 223
Murray, M. 78
MuSeele, Germany 282
Museu da Vida, Brazil 282
Museum Dr Guislain, Belgium 282
Museum of Fine Art, Boston, USA 282
Museum of Hartlepool, England 284
Museum of Liverpool, England 282
Museum of Modern Art (MOMA),
    New York 41
Museum Ovartaci, Denmark 282
museums 281–7
  cultural consumption in general
      population 56
  examples 282–3
  impact measurement 283–5
  understanding museums in health 285–6
Museum Victoria, Australia 282
Museum Wellbeing Measure and
    Toolkit 284
Museveni, Yoweri 125
music
  Australia, doctor's orchestra 137
  children and young people 203
    Art Talks project, Pune, India 207
    Usinga World Centre for Dance and
        Music, Bagamoyo, Tanzania 206–7
    China 165–8
  criminal justice settings 187–90, 293

Culture Palette in Healthcare Centres,
    Stockholm, Sweden 173
dementia 172, 240–2
emotional competence 66, 67
female sex workers, Mumbai, India 325–9
Grupo Cultural AfroReggae, Rio de Janeiro,
    Brazil 181
health music(k)ing 194, 195, 197
health professional education and
      practice 310, 311
India 151, 153–4
intergenerational music-making 259–65
  benefits 259–60
  challenges 264
  cooperative programmes 261–4
  future 264
  older people assisting younger 260
  younger people assisting older 260–1
mirror neurons 67
narrative analysis 77
neurobiology 115
Norway 172–3, 175
psychoneuroendocrinology of musical
      behaviours 213–14
psychophysiology 67–70
public health 211–15
  cultural consumption in general
      population 56, 57
  dancing 215
  evolutionary perspective 55
  life span perspective 58–9
  listening to music 214
  measuring the value of music 212
  modelling the value of music 213
  playing an instrument 215
Sistema programmes 193–7
social competence 66
Sweden 173
therapeutic powers, natural belief in 12–13
Uganda 123, 124
  HIV/AIDS 125
USA
  healthcare settings 114
  prisons 187–90
see also singing
Music Basti, Delhi, India 154
Music for Life project, London,
    England 261–4
Music in Prisons 295
music therapy 272
  case study 276
  foundational principles 273
Music Therapy Trust of India, New Delhi 158
Myers, D. 264
Myskja, Audun 172

N
Nabulime, Lilian 126
Nada, Chennai, India 158
Nalumaansi, Princess 124
Names Project, California, USA 108
Nanda, U. 113
Nandikeshwar, Acharya, Abhinay Darpan 154
narrative analysis (NA) 75, 77–8
  data collection 74
Nasyashala Charity Trust, Mumbai, India 156
National Air and Space Museum, Washington,
    DC, USA 285
National Alliance for Arts, Health and
    Wellbeing 4

National Alliance for Arts in Criminal
    Justice 291, 292, 295
National Books on Prescription Scheme 37
National Children's Bureau 42
National Council for Education Research
    Trust (NCERT, India) 158
National Gallery, London, England 292
National Gallery of Australia 41, 283, 284
National Museums Liverpool (NML),
    England 282, 283
National Offender Management Service
    (NOMS) 291, 292–3, 295
Native Americans 13–14
nature, design for 300, 301, 302
nature-based rehabilitation 173
nausea following chemotherapy 154
Navajo 'night chant' 13–14
Neanderthals 55
Neehar, Pune, India 325
networks for arts and health 3, 4
neurobiology 65, 115
New Economics Foundation (NEF) 96, 284
Newman, S. 259, 264
New York Museum of Modern Art,
    USA 281–2, 283
New Zealand, Hip Op-eration Hip Hop Crew,
    Waiheke Island 105
NHS Choices 252
Nightingale, Florence 310
Noble, G. 281, 282, 283, 287
Nojeza, Celani 129
Northern Ireland
  Arts and Older People Programme 238–9
  ArtsCare 106
  Rowan, Antrim 106–7
Northside Seniors, Pittsburgh 247
Norway: culture and public health
    activities 171–6
  context 172
  cultural consumption in general
      population 57–8
  life span perspective 59, 174–6
  music therapy 172–3
  national statistics 172
Not Shut Up 295
NSW Ageing Strategy 140
Ntuuha Drama Performers 125
nursing education and practice 309–14
Nussbaum, Martha C. 15
Nutbeam, D. 107

O
obesity 20, 21
Obote, Milton 124
Office for Standards in Education (Ofsted) 43
older age 235–42
  Active Energy project, London,
      England 245–8
  Australia 139
    NSW Ageing Strategy 140
  China 164, 167
  community health and education, arts in 41
  cultural and social capital 235
  dance 70
    Dance for PD, Pune, India 237–8
    Hip Op-eration Hip Hop Crew, New
        Zealand 105
  global demographics 235, 236
  intergenerational music-making 259–65
  Norway 176

participatory arts 235, 236
   Arts and Older People Programme,
     Northern Ireland 238–9
   case studies 237–42
   Dance for PD, Pune, India 237–8
   dementia 240–2
   evidence, opportunities, and
     challenges 236–7
   USA 239–40
   public health and cultural experiences 60–1
   residential care homes 301–2
   singing 253–4
   Silver Song Clubs 253
   social determinants of health 31–2
   Sweden 176
   USA 113, 115, 239–40
   watching life 301
   see also ageing of population
Olympic Games, London (2012) 41, 245
Omugelegejo ceremony (Uganda) 123–4
O'Neill, D. 118
One Land, Many Faces programme 51
Ono, Yoko 37
Open Museum, Glasgow, Scotland 283
Operation Oak Tree, USA 117
orchestras see music
Oriel Ynys Môn, Anglesey, Wales 282
origins of 'arts and health' 14–16
Orquesta Sinfónica Infantil de Carora 193
Ottawa Charter 5–6, 119, 137, 187–8
Oxford University Museums, England 283
oxytocin 68, 252

P
Pacheco, Roberto 182–3
Pacification Police Units, Rio de Janeiro,
   Brazil 180–1
Padt, Renee 132
Paes, Eduardo 179
Pagan, J. 135
painting see art
palliative care 115–16
papermaking 117
parades
   bonfire night parade, Rye, East
     Sussex, UK 52
   community health and education, arts
     in 43, 44, 45–7
parietal cortex 69
Parkinson Mitra Mandal 237
Parkinson's disease (PD), dance for 114,
   215, 273
   India 155, 156, 237–8
   USA 104–5
participation in society 30–2
participatory action research (PAR) 78
partner violence, photovoice study with
   women experiencing 85–6
Passos, Pereira 179, 185
Pasteur, Louis 19
Patanjali 156, 157
Paul, L.K. 69
Pauwels, L. 84
Pawar, Hrishikesh 155, 156, 237
Pawson, R. 97
Pearce, D. 299
Pearce, S.M. 285
Pelletier, K.R. 118
Peña Hen, Jorge 193
Pence, G.E. 309

People with AIDS Development Association
   (PADA), Iganga, Uganda 125
Perana, Mumbai, India 325
Perim, Junior 184–5
Perkins 202
Perrier, Eileen 310
Perry, Bruce 42
Perry, Grayson 3, 295
Petticrew, M. 7
Philadelphia, USA: community-based arts for
   health 104
Phiri, M. 300, 303
photography/photovoice projects
   children's perceptions of vintage
     photographs 113
   ethical issues 83, 85–6, 87
   From War to Home, USA 117
   heart surgery, patient narratives of 87
   women experiencing partner violence 85–6
Piaget, Jean 202
Pickett, K. 21
Pierson, J. 104
Pimlico Opera 295
Plato 3, 13, 14, 22
Please Touch Museum, Philadelphia, USA 282
Pleiman, Tia 152
poetry
   Ancient Greece 14
   criminal justice settings 189–90, 293, 296
   emotional competence 66
   health research participation 85, 86–7
   heart surgery, patient narratives of 87
   life span perspective 60
   therapy
     case study 276
     foundational principles 273, 274
Pomegranate Workshop, India 158
Ponic, P. 85
population
   ageing see ageing of population
   global growth 21
portraiture 187
positive regard theory 42
Potter, Laura 310
poverty
   health inequalities 8
   social determinants of health 27, 29, 30
   South Africa 130
pregnancy, Grupo Cultural AfroReggae, Rio
   de Janeiro, Brazil 183
prematurity 108
premotor cortex 69
Press Ganey 114
Preston-Whyte, E. 131
Price, Neal 139
primary generators in design 303
primary motor cortex (M1) 69
Prince Charles Hospital, Brisbane,
   Australia 136
Prior, Ross 3
prisons see criminal justice settings
privacy, design for 300, 301, 302, 303
procedural ethics 84, 88
Projeto Casa Viva, Rio de Janeiro, Brazil 179
proportionate universalism 29, 32
prostitution 325–9
psychological health and wellbeing,
   children 202–3
psychoneuroendocrinology (PNE) of musical
   behaviours 213–14

psychophysiology see public health:
   and cultural activities,
   psychophysiological links between
psychosis 85, 86
public health
   Brazil 179, 180, 184
   China see China: creative arts and
     public health
   creativity's importance to 41
   and cultural activities, psychophysiological
     links between 65–70
     art therapy in rehabilitation 70
     dance 69–70
     emotional and social competence 65–7
     music 67–70
     neurobiological background 65
   and cultural experiences, epidemiological
     studies of relationship between 55–61
     cultural participation and health across
      the life span 58–61
     general population, cultural consumption
      in the 56–8
     issues and concepts 55–6
   cultural participation 211
   definition 19, 118
   embedding participatory arts in a public
     health programme 95–100
   ethics 23
   group singing as public health
     resource 251–6
     De Haan Centre 252–6
   museums and art galleries 281–7
   music, value of 211–15
     dancing 215
     listening to music 214
     measurement 212
     modelling 213
     playing an instrument 215
     psychoneuroendocrinology 213–14
     singing 214–15
   'new' 47
   Norway see Norway: culture and public
     health activities
   prisoners 190
   Sweden see Sweden: culture and public
     health activities
   Uganda 124
   USA 118–20
   waves
     first 19, 20
     second 19, 20
     third 19–20
     fourth 20
     fifth 22–4
public opinion 12–13
Pulford, Paul 37
purposive sampling 74
Putland, Christine 135, 138
pyramidal tract 69

Q
qualitative research 73–80
   arts-based methods 78–9
   Australia 138
   data analysis 75–7
   data collection 74–5, 79
   ethics 74, 75, 79–80
   focus groups 74–5
   interviews 74–5
   narrative research 77–8

Qualitative research (*Cont.*)
  participatory action research 78
  purpose 73–4
  quantitative research combined with *see* mixed-methods research
  sampling 74
  state of the art 73
  USA 113, 114
    palliative care 116
Quality Framework 80
quality of life (QoL)
  architecture 300, 301, 302
  China 164
  defined 248
  measures 299
  singing 252
    homeless men 317
    in hospitals 318, 322
quality of place and wellbeing 299–306
  current design practice 302
  problems of implementation in design practice 302–3
  research findings 300–2
  ways forward 303–6
quantitative research combined with qualitative research *see* mixed-methods research
Queensland Artsworkers Alliance 136
Queensland Children's Hospital, Australia 135
quilting 108
Quiroga Murcia, C. 70, 215

R
race factors, mortality in Brazil 180
Ramamani Iyengar Memorial Yoga Institute, Pune, India 157
Ramamoorthi, Parsuram 156
randomized controlled trials (RCTs) 6, 13
rape and sexual violence
  of male prisoners 190
  Rowan, Antrim, Northern Ireland 106–7
  South Africa 130
Raum, O. 130
Rauscher, Frances 12
reading 56
Reading Agency, The 37
Reading Museum, England 283
realism 74
Reason, P. 78
Red Cross USA 117
Red Door, India 156
reductionism 23
relational aesthetics 88
relaxation
  BrightHearts App 136
  dance 215
  music 214
  singing in hospitals 320
religion *see* spirituality and religion
Repton, John 45, 46
research
  arts-based health research (ABHR) 83–9
    benefits 83–4
    challenges 84
    ethical issues 84–9
  evidence question 12
  found poetry about participation in health research 85, 86–7
  India 158–9
  qualitative *see* qualitative research

role 6–7
USA 113–14
research ethics boards *see* ethics committees
residential care homes, architecture 301–2
resilience 145, 163
  arts therapies 271
  Australian Aboriginal and Torres Strait Islander people 146–7, 148, 149
  children and young people 224
  China 166, 167, 168, 169
Resilience Survey, China 166
Rethink Mental Illness 230
Rhodes, J. 227
Riqueime, L. 202
Risse, Guenter 115
Roberts, C. 75
Roberts, H. 7
Robson, Mary 42, 46
Rock Choir 251
Rock City, Namsos, Norway 175
Rogers, Carl 42
Rojcewicz, Stephen 14
Rollins, J. 113, 117
Rolvsjord, Rune 173
Romanowska, J. 60, 66
Roots and Wings project, Chickenley, West Yorkshire 42–4, 45, 47
Rosas, J. 202
Ross, Alex 38
Rowan, Antrim, Northern Ireland 106–7
Royal College of Music, Stockholm, Sweden 173
Royal Melbourne Children's Hospital, Australia 135
Royal Melbourne Hospital, Australia 136
Royal Melbourne Institute of Technology (RMIT), Australia 139
Royal Society for Public Health (RSPH) 119
Rubinstein, R.L. 260
Rumbold, J. 79
rural communities
  health inequalities 103
  Siyazama Project, South Africa 129–32
  Uganda, HIV/AIDS 126
  USA
    Arts in Healthcare for Rural Communities, Florida, USA 109
    arts in healthcare settings 116–17
Russia, life expectancy 30
Ruud, Even 172
Rwanda
  Barefoot Artists, Gisenyi 107
  coffee industry 108
  SPREAD theatre programme 108
Ryff, C. 236

S
Safe Ground 293
safety issues 85
Sagan, O. 6
Sage Gateshead 41
St George's Respiratory Questionnaire (SGRQ) 256
St John, P.A. 264
Samaritan Health Services 116
sampling in qualitative research 74
Sampoorna Music Therapy Centre (SMTC, India) 154
Sancheti, Parag 238

Sancheti Institute for Orthopaedics and Rehabilitation (SIOR) 237, 238
Sanford arts programme, South Dakota, USA 116
Sanlaap, Kolkata, India 325
Schellenberg, E.G. 66
Schibbolet 60
Schlaug, G. 69
schools 202
  architecture 299–300, 301, 302, 303, 304, 305
  community health and education, arts in 42–7
  public health and cultural experiences 58–9
  Malaysia 207–8
  USA 115
Science Museum, London, England 282
Scotland
  Big Noise 196
  criminal justice settings 291, 295
  museums and art galleries 283
SCREAM programme, International Labour Organization 207
sculpting *see* art
Seedhouse, David 41
Self, Will 295
Selig, Franz Josef 318
Seltzer, K. 237
semantic meaning 75
Sen, Amartya 30
Senior, Peter 135, 137
sexual violence *see* rape and sexual violence
sexually transmitted infections 109
sex workers, female 325–9
shamanism 13, 14
Shaw, George Bernard 309
Shekar, Devika 152
Short Warwick–Edinburgh Mental Well-being Scale (WWEMWBS) 284
Sidney De Haan Centre, Canterbury Christ Church University, England 251, 252–6
Sierra Leone
  child soldiers 203
  life expectancy 27
Silverman, D. 79, 80
Silverman, Lois 281
Silver Song Clubs 253
Sing a Smile, Mumbai, India 154
Singer, B. 236
Sing For Your Life 253
singing
  adverse effects 56
  Australian Aboriginal and Torres Strait Islander people 145–9
  breathing techniques 68
  China 166–8
  cognitive effects of training 69
  community health and education, arts in 41
  cultural consumption in general population 57
  Culture Palette in Healthcare Centres, Stockholm, Sweden 173
  dementia 241
  female sex workers, Mumbai, India 326
  health professional education and practice 310, 311–14
  in hospitals 317–23
    benefits 318
    certification 318–19
    history 317

international collaboration and musical ambassadors 318
mission and dissemination 317–18
quality control 318
research 319–22
India 151–3
intergenerational 261, 262
life span perspective 59–60, 61
prisoners 188–9
psychoneuroendocrinology 214
psychophysiology 68, 69
as public health resource 251–6
De Haan Centre 252–6
resilience 145
Sistema programmes 193–7
Sweden 173
television programmes 41, 251
value of 214–15
Singing as Health Promoting Work (Norway) 172
Singing for Health Project, east Kent, England 254–5
Singing Hospitals Association 317–23
Sinha, Aarti 152
Sistema programmes 8, 193–7
background 193
community health and wellbeing, framework for understanding 194–6
global setting 193
principles and practices 193–4
transferability 196–7
Siyazama Project, KwaZulu-Natal, South Africa 129–32
Skaife, S. 13
smallpox 123
Smith, Katherine 12
Smith, P. 51, 53
Smith, Richard 11
Snehalaya, India 325
Snyder-Young, Dani 15
social capital 30–2
older age 235
public health and cultural experiences 57
singing 147
social change, model of 294–5
social competence 65–7
social contact 30–2
social determinants of health 27–32
control, stress, and empowerment 30
health inequalities 27
life course approach and intergenerational equity 29–30
literacy 44
previous work 27–8
social contact, social capital, and participation 30–2
social gradient 29
USA
public health 119, 120
rural communities 116
social engagement
children and young people 207
China 167, 169
community-based arts for health 104
social gradient 29, 32
social health, children 203
social inclusion
Australian Aboriginal and Torres Strait Islander population 148
Tanpopo-no-ye, Nara City, Japan 107

social interaction 147, 149
socially engaged art 51
social medicine 19
social utility of the arts 35–9
Society for Culture and Health (Sweden) 171–2
Society of Chief Librarians 37
socio-economic factors, public health and cultural experiences 56, 57, 59
South Africa
46664 campaign 8
Siyazama Project, KwaZulu-Natal 129–32
Southbank Centre London, England 35–9, 295
South London and Maudsley NHS Foundation Trust (SLaM) 229–30
Southmead Hospital, Bristol, England 303
SPACE Studios London 245–6
spatial legibility, design for 300–1, 302
special needs populations, India 156
speech and language, children and young people 203
Speech Bubbles programme 204–5
Speech Bubbles programme, England 204–5
spirituality and religion
India 156–7
yoga 151
South Africa 130, 131–2
Uganda 123, 124
Splash Studios, Melbourne, Australia 136
SPREAD theatre programme, Rwanda 108
Spychiger, M. 58
staff, design for 301
Stanislavski, Konstantin 15
Stanworth, R. 116
Staricoff, Rosalia 138
Statistics Sweden 172
Stegemann, T. 214
Steinmuller, Ellen 230
Stickley, T. 12, 78
stigma
ethical issues 85, 86
female sex workers, India 326
mental health disorders 230, 231, 317
Storor, Mark 88
story-telling 105
Strauss, A. 75
Strauss, Paul 228
stress
Australian Aboriginal and Torres Strait Islander population 146–7
childhood adversity 223
China 164
community-based arts for health 104
dance 215
India 153
mindfulness-based stress reduction 273
music 214
neurobiology 65
in pregnancy 66
resilience 163
social determinants of health 30, 32
Studio for Movement Arts and Therapies, Begaluru, India 158
Suet Li, Liew 207–8
Sufism 151
Sumner, Allan 140
Sun, J. 146
Sur Sanjeevan Centre for Music Therapy 154
Sustaining Partnerships to Enhance Rural Enterprise and Agribusiness

Development (SPREAD) programme, Rwanda 108
Swadhar, India 325
Swami Vivekananda Yoga Anusandhana Sansthana, Bengaluru, India 157
Sweden
culture and public health activities 171–6
context 171–2
cultural consumption in general population 56–7
life span perspective 59, 60–1, 174–6
music therapy 173
national statistics 172
women 173
dementia 240–1
Swedish Organization for Concerts 172
Swedish Twin Registry 172
Switzerland
public health and cultural experiences 58
singing in hospitals 318
Synergy Theatre 295
systematic reviews 6
Sze, Szeming 5
Szmedra, L. 67

T
Taal Inc. (India) 154, 325, 326–7
Tagore, Radindranath 158
Tai Chi 164–5, 166–8
TaMHS (Targeted Mental Health in Schools) initiative 44
Tanpopo-no-ye, Nara City, Japan 107
Tanzania, Usinga World Centre for Dance and Music, Bagamoyo 206–7
Tasmanian Museum and Art Gallery, Australia 282
Tate Modern, London, England 41, 282
Taylor, M. 100
Teach for Malaysia 207–8
technology
Active Energy project, London, England 245–8
cultural consumption in general population 56
television programmes 41, 251
testosterone 68, 70
Thackray Medical Museum, Leeds, England 282
thalamus 65
theatre
Arts in Healthcare for Rural Communities, Florida, USA 109
Asociación Ak'Tenamit, Guatemala City, Guatemala 109
Australia 139
catharsis 15–16
cultural consumption in general population 56
Culture Palette in Healthcare Centres, Stockholm, Sweden 173
ethical issues 83
life span perspective 59
risky moments in applied theatre with children 85, 88
social competence 66
SPREAD programme, Rwanda 108
Uganda 125
US military-based programmes 117–18
see also drama
thematic analysis 75, 77

Theorell, T.  67, 70
theoretic sampling  74
Thomas, Dylan  35
Thomson, L.  284
Thorpe, Jo  131
Tiger Monkey's '100 Angels' project,
    Edmonton, London  98
Tilery lanterns project, Stockton-on-Tees  45–7
Tilley, N.  97
Time Being 2 project  12
TimeSlips, Wisconsin, USA  105
Todd, Cecil  124
Tolfree, Elinor  311
tone deafness  55, 211
Torres Strait Islanders see Australian
    Aboriginal and Torres Strait
    Islander people
Torrington, Judith  301
Tower of London, England  291
traditional healing practices
    South Africa  129, 130, 131–2
    Uganda  123–5
training
    in arts therapies  272
    India  158–9
    singing in hospitals  318
tribal art, India
    dance  155
    drama  156
Trondheim University, Norway  172
Trowell, Margaret  124
Tullie House Museum and Art Gallery,
    Carlisle, England  282, 283
Tyne and Wear Museums, England  283

U
Uganda
    arts in healthcare  123–6
        colonialism  124
        HIV/AIDS  125–6
        post-colonialism  124–5
        pre-colonialism  123–4
    HIV/AIDS  8, 125–6
    Ministry of Health  124, 125, 126
    National Association for Mental Health  124
Uganda Art Consortium  125, 126
Ulrich, Roger  135, 300
UNAIDS  108
unemployment  30
UNESCO
    Creative Cities Network  50–1
    health education  108, 109
        HIV/AIDS  109
    Observatory  139
    World Decade for Cultural
        Development  172
UNICEF
    India  158
    Uganda  124
Unidades de Policia Pacificadora (UPPs), Rio
    de Janeiro, Brazil  181
United Kingdom
    arts and health, support for  11
    Arts on Prescription programme  78
    children and young people
        Dance United  227–32
        development  202
    chronic obstructive pulmonary disease  255
    Civil Service  30
    colonialism  124

community cultural development  53
community health and education, arts
    in  41, 42–7
consumerism  22
criminal justice settings  291
Culture, Health and Wellbeing
    Conference  7
Department for Education and Skills  42
Department of Culture, Media, and Sports
    (DCMS)  11
Department of Health  11
    A Prospectus for Arts and Health  11
food  22–3
health improvements, waves of  19–20,
    21, 22–4
health inequalities  21
Health Research Authority  79
intergenerational practice  260
Medical Research Council see Medical
    Research Council
museums and art galleries  282, 283–4
National Health Service (NHS) ethics
    approval  79
National Network for Art and Health  137
new public health movement  41
older age  31, 236
public health  119
quality of place and wellbeing  299, 301, 302
singing
    Military Wives choirs  251
    Rock Choir  251
    Young Voices  251
social determinants of health  29, 31
Whitehall studies  30
see also England; Northern Ireland;
    Scotland; Wales
United Nations (UN)
    child health and wellbeing  202, 203
    Children's Fund see UNICEF
    community-based arts for health  108
    Convention on the Rights of the
        Child  202, 203
    Educational, Scientific and Cultural
        Organization see UNESCO
    Programme on HIV/AIDS  108
United States of America
    Alliance for Arts and Health Alliance  3, 4, 8
    arts in healthcare settings  113–20
        credentialling  118
        health education  118
        life span perspective  115
        military-based programmes  117–18
        new directions  114–15
        overall state of the field  113
        palliative care  115–16
        public health  118–20
        research  113–14
        rural communities  116–17
    arts in medicine  274
    arts therapies  274
    child development  203
    community-based arts for health  104
        Artes y Salud en Immokalee, Florida  107
        Arts in Healthcare for Rural
            Communities, Florida  109
        Barefoot Artists, Pennsylvania  107
        Dance for PD programme, Brooklyn,
            New York  104–5, 114, 237
        Names Project  108
        TimeSlips, Wisconsin  105

community cultural development  49, 50
    Animating Democracy  51–2
    ArtPlace America  52
Department of Defense  117
Department of Health and Human Services
    (USDHHS)  113, 119
Department of Veterans Affairs  117
Federal Interagency Task Force in the Arts
    and Human Development  115
health literacy  107–8
Hospital Audiences Incorporated  137
Institute of Medicine  107
museums and art galleries  281–2, 283, 285
music
    intergenerational music-making  259
    prisons  187–90
    training of music therapists  272
National Academy of Sciences  115
National Center for Creative Aging
    (NCCA)  115, 117
National Endowment for the Arts
    (NEA)  113, 115, 116, 118
National Initiative for Arts and Health in
    the Military  117
National Intrepid Center of Excellence
    (NICoE)  117
National Wellness Institute  104
Northside Seniors, Pittsburgh  247
older age  235
    Cohen, Gene  239–40
    prisons  187–90
    public health and cultural experiences  61
    Sistema programmes  194, 195, 196
    urban bias in health planning and
        assessment  103
United Way  108
Universal Declaration of Human Rights  295
University College London (UCL) Museums,
    England  283–4, 285–6
University of Gothenburg, Centre for Research
    on Culture and Health  172
University of Melbourne, Australia  139
University of Newcastle, Australia  139
University of South Australia  139
urbanization, China  164
Usinga World Centre for Dance and Music,
    Bagamoyo, Tanzania  206–7
Uy, M.  195

V
Väänänen, A.  57
Vaccine Revolt, Rio de Janeiro, Brazil  179
Valliappan  156
values and wellbeing  201–2
Vanchit Vikas, India  325–6
Van Huynh, Dam  229, 230, 231
Västfjäll, D.  213, 214
Västra Skådebanan, Sweden  176
Velvi (India)  156
Venezuela, El Sistema Project  8, 37, 193,
    195–6, 197
Venkit, Varun  154
Veshya AIDS Mukabla Parishad, Sangli
    (VAMPS), India  325, 326
Veterans Administration Medical Centers
    (VAMCs), USA  117
Veterans in Art initiative, Los Angeles,
    USA  117–18
VicHealth  138
Vickhoff, B.  252

Vietnam veterans  117
views, design for  300, 301, 302, 303
village fêtes  52–3
Viva Rio, Brazil  179
VOLCO  245
Voluntary Service Trust Team, Lowero
    district, Uganda  125
volunteering
    arts in medicine programmes  274
    health benefits of  32
    Norway  173
Vries, P. de  260
VVM Research Centre, India  158
Vygotsky, L.  285

W
Wales
    criminal justice settings  291, 292, 294, 295
    museums and art galleries  282, 284
Wali, A.  235
Walker, A.  259
Walk the Plank Theatre  41
Walsh, A.  88
Walsh, Fintan  15–16
Walter and Eliza Hall Institute (WEHI),
    Melbourne, Australia  136–7
Walter Reed National Military Medical Center
    (WRNMMC)  117
Wan, D.Y.  251
Warwick–Edinburgh Mental Well-being Scale
    (WEMWBS)
    dance  231
    museum evaluation  284
Watt, J.A.  16
We beat drums project, Skåne, Sweden  174–5
Wecker, Konstantin  318
Welch, Jonathan  148
Welfare State Arts Company  41
wellbeing

definition  104
loss of  20, 21
Wellcome Foundation  282, 310, 311
Well London programme  95–100
West, Susan  261
Westmead Hospital, Sydney, Australia  135–6
white matter  69
White, Mike  6, 11, 12, 41
White, V.  84
Whitworth Art Gallery, Manchester,
    England  283
whole person concept  115
Wikström, B.M.  176
Wilkinson, R.G.  21
Wilson, Michael  47
Winslow, C.A.  118
Wojcicki, Janet Maia  130
women
    burnout syndrome  173–4
    Grupo Cultural AfroReggae, Rio de Janeiro,
        Brazil  183
    prisoners, USA  188, 189
    sex workers, Mumbai, India  325–9
    see also gender factors
Women of the World (WOW)  38
working age
    public health and cultural
        experiences  59–60
    social determinants of health  30, 31
    Sweden  175–6
World Centre for Creative Learning
    Foundation (WCCLF), Pune,
    India  154, 158
World Health Organization (WHO)
    access to healthcare  106
    Active Ageing Policy Framework  236
    Alma Ata Declaration  187–8
    Commission on the Social Determinants of
        health  8

community
    cultural development  51
    definition  103
    health and education, arts in  47
Constitution  187
depression  21
health
    definition  5, 104, 211, 236, 299, 317
    India  153
    inequalities  42
    promotion  6, 137
    public  119, 211
Ottawa Charter  5–6, 119, 137, 187–8
public health  119, 211
quality of life indicators  299
social determinants of health  28, 119
    literacy  44
writing  57
Writing for Life (Norway)  172

Y
yoga  156–8
Yogavidyadham, Nashik, India  157
Yokoyama, Ikko  132
York SF-12  253, 254
Youn, Samuel  318
Young and Well Cooperative Research Centre
    (YAWCRC, Australia)  139
young people see children and young
    people
Young Person's Guide to East London  245
Young Voices  251
Yousafzai, Malala  39
Youth Music Lullaby Project, London,
    England  205–6
Yung, R.  49

Z
Zuma, Jacob  130

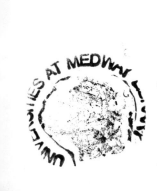